Intelligent Systems for Healthcare Management and Delivery

Nardjes Bouchemal
University Center of Mila, Algeria

A volume in the Advances in Healthcare Information Systems and Administration (AHISA) Book Series

IGI Global
DISSEMINATOR OF KNOWLEDGE

Published in the United States of America by
IGI Global
Medical Information Science Reference (an imprint of IGI Global)
701 E. Chocolate Avenue
Hershey PA, USA 17033
Tel: 717-533-8845
Fax: 717-533-8661
E-mail: cust@igi-global.com
Web site: http://www.igi-global.com

Library of Congress Cataloging-in-Publication Data

Names: Bouchemal, Nardjes, 1977- editor.
Title: Intelligent systems for healthcare management and delivery / Nardjes Bouchemal, editor.
Description: Hershey, PA : Medical Information Science Reference, [2019] | Includes bibliographical references.
Identifiers: LCCN 2018014972| ISBN 9781522570714 (hardcover) | ISBN 9781522570721 (ebook)
Subjects: | MESH: Artificial Intelligence | Health Information Systems | Medical Informatics Applications | Diagnosis, Computer-Assisted
Classification: LCC R858.A2 | NLM W 26.55.A7 | DDC 362.10285--dc23 LC record available at https://lccn.loc.gov/2018014972

This book is published in the IGI Global book series Advances in Healthcare Information Systems and Administration (AHISA) (ISSN: 2328-1243; eISSN: 2328-126X)

British Cataloguing in Publication Data
A Cataloguing in Publication record for this book is available from the British Library.

Advances in Healthcare Information Systems and Administration (AHISA) Book Series

Anastasius Moumtzoglou
Hellenic Society for Quality & Safety in Healthcare and P. & A. Kyriakou Children's Hospital, Greece

ISSN:2328-1243
EISSN:2328-126X

Mission

The **Advances in Healthcare Information Systems and Administration (AHISA) Book Series** aims to provide a channel for international researchers to progress the field of study on technology and its implications on healthcare and health information systems. With the growing focus on healthcare and the importance of enhancing this industry to tend to the expanding population, the book series seeks to accelerate the awareness of technological advancements of health information systems and expand awareness and implementation.

Driven by advancing technologies and their clinical applications, the emerging field of health information systems and informatics is still searching for coherent directing frameworks to advance health care and clinical practices and research. Conducting research in these areas is both promising and challenging due to a host of factors, including rapidly evolving technologies and their application complexity. At the same time, organizational issues, including technology adoption, diffusion and acceptance as well as cost benefits and cost effectiveness of advancing health information systems and informatics applications as innovative forms of investment in healthcare are gaining attention as well. **AHISA** addresses these concepts and critical issues.

Coverage

- Telemedicine
- Measurements and Impact of HISA on Public and Social Policy
- Decision Support Systems
- IT security and privacy issues
- IT Applications in Physical Therapeutic Treatments
- Virtual health technologies
- Pharmaceutical and Home Healthcare Informatics
- Management of Emerging Health Care Technologies
- IS in Healthcare
- IT Applications in Health Organizations and Practices

IGI Global is currently accepting manuscripts for publication within this series. To submit a proposal for a volume in this series, please contact our Acquisition Editors at Acquisitions@igi-global.com or visit: http://www.igi-global.com/publish/.

The Advances in Healthcare Information Systems and Administration (AHISA) Book Series (ISSN 2328-1243) is published by IGI Global, 701 E. Chocolate Avenue, Hershey, PA 17033-1240, USA, www.igi-global.com. This series is composed of titles available for purchase individually; each title is edited to be contextually exclusive from any other title within the series. For pricing and ordering information please visit http://www.igi-global.com/book-series/advances-healthcare-information-systems-administration/37156. Postmaster: Send all address changes to above address.

Titles in this Series

For a list of additional titles in this series, please visit: www.igi-global.com/book-series

Contemporary Applications of Mobile Computing in Healthcare Settings
R. Rajkumar (VIT University, India)
Medical Information Science Reference • copyright 2018 • 259pp • H/C (ISBN: 9781522550365) • US $205.00 (our price)

Handbook of Research on Emerging Perspectives on Healthcare Information Systems and Informatics
Joseph Tan (McMaster University, Canada)
Medical Information Science Reference • copyright 2018 • 641pp • H/C (ISBN: 9781522554608) • US $355.00 (our price)

Big Data Analytics in HIV/AIDS Research
Ali Al Mazari (Alfaisal University, Saudi Arabia)
Medical Information Science Reference • copyright 2018 • 294pp • H/C (ISBN: 9781522532033) • US $215.00 (our price)

Advanced Systems for Improved Public Healthcare and Disease Prevention Emerging Research and Opportunities
Thierry Oscar Edoh (Technical University of Munich, Germany)
Medical Information Science Reference • copyright 2018 • 262pp • H/C (ISBN: 9781522555285) • US $185.00 (our price)

Global Perspectives on Health Communication in the Age of Social Media
Seif Sekalala (Kean University, USA) and Brandon C. Niezgoda (Drexel University, USA)
Medical Information Science Reference • copyright 2018 • 348pp • H/C (ISBN: 9781522537168) • US $225.00 (our price)

Healthcare Administration for Patient Safety and Engagement
Aleksandra Rosiek-Kryszewska (Nicolaus Copernicus University, Poland) and Krzysztof Leksowski (Military Clinical Hospital, Poland & Nicolaus Copernicus University, Poland)
Medical Information Science Reference • copyright 2018 • 343pp • H/C (ISBN: 9781522539469) • US $235.00 (our price)

Big Data Management and the Internet of Things for Improved Health Systems
Brojo Kishore Mishra (C. V. Raman College of Engineering, India) and Raghvendra Kumar (LNCT Group of Colleges, India)
Medical Information Science Reference • copyright 2018 • 312pp • H/C (ISBN: 9781522552222) • US $255.00 (our price)

IGI Global
DISSEMINATOR OF KNOWLEDGE

701 East Chocolate Avenue, Hershey, PA 17033, USA
Tel: 717-533-8845 x100 • Fax: 717-533-8661
E-Mail: cust@igi-global.com • www.igi-global.com

Table of Contents

Detailed Table of Contents

The drug development phase is one of the most time-consuming and expensive stages in the lifecycle of a drug. Marred by patent expirations, price regulations, complexities in disease conditions, life sciences companies are facing a daunting task to bring new molecular entities into the market. Digital health technologies are playing a critical role in addressing some of the challenges faced during drug development. In this chapter, the author talks about the challenges and key trends in the world of drug development, use of new digital health technologies, and the future of drug development. As an example, the author dives into a specific case study on the use of virtual assistants in clinical trials and the benefits of its usage on patients, healthcare professionals, and life sciences companies.

For the past few decades, an increase in experimental research has been carried out in enhancing the quality-of-life of the persons with different levels of disabilities. To enhance the lifestyle of differently disabled in terms of their mobility or movement or transportation, a proper aid with appropriate human-computer interface system is needed. So, in this chapter, a hybrid classification model is proposed, which combines and uses hM-GM and ANN models, for classifying human speech signal, especially the word for driving a wheelchair for helping the people, who seek transportation. For classifying the correct word from the phase of sentence (i.e., the human speech signal) to corresponding trigger command for an electrically powered wheelchair prototype, under the certain experimental condition, the hM-GM model yields good recognition of words, but they suffer major limitations as it relies on strong statistical properties and probability. Hence, by combining hM-GM and ANN model-based classifier for enhancing the accuracy of classifying the word to corresponding trigger command.

Chronic diseases are a major cause of death in the world. Thus, many guidelines have been proposed to prevent these diseases. In addition, various systems have been developed to ease health monitoring. However, they are generally behaving as reminders or as anomaly detection systems. After giving an overview of the existed solutions and discussing their drawbacks, the authors present their system which is called ambient healthcare monitoring system (AHMS). It provides a continuous, unobtrusive, and mobile health monitoring of patients with chronic diseases. It is based on the multi-agent paradigm that allows devices to be distributed and autonomous. In addition, it benefits from the characteristics of ambient intelligence (AmI) such as ubiquity and context-awareness. So, AHMS is a promising solution for unobtrusive healthcare monitoring, in which it offers efficient medical services, with less energy consumption, that can significantly reduce the healthcare cost by automating some routine tasks. Consequently, it reduces the latency as well it minimizes the overload on the caregiver.

Big data has unlocked a new opening in healthcare. Thanks to the considerable benefits and opportunities, it has attracted the momentous attention of all the stakeholders in the healthcare industry. This chapter aims to provide an overall but thorough understanding of healthcare big data. The chapter covers the 10 'V's of healthcare big data as well as different healthcare data analytics including predictive and prescriptive analytics. The obvious advantages of implementing big data technologies in healthcare are meticulously described. The application areas and a good number of practical use cases are also discussed. Handling big data always remains a big challenge. The chapter identifies all the possible challenges in realizing the benefits of healthcare big data. The chapter also presents a brief survey of the tools and platforms, architectures, and commercial infrastructures for healthcare big data.

Deep learning (DL) is a special type of machine learning that attains great potency and flexibility by learning to represent input raw data as a nested hierarchy of essences and representations. DL consists of more layers than conventional machine learning that permit higher levels of abstractions and improved prediction from data. More abstract representations computed in terms of less abstract ones. The goal of this chapter is to present an intensive survey of existing literature on DL techniques over the last years especially in the medical imaging analysis field. All these techniques and algorithms have their points of interest and constraints. Thus, analysis of various techniques and transformations, submitted prior in writing, for plan and utilization of DL methods from medical image analysis prospective will be discussed. The authors provide future research directions in DL area and set trends and identify challenges in the medical imaging field. Furthermore, as quantity of medicinal application demands increase, an extended study and investigation in DL area becomes very significant.

In this chapter, the authors propose Medi-Ring, a compact system to carry all the medical records for senior citizens to avoid improper medication, delay in treatment in emergency situation. The three main aspects of Medi-Ring are NFC technology, system memory, and a controller. NFC technology is used for transferring the data, the system memory is used to store the medical records which includes patient's details, doctor's prescription, and all other medical details. A controller is used to control the whole system. As the proposed Medi-Ring is wearable, compact, and flexible, it can be used as a medical companion for senior citizens.

Digital fundus imaging is becoming an important task in computer-aided diagnosis and has gained an important position in the digital medical imaging domain. One of its applications is the retinal blood vessels extracting. Object detection in machine vision and image processing has gained increasing interest due to its social and security potential. Plenoptic imaging is a promising optical technique. This technique computes the location and the propagation direction information of the object light, which are used as efficient descriptors to detect and track the object displacement. In this chapter, the authors use an edge detection technique to extract and segment blood vessels in the retinal image. They propose a novel approach to detect vessels in a simulated light fields fundus image, based on the image representation with the first and the second order derivative, well known as gradient and Laplacian image descriptors. Since the difficulties to get a light field image of a fundus in the retinal image, the authors test their model in the image provided by Sha Tong et al.

Generally, distributed computing through a handheld/mobile device has to be considered with care because of the limited capabilities on these devices. Especially in ubiquitous telemonitoring healthcare, which refers to the disposition of any type of health services, such that medical staff members (physicians, emergency workers, other healthcare providers, etc.) through mobile computing devices can access them and expect data to be made available. In this chapter, the authors present a new system based on ubiquitous agents to assist telemonitoring employees, not only anytime and anywhere but also on any device.

Interdisciplinary research on autism diagnosis and training for the autistic children are current requirements. Behavioral analytics are the techniques followed by pediatricians for identifying ASD in children. However, the techniques successfully accepted by the pediatricians worldwide would be useful for the parents and pediatricians only for the elementary school-aged children, and the system is not helping for early diagnose among children of age 2. Machine learning, image processing, and pervasive techniques are trending for early diagnosis of ASD. Hence, the chapter has done a research-based survey and detailed analysis on behavioral analytics algorithms, neuro imaging, and eye tracking techniques for early diagnosis. The behavioral analytics survey mainly focuses on social and meta-cognitive skills, and the input dataset has been taken from parents, trainers, teachers, and peer groups. The chapter also identifies that computing technologies with neuro-imaging and pervasive techniques are better than the behavioral skill analysis for early diagnosis.

Healthcare providers treat a plethora of conditions associated with the human body for a patient to achieve optimal healthiness. However, aspects of a patients' entire wellbeing can often be overlooked, which leads to issues such as drug interactions, missed diagnoses, and other gaps in care. Healthcare can benefit from implementing better data management and integration to improve data analysis, which could bridge gaps in care. This chapter will explain data analysis and data integration, why they are pertinent in the healthcare system, and their associated rewards and challenges. After analyzing these healthcare facets, this chapter will conclude with a proposal for healthcare providers to leverage technology for patients' general wellbeing and a healthier population.

The internet of things (IoT) revolution is improving the proficiency of human healthcare infrastructures, and this chapter analyzes the applications of IoT in healthcare systems with diversified aspects such as topological arrangement of medical devices, layered architecture, and platform services. This chapter focuses on advancements in IoT-based healthcare in order to identify the communication and sensing technologies enabling the smart healthcare systems. The transformation of healthcare from doctor-centric to patient-centric with the diversified applications of IoT is discussed in detail. In addition, this chapter examines the various issues to be emphasized on designing an effective IoT-based healthcare system. It also explores security in healthcare systems and the possible security threats that may be vulnerable to the security essentials. Finally, this chapter summarizes the procedure of applying machine learning techniques on healthcare streaming data which provides intelligence to the systems.

Emergency departments (EDs) are one of the most valuable departments of healthcare management systems. Patient arrivals at the EDs are crucial for planning of the future. Accurate forecasting of patient arrivals contributes to better organized human resources and medical devices in the EDs. Therefore, in this chapter, the authors aim to develop a hybrid model including the methods of autoregressive integrated moving average with external variables (ARIMAX) and artificial neural network (ANN) in a hospital ED. The arrival data was collected from the hospital information system of a public hospital in eastern Turkey. The model incorporates factors related to ED arrivals such as climatic and calendar variables. By the aid of the proposed model, an insight to arrangement and planning of ED resources can be provided in a better way.

Epidemiology is the study of dynamics of health and disease in human population. It aims to identify the occurrence, pattern, and etiology of human diseases so that the causes of these diseases can be understood, which in turn will help in preventing their spread. In traditional epidemiology, the data is collected by various public health agencies through various means. Many times, the actual figures vary a lot from the one reported. Sometimes this difference is due to human errors, but most of the time, it is due to intentional underreporting. Big data techniques can be used to analyze this huge amount of data so as to extract useful information from it. The electronic health data is so large and complex that it cannot be processed using traditional software and hardware. It is also not possible to manage this data using traditional data management tools. This data is huge in terms of volume as well as diversity and the speed at which it is being generated. The ability to combine and analyze these different sources of data has huge impact on epidemic tracking.

Preface

INTRODUCTION

Populations are increasingly inclined to integrate Artificial Intelligence (AI) into their daily lives. Although considered a science fiction a few years ago, the AI and its technological advances are already in the process of upsetting whole sections of society, notably healthcare domain.

Indeed, the use of artificial intelligence and new technologies in healthcare systems improves the quality of services and allows better coordination of care.

With the various techniques of AI and the growing use of new technologies, intelligent systems for healthcare manages huge amounts of existing data. Surgeons, hospital medical and emergency staff, etc. will soon be able to refer the best medical practices performed on rare diseases. These innovations will help as many people and will help reduce the costs of time spent searching for solutions that take years or even decades before result on concrete solutions.

In the fields of healthcare intelligent systems management, there exists a need for an edited collection of original research in this area.

The *Intelligent Systems for Healthcare Management and Delivery* book will aim to provide relevant and advanced methodological, technological and scientific approaches related to the application of sophisticated exploitation of artificial intelligence in Intelligent Systems for Healthcare Management and Delivery.

The principal objective is to foster a scientific debate for the new era of Healthcare Intelligent systems; requiring sophisticated approaches for enhanced healthcare services.

Intelligent Systems for Healthcare Management and Delivery book will provide an insight of the technologies and intelligent applications that have received growing attention in recent years from various perspectives.

The target audience of this book will be composed of professionals and researchers working in the field of information management in healthcare domain, biomedical engineering, rehabilitation engineering, electronic devices in drug delivery technology.

Furthermore, it will be an excellent reference book for the students studying intelligent systems and new technologies.

It will also be of interest to the persons working in healthcare centers, hospitals and rehabilitation centers.

To meet these challenges and to satisfy the target audience, we have worked over a year on this book, and we had the honor of selecting the best chapters, presented below:

Chapter 1: Evolution of Digital Technologies and Use of Virtual Assistants in Drug Development

It is a common knowledge in the Life Sciences Industry that conduct of clinical trials and their approvals by regulatory authorities as part of the drug development journey takes a major share of the time and cost spent by pharmaceutical companies in their attempt to bring a new drug into the market. While there have been big advances in improving the operational and process efficiencies in drug development, there are still ample avenues to further automate and reduce the cost and schedule burden on the pharma companies. Information technology have been on the forefront in this journey and have been enabling companies to move away from traditional business models to more patient centric models in drug development.

The chapter begins with an understanding of the current state of drug research and development, various challenges faced and key trends. It then goes through the evolution and use of various technologies that have shaped drug development. It introduces new technologies like artificial intelligence, machine learning, automated / virtual reality, blockchain and how they can be adopted to change the way various functions in the research and development operate today. The chapter provides an overview of the ongoing developments taken up by regulatory authorities favouring the adoption of new technologies by industry players. As an example of use of AI technology, the chapter deep dives into a conceptual model and few use cases of how virtual assistants or chatbots can benefit the main stakeholders in clinical trials – the subject, the investigator and the sponsor. The chapter concludes by providing the reader with a view into the future of clinical development – a digital convergence.

Chapter 2: Development of Human Speech Signal-Based Intelligent Human-Computer Interface for Driving a Wheelchair in Enhancing the Quality-of-Life of the Persons

The real-time processing of speech signal generally deals with analysing the nature and characteristics of the signal(s) produced to the corresponding observable outputs. The signals used can either be discrete or analog/continuous in nature and either it can be stationary or non-stationary signals. If the signals are stationary then, the signal's statistical properties won't change with respect to time, but if it is non-stationary signal then, the signal's statistical properties will get change depending upon the time. By analyzing this, we can able to develop a "signal model". The signal model developed is nothing but a theoretical description of the system. Speech signals are basically one-dimension signals which vary over the time period and can be related to a source-filter system.

The source filter system consists of respiratory mechanism as a source and filtering are caused due to change in air pressure when the air starts to flow from lungs with pulmonary pressure. The air pressure gets change as it reaches the larynx in the throat and produces vibration, and the hissingness. Vibration and hissingness is the primary cause of speech production.

Chapter 3: An Ambient Multi-Agent System for Healthcare Monitoring of Patients With Chronic Diseases

Chronic diseases are among the most widespread diseases in the world. According to the World Health Organization (WHO), in 2015 an estimated 1.6 million deaths were directly caused by diabetesand17.7 million people died from cardiovascular diseases (CVDs). Thus, healthcare organisations provide various guidelines and recommendations to help patients to deal with these chronic diseases. They recommend respecting diet, controlling vital signs, taking medications and doing physical activitiesto treat chronic diseases. But, these guidelines limit the patients' lifestyle where a patient should frequently measure his/her physiological parameters and he/she should often visit his/her doctor.

During the past decade, technology had been moving gradually towards Ambient Intelligence (AmI) environments aiming to help inhabitants in everyday life. AmI tries to adapt the technology to the peoples' needs using omnipresent computing elements, which communicate amongst them in a ubiquitous way. In particular, AmI systems can considerably enhance the healthcare domain. Due to the fact that health monitoring of patients within a controlled environment (e.g. hospitals) will disturb them, researchers have proposed to monitor the patients within smart environments, which use AmI technologies. However, previous work has only focused on facilitating the vital sign measuring task, detecting any occurred abnormal situation, and helping caregivers to make suitable decisions. So, these systems can be viewed as reminders (e.g. they remind the patient when the time of taking a drug has arrived) or as anomaly detection systems (e.g. they alert caregivers when a patient is on a critical health situation) or as decision support systems (e.g. they provide to doctors clinical analyses and documentation that assist them to make decisions).

Although the previous solutions are interesting, they don't have mechanisms to apply treatments, in which these systems need for a direct intervention of caregivers. Moreover, patients in critical health situation need for an immediate intervention, where any unnecessary delay can cause the death of the patient. In this purpose, the authors present a multi-agent system named Ambient Healthcare Monitoring System (AHMS), which allows patients to control their health everywhere, at any time, and in an unobtrusive manner without limiting their lifestyle. So, the patient doesn't need to measure his/her vital sign regularly. Instead, the system measures them in a transparent manner using wearable sensors. Also, AHMS helps doctors to remotely monitor the patients' health in real-time by providing a detailed medical information about them. Besides, it uses the guidelines of caregivers (which are saved on the knowledge base) to make instantaneous decisions. These decisions will be directly applied by actuator devices(i.e. it don't need a physical intervention of caregivers). Especially in emergency situations where a delay is not accepted.

The remainder of this chapter is organised as follows: Section 2 presents an overview of the existing systems for health monitoring. Section 3 describes the proposed system, by presenting its objectives, its general architecture, and describes its various agents. An experimental scenario is presented in Section 4, to deepen the understanding of the AHMS operation. Finally, a conclusion and some future works are mentioned in Section 5.

Chapter 4: Healthcare Big Data – A Comprehensive Overview

Healthcare industry is going through a trailblazing makeover. Due to the significant advancement in digitised and open and pervasive healthcare systems, it is generating a massive amount of data. This healthcare data is truly comparable to the Big Data both in size and nature, hence termed as healthcare Big Data. Though compared to other industries, the healthcare industry has been lagging behind in the adoption of Big Data technologies, the changed medical and clinical landscape has forced the stakeholders to delve into the development quickly. Suddenly, Big Data has become crucial for almost every operational, clinical, and management task. The healthcare people are now convinced of the benefits of Big Data and persuading themselves to analyse the data for extracting new insights that have given them the access to promising new threads of knowledge which are being transformed into innovative and purposeful actions.

Several healthcare use cases are well-suited for incorporating Big Data technologies. The healthcare Big Data analytics has opened up many exciting avenues in different healthcare operations including diagnosis and medical care, clinical decision support, population health management etc. The success of healthcare Big Data is mostly dependent on the efficient collection and storage of massive quantities of disparate data acquired from diverse sources and also running it through an in-depth analysis. The effective utilization of healthcare Big Data and obtained knowledge through analytical processes has the potential to save a significant amount of money and most importantly, people's lives.

This chapter provides a preliminary and overall understanding of healthcare Big Data. The rest of the chapter is organised as follows. Section 2 discusses the 'big' aspect of the healthcare data including the ten 'V's of healthcare Big Data. It also covers the basics of healthcare Big Data analytics as well as the present healthcare Big Data market. Section 3 identifies several advantages of Big Data in healthcare. Section 4 mentions some application areas while Section 5 lists some specific examples of healthcare Big Data. The associated challenges are discussed in Section 6. Section 7 provides a brief survey of the different platforms and tools, architectures, and practical infrastructure for healthcare Big Data. Section 8 concludes the chapter.

Chapter 5: Deep Learning and Medical Imaging

Deep learning is a developed direction in general data analysis, and has been entitled one of the year 2013 ten-breakthrough technologies. It is a significant subfield of Artificial Intelligence (AI) that linked various topics like Machine Learning, Neural Networks, and Classification. Figure 1 represents the connections between the diverse AI fields. This discipline has advanced significantly over the years due to the huge works of scientists like Andrew Ng, Geoff Hinton, Yann LeCun, Adam Gibson, and Andrej Karpathy.

For decades, attaining and extracting the well-founded and distinguishable features is always a pivotal step to complete the task of image recognition and computer vision. Engineering expertise is required in the domain to model a feature extractor that mutated raw data (i.e., such as pixels in the image) into a suitable internal representation or feature vector from which the classical machine learning subsystem could complete its work either classification, prediction, or clustering of the input. An interest and research venture in feature extraction is a key concern in a lot of researches in various applications. Representation learning is a set of procedures that provides a machine to be fed with raw data and to automatically determine the portrayals needed for recognition or grouping. Deep learning techniques are representation learning techniques with multiple levels of portrayal, prevailed by composing simple but non-linear modules that each transmuted the representation at one level (starting with the raw input) into a representation at a higher, slightly more abstract level. With the composition of enough such transmutations, very complex functions can be learned. Figure 2 demonstrates stream outlines for the disparate parts of an AI system relate to each other within different AI disciplines. Shaded boxes indicate components that are able to learn from data.

A deep learning framework is a multilayer heap of simple modules, all (or most) of which are liable to learning, and many of which calculate non-linear input–yield mappings. Each module in the load transforms its input to elevate both the selectivity and the invariance of the representation. With multiple non-linear layers, a framework can implement extremely sophisticated functions of its inputs that are altogether sensitive to minute details and unkind to large unrelated variations such as the background, pose, lighting and surrounding objects. The hidden layers of a deep multilayer neural network learn to represent the network's inputs in a way that makes it easy to predict the target outputs.

Deep learning is known of sundry hundred years as modern neural networks with multiple hidden layers. Back in the nineteen eightieth, the researchers were excited about the prospect of using neural networks with many layers of hidden neurons, but it was hard to get networks to learn well using standard techniques (i.e. Backpropagation "especially with the problem of gradient descent over the loss function" more details are discussed in sub-section 2.1). Neural nets fell out of favor as other machine learning approaches with comparable better results stemming from statistical machine learning in 1990s and 2000s. In the previous couple of years the deep learning has become more useful and gained the attention as the development of the methods of training networks (i.e. good weight regularization/dropout), amount of available training data has increased, its models have grown in size over time as computer hardware (i.e. compute power of the parallel hardware graphical processing units [GPUs], computer clusters) and software infrastructure has improved.

Chapter 6: Medi-Rings for Senior Citizens – Distributed EMR System

Mostly in medical emergency, a patient can be treated with a proper medication if and only if the previous medical records of the patient are available. In developing countries such as India such records are not accessible during medical emergency because of the lack of infrastructure. In western countries, several Electronic Medical Record (EMR) options such as object storage systems, compliance WORM storage, IBM's Hippocratic databases etc. available to maintain the medical records where the data is loaded into a centralized network. EMR is a real time transaction processing database for clinical patient information. EMR is a record in digital format which requires resources such as internet to synchronize with central network and needs technical persons to maintain it. In developing countries such as India, medical records are mostly handwritten. Handwritten paper medical records have their own set of advantages and disadvantages. The main advantages are that they are very cost effective, gives more leeway for the doctor to represent the symptoms in form of diagrams etc. for easy understanding, to increase speed of diagnosis common elements can be typed and can have boxes for selecting etc. Along with the advantages they have disadvantages such as storage problems, accessibility issues, fragmentation of manual medical records if the patient visits different Doctors for multiple aliments, difficulty in transfer of medical records from one hospital to another and also manual records can be associated with poor legibility which can contribute medical errors. In India medical records in most of the hospitals are manual in nature. 50% of medical records in India are unusable or partly usable as they are not properly stored or the handwriting of the medical practitioner is not legible. As mentioned in article of Times of India, World Health Organization lists India among the top 10 killers in the world due to medical errors. While a British National Health system survey in 2009 reported that 15% of its patients were misdiagnosed.

Due to the manual medical records, during medical emergency, patients in India have to be taken to the same hospital for treatment. If patient is taken to another hospital, physician or doctor will have no access to patient's previous medical records leading to re-simulate all the treatments which consumes lifesaving minutes. To overcome the problems associated with manual medical records, some hospitals have migrated to electronic medical records to serve patients better. Some of the challenges faced by the hospitals in India due to electronic medical records are high installation cost, need for reliable internet facility, and need for uninterrupted power supply. Due to high patient to doctor ration in India EMR implementation which requires a centralized network, becomes very expensive in terms of cost of installation. In addition to this EMR are associated with another problem –data security. An article from NDTV gadgets beta, "Your medical Record is worth more to hackers than your credit card", The FBI warned health care providers to guard against cyber-attacks after one of largest U.S. hospital operators, community Health system Inc., said Chinese Hackers had broken into its computer network and Stolen the personal information of 4.5 million patients. This article clearly states that the centralized networks are more prone to security threats and very expensive for implementation.

To address the problems discussed, the medical records can be stored locally than global, which can be accomplished with a wearable gadget "Medi-Ring". As every person in his life has to visit the hospital for a regular check-up, each time it is required to carry necessary report or previous check-up report. There may be chance that some patients may forget to carry reports and some may have lost the report. In such case the patient as well as doctor will face a problem, and this may insist them to take another check-up which will be burden to the patient. So in order to avoid such problems, proposed medi-ring, which can store the file and transfer the files to other system.

Chapter 7: Edge Detection on Light Field Images – Evaluation of Retinal Blood Vessels Detection on a Simulated Light Field Fundus Photography

As a crucial technique in computer vision and image processing, object detection has often been used for object segmentation and tracking for computer vision systems. It is based on the detection of instant objects like the human body, face, car, bicycles, or buildings. This approach plays an important role in visual surveillance applications, pedestrian detection and tracking, image retrieval, and face recognition.

Different techniques and methods have been proposed to yield an efficient solution, as we can cite the background subtraction, the saliency detection, and many other ones.Earlier measurement methods suffer from drawbacks due to complexes scene properties (geometrics, illumination, etc.).

To improve these limits, new optical methods for describing objects are efficiently and largely invaded in computer vision and machine learning. Quite recently, considerable attention has been paid to plenoptic imaging, this approach captures information on the three-dimensional light field of appropriate scene and records, simultaneously, the location information and the propagation direction of the object light plane. These computed measures are used as efficient descriptors to detect and track moving objects.

In this chapter, we propose a new sensing strategy for blood-retinal vessels detection and extraction based on, first, the extraction of visual information of a frame image such as a discrete object, specifically: edges. At this level, we focus on the description of light field images based on the detection and the localization of significant intensity variation, or what it is called: edge.

First and the second derivative, well known as Gradient and Laplacian, will be used to compute the edge image, that we will use to extract retinal blood vessels in retinal images.

Chapter 8: Telemonitoring Healthcare System-Based Mobile Agent Technology

Several studies point to the aging of population during the next decades. While being a good result of increasing of life expectation, this also implies some problems. The percentage of population with health problems will increase and it will be very difficult to Hospitals to maintain all patients. Our society is faced with the responsibility to care for these people in the best possible social and economic ways.

Thus, there is a clear interest to create Ubiquitous Telemonitoring Healthcare, where devices and environments allow patients to be followed in their own homes or during their day-by-day life.

Ubiquitous telemonitoring healthcare refers to the disposition of any type of health services such that individual consumers through mobile computing devices can access them.

Patients will be monitored at long distance, and medical control support devices may be embedded in clothes, like T-shirts, collecting vital-sign information from sensors (blood pressure, temperature, etc.).

Telemonitoring healthcare systems work with two important components; the system itself and network construction. The systems have the following important goals:

- Provides an electronic healthcare record for the patient conditions in the past and in the present time.
- Issues and alarm if there is anything wrong with the patient's vital signs or if one of his/her family member's see something is wrong.
- Sends a report, to include general information about the patient's health status.
- Presents the patient's health status such as temperature and other vital signs to the medical experts to analyze and they can offer advice.
- Offers support service in emergency situations (first-aid).

It is clear that these systems must be permanently connected with the medical staff, which is not evident in the context of ubiquitous environments where devices have reduced energy autonomy and can be off-line at any time.

One key aspect in any ubiquitous system, and especially in healthcare systems, is the use of context-aware technologies. Therefore, a correct information management is vital. It is not enough to gather information about the context, but that information must be processed by self-adaptable and dynamic mechanisms and methods that can react independently of each particular situation that arises.

In this sense, agents and Multi-Agent Systems comprise one of the areas that can contribute expanding the possibilities of ubiquitous healthcare systems and telemonitoring systems. An agent can be defined as a computational system situated in an environment and is able to act autonomously in this environment to achieve its design goals.

On the other hand, such as many other users, medical staff members are surrounded by many mobile and ubiquitous devices. We want to take advantage of this diversity to let them always connected.

For that, we propose in this chapter an approach based on Ubiquitous Mobile Agent System. Its goal is to recognize medical staff devices; with the ability to migrate from one device to another.

The rest of the chapter is organized as follow: section 2 summarizes some works based on the use of agents in telemonitoring systems. We present in section three our contribution, the implementation and experimentations on JADE-LEAP. Finally, some conclusions are drawn.

Chapter 9: Research Investigation and Analysis on Behavioral Analytics, Neuro Imaging, and Pervasive Sensory Algorithms and Techniques for Autism Diagnosis

Interdisciplinary research on Autism diagnosis and training for the autistic children are current requirements. Behavioural Analytics are the techniques followed by pediatricians for identifying ASD in children. However the techniques successfully accepted by the pediatricians worldwide, the techniques would be useful for the parents and pediatricians only for the Elementary school aged children and the system is not helping for early diagnose among children of age 2 or < 2. Machine learning, Image processing and pervasive techniques are trending for early diagnose of ASD. Hence, the chapter has done research based survey and detailed analysis on behavioural analytics algorithms, neuro imaging and eye tracking techniques for early diagnosis. The behavioural analytics survey mainly focus on social and meta-cognitive skills and the input dataset has been taken from parents, trainers, teachers and peer groups. The paper also identified that computing technologies with Neuro-imaging and pervasive techniques are better than the behavioural skill analysis for early diagnosis.

Chapter 10: Data Analysis and Integration in Healthcare

There has been ample research about the influence and role of information technology in medical systems. Technology is increasingly used in pertinent roles, such as acquiring data, processing data, communicating collaborative data to caregivers, as in nurses and doctors, and administering treatment to patients. The increase in the use of technology is accounted for by various reasons. These rewards have motivated hospital systems to increase their technological prowess. However, while the available technological aspects of healthcare advance in some hospital systems, others have been left in an antiquated state, which could be detrimental as information technology continues its rapid improvements. Many medical systems continue using relational databases for both patient information and general business information, while higher end medical systems are migrating to much more fluid forms of data management. However, both types of systems need to continue or begin to apply data analysis and data integration to truly make the most of the vast amounts of data collected by medical practitioners. Herein will serve as an encouragement for healthcare providers to continue their pursuit of new technologies for both caregivers and patients, primarily by recognizing the importance of data analysis and integration in modern medical systems.

Herein, the current uses and possibilities of data integration will be explored in medical fields, specifically with federal initiatives to incorporate data analysis in the healthcare system. The chapter will divulge several benefits and challenges associated with incorporating data analysis and integration in healthcare systems. Benefits include: improved diagnosis, preventative diagnoses, accurate records of prior and current treatment, protection from drug interactions, overdoses, and allergies, real time diagnoses and treatment, a more cost effective system, and enhanced research for future improvements. Some challenges include: data security, patients' privacy concerns, the learning curve for clinicians, incentives for data integration, analysis, and sharing, implementing a standard for integration and sharing, and maintaining a patient-centric practice. This chapter will end with a proposal for healthcare providers to collaborate on medical analysis and integration across health professions, and the associated risks and rewards with an application on that scale.

Chapter 11: Healthcare IoT Architectures, Technologies, Applications, and Issues – A Deep Insight

The idea of the IoT was originated and devised with the context of Radio Frequency Identification (RFID), which is used for tracking the objects in various domains like logistics and supply chain management. For example, Automated Teller Machines (ATMs) are interconnected to the bank network, which enables the payments with ATM cards at the point of sales depots. ATM uses the machine-to-machine (M2M) networks and these established a basement for IoT through network connected systems and data. The probability of connecting the objects to the network provides tagging, tracking and reading of data from objects that goes hand in hand with greater efforts which would become a promising technology of this era called as IoT.

IoT was first coined by Kevin Ashton in 1999 and developed in analogous to Wireless Sensor Networks (WSN). The term IoT refers to the physical devices that are interconnected to gather and share the data with each other via communication technology and cloud computing enables to collect, record and to analyze the data stream more accurately within short span of time. The term "Things" in IoT specifies variety of devices includes sensors, automobiles, buildings, industries, human beings, animals, plants any type of goods. WSNs are assumed to rely on wireless communication technologies whereas IoT does not assumed to rely on specific communication technology. The characteristics of wireless sensors like tiny, rugged, inexpensive and low powered renovated the IoT, facilitates the smallest objects can be integrated with different environments. IoT can be considered as an upcoming evolution of the internet which uses many existing features including machine-to-machine communication (M2M), radio frequency identification (RFID) and sensors.

IoT is defined as an ever growing technology through which computing devices, mechanical and digital machines, physical objects, animals or human beings are interconnected via communication medium provides the ability to exchange information and automate the tasks without human-interaction.

IoT is being labeled by different applications, protocols, standards and architectures. IoT is not just a technology but certainly comprising of different things like data analytics, actuators, hubs, artificial intelligence, communication, wide range of sensors, IoT nodes, gateways, networks, cloud computing, edge computing, processing, optimization, IoT platforms and so on. Connecting the physical things through networks and data stream processing increases the potentiality of IoT by adding intelligence to the systems. The common technologies driving the IoT applications are depicted in the Figure 1.

As IoT can be considered as a fully dependent on the potentials of sensors and other technologies, IoT devices must possess three basic qualities such as:

- **Sensable:** IoT devices must be able to sense and aggregate the data. For example, in healthcare field aggregating the blood glucose, pulse rate and body temperature data via sensors. The data aggregated must be self-directed.

- **Communicable:** The data aggregated must be transmitted to data centers or other devices upon specific conditions via communication medium (i.e. Wireless Technologies).
- **Actionable:** The data aggregation itself doesn't make any sense or change behavior. It must exhibit some actions. For example, if a patient's pulse rate or blood level exceeds its normal range, the IoT system must automatically send an alert message to the healthcare providers for further interventions.

Chapter 12: A Forecasting Model for Patient Arrivals of an Emergency Department in Healthcare Management Systems

Forecasting can be expressed as making predictions at times when the results are not observable in the present situation. Forecasting play an important role in making short and long-term decisions. In all societies, the level of population access of health resources is directly related to the well-being of the community. One of the most important part of the National Health System is hospitals which has special technologies, advanced equipment and also healthcare personnel. Emergency departments (EDs) are one of the most valued parts of the healthcare management systems. It has to provide adequate, immediate and accurate healthcare management. Performance determiners for service quality through EDs are related with length of stay (LOS) and waiting times, which are affected by high levels of ED arrivals. The number of patients who will come to the EDs and the waiting times will be one of the most important input parameters in the planning of the investments and arrangements to be made in the ED in the future. Compared with other departments of the hospitals, the ED is clearly the more crowded than other departments. One of the most important factors that cannot predicted in emergency services is the time of arrival of the patients. The number of future patients which need to health care to the ED service is directly related to the various independent variables and the number of patients coming in per day in the past period. Accurate forecasts of patient arrivals which need immediate health care contribute to better organized human resources and medical devices in EDs.

On the other hand, time has important effects on the performance of EDs. It is measured and analyzed for suitable evaluation of ED performances. Patient arrivals are one of the important process of EDs in healthcare management systems. Long wait and overcrowding in ED processes is increased in recent years which directly affect the quality of ED performances. These processes have the potential to improve ED throughput and patient pleasure if these are efficiently fulfilment. Because of delay within time related processes have potential to effect overcrowding in the EDs, it gets significant must to be forecasted and known time by means of prevent from the delays. Statistical forecasting considered as an operation research technique that uses time series data and a kind of statistical formulae and data mining approaches to forecast different types of ED processes. The more researches are needed for more exact planning due to improvement of forecasting models. It helps to decrease of overcrowding linked to other hospital units and external world.

In this chapter, we aim to develop a hybrid model including the methods ARIMAX and ANN for patient arrivals of a hospital ED. By the aid of the proposed model, an insight to the doctors and administrator staff for planning of ED resources will be provided in a better way. Our ultimate goal is to provide ED stakeholders with a background on the ED as healthcare management systems and a hybrid statistical forecasting method that can be practically applied to various ED processes. This chapter will contribute to the literature by the following aspects: (1) To the best of our knowledge, there is no studies that have used the ARIMAX-ANN hybrid model to forecast ED arrivals in Turkey, (2) The model includes not only calendar factors but also climate factors and some special factors (weekend and public holidays) in forecasting ED arrivals, (3) By the proposed model, it will be proved that using the ARIMAX-ANN hybridization is applicable for forecasting of ED patient arrival forecasting and helping in arrangement and planning of ED resources.

The study is structured as follows: Section 2 details related literature and background for forecasting of patient arrivals. Section 3 analyzed data source and provides detail of ARIMAX and ANN methods. In section 4, application of the hybrid approach is investigated for the case of public hospital ED arrivals in Turkey. Finally, Section 5 presents conclusion, limitations, and future remarks.

Chapter 13: Application of Big Data in Digital Epidemiology

The power of technology in this era is so huge that anyone can track your whereabouts just by using your cell phone location. They can even predict where you can be at some later point of time by using various analytics. This information may be used by a security agency for nabbing the criminals. But not only this! There is a Swedish project by the name of Flowminder which tracks the movement of population during any natural disaster and can use it for the sake of relief and rescue.

This is just one of the examples of a project in the field of digital epidemiology. Epidemiology is a field which deals with the study and analysis of various patterns, their reasons and how they affect the health and disease in any geographical area or a defined population. Traditionally the data has been collected from various sources by different agencies and it is analyzed using tools to get some insight into the reasons for the spread of diseases. The new field of digital epidemiology relies on collecting the data using digital techniques such as getting data from various social networking sites and then using computational methods to measure health and the spread of disease. Governments of various countries are supporting projects which use big data for digital epidemiology. Air quality data is being captured by environmental scientists from the polluted areas and then it is compared with the health status of the people living in those areas. This can give an insight into the correlation between the environmental hazards and the diseases present there. Information on sexual and social networks are gathered by Epidemiologists which helps them predict the signs of spread of diseases so that early warning signs can be issued.

Big data analytics helps in predictive modeling in healthcare sector which provide faster, better and more targeted results in digital epidemiology which helps to develop better vaccines faster. It also helps in analysis of disease patters which helps track disease outbreaks which results in faster disaster management.

Chapter 14: Artificial Intelligence in Medical Science

Any device or machine having its own computation ability is considered as intelligent. With the advancement of technology, many intelligent devices are developed with less expense having high computational and analytical ability. These characteristics of intelligent devices have increased the demand of these devices in engineering, medical science, space research, geological survey, automobiles, traffic control and many more. The intelligent devices have the capability to learn like a human being and solve many real-world problems in an intelligent manner. In many cases, they are replacing human beings and giving more accurate and faster results than humans. Such type of systems have the ability of learning from past experience, communicating with other devices to gather and share information. The storage capacity and processing speed of these devices are much higher than the human brain which has increased the popularity of these devices. These devices are used to solve many sensitive and sophisticated problems in medical field. The systems also have the capability to solve many problems using past information and data stored in the form of a knowledge base.

Intelligent systems consist of devices which are intelligent in nature and have the capability to work on software designed using the concepts from Artificial Intelligence as well as having network connectivity.

Intelligent devices use their analytical ability on the defined set of information in the form of rules to obtain a conclusion. Humans learn from experience, machines derive new rules from existing rules using inference mechanism. Machine also have the analytical and reasoning ability like human beings. The computing capability of machine is more as compared to humans. Machine also has the ability to process different languages so that they can interact with people and can store and analyse the information stored in different languages.

In short, the book will provide insights and support executives concerned with the management of expertise, knowledge, information and organizational development in different types of healthcare work communities and environments.

Nardjes Bouchemal
University Center of Mila, Algeria

Chapter 1
Evolution of Digital Technologies and Use of Virtual Assistants in Drug Development

Manu Venugopal
Independent Researcher, India

ABSTRACT

The drug development phase is one of the most time-consuming and expensive stages in the lifecycle of a drug. Marred by patent expirations, price regulations, complexities in disease conditions, life sciences companies are facing a daunting task to bring new molecular entities into the market. Digital health technologies are playing a critical role in addressing some of the challenges faced during drug development. In this chapter, the author talks about the challenges and key trends in the world of drug development, use of new digital health technologies, and the future of drug development. As an example, the author dives into a specific case study on the use of virtual assistants in clinical trials and the benefits of its usage on patients, healthcare professionals, and life sciences companies.

INTRODUCTION

It is a common knowledge in the Life Sciences Industry that conduct of clinical trials and their approvals by regulatory authorities as part of the drug development journey takes a major share of the time and cost spent by pharmaceutical companies in their attempt to bring a new drug into the market. While there have been big advances in improving the operational and process efficiencies in drug development, there are still ample avenues to further automate and reduce the cost and schedule burden on the pharma companies. Information technology have been on the forefront in this journey and have been enabling companies to move away from traditional business models to more patient centric models in drug development.

DOI: 10.4018/978-1-5225-7071-4.ch001

The chapter begins with an understanding of the current state of drug research and development, various challenges faced and key trends. It then goes through the evolution and use of various technologies that have shaped drug development. It introduces new technologies like artificial intelligence, machine learning, automated / virtual reality, blockchain and how they can be adopted to change the way various functions in the research and development operate today. The chapter provides an overview of the ongoing developments taken up by regulatory authorities favouring the adoption of new technologies by industry players. As an example of use of AI technology, the chapter deep dives into a conceptual model and few use cases of how virtual assistants or chatbots can benefit the main stakeholders in clinical trials – the subject, the investigator and the sponsor. The chapter concludes by providing the reader with a view into the future of clinical development – a digital convergence.

DRUG RESEARCH AND DEVELOPMENT OVERVIEW

It takes 10-15 years for a single drug to reach the market. The overall cost for this process increases every few years and currently stands at around $1.4 billion. It is not just the time and cost involved but also the success rate of the compound that makes development of a drug one of the most complex and risky process in the whole pharma value chain. If one starts to screen 10,000 compounds during the initial discovery phase, there is a chance of just 1 compound to get a market approval from a regulatory authority. Hence, both from a social and economic perspective, it is quite natural that drug research and development phase is a key focus area to implement process and operational efficiencies, automation and risk reduction techniques.

Drug research and development comprises of four major stages namely, discovery, pre-clinical, clinical development and pharmacovigilance. As the drug passes through these phases in the development life cycle, there are important regulatory milestones that defines the progress of the compounds till market approval. Figure 1 depicts the various R&D phases and regulatory milestones.

During the drug discovery phase, the scientists get involved in understanding the mechanisms of the disease, identifying the disease targets, screening the potential compounds that can bind with the target and selecting the most promising compounds that exhibit good potency with minimal toxicity. Most of the work is done in the laboratory through in silico (using computer simulation and modelling) and in-vivo (in test tubes) methods.

The high potential compounds enter the pre-clinical phase where they are tested on animals whose animal models are analogous to humans and appropriate for the tests being conducted. The main objectives of the pre-clinical testing are to arrive at the right dosages of the compound that are safe for human

Figure 1. Drug research and development process

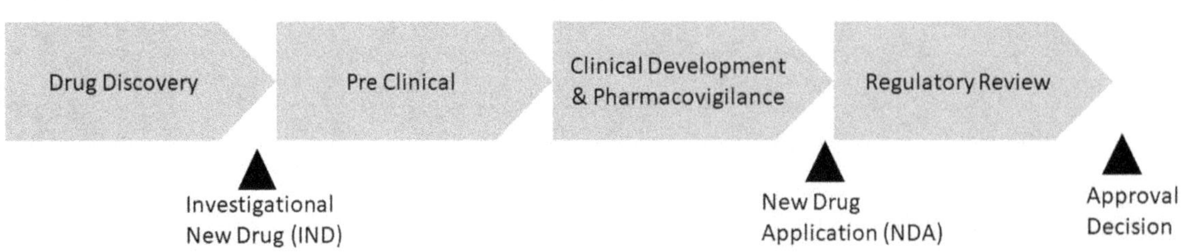

consumption, evaluate the pharmacokinetics properties measured by ADME (Absorption, Distribution, Metabolism, Excretion) tests and determine the toxicity profile of the compound. Once the compound is found to achieve the objectives, the trial sponsor files an Investigational New Drug (IND) application to FDA. This application is to seek approval for conducting clinical trials on humans.

Clinical development involves testing the compound on humans and collecting evidences for efficacy and safety. Clinical trials are conducted in three phases namely, Phase I, Phase II and Phase III each differing in the type and number of trial subjects, trial duration and objectives. Different dosages of various compounds that passed the pre-clinical tests go through clinical trials. The trials are conducted in clinical sites which could be a hospital, primary health clinic or research site. Each site has a primary investigator responsible for the trial conduct supported by site staff. Trial subjects are recruited at each clinical site and they go through the treatment as prescribed in the clinical trial protocol. Once the subjects have completed the study, data is collected and analysed to verify if they meet the trial objectives. The clinical data and outcomes are submitted to FDA along with the New Drug Application (NDA). NDA application is to seek approval from FDA to market the drug in United States.

FDA conducts a thorough review of the data submitted that could take around 18 to 24 months. Upon receiving approval, the trial sponsor decides to setup the manufacturing units for mass production. Throughout the clinical development phase and even after gaining regulatory approval, the safety parameters of the drug are continuously monitored, recorded, reviewed and submitted. Broadly known as pharmacovigilance, it is the responsibility of the trial sponsor to ensure that safety of the patients participating in the trial and those consuming the drug after launching the drug into the market. Regulatory bodies have stringent regulations by way of adverse event reporting and signal management to minimize the health risks in patients.

Challenges in Drug Development

Over the last 50 years, one has witnessed major advancements in the field of medicine and technology. However, the numbers indicate that the productivity of the pharma R&D is on the decline. There are many economic and geopolitical factors at play. Firstly, is the increasing number of patent expirations or commonly known as the patent cliff that indicates the huge drop in drug sales after a patent expiration. In the year 2018 alone, 26 drugs will go off patent which translates into an estimated $31 billion in losses. According to EvaluatePharma World Preview 2017, Outlook to 2022 report during the period 2017-2022, $194 billion of drug sales is at risk (EvaluatePharma, 2017). Such huge losses can shake even the big pharma companies. Secondly, the golden era of blockbuster drugs (drugs that make more than $1 billion in revenue) has come to an end. It is increasingly difficult to find new molecules for common health issues and the competition is so fierce that chances of one drug raking in billions of dollars is daunting. Pharma companies cannot depend on blockbusters to drive up their revenue numbers. Thirdly, in recent years pharma companies have been put to lot of public pressure in controlling the pricing of drugs. The US government has stressed on reforms in healthcare to contain health care costs and make drugs affordable. The drug pricing challenge further pulls down the chances of companies to recoup its R&D and marketing expenses and remain profitable. Another issue that does not favour R&D is the rising development costs and changing regulatory environment. Clinical trials have become more complex but at the same time they continue to follow traditional approaches that are inefficient and time consuming. Rigid trial designs, lack of better patient recruitment and retention strategies, inefficient and redundant ways of trial management do not yield the right outcomes leading to cost overruns.

It is imperative that companies need to devise strategies to overcome some of these challenges in order to stay relevant in the marketplace.

Changing Business Models in Pharma R&D

It is good news that Life Sciences players are responding positively to the changing business conditions and many are in the process of transforming their business models and strategies to ride on the next wave of growth. Following are some of the interesting trends that companies have tuned into:

- **From Primary Care Drugs to Specialty Medicine:** The focus of companies is shifting from developing drugs for common problems such as hypertension, diabetes, gastric disorders to drugs for patient's unmet needs (called novel drugs) and for rare medical conditions (called orphan drugs) that affect a small number of patients. The trend is driven by factors such as high price and high profit margin through the sale of such drugs, accelerated regulatory approvals and lesser competition.
- **Shift to Patient Centricity:** With internet, social media and mobile devices becoming ubiquitous, patients have better access to information making them more informed to take decisions of their health. Patient experiences and opinions are voiced through public domains. Insights from such experiences help companies to provide patients with products and services that matter to them most. Known as 'Beyond the pill' services, companies use digital technologies to offer services to the patients and connect them with overall health care ecosystem.
- **Personalised Medicine:** All patients do not respond to a drug in the same manner but drugs have been developed assuming a 'one size fits all' approach. With the advancements in genetic testing and diagnostic methods coupled with real world data about patients, scientists can now identify the target population that is best suited for the drug. Known by different names such as precision medicine, personalized healthcare, targeted therapies, it drives the success rate for the drug manufacturer as well as helps the patient by receiving the right treatment.
- **Develop Combination Therapies:** Combination drug is to combine two or more approved drugs that can help fight diseases more effectively than single drugs. This is particularly useful in treating cancer since cancer can metastatize and become resistant to therapies over time. Combination product also improves scientific collaboration as it could involve combining drugs from multiple drug manufacturers.
- **Leaner and Focused Model:** For more than a decade, pharma industry has seen a lot of consolidation through mergers and acquisitions. Acquisition targets were mostly those companies that has specialized expertise or products that the parent company lack such as biotechnology firms, firms specializing in certain therapeutic areas such as oncology. In recent years, there is another phenomenon seen mainly in Big pharma – to go leaner in their portfolio by divesting their low growth assets. For example, GSK swapped their oncology division for consumer health and vaccines division from Novartis and vice versa. AstraZeneca is narrowing their focus on few core therapeutic areas. Companies like Abbott split its company into 2 companies to have a better focus on both businesses (Gautam, 2016).

TECHNOLOGIES SHAPING THE DRUG DEVELOPMENT ECOSYSTEM

Information technology has been reinventing itself and taking up different roles over past few decades. From a mere support function, IT has come to the forefront in transforming the way businesses are run. Though pharma industry is known for its late adoption of technology, the digital wave caught up early and has influenced in building new business models focusing more on patient centricity.

Early Digital Technologies: SMAC and Big Data

It wasn't that early when technologies like the Social, Mobility, Analytics, Cloud, together known by the acronym S-M-A-C were known as new age digital technologies. Also, it does not imply that these technologies are phased out completely. These technologies have now become more mainstream and other newer technologies have taken their place. The drug development phase has immensely benefited with the usage of SMAC and big data and pharma industry continue to invest in these technologies. Following gives a brief overview of how these technologies are helping companies to solve many of the challenges faced during drug development.

- **Social Media**: Social media platforms such as Facebook, online communities like PatientsLikeMe, AskaPatient and microblogging sites are used for recruiting patients for participating in clinical trials, providing disease management and wellness tips, collaborating with fellow trial participants to share experiences as well as with investigators and site staff to improve quality of care.
- **Mobility**: Mobile devices and mobile health apps combined with wearables are being considered as medical devices. Smart inventions such as the 'digital pill' use mobile devices to transfer patient data to health care providers. Many health apps help trial subjects to understand and manage the disease condition, trial procedures and treatment options. There are gamification health apps used for specific purposes such as pain relief and drug adherence measurements. B Braun's NuTRIscreen app, Sanofi's iBGStar Diabetes Manager app are some examples of health apps targeted at patients and general public.
- **Analytics**: Clinical trials generate large amount of data, both patient and operational data, which contain wealth of information. Using this data, analytics can unlock interesting insights about trial procedures, patient expectations and trial issues. Predictive modelling and simulation to identify the right target and compound slashes the time taken for drug discovery. Optimization algorithms for better utilization of CRAs increases the quality and on time delivery of a trial. Analytics to assess the site risks and remotely monitoring the trial progress helps in identifying risky sites earlier and enables trial team to take corrective action sooner.
- **Cloud:** With health care and pharmaceutical industries put together, the global health care computing market will reach $9.5 billion by 2020 (McCarthy, 2015). Like other industries, the benefits of cloud computing such as reduced capital expenditure, higher scalability, broader access, efficient data storage has pushed pharma to move to cloud based solutions. Though pharma companies showed resistance in cloud adoption in the initial stages due to data privacy, data security issues and lack of proper regulatory guidance, now most of them have cloud strategy defined and implemented across the technology stack. Different cloud service models such as SaaS (software as a service), PaaS (Platform as a service) present companies the flexibility to adopt a model that best suits their business operations.

- **Big Data:** The term Big data refers to high availability of digitized data. The value of Big data is best realized when it is used with proper analytics that generate deep insights which was not possible earlier due to the volume, variability and structure of data. One example of a big data application is in drug discovery where petabytes of unstructured data are generated through next generation sequencing solutions. Another application is in real world evidence (RWE) where data comes from prescription data, claims data and electronic health records (EMRs). RWE can provide good insights about patients, their demographics and drug effects to the pharma R&D team. Since this data comes in different formats from disparate systems, data aggregation requires a big data platform powered by an analytics engine or even more better by artificial intelligence.

Newer Digital Technologies

An analysis by a leading IT consulting group, revealed that digitization in the pharmaceutical market will fuel almost one-third of the growth and an estimated 40 percent of the profitability by 2020 (Accenture, n.d.). Digitization wave took off with SMAC, big data and Internet of things but has now shifted gears to propel even faster with emerging technologies namely artificial intelligence (AI), virtual and augmented reality (VR/AR) and blockchain. It is important to first understand what do these technologies comprise and what benefits do they offer before going into the applications in the drug development space.

Artificial Intelligence (AI)

Artificial Intelligence in simple terms is enabling a machine to think, comprehend and act like a human in a given context. Also known as cognitive computing, AI is an umbrella term encompassing multiple technologies such as expert systems, machine learning (ML), natural language processing (NLP) and robotics. While this concept existed as early as in the 1950s, it was only in the last 5 years that prominence of AI is felt across multiple industries. Majority of the applications that are seen around us comes under Artificial Narrow Intelligence (ANI) or called 'Weak AI'. It means that it can handle simple to complex tasks based on large set of algorithms but it lacks human intuition and self learning capabilities. Virtual personal assistants, chatbots, robotic process automation fall under this category. Machine learning enables the machine to learn by itself and improve its output based on prior experiences. Natural language processing enables machines to comprehend a human language and respond in a similar fashion. Such technologies, grouped as 'Strong AI', are still in different stages of evolution.

AI will soon get fully integrated in the overall drug development process since AI technology can address some of the main challenges notably reducing the time taken to bring the drug to market and reducing the failure rate of a compound in discovery and clinical trials. Through the application of deep learning and neural networks, one can analyse the complex disease pathways and the effect of various demographic, genetic and phenotypic variations on the efficacy of a drug. Through AI, the scientists can predict which section of population will experience a positive effect of the drug when compared to other sections of the population. This helps in the discovery of targeted therapies which forms the basis of personalized medicine. Since the technology suggests the potential success molecules, scientists can spend lesser time and money by avoiding trial and error tests on large number of molecules. During the clinical trial phase, AI will be useful in engaging patients and providing them with a more personalized experience. One such application where virtual assistants powered by AI improve patient engagement is illustrated in greater detail in the next section of this chapter. The applicability of AI is also high in the other phases of the drug development such as management of safety reports and safety signals, regulatory operations and in clinical trial supply planning and distribution.

There are many real-world examples of the use of AI in drug development. BERG, a pharmaceutical startup has developed a cancer drug based on the insights from a AI program. The AI program takes over 14 trillion data points from a single human cell that changes from healthy to cancerous. Another bioinformatics firm, Insilico Medicine, has developed an AI solution which predicts the therapeutic area of new drugs. It helps scientists to identify secondary and tertiary therapeutic uses which is difficult to find out from the preliminary in-vitro tests during discovery (Pharmaceutical Online, 2017). IBM's artificial intelligence platform, Watson, is making great strides by partnering with multiple pharma majors such as Pfizer, Novartis, Teva, Otsuka, Novo Nordisk in the areas of oncology, psychiatric disorders and diabetes.

Virtual Reality (VR), Augmented Reality (AR), and Mixed Reality (MR)

Together known as 'immersive technologies', VR/AR/MR provides the user an immersive experience. In other words, these technologies provide a perception to the user that he/she is physically present in a non-physical world or a real world supplemented by virtual objects. There isn't a universal agreement on the definition of various immersive technologies and hence one will find different interpretations of each technology in the public domain.

- **Virtual Reality (VR):** The most popular among all and it refers to an experience of a virtual world created using real world content or computer-generated content or a combination of both. To experience VR, one requires a head mounted displays (HMD) such as a simple Google cardboard, HTC Vive, Occulus Rift and so on. An example of VR application is to virtually view the interiors of a car and perform actions such as opening the car door, sitting inside the car and operating the dashboard controls. The view can be generated either using a real video recording or computer graphics.
- **Augmented Reality (AR):** Provides the user an immersive experience by supplementing or overlaying virtual content on the real-world content. Imagine a surgeon performing an operation, getting the latest information of the patient's vitals and details of the surgical procedures right in front of his eye. Google Glass, Microsoft Hololens attempt to provide an AR experience and there are many use cases built using these gadgets. The popular video game, Pokeman GO is a great example of AR.
- **Mixed Reality (MR)**: More advanced when compared to VR and AR. It is truly immersive since it blurs the barrier between an imaginary and real world. In an MR, both real world content and a synthetic/ computer generated content co-exist and respond to each other. Imagine you are sitting across the table with a computer generated human character and when you offer a real glass of water, you see the character extending the hand for the glass.

Global Industry Analysts predict that the worldwide market for VR in healthcare will reach $3.8 billion by 2020. In the field of drug development, one can think of many applications for VR, AR and MR. Scientists working on a group of compounds need not sift through lot of literature physically when an AR device can fetch the relevant information of the compound after identifying it using the compound structure or name. A VR setup showing a recently enrolled patient all the clinical procedures expected to be performed is another useful application which improves the patient's awareness and confidence to participate in the trial. VR and AR applications can make the education and training of investigators and site staff more engaging and interesting.

Blockchain

Blockchain technology has been touted as the best invention in the recent years after Internet. What started with a use case for financial transactions, blockchain usage has touched all industries in the past couple of years. It is particularly attractive to the Life Sciences industry because its fundamentals are built on creating a 'trusted' network. With intellectual property, patient confidentiality, data privacy, regulatory policies being critical aspects that Life Sciences companies must adhere to, having an efficient, cost effective trusted mechanism to manage operations seems to be the most ideal way to run the business.

In simple terms, Blockchain is a shared or distributed ledger that is not owned by a single authority, an organization or a person and is used to store and transact assets among multiple parties. The ledger maintains a permanent record of a transaction that cannot be tampered. Computers communicating over a peer to peer (P2P) network ensures that any new transaction happening over the network is validated for authenticity before adding it to the ledger. The term blockchain comes from the way the data is stored and linked. The transactions happening at a specific time period are placed in a block which is linked to a previous block after validation forming a chain of transaction blocks. The first use case for blockchain was the bitcoin, which is a digital currency also called as cryptocurrency. While transacting in cryptocurrency is still illegal in many countries, the idea of bitcoins triggered a new wave of applying the underlying blockchain technology to several business contexts.

Within Life Sciences, blockchain technology is slated to provide a $3 billion opportunity by 2025 (Guenther, Pierson & Modi, 2018). By virtue of the very functioning of blockchain, it has a very high applicability in drug supply chain. The serialization track and trace to track down counterfeit drugs can be best achieved by implementing a blockchain enabled logistics network. In drug development, blockchain can be employed in securely transferring anonymized clinical trial data and results and tracking its usage to prevent misuse. One of the challenges in clinical trials is the incidence of data manipulation at the site level and at the program level. When data gets collected from multiple CROs and associated sites, there needs to a robust mechanism to track the data from the source to destination and detect any data pilferage or corruption. Blockchain can prove very beneficial in this regard. Another possible use case in clinical trials is creating a trial document such as a trial protocol as a smart contract in the blockchain network. Any changes to the trial document gets notified to the stakeholders permissioned with the access which can then be validated using a proof of existence algorithm and accepted by all stakeholders.

Several companies including pharma majors such as Pfizer, Amgen, Sanofi are eyeing on blockchain to provide a streamlined process in developing and testing of their drugs. It is also interesting to note that companies are coming together to collaborate on aspects that has an industry wide relevance. In the coming years, one can witness lot more traction in terms of investment in blockchain from companies as well as from industry consortiums.

REGULATOR'S PERSPECTIVE ON THE USE OF DIGITAL HEALTH TECHNOLOGIES

The advancement of digital technologies and its acceptance by patients and health care providers have led regulatory authorities around the world to modify their guidance for approvals of digital health technologies. The context of medical devices in the Federal Food, Drug, and Cosmetic Act (FDCA) were more hardware dependent and followed the traditional approach of device development. With mobile applications, software as a medical device and AI powered wearables, the scope changed significantly resulting in the need for changes to regulatory guidance. While pharma industry is ready to adopt the technologies and transform their business models to be patient focused, lack of clear guidance from regulators remains a hinderance for implementation.

Over the last many years, FDA has taken several steps in addressing the fast changing technology environment because it realizes the potential of digital technology driving a revolution in health care. Some of the recent regulatory activities undertaken by FDA have been mentioned below.

- **Digital Health Program:** The aim is to develop and implement regulatory strategies, policies and processes for certain digital health products and help foster collaboration with digital health developers, patients and providers. In December 2017, FDA came up with the Digital Health Innovation Action plan which includes increasing the number and expertise of digital health staff at the FDA, launching the digital health software precertification pilot program ("Pre-Cert") and issuing guidance to modernize the policies (FDA, 2017).
- **21st Century Cures Act:** In this law that the United States Congress enacted in December 2016, the definition of 'device' was amended to exclude certain medical software used for storing and displaying electronic health records, supporting administrative functions or providing limited clinical decision support. Also, clinical decision-making software (CDS), the category in which artificial intelligence algorithms falls into, is excluded from FDA's jurisdiction as long as health care professional does an independent review on the basis of the clinical recommendation produced by the software (Jones Day, 2018).
- **Release of new draft guidance:** FDA has issued many final and draft guidance over the last couple of years and plans for many more draft guidance for the provisions mentioned in the 21st Century Cures Act. This includes policy on Mobile medical applications, Clinical and Patient Decision Support Software, General Wellness and Mobile Medical Applications, Medical image storage devices used to store or retrieve medical images electronically and Software as a Medical Device: Clinical Evaluation.

In the EU, the regulatory authority has made significant changes to the current regulatory structure by publishing the new Medical Device Regulation (EU MDR) in May 2017. The regulations specifically address the classification of software as medical devices. A software with a medical purpose of "prediction and prognosis" will fall within the scope of the Regulation. This means that an AI software that do not provide a treatment recommendation but only a disease risk prediction falls in the scope of medical devices. EU has also modernized its data protection framework by adopting a General Data Protection Regulation (GDPR).

With more health applications being introduced through digital technologies, the regulatory regime of FDA, EU and other parts of the world continue to widen their scope and evolve their policies to provide the oversight as well as enable the advancement of health innovations beneficial for the consumer.

AI POWERED VIRTUAL ASSISTANTS: A TRUE COMPANION FOR PATIENTS AND PHYSICIANS

This section talks about a practical implementation of an AI use case in clinical trials. The intent is to provide the reader with how can virtual assistants be used in the clinical context by delving into the business problem, conceptual model for implementation and the business benefits.

Overview of Virtual Assistants and Chatbots

Gartner defines Virtual Assistant (VA) as "a conversational, computer-generated character that simulates a conversation to deliver voice- or text-based information to a user via a Web, kiosk or mobile interface". While a virtual assistant encompasses conversation with a virtual character in any form (speech or text), people associate it more with voice conversations. Apple's Siri, Microsoft's Cortana, Google's Google Now, Amazon's Alexa which have the capability to understand, interpret and respond in natural language are referred to as popular examples of virtual assistants. Chatbot, on the other hand, is associated with textual conversations. Chatbots are the first generation of virtual conversational agents and are primarily rule based systems with some involvement of machine learning. Chatbots can be employed in any customer facing environment and can either be a standalone app or integrated with other messenger apps such as Facebook Messenger, Slack, Telegram to name a few.

Virtual assistants work with internet connected devices which could be a smartphone app or a dedicated device like Amazon's Echo. In most of the cases, the virtual assistant software is deployed on the cloud which gets connected to other devices over internet. Technologies that drive the software must be capable of handling and analysing huge amounts of data. Machine learning and natural language processing are used many a time to understand the requests from the user, learn their needs over time and provide appropriate responses hence creating a personalized user experience.

As mentioned earlier, the main benefit of the use of virtual assistant is to drive customer engagement which in turn leads to enhanced customer loyalty and revenue growth. Some of the other benefits that make VA a huge business opportunity are:

- Provides a more personalized experience than other online interfaces
- Helps to understand the customer preferences better
- Provides 24/7 support to customers by addressing queries and concerns round the clock
- Reduces the dependency on human workforce online thereby reducing operational costs
- Enables handling of multiple conversations in parallel driving overall productivity
- Freeing up time of human agents to perform more sophisticated tasks

Virtual Assistants in Clinical Development

It is worthwhile to revisit some of the main challenges the pharma industry faces in clinical development phase. Patient recruitment for participating in clinical trials is one of the top 3 reasons for delays in clinical trial completion. 80% of the trials fail to finish on time due to recruitment issues. Recruitment relies heavily on the capability of the clinical site and the investigator to draw enough patients into the study. But statistics indicate that 50% of the sites end up enrolling less than 1 patient to their studies. With about 40% of the total US pharmaceutical clinical trial budget is spent on patient recruitment, it is an expensive activity (Diamond, 2015). Enrolling patients in a clinical trial is just one step towards a successful start of the clinical trial. To achieve the desired results from clinical trial, it is equally important to have the enrolled subjects adhere to the clinical protocol procedures and remain in the study until its end. However, retaining an enrolled patient is yet another important challenge faced by sites. If the trial does not produce sufficient patient data, it cannot meet the statistical significance in its results leading to further delays in trial completion and a risk of not getting approval from the regulatory authorities. 85% of the clinical trials fail to retain enough patients and as high as 30% of the patients drop out during the trial (Diamond, 2015). There are many reasons for such staggering numbers in recruitment and retention. It turns out that lack of awareness in patients and proper engagement in the trial are the main causes.

Turning the focus on clinical sites, there are many issues around experience and workload of site staff, process adherence, site infrastructure that impacts trial progress. A majority of the site's success is attributed to the principal investigator. An experienced investigator with a large patient base and good site facilities is an ideal candidate. Such investigators are always in demand and are approached by multiple study sponsors. Workload along with legal and regulatory burden are immense for the investigator since he/she has to handle multiple aspects of the trial proceedings along with the regular clinical practice. Corneli et al (2017) conducted a survey to understand why many principal investigators chose to participate in only one FDA regulated trial. Among the barriers identified as challenging for investigators, close of two thirds of the investigators cited lack of proper workload balance and almost the same proportion of investigators indicated the pressure on time requirements for many trial activities.

Creating a collaborative and personalized experience both for patients and investigators will drastically improve the current situation leading to better trial outcomes and patient care. In other industries such as retail and financial services, virtual assistants are being increasingly accepted as a platform to drive customer engagement and manage medium to complex tasks. In the clinical trial setup, this platform can open new ways of interacting with the patients at the same time support in many of the administrative and regulatory activities handled by the investigator and site staff. One of the subsequent sections will go through several potential use cases that employ the virtual assistant platform.

Conceptual Model

Before delving into the use cases, it is important to understand what does a VA environment comprise of and how the data flow between the system and the users in the context of a clinical trial. Figure 2 depicts the VA conceptual model and the interactions with the various internal/ external systems and with the stakeholders.

The model has three broad architecture layers – namely, UX or the client layer, AI processing engine or business layer and Information sources or data/ data access layer. Each of these layers are described below:

Figure 2. Conceptual model for virtual assistant-based clinical trial

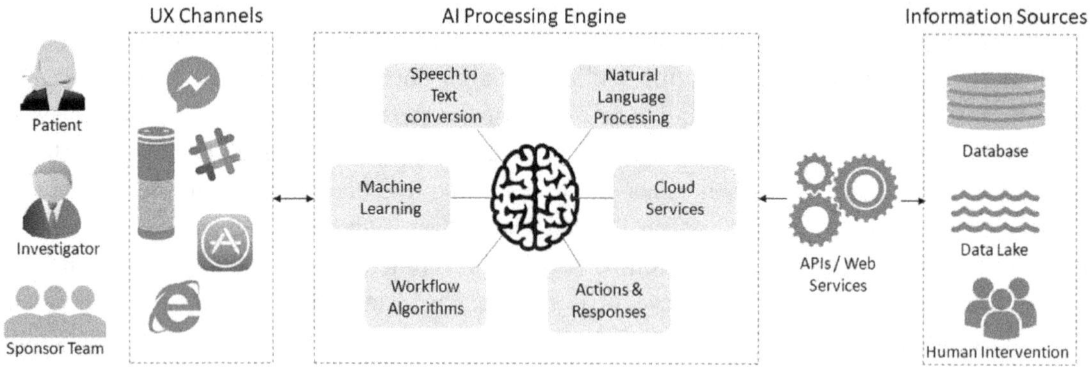

- **UX Layer:** This layer is the top most layer that interacts with the user, in this case, the patient or investigator or in some cases the clinical sponsor team members. The main function of this layer is to provide an intuitive interface that can efficiently communicate with the user, accept his/her request, send the response processed by the AI engine to the user. In a clinical trial, choosing an appropriate UX channel depends on the type of trial and subject. For example, in a trial with geriatric population, using a virtual assistant through a smartphone might be challenging when compared to the large screen desktop computers. In case of a paediatric study, it is not the patient but the caregiver who will be using the services of VA. There are multiple UX channel options available such as text based Facebook messenger, slack or voice based Amazon Alexa, Microsoft Cortana.
- **AI Processing Engine:** This is the heart of the VA system where bulk of the processing occurs. There are many services at play within the AI engine that processes the user requests. The services typically used in a VA application are:
  - **Speech to Text Conversion:** This is used for voice based conversations where a patient's voice request is translated to textual form that can be understood and processed.
  - **Machine Learning:** This is primarily used where there is a need for the system to continuously learn new user inputs and improve on the response. The system undergoes supervised learning for new queries and enhance its pattern matching capabilities.
  - **Natural Language Processing:** NLP is an important component of AI which converts a human language into a machine understandable language. Human language can convey an information in different ways and NLP attempts to understand the intent of the conversation and take appropriate action.
  - **Workflow Algorithms:** The algorithms are procedures that guide the chatbots to engage in a conversation and provide responses intuitively. Based on the requests from the user, the algorithms direct the requests to the appropriate services and seek responses.
  - **Cloud Services:** Machine learning, NLP and speech processing require significant compute power which is best provided by a cloud based platform. Cloud services can efficiently manage the large amount of structured and unstructured data emerging from user conversations.

    - **APIs for Action and Response Services:** In order to communicate with the other layers, the system exposes a host of APIs to input and output data. Many of the UX channels such as Facebook, Amazon, Google provide API services to integrate their products with other business applications. The communication between AI processing engine and the information sources layer is also enabled through custom build APIs.
- **Information Sources:** This layer forms the back-end layer that feeds raw data to the processing engine. Information sources can either be a repository of data such as a database or be a human providing appropriate information based on the user request. For example, when a patient enquires about a specific medical condition he experiences, it requires a medical practitioner to respond to the query. In this case, query gets directed to the site staff or the investigator who can provide the necessary advice.

Use Cases Applicable to Clinical Trials

This section introduces few important use cases where virtual assistants can be employed in the clinical trial context. The virtual assistant service will be specific to a study typically owned by the trial sponsor. Once the patient logs into the virtual assistant, it can be accessed anytime and will remain as a virtual companion throughout the trial journey. As mentioned earlier, while the main beneficiaries and users are the clinical trial participants and the site personnel, the benefits extend beyond to other stakeholders such as trial sponsors, regulators and service providers.

Electronic Informed Consent (eConsent)

Regulatory authorities across the globe have been actively working on developing guidance for the usage of digital technologies in drug development. One of the latest advancements in this direction is the final guidance released by FDA on eConsent in December 2016 (FDA, 2016). eConsent is the use of electronic means to obtain informed consent by trial participants. As per the regulations, before a subject participates in a clinical trial, the investigator must provide the details of the study, trial procedures, risks and benefits and obtain the subject's consent in the Informed Consent form. With eConsent, FDA emphasizes the need to use multimedia and digital means to make the trial subjects understand the study objectives and obtain the consent remotely.

Applicability of a virtual assistant/ chatbot in this process is extremely high. A potential trial participant interested in a specific study can interact with the study specific chat bot via a Facebook Messenger or a custom app. The chatbot guides him in a step by step fashion on how to obtain the informed consent. The description of the trial objectives and other details are provided through videos via the chatbot screen. At regular intervals during this process, the chatbot tests the understanding gained by the subject using knowledge checks. The chatbot answers any queries that the trial subject may have regarding the trial. Also at any point, if the chatbot is unable to answer, it notifies the investigator who can provide the response either real time or at a scheduled time. In the end, the chatbot requests for an electronic signature to obtain the consent. Electronic signature can be authenticated through username -password combination or a unique token mechanism. Once the chatbot receives the consent remotely, it shares the copy of the signed consent and patient information sheet (PIS) to the trial subject for reference.

Employing this technology eliminates the trial participants to travel to the research sites for obtaining the informed consent. Travel to the sites is a big challenge for those patients who are aged or whose disease condition restricts mobility. Having a chatbot to answer their concerns anytime anywhere helps subjects to gain more confidence and increases the possibility of giving the final consent thus helping drive up the patient recruitment numbers. On the other hand, investigators need not spend time to sit through the entire informed consent process for each potential trial participant. This enables him to focus his time on his clinical practice and other trial priorities.

Trial Subject Adherence

Trial subject adherence includes medication adherence, study visit compliance, study procedure adherence and so on. Medication adherence means following the medication regimen by patients as prescribed in the trial protocol. In a study conducted across 95 clinical trials, about 40% of the patients became non-adherent to the drug after 150 days into the trial. Not adhering to this regimen leads to invalid subject outcomes. Invalid subject data results in trial not meeting the statistical significance to prove the trial endpoints leading to further trial delays. For example, a 20%-30% decrease in medication adherence requires an increase of patient sample size by 50% in order to maintain the statistical significance (Al-sumidaie, 2017). Study visit compliance relates to the site visits made by the subjects at specific intervals of time as defined in the visit schedule in the trial protocol. The data collected from subjects who have either delayed or missed their visits introduces data variability in the overall trial results.

Use of virtual assistants can improve the overall adherence among patients. A trial virtual assistant knows the visit schedule and dosing regimens of the subject it interacts with. It sets a reminder for the subject to take the medication dose as prescribed in the protocol. It seeks a response from the subject once the drug has been consumed. This real time information can be used to calculate the medical adherence in a more accurate manner. Virtual assistant looks up the visit schedule and sets reminders for an upcoming site visit. It gives additional information such as sharing pre-visit procedure to be followed by the subject, trial procedures to be expected at the site, Google Maps showing the site address and so on.

The probability of a subject becoming nonadherent despite a constant follow up by the virtual assistant is less. This approach works better than the traditional ways of reminders (phone calls, SMS reminders) since the virtual assistant also receives inputs from the subject and responds accordingly in real time. It also reduces the burden of the clinical co-ordinator at the site who otherwise should keep sending reminders to every subject before an upcoming visit. Another benefit is that the data collected is used to analyse the compliance rates and a deviation from the desired levels is flagged to the investigator and site staff.

Query Redressals

Addressing questions from patients promptly in a satisfactory manner and addressing their issues is one of the most effective ways to build their confidence and better engagement. Some of the clinical trials especially those related to cancer and central nervous system treatments involve patients who undergo a lot of pain and anxiety about their disease condition and treatment procedures. Responding to their queries on time not only brings immediate relief to them but also reduces the psychological effects on the treatment.

Virtual assistants help in addressing patient queries and receiving feedback in a timely manner. It is important to note that virtual assistants cannot replace a medical practitioner by providing medical advice. The use of virtual assistants is restricted to providing general and commonly asked information. However, it still ensures that questions related to a patient's medical condition are alerted to the site staff who can address them by reaching out to the patient promptly. Through supervised learning of the AI engine, the system can learn the responses to the commonly asked queries and engage the patient in an intuitive manner.

Trial Adverse Event Reporting

Adverse events are untoward medical occurrences experienced by the patient. Adverse events may or may not be causally associated with the treatment drug. It is mandated by regulations that all adverse events reported in a clinical trial and beyond must be reported to regulatory authorities and Institutional Review Board (IRB) that oversees the safety of the trial participants. In the event of an adverse event, it must be submitted to the FDA within 15 days of an issue arising. In a typical trial setup, if a patient experiences an adverse event, he/ she will call up the trial co-ordinator at the site and fix an appointment with the investigator. An unscheduled AE visit is opened and the patient travels to the site to meet the investigator. The investigator then records the adverse event and submits it to the trial sponsor who in turn reports as an expedited safety report to FDA.

It is more efficient and accurate when a patient reports the adverse event at the time when the event occurred. Various platforms such as websites and social media where the patient can report the event directly. Virtual assistant is a better alternative for patient reporting the event due to couple of reasons. Firstly, it guides the patient to enter the correct information such as selecting the correct drug information, identifying the correct adverse event thus improving the quality of data collected. Secondly, if the event is a commonly occurring one, it recommends possible ways approved by the investigator to reduce the effect of the event thereby providing relief to an anxious patient. On the other hand, the investigator does not need to record the adverse event in an EDC system during the site visit. Instead, the data recorded by the virtual assistant can get transmitted to EDC and safety system directly increasing the compliance of safety reporting mandated by regulatory authorities.

eCOA Assessments

According to the FDA, "Clinical outcome assessments (COAs) measure a patient's symptoms, overall mental state, or the effects of a disease or condition on how the patient functions. COAs can be used to determine if a drug has been demonstrated to provide treatment benefit." Electronic COA (eCOA) is the use of electronic technology to report the outcomes by patients, clinicians or caregivers. Utilizing COA in a clinical trial is beneficial especially in certain category of ailments such as neurological disorders, cancers since it captures the state of the patient at a specific point in time. However, there are many challenges in using COA primarily being noncompliance by patients leading to missing data. Hence, the success of COA is heavily dependent of real time monitoring of compliance and ensuring that patient is motivated to participate in the tests within the stipulated time.

Virtual assistants present an intuitive way of capturing the eCOA data from patients. It is easier and interesting for the patient to provide information in a conversation format than filling up a long form with multiple questions. In a VA setup, COA can be designed in a way to encourage the patient to provide responses and at the same time meet ALCOA standards (Attributable – Legible – Contemporaneous – Original – Accurate) mandated by FDA. Another benefit of using virtual assistants is the ease of monitoring the compliance in real time. If the virtual assistant does receive any response even after multiple reminders then it can alert the site co-ordinator who can reach out to the patient. It also benefits the investigator site since it reduces the burden of actively monitoring and reminding patients to fill COA assessments.

Knowledge Dissemination

Patients participating in clinical trials experience lot more anxiety when compared to those receiving standard of care treatments. Firstly, they have been treated using a drug / procedure that are yet to deliver expected results in humans. Secondly, in randomized blinded trials there is a good probability that they are administered a placebo which means they are not treated for the disease condition. Thirdly, there could be a chance of developing other symptoms because of an adverse reaction of the drug. Hence, it is the responsibility of the trial sponsor and sites to share as much knowledge as possible to the participating patients. It is also known that lack of proper communication from the trial team is a major factor leading to patient disengagement and subsequent withdrawals from trials. Using a virtual assistant system, patients can be kept abreast with some of following information:

- Disease understanding and new developments in treatments
- Wellness and health tips to manage the disease condition better
- Periodic reports on the trial progress and milestones
- Awareness on trial procedures and their importance
- Patient experiences about the trial, its procedures and the benefits

When patients are fed with relevant information frequently, it increases the overall engagement and motivation. This keeps the patients well informed and thereby increases their chances of being associated to the trial till the trial closure.

FUTURE OF DRUG DEVELOPMENT: A DIGITAL CONVERGENCE

Multiple companies ranging from life sciences players, technology giants to angel investors are placing their bets on bringing technological innovations in medicine. For most part of this chapter, we discussed about how digital health technologies can be beneficial in drug research and development. While life sciences companies are trying out newer digital technologies in a specific function or area, the future lies in embracing digital innovations across the value chain blurring the silos that exist among business functions and technologies used. In drug development, digital convergence can happen in multiple ways:

- When digitization of major activities happens right from understanding a disease through clinical studies to a patient administering the drug
- When all stakeholders are empowered through digital channels to contribute and be connected throughout the drug lifecycle
- When technology goes beyond the realm of providing data insights to replacing traditional medicines and devices, commonly called as 'digital therapeutics' or 'digital medicine'

Some of the innovations in the R&D space clearly indicate the shift towards the digital convergence phenomenon. The changing business models that are described in the beginning of this chapter also suggest the movement in this direction. Translation research where real world patient data is utilized for scientific research, simulation based drug discovery where historic data of drug test profiles are used for simulating efficacy and toxicology tests of new compounds, digital clinical trials where a digital devices and software applications are used to overcome many challenges in patient recruitment, patient engagement, trial monitoring, data collection, analysis and reporting, connected patient services where patient groups contribute from early stages of drug development to market launch are some broad shades where digital convergence is seen to take action. Many technology start-ups are investing in digital therapeutics where technology being used as medicinal treatment such as a mobile application to treat substance abuse that was approved by FDA in late 2017 and a technology to filter out certain frequencies from music collection as a treatment for tinnitus.

For such digital disruptions to bring about transformations in the way life sciences companies operate, they must adopt new strategies in the following areas:

1. **Make Digital Adoption a Top Business Priority**: The journey to digital transformation must be the priority of the business and not restricted to the IT function
2. **Be Patient-Centric and Stay Connected With Stakeholders**: Define products and services that give an enriched experience to the patient. Build a connected ecosystem with payers, patients and providers playing an important role in the drug life cycle.
3. **Forge Partnerships With Technology Companies and Build New Competencies**: Innovating on new technologies is not a core competence of a Life Sciences organization. Build competencies through partnerships or acquisitions.
4. **Align the Organization for Non-Linear Growth**: Digital solutions do not follow the traditional revenue streams and growth patterns that life sciences companies are used to. Build organizational and operational controls to handle such uncertainties.

CONCLUSION

Technologies are changing rapidly. When Life Sciences companies are reacting to SMAC, big data and Internet of Things, there is another wave of digitization already disrupting the marketplace in a much more stronger fashion. Artificial Intelligence, Virtual and Augmented reality, blockchain are opening up new avenues which have never been explored before.

Life Sciences and specifically the drug research and development are big generators of data. It is a good playing ground for the digital technologies because quality data is the main ingredient for such technologies to realize outcomes of significant business value. The new digital health technologies enable scientists to discover newer products, provide personalized experience for the patients and allow physicians, payers and providers to be better connected. Many of the newer technologies are still in the path of evolution and Life Sciences will take a longer time to adapt them. On the other hand, global regulatory bodies are tailoring their policies and developing new guidelines for the industry players to become digitized. Drug development will witness a major transformation and a shift from traditional business and operational models when the entire value chain from discovery, to development and to post marketing embrace digital means. For this digital convergence to happen and start yielding value, life sciences companies must be open to radical changes in the way they operate within and with the outside world.

REFERENCES

Accenture. (n.d.). *Pharmaceutical companies that digitize grow more*. Retrieved January 25, 2018 from https://www.accenture.com/in-en/insight-highlights-life-sciences-pharmaceutical-grow

Allen-Vercoe, H. (2017). Prepare for the VR and AR healthcare revolution. *Pharmaphorum*. Retrieved February 15, 2018 from https://pharmaphorum.com/views-and-analysis/vr-ar-healthcare-pharma/

Alsumidaie, M. (2017a). *Non-Adherence: A Direct Influence on Clinical Trial Duration and Cost*. Retrieved March 10, 2018 from http://www.appliedclinicaltrialsonline.com/non-adherence-direct-influence-clinical-trial-duration-and-cost

Alsumidaie, M. (2017b). *Technology Tips on Improving Clinical Trial Patient Adherence*. Retrieved March 10, 2018 from http://www.appliedclinicaltrialsonline.com/technology-tips-improving-clinical-trial-patient-adherence

Arthur.D.Little. (2016). *Impact of Digital Health on the Pharmaceutical Industry*. Retrieved March 23, 2018 from http://www.adlittle.com/sites/default/files/viewpoints/ADL_HC_2016_Digital-Health_01.pdf

Ascione, A. (n.d.). *The convergence of healthcare: when digital and medical collide*. Retrieved March 23, 2018 from http://deep-dive.pharmaphorum.com/deep-dive-future-pharma-july-2017#!/the-convergence-of-healthcare-when-digital-and-medical-collide

Clinical Leader. (n.d.). *Considerations For Improving Patient Recruitment Into Clinical Trials*. Retrieved March 10, 2018 from https://www.clinicalleader.com/doc/considerations-for-improving-patient-0001

Corneli, A., Pierre, C., Hinkley, T., Lin, L., Fordyce, C. B., Hamre, G., & Roe, M. T. (2017). One and done: Reasons principal investigators conduct only one FDA-regulated drug trial. *Contemporary Clinical Trials Communications, 6*. Retrieved March 10, 2018 from https://www.sciencedirect.com/science/article/pii/S245186541630093X

Diamond, O. (2015). *Overcoming Patient Recruitment and Retention Hurdles*. Retrieved March 10, 2018 from http://medrio.com/partners/overcoming-patient-recruitment-and-retention-hurdles/

EvaluatePharma. (2017, June). World Preview 2017 *Outlook to 2022*. Retrieved from http://info.evaluategroup.com/rs/607-YGS-364/images/WP17.pdf

Food and Drug Administration. (2009). *Guidance for Clinical Investigators, Sponsors, and IRBs*. Retrieved March 18, 2018 from https://www.fda.gov/downloads/regulatoryinformation/guidances/ucm126572.pdf

Food and Drug Administration. (2015*). Mobile Medical Applications: Guidance for Industry and Food and Drug Administration Staff.* Retrieved March 7, 2018 from https://www.fda.gov/downloads/MedicalDevices/.../UCM263366.pdf

Food and Drug Administration. (2015). *Digital Health Innovation Action Plan*. Retrieved March 7, 2018 from https://www.fda.gov/downloads/MedicalDevices/DigitalHealth/UCM568735.pdf

Food and Drug Administration. (2016). *Use of Electronic Informed Consent*. Retrieved March 10, 2018 from https://www.fda.gov/downloads/Drugs/GuidanceComplianceRegulatoryInformation/Guidances/UCM436811.pdf

Food and Drug Administration. (n.d.). *Clinical Outcome Assessment Qualification Program*. Retrieved March 18, 2018 from https://www.fda.gov/Drugs/DevelopmentApprovalProcess/DrugDevelopmentToolsQualificationProgram/ucm284077.htm

Foundry. (n.d.). *VR? AR? MR? Sorry, I'm confused*. Retrieved February 12, 2018 from https://www.foundry.com/industries/virtual-reality/vr-mr-ar-confused

Gartner. (n.d.). *Gartner IT Glossary: Virtual Assistant*. Retrieved March 10, 2018 from https://www.gartner.com/it-glossary/virtual-assistant-va/

Gautam, A., & Pan, X. (2016). The changing model of big pharma: Impact of key trends. *Drug Discovery Today*, *21*(3), 379–384. doi:10.1016/j.drudis.2015.10.002 PMID:26477304

Gilbert, M. R., Rubinstein, L., & Lesser, G. (2016). Creating clinical trial designs that incorporate clinical outcome assessments. *Neuro-Oncology, 18*(Suppl 2). Retrieved March 18, 2018 from https://www.ncbi.nlm.nih.gov/pmc/articles/PMC4795995/

Global Industry Analysts, Inc. (2018). *Virtual Reality (VR) in Healthcare – A Global Strategic Business Report*. Retrieved March 01, 2018 from http://www.strategyr.com/MarketResearch/Virtual_Reality_VR_In_Healthcare_Market_Trends.asp

Guenther, C., Pierson, M., & Modi, N. (2018). In Blockchain We Trust: Transforming Life Sciences with blockchain. *Accenture Life Sciences*. Retrieved March 10, 2018 from https://www.accenture.com/t20180406T080254Z__w__/us-en/_acnmedia/PDF-71/Accenture_Blockchain_Innovations_Life_Sciences.pdf#zoom=50

Intel. (n.d.). *Demystifying the Virtual Reality Landscape*. Retrieved February 12, 2018 from https://www.intel.com/content/www/us/en/tech-tips-and-tricks/virtual-reality-vs-augmented-reality.html

Jones Day. (2018). FDA's Evolving Regulation of Artificial Intelligence in Digital Health Products. *Lexology*. Retrieved March 7, 2018 from https://www.lexology.com/library/detail.aspx?g=cf6351a3-a944-4468-9214-d141a689955e

McCarthy, J. (2015). Hospitals to triple use of cloud services. *HealthcareIT News*. Retrieved January 20,2018 from http://www.healthcareitnews.com/news/hospitals-triple-use-cloud-services

Petre, A. (2017). *Blockchain Use Cases in Healthcare*. Retrieved March 10, 2018 from https://www.intelligenthq.com/innovation-management/blockchain-use-cases-in-healthcare/

Pharmaceutical Online. (2017). *What To Expect From Artificial Intelligence In Pharma — And How To Get There*. Retrieved March,01, 2018 from https://www.pharmaceuticalonline.com/doc/what-to-expect-from-artificial-intelligence-in-pharma-and-how-to-get-there-0001

TechTarget. (n.d.a). *Definition: AI (Artificial Intelligence)*. Retrieved March 01, 2018 from http://searchcio.techtarget.com/definition/AI

TechTarget. (n.d.b). *Definition: Virtual Assistant (AI assistant)*. Retrieved March 10, 2018 from http://searchcrm.techtarget.com/definition/virtual-assistant

Tsang, L., Kracov, D. A., Mulryne, J., Strom, L., Perkins, N., Dickinson, R., … Jones, B. (2017). The Impact of Artificial Intelligence on Medical Innovation in the European Union and United States. *Intellectual Property & Technology Law Journal*. Retrieved March 7, 2018 from https://www.arnoldporter.com/~/media/files/perspectives/publications/2017/08/the-impact-of-artificial-inteelligence-on-medical-innovation.pdf

Venugopal, M. (2016). Application of SMAC Technology. In P. Chakraborty & A. Nagal (Eds.), *Software Innovations in Clinical Drug Development and Safety* (pp. 90–126). Hershey, PA: IGI Global. doi:10.4018/978-1-4666-8726-4.ch006

KEY TERMS AND DEFINITIONS

Clinical Trial: It is a scientific study where new investigational medicinal product is tested on human beings for efficacy and safety. Only products passing clinical trials can be launched to the market for use by wider patient population.

FDA: Food and Drug Administration is the regulatory body of United States that regulates the use of any food and medicinal products in the United States.

IND: Investigational new drug is a formal application requesting the Food and Drug Administration (FDA) to approve the conduct of clinical trials with the drug under investigation.

Investigator: Investigator is a person practicing medicine and is responsible for all clinical trial activities in the hospital site.

NDA: New drug application is a formal process of requesting the Food and Drug Administration (FDA) to approve the use of a medicinal drug in the United States.

R&D: Research and development is the first phase in the life cycle of a drug. It is further divided into discovery, pre-clinical, clinical, and pharmacovigilance.

SMAC: It is an acronym for four digital technologies, namely social media, mobility, analytics, and cloud computing.

Subject: Trial subject is a person participating in a clinical trial. He/she could be a healthy patient or a patient with a disease condition.

Chapter 2
Development of Human Speech Signal-Based Intelligent Human-Computer Interface for Driving a Wheelchair in Enhancing the Quality-of-Life of the Persons

Uvanesh Kasiviswanathan
Indian Institute of Technology (BHU), India

Abhishek Kushwaha
Indian Institute of Technology (BHU), India

Shiru Sharma
Indian Institute of Technology (BHU), India

ABSTRACT

For the past few decades, an increase in experimental research has been carried out in enhancing the quality-of-life of the persons with different levels of disabilities. To enhance the lifestyle of differently disabled in terms of their mobility or movement or transportation, a proper aid with appropriate human-computer interface system is needed. So, in this chapter, a hybrid classification model is proposed, which combines and uses hM-GM and ANN models, for classifying human speech signal, especially the word for driving a wheelchair for helping the people, who seek transportation. For classifying the correct word from the phase of sentence (i.e., the human speech signal) to corresponding trigger command for an electrically powered wheelchair prototype, under the certain experimental condition, the hM-GM model yields good recognition of words, but they suffer major limitations as it relies on strong statistical properties and probability. Hence, by combining hM-GM and ANN model-based classifier for enhancing the accuracy of classifying the word to corresponding trigger command.

DOI: 10.4018/978-1-5225-7071-4.ch002

1. INTRODUCTION

The real-time processing of speech signal generally deals with analysing the nature and characteristics of the signal(s) produced to the corresponding observable outputs (Schultz et al., 2017). The signals used can either be discrete or analog/continuous in nature and either it can be stationary or non-stationary signals (Gannot & Burshtein, 2001). If the signals are stationary then, the signal's statistical properties won't change with respect to time, but if it is non-stationary signal then, the signal's statistical properties will get change depending upon the time. By analyzing this, we are able to develop a "*signal model*" (Mermelstein, 1973; Huang et al., 2001). The signal model developed is nothing but a theoretical description of the system. Speech signals are basically one-dimension signals which vary over the time period and can be related to a source-filter system (Bell-Berti & Harris, 1981).

The source filter system (Galas & Rodet, 1991) consists of respiratory mechanism as a source and filtering are caused due to change in air pressure when the air starts to flow from lungs with pulmonary pressure. The air pressure gets changed as it reaches the larynx in the throat and produces vibration, and the hissingness. Vibration and hissingness is the primary cause of speech production (Mermelstein, 1973; Deller et al., 1993).

1.1. The Anatomical Structures Responsible for Speech Production

- **Alveolar Ridge**: A bony ridge located on the roof of the mouth (a half-inch behind upper teeth).
- **Glottis**: A hole/space present in between the vocal folds of the throat.
- **Larynx (or Adam's Apple)**: Made of cartilage that holds the vocal folds of the throat.
- **Lips**: Are used to form consonants.
- **Palate**: The roof, divided into hard (front region) and soft (back region) palate present in the mouth.
- **Pharynx**: A tube that connects the larynx to the mouth region (oral cavity), located at backside in the throat.
- **Tongue**: Where the speech is originated. It is a large muscle, which can change its shape to generate different sounds.
- **Uvula**: Present at soft palate (the velum) that is responsible for the articulation of consonants.
- **Vocal Folds/Cords**: A small flap of muscle in the larynx, vibrates to generate different sounds (Isshiki 1989).

1.2. The Flow of Speech Production

A steady flow of air is supplied from the lungs with some pulmonary air pressure through the trachea, larynx, and pharynx. Then, the vocal folds/cord present in the larynx gets vibrated and generates a fluctuations/variations in air pressure, due to which sound waves generate (Mermelstein, 1973). The significate changes in the vocal tract modify the wave according to the position and shape of the speech organs to produce voiced/tone sound waves. Thus, through the mouth and nose openings, the sound waves radiate out into the environment (Mermelstein 1973; Rabiner & Juang 1993; Bogdashevsky et al., 1999).

The speech signal generated/produced has the bandwidth of about 4000Hz as per telephonic speech. Whereas as generally, speech signal falls below 10,000 Hz and to match the Nyquist rate criteria 20,000 Hz (general) and 8000 Hz (telephonic) sampling frequency is necessary to choose (Schwartz et al., 1985; Juang & Rahim, 1996; Brandstein & Ward, 2013).

It is important aspect to map a particular word(s) to its corresponding speech signal(s) in any Speech or pattern recognition system development. For the last few decades, researchers all around the world trying hard to develop a pattern recognition system which can be used as a matching/recognising and mapping platform to recognise the speech without any loss (Schwartz et al., 1985). For developing such an automatic pattern recognition system, many unique features are needed to be extracted from processed/digital speech signal and this can be termed as '*acoustic features*'. The acoustic features (Junqua, 1996) represent the characteristic behaviour of the speech signal. The acoustic feature vectors are directly proportional to the original underlying information of the speech which is processed or digitalized. If it get fails, then the information gets mismatched. Hence, it is important to develop such a system with higher performance to match the extract underlying information. To achieve this one must select the proper acoustic feature and the property to be used. One has to select involvement of a proper acoustic feature extraction method, with anticipate reduction in the complexity over classification and representation of the particular speech signal (Pickett, 1999).

In general, Speech recognition (SR) system (Pickett, 1999) involves two important steps: (i) feature extraction method, the process by which the unique properties of a particular signal are analysed/measured but it is not possible to reconstructing the original signal using the features, as the feature extraction method is non-invertible and lossy transformation method to analyse the characteristic property of the particular signal. Furthermore, Feature extraction method is generally made up of either temporal and/or spectral analysis technique. The temporal analysis technique uses the input signal/waveform itself, whereas the spectral analysis technique uses the spectral representation of input signal/waveform given, for the analysis of the characteristic properties (Furui, 1981). (ii) Classification algorithm for classifying them into their corresponding speech signal using an appropriate pattern recognizing method. The classification accuracy, robustness, and complexity of the algorithm developed are needed to be measured for evaluating the performance of such a classification algorithm method to be used (Atal & Rabiner, 1976; Stowell et al., 2015). In Speech recognition systems, Linear Predictive coding (LPC) (Nair et al., 2016), Mel-frequency Cepstral Co-efficient (MFCC) (Murty & Yegnanarayana, 2006), and Perceptual linear Prediction (PLP) (Hermansky, 1990; Hwang & Hu, 2001) are widely used to extract acoustic features of the original raw speech signal.

In this chapter, our concern will be strictly with using Mel-frequency Cepstral Co-efficient (MFCC) for extracting the feature of the original raw digitalized speech signal and for classification, we used hidden Markov model (HMM) and Gaussian Mixture Model (GMM) (Reynolds, 1995; Reynolds et al., 2000), together as a stochastic signal model, namely the hidden Markov- Gaussian Mixture model (HM-GMM) (Bahl et al., 1990) with Artificial Neural Network (Hwang & Hu, 2001) as a classifier for classifying the speech signals using the Mel-frequency Cepstral Co-efficient (MFCC) feature extraction process (Murty & Yegnanarayana, 2006).

2. BACKGROUND

2.1. Speech

The process of communication between animals in any vocalic form is termed as "Speech," and it is generated due to a syntactic combination of stress (sound) and strain (vibration) developed, depending on their vocabulary/lexicon (Atal & Rabiner, 1976). Each word represents the phonetic combination of vowels and/or consonant sounds, which is referred as phonemes. The phonemes with different syntax structure's them into a specific set of speech, in thousand ways creates thousand different languages (Soliman & Hsue, 1992).

2.1.1. Speech Production

The process by which the thoughts are translated/converted into a word or group of continuous words (i.e., phase or sentence) represents the speech and the process of production is called as "Speech production." The spoken words or the group of words can be of unorganized or organized grammatical forms.

Speech is normally produced due to the creation of pulmonary pressure by the lungs. The pulmonary pressure is converted into the sound by generating phonation. The phonation is developed at the glottis in the larynx, which is later modified into different vowels and consonant sounds by vocal tract. Thus, here the speech production is due to pressure developed by lung but whereas the speech can also be formed without using lungs, which is termed as "alaryngeal speech." The speech produced at glottis in the larynx using only the upper position of the vocal tract shown in Figure 1 (Guenther, 1994).

2.1.2. Motor Area Responsible for Speech Production

Left cerebral hemisphere controls the production of speech through the supplementary motor area (SMA). The SMA includes the bilateral supplementary motor area (BSA), the opercular parts of the precentral gyrus with left posterior inferior frontal gyrus (mainly Broca's area), the left insula, the left primary motor cortex (mouth region) and temporal cortex with other subcortical areas (like the basal ganglia, thalamus and cerebellum). The other areas like superior temporal gyrus and lower parietal areas also play a vital role during hemodynamic responses (Ackermann, 2008; Ackermann & Riecker, 2010).

2.1.3. Characteristics Models in Speech Production

Speech production is broadly processed in three different levels namely: *conceptualization, formulation,* and *articulation* (Hagoort et al., 1999; Hwang & Hu, 2001).

1. Conceptualization level deals with speech (concept) creation/identification such as formulation of a particular word(s)/concepts which need to be expressed.
2. Formulation level deals with encoding/structuring of desired linguistic form which needed to be expressed for a desired concept, this includes grammatical encoding, morpho-phonological encoding, and phonetic encoding.
    a. Grammatical encoding focusses on selection/structuring of the appropriate syntactic frame for the conceptualized/identified concept.

Figure 1. The speech production model

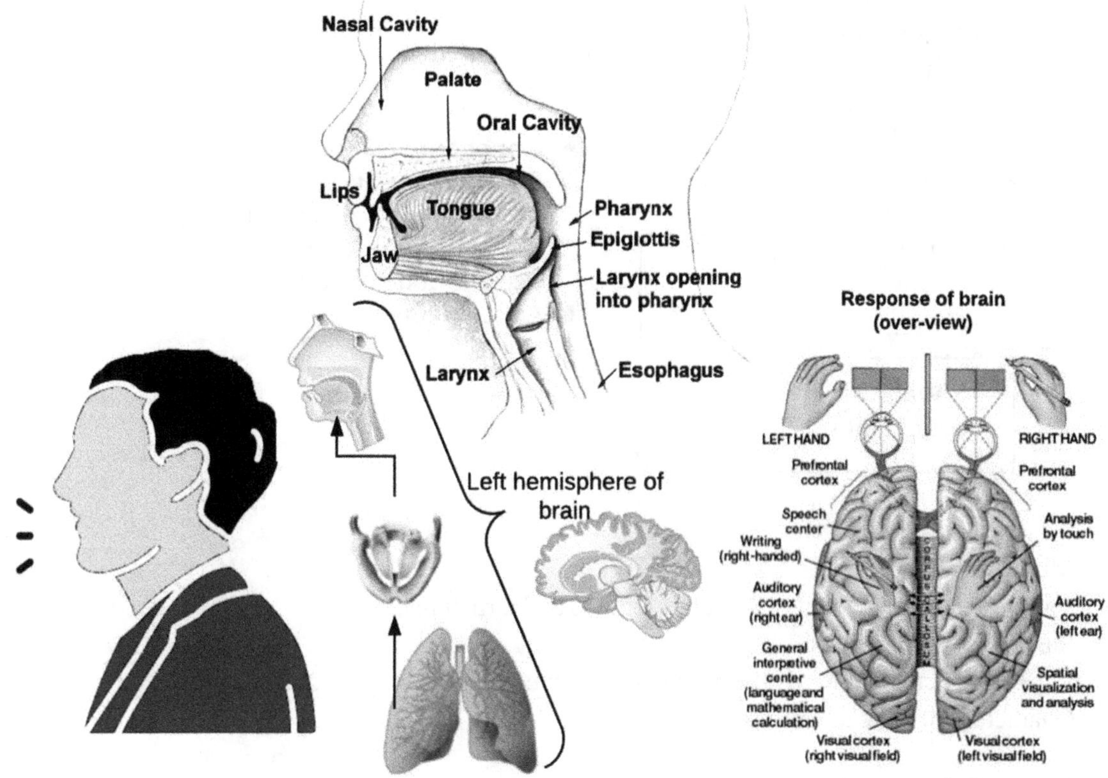

b. Whereas, the Morpho-phonological encoding breaks the words down into syllables which to be expressed in overt speech based on the meaning.

c. Then, the phonetic encoding syllabifies the conceptualized/identified concept or articulatory gestures into the speech-like form, dependent on the selected syllables.

3. Articulation or phonetic stage creates the commands/instructions which needed to be sent to activate the muscles of articulations to produce the speech through lungs, glottis, and larynx of the vocal apparatus.

2.1.4. Vocal Apparatus or Place of Articulation

In articulatory phonetics, a dynamic airflow through the vocal tract gets transformed into sound waves due to change in air pressure when it passes from articulatory gesture to an active articulator and a passive location. Here, some part of tongue referred as "an active articulator," and some part of mouth referred as "a passive location." It is observed that the speech signal of every individual is different due to variation in the physical structure of the human system (such as nose, throat, vocal cords, etc.), which an essential role in the production of a unique speech signal shown in Figure 2 (Flanagan, 2013).

Speech characteristics (Spencer, 1988; Hazan & Baker, 2011) based on sense of hearing can be determined by:

Figure 2. Shows process involved in speech production model

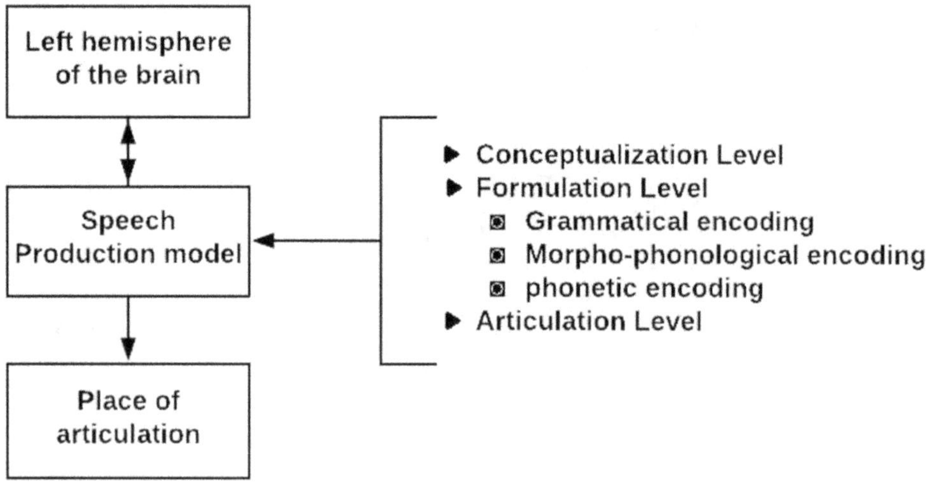

1. Muscle tension level,
2. Variation and movement of muscle's lengths and structures,
3. Shape of the vocal tract,
4. Place of articulation (overall aerodynamic events happens at that point),
5. Characteristics sound wave produced.

2.2. Speech Signal Processing

Speech signal processing is used to study the characteristic of the audio signal quantitatively. Here, the speech signals are acquired using the microphone (Huang et al., 2001; Gay & Benesty, 2012). The microphone converts the sound/acoustic energy into corresponding electrical energy and therefore using certain digital processing methods, the analog signal is converted into a digital signal with other functions (such as amplification, de-noising, feature extraction, classification, etc.) for analysis (Hossan et al., 2010; Ai et al., 2012; Barchiesi et al., 2015).

2.2.1. What Is the Need of Intelligent System Using Speech Signal Processing for Assisting Rehabilitative Device

Motor impairment is the serious cause that affected the human body part (the limbs). Usually, motor impairment is due to weakness in the muscle, lack of stamina, loss of control over muscles, and/or total or partial paralysis. Motor impairment is a serious neurological condition occurs after any of this diseased condition such as cerebral palsy, Parkinson's disease, stroke and/or multiple sclerosis (Sussman & Tjaden 2012; Miller, 2013). The level of impairment shows whether any system such as any biological (EMG, EOG, EEG, etc.) signal driven system and/or electromechanically or electronically (joystick based, GPS based, etc.) driven system has to be employed for replacing the particular muscle impairment to aid the person towards his/her locomotion/travel (Ahamed et al., 2013).

2.2.2. Biosignal Based Intelligent System for Assisting Any Rehabilitative Device

An increase in experimental research has been witnessed in last few decades towards the development of biosignal system driven assistive devices or aids towards enhancing the Quality-of-life of persons with the different level of different inabilities. The use of biosignals towards controlling the functionalities of any assistive devices has attracted the researcher, to incorporate the biological and Machine system interaction, which is termed as "Body-Computer Interface" (BCI) or "Human-Computer Interface" (HCI) or "Human-Machine Interface" (HMI). This type of interfacing studies uses the residual signals of the in-abled persons for controlling the assistive devices such as a motorized wheelchair for their movement. Such type of devices has shown great improvement towards the quality of the life of the persons with the different level of different inabilities by reducing their dependence others (Ahamed et al., 2013). As per the literature, the researchers have used biosignal like electroencephalogram (EEG) (Moghimi et al., 2013; Ang et al., 2015), electrooculogram (EOG) (Banerjee et al., 2012) and electromyogram (EMG) (Uvanesh, 2015) for developing HCI based control systems. For neural interfaces and EEG based system, have been successfully explored to the patients for restoring functionality of severely motor-impairment though implanting devices in a particularly active area of the motor cortex, and the active signals are used to construct the HCI for communicating or moving a motorized wheelchair. Whereas, EMG and EOG based system used surface electrode for acquiring the biological activities and classified them to corresponding movement of a motorized wheelchair. EMG signal based HCI system can be successfully employed if the person is suffering from Tetraplegia, or paraplegia, hemiplegic, etc. where the EMG signal can be acquired from hand and used for to the corresponding movement of a motorized wheelchair (Uvanesh, 2015; Uvanesh et al., 2016). EOG signal based HCI system can be successfully employed if the person is suffering from Tetraplegia, or paraplegia, where the EOG signal can be acquired by placing the electrode on the horizontal and vertical direction across the eye and used for to the corresponding movement of a motorized wheelchair (Banerjee et al., 2012). But, the use of biological signal driven system for developing Human-Computer Interface (HCI) system has restriction, and it is not advisable for the patients, who has progressive motor-neuron degenerative diseases (NMD) (Moghimi et al., 2013) such as multiple types of sclerosis which generally occurs after 40 years in both men and women and it tends to affect the total body parts or partial body parts like trunk, legs, and arms (Miller, 2013).

2.2.3. Advantage of Speech Signal Based Intelligent System for Assisting Any Rehabilitative Device

Biosignal driven assistive devices or aids cannot be used if the level of impairment is higher, (i) where it is difficult to pick-up/acquire the residual muscular activities of the remaining active limb (Weismer & Kim, 2010), (ii) where the training given to activate that particular residual muscular activities, again and again, is difficult (Miller, 2013). Whereas, the speech signal of any word(s) (which the in-abled person can speak easily) can be acquired using a microphone and by employing that word(s) for classifying directly to the corresponding movement of a motorized wheelchair is easy (Uvanesh et al., 2016). Combining these advantage with the field of robotics has allowed the researchers to use the robotic technologies with speech signal for improving the Quality of life of the motor disabled patients. Hence, this devices will highly improvise the independence of these motor disabled persons with various level of impartment (Miller, 2013).

Human Machine or Computer interface is the tool, which allow the researchers to modify/construct the interfacing system with desired need depending upon the requirement for the betterment of Quality of life of the motor disabled patients (Weismer & Kim, 2010). The main theme of interfacing/using HCI/HMI system is to reduce the need of normal persons and also to provide physical and mental support to the person with motor disabilities to enhance their day to day activities related to locomotion/movement (Uvanesh et al., 2016).

3. MAIN FOCUS OF THE CHAPTER

The main focus of the work is to develop a speech signal based human computer/machine interface to drive/control a motorized wheelchair (prototype), which reduce the dependence of the motor imparted patients on the other. Here, in this work, we have combined Mel-frequency Cepstral Co-efficient (MFCC) feature extraction method with both hidden Markov - Gaussian Mixture model (HM-GMM) (Veaux et al., 2012) and Artificial Neural Network (ANN) to build an efficient classify model for controlling the motorized wheelchair directly.

4. METHODS

Process of interfacing speech signal for controlling the assistive device in short given below and pictorially in Figure 3:

- Speech signal is acquired through using microphone or mic (Brandstein & Ward, 2013), a transducer which converts sound/acoustic energy into analogue electrical signal over the time.
- The analogue electrical signal is then converted into digital domain and preformed pre-processing (such as amplification, de-noising, envelope creation, thresholding, etc)
- Then, the signal's unique feature were extracted using MFCC feature extraction method.
- Using the extracted (feature) parameter, the HM-GMM algorithm (Veaux et al., 2012) & ANN classifiers are used classify the speech signal or words into corresponding action/command to drive a motorized wheelchair.

Commercially available, SAMSUNG's mobile Headphone with Mic (Model: EHS61ASFWE, Samsung Electronics Co. Ltd, South Kr), HP Pavilion dv6 Laptop [2nd gen Core i5, 4 GB RAM, Windows 10], and Matlab software (ver. 2010, MathWorks, USA) were used in this study (Brandstein & Ward, 2013).

5. RESULTS AND DISCUSSION

5.1. Acquisition of Speech Signal

Frequencies lesser than 4 kHz can only be able to transmit via telephone due to filtering at switching network. Hence, about 8 kHz samples/second is sufficient to analysis Speech signal transmission line. Whereas in microphone 16 kHz samples/second is used (has it falls under wide bandwidth) to analysis

Figure 3. Overview of the proposed work

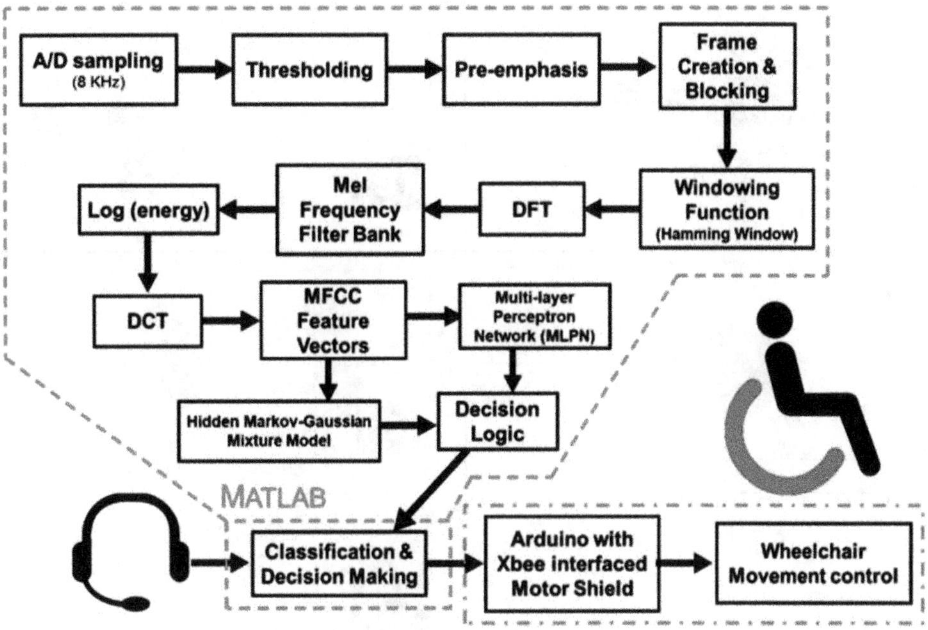

Speech signal. Figure 4 shows speech source model while equation 1 shows the system response when y(n) represents raw speech signal developed and s(n) represents the source of speech production (Bell-Berti & Harris, 1981; Gay & Benesty, 2012; Brandstein & Ward, 2013).

$$s(n) = y(n) - \sum_{n=1}^{M} \alpha_n x(z-n) \quad (1)$$

For acquiring the Speech signal, we connected Samsung headphone to the sound/audio jack of the HP laptop. Using Matlab software, recording the words such as Forward, Reverse, Right, Left, and Stop were performed. The Figure 5 shows the raw input speech signal of each words used.

5.2. Feature Extraction

Feature extraction relies on estimation of spectral analysis of a signal for a short period of time. Spectral analysis is used to estimate frequency components of a non-stationary or continuous time varying signal and it is determined by energy or power spectrum of the signal (Li & Huang, 2010; Ghoraani & Krishnan,

Figure 4. Speech source model

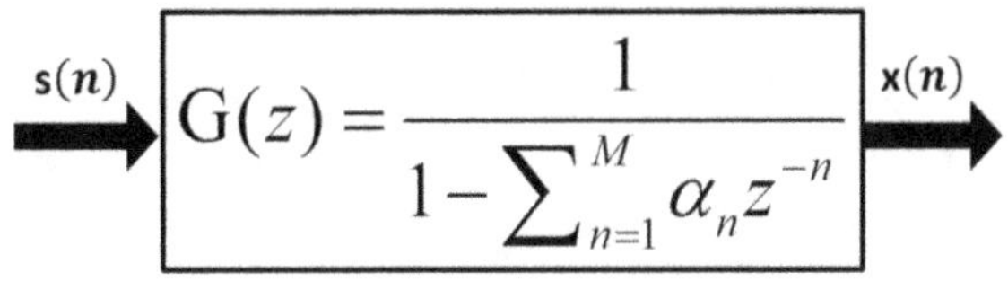

Figure 5. Shows the original speech signals

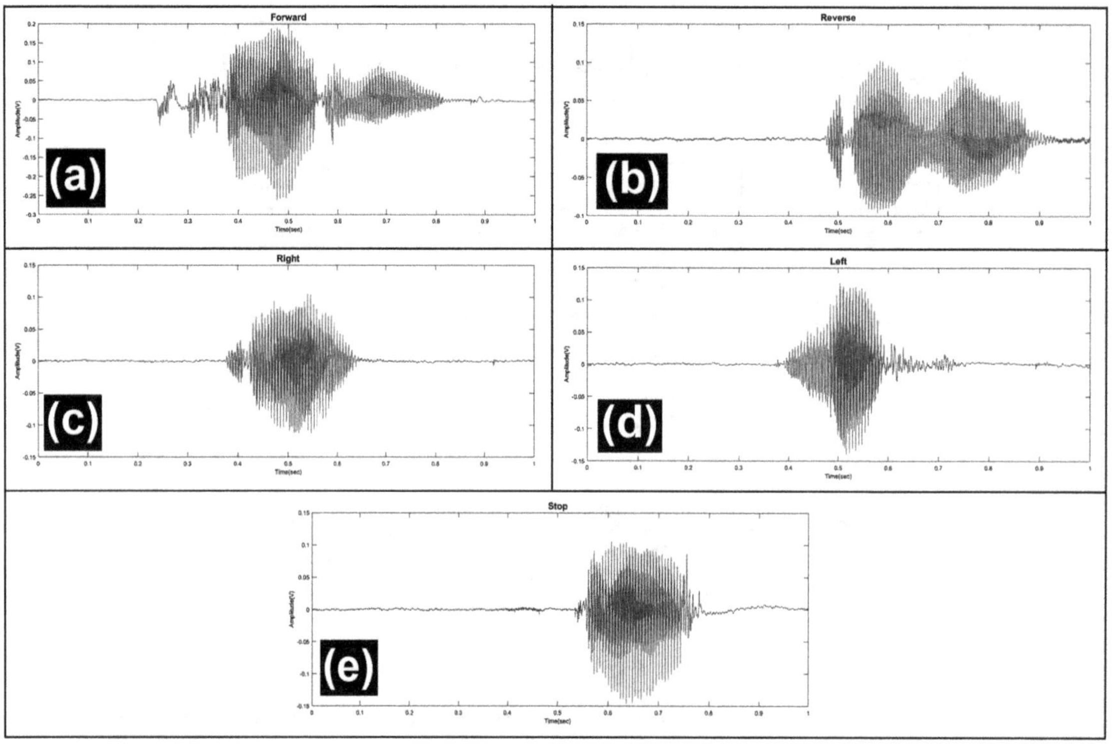

2011). Generally, Speech signal is segmented into overlapped fixed-length frames over a short period of time and for each segmented frame, a corresponding parameters are estimated using either frequency/ cepstral domain to form, the feature vector.

5.2.1. Pre-Emphasis (Spectral Flattening)

Pre-emphasis is the process by which, the magnitude/amplitude of higher frequencies gets increased, while the magnitude/amplitude of lower frequencies gets supressed artificially but it will be within the frequency band. Pre-emphasis uses first order FIR filtering technique (equation 2), in-order to improve the overall signal-to-noise ratio of the speech signal, (Heckmann et al., 2011).

$$\mathrm{G}\left(z\right) = 1 - \alpha * z^{-1}; \quad 0 < \alpha \leq 1 \tag{2}$$

By considering the transfer function (equation 2), then the output of the pre-emphasised signal $\overline{y}\left(n\right)$ will be expressed as in equation 3

$$\overline{y}\left(n\right) = y\left(n\right) - \alpha * y\left(n-1\right) \tag{3}$$

Where, the input signal is represented by $y(n)$, and α is pre-emphasized parameter (normally α ≈ 0.95).

An increase of about 20 dB in the spectrum magnitude of $\overline{y}(n)$ with a 32 dB increase in Nyquist frequency in the upper frequencies can be observed. Figure 6 shows the pre-emphasized output of the speech signal processed.

5.2.2. Frame Blocking and Windowing Function

The pre-emphasized speech signal, $\overline{y}(n)$ is a non-stationary signal. Hence, keeping the frame length short will preserve spectral properties of the signal across the window over the time. So, the signal is subdivided into a frame of about 25 millisecond each with length of about 200 samples/frame, and kept frame shift of about 80 samples for 10 milliseconds with an overlap frame of about 60%. So, the information to be captured will be within the respected frame boundaries.

Presence of discontinuities at both the ends of the available frames may have some unwanted things in the frequency response. So, we need to limit the signal in short period of time. So that we can able to create non-zero values at frequencies other than ω in each frame, by multiplying each frame with a fixed frame length to preform windowing function (equation 4) and it is otherwise called as silence removal (Figure 7).

Figure 6. Shows the pre-emphasized speech signals

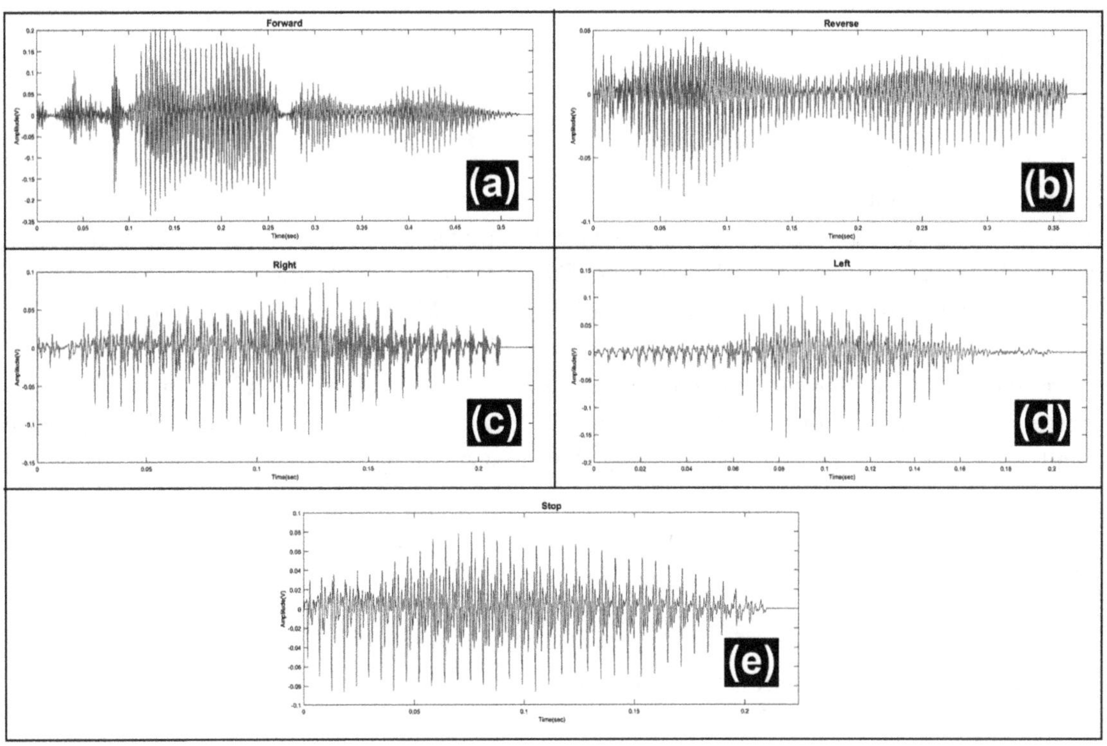

Figure 7. Shows the speech signal after removal of silence from the pre-emphasized speech signal

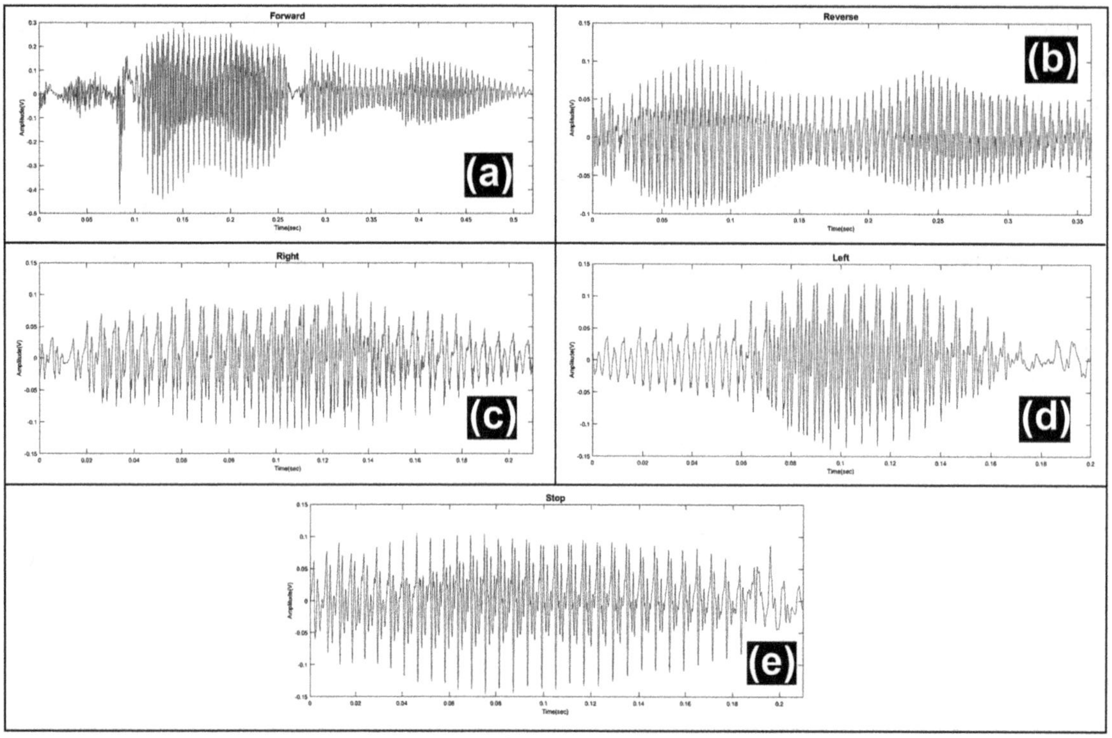

$$\left[g\left(n\right)\right]_{n=0}^{L-1} \tag{4}$$

where L is length of the frame.

It is observed that the leakage will be higher at the frequencies near ω and lower at frequencies, which are far away from ω. In the telephonic channels, Hamming and Hann windows are used to minimize the signal discontinuities in the edge of each frame, (Podder et al., 2014) as it is used to match the signals having nearly zero values at both the ends of each frame.

Here in this work, we have used the hamming window as the preferred windowing function and the hamming window (Podder et al., 2014) is defined by equation 5 and Figure 8 shows the stepwise corresponding change happened to the speech signal using windowing function.

$$w(n) = \begin{cases} 0.54 - 0.46 * \cos(2\pi n \,/\, L); & 0 \le n \le L \\ 0; & otherwise \end{cases} \tag{5}$$

The output after windowing function will be expressed as equation 6

$$X(n) = \overline{y}(n) * w(n); \quad 0 \le n \le L \tag{6}$$

Figure 8. Shows response before and after applying windowing function on frame no 15

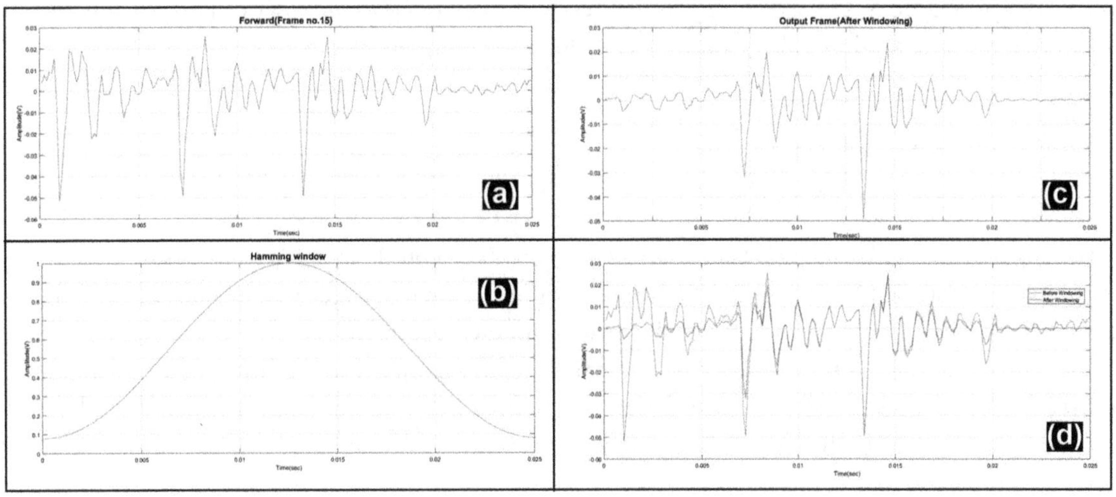

5.2.3. Spectral Analysis With the Discrete Fourier Transform (DFT)

Using Fourier analysis method, DFT converts a set of equally spaced time domain data to a corresponding complex data of same length in frequency domain. Here, DFT converts the speech signal present in time-domain to frequency-domain using equation 7 for preforming spectral analysis (Harrington, 2010).

$$X(k) = \sum_{n=0}^{L-1} X(n) * e^{\frac{-j2\pi nk}{L}}, 0 \leq k \leq L-1 \qquad (7)$$

In our work, we have used 200 point FFT algorithm (expressed in equation 7) to get 200 data from each frame and converted it into its corresponding DFT data, where the output of the 200 point FFT algorithm will have the complex value of each and every data. In our case, processing of speech signal can be done only by using real part, so, we discarded the imaginary part/data's using equation 8. Then, the spectrum of each frame representing only real values were stored in a single matrix (number of row represents number of frame and number of column represents the total number of samples present in speech signal).

$$|X(k)| = \sqrt{\left[\mathrm{Re}\{X(k)\}\right]^2 + \left[\mathrm{Im}\{X(k)\}\right]^2} \qquad (8)$$

5.2.4. Critical Band Filter Bank Analysis

As per literature, Human auditory system are used to emphasize the low frequency then that of higher frequency (range 20 Hz to 20 kHz) (Wang et al., 2011). Depending on this, the Critical Band Filter Bank Analysis was proposed and it is built on the basis of initial transduction phenomenon. Spectral representation of speech signal, uses linear phased FIR bandpass filters (BPF) on the Bark or Mel scale of a simple bank for feature extraction (Zhou et al., 2011) but the speech signal is not a linear frequency as like in FFT. Whereas, the speech signal is directly proportional to the log of linear frequency and it is respected by the equation 9 depending on the Mel-scale frequency.

$$M_f(f) = 2595 * \log_{10}\left(1 + \frac{f}{700}\right) \tag{9}$$

Then, a triangular overlapping filters are used to create spectral envelope to represent the dominating components present in that particular (speech) signal (shown in Figure 9). The process of envelope creation on the signal using Mel-filter bank is shown in the Figure 10.

The triangular filter is used to distribute the spectral components to the linear-scale frequency and uniformed components to the *Mel-scale* frequency, by placing more number of filers in the lower frequency region then the higher frequency region ($f_h < filter < f_l$), which is represent by equation (10) and it must satisfy equation (11):

Figure 9. Triangular overlapping filter and the change in Mel frequency

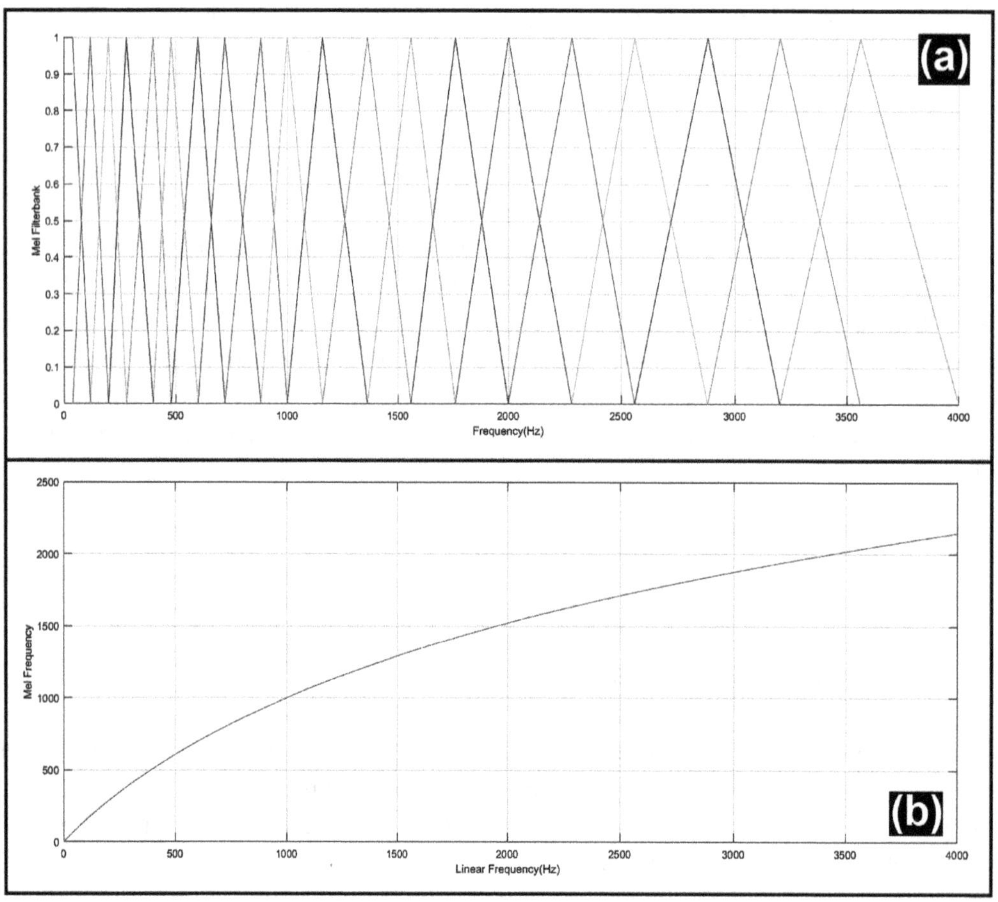

$$S(k)=\begin{cases}0 & ;for\ k<f(n-1)\\ \dfrac{k-f(n-1)}{f(n)-f(n-1)} & ;for\ f(n-1)\leq k\leq f(n)\\ \dfrac{f(n+1)-k}{f(n+1)-f(n)} & ;for\ f(n)\leq k\leq f(n+1)\\ 0 & ;for\ k<f(n+1)\end{cases} \tag{10}$$

$$\sum\nolimits_{n=0}^{L-1} S(k)=1 \tag{11}$$

Where, *n* represents number of filter in filter bank. We have used 20 filter to compute the *Mel* spectrum. To calculate centre frequency f_c of filter bank is defined by equation 12:

$$f_c(n)=\left(\frac{M}{f_s}\right)Mel^{-1}\left(Mel(f_l)+n*\left[\frac{Mel(f_h)-Mel(f_l)}{L+1}\right]\right) \tag{12}$$

where, Sampling frequency (f_s) in Hz), *M* and *N* are the number of filters and size of FFT. The inverse *Mel*-scale frequency is defined by equation 13

$$Mel^{-1}(a)=700*(10^{\frac{a}{2595}}-1) \tag{13}$$

5.2.5. Log Energy Estimation of Filtered Bank

This *log energy* $E\left(s\right)$ resemble the process of smoothening of spectrum for approximation of log-scale, which is basically done by human ears (Zhou et al., 2011). The equation 14 is used to computes $E\left(s\right)$, to describe logarithmic sum of spectral magnitudes of filtered components present in each filter bank (i.e. each bins per frame per filter will have $E\left(s\right)$. Here, we will be getting 20 numerical values for each frame at the output of filter-bank.

$$E(s)=\log_{10}\left[\sum\nolimits_{k=0}^{K-1}\left|X(k)\right|^2\cdot S(k)\right];\ for\ 0\leq s\leq S \tag{14}$$

5.2.6. Discrete Cosine Transformation

DCT collects maximum information from the signal that's lower order coefficients, by ignoring the higher order coefficients. This, further significantly reduces the computational cost. Whereas, inverse DFT (IDFT) converts the log power spectrum of Mel-frequency into time domain using diagonal covariance matrices of Gaussian function to reduce the complexity and computational cost. DCT especially

Figure 10. Mel-filter bank creation

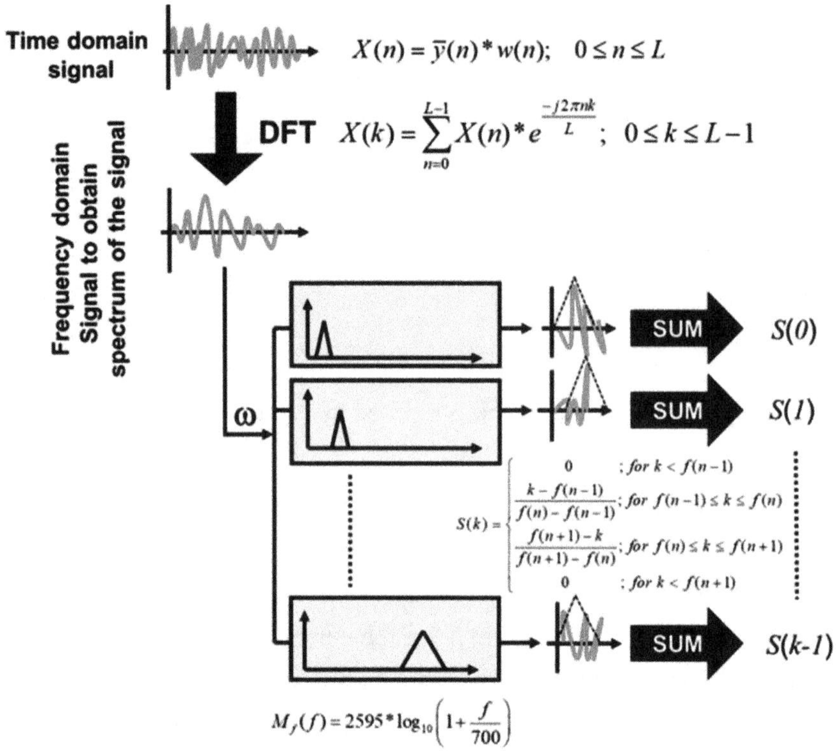

useful for speech recognition systems due to its simplicity. DCT is defined as a sum of cosine function fluctuating at each and every frequencies to get a finite sequence of data points, which is expressed as in equation 15:

$$c(n) = \sum\nolimits_{x=0}^{X-1} E\left(s\right) \cdot \cos\left[\frac{\pi n\left(x + 1/2\right)}{X}\right]; \quad for\ 0 \le n \le N \tag{15}$$

where, n is varied (8 to 13) but in our case we have used 13 to get 13 coefficients for each frame. Thus, cepstral analysis is used to calculate Mel-frequency cepstrum coefficients (MFCC) feature vector on Mel-spectrum.

5.2.7. Delta and Acceleration Coefficient Estimation (Derivative Operation)

In addition to the MFCC coefficients, the time domain approximations are also an important feature vectors used to represent the dynamic characteristic of speech signal (Murty & Yegnanarayana, 2006; Hossan et al., 2010). So, to combine the dynamic characteristics of speech signal, the 1st order (Delta coefficients) & 2nd order (Delta-Delta or Acceleration coefficients) differences of these MFCC coefficients are used. Further incorporation of these two coefficients enhanced the performance of speech signal recognition dynamically. Simply, the Derivative operation [delta ($d_{t,k}$) & Acceleration ($a_{t,k}$)] are used to find the temporal data with respect to time are defined as equation 16 & 17 respectively and the process flow of derivative operation is pictorially shown in Figure 11.

$$d_{t,k} = \frac{\sum_{n=1}^{N} n\left[c(t+n,k) - c(t-n,k)\right]}{2\left[\sum_{n=1}^{N} n^2\right]} \tag{16}$$

$$a_{t,k} = \frac{\sum_{n=1}^{N} n\left[d(t+n,k) - d(t-n,k)\right]}{2\left[\sum_{n=1}^{N} n^2\right]} \tag{17}$$

Where, k represents cepstrum coefficient at frame t after performing DCT. Now, we will be having 39 feature vector totally (MFCC, Delta and Acceleration coefficients) and the overall flow of feature extraction process is shown in Figure 12.

5.3. Speech Signal Classification

Classification is a process by which a particular signal/data is assigned to a particular class by defining a set of boundary conditions in the feature space (Ghoraani & Krishnan, 2011).

Based on their capabilities, the classifiers are divided into (i) Real-time classifiers and (2) Non-real-time classifiers. Real-time classifier has the ability to update the classification outcome frequently over vary milliseconds to provide a classification result. Whereas, the non-real-time classifiers uses a long portion/length of signal to provide a classification result. In terms of accuracy, the non-real-time classifier provide better classification result than that of real-time classifier (Huang et al., 1990).

Figure 11. Derivative operation over time to get MFCC feature vector

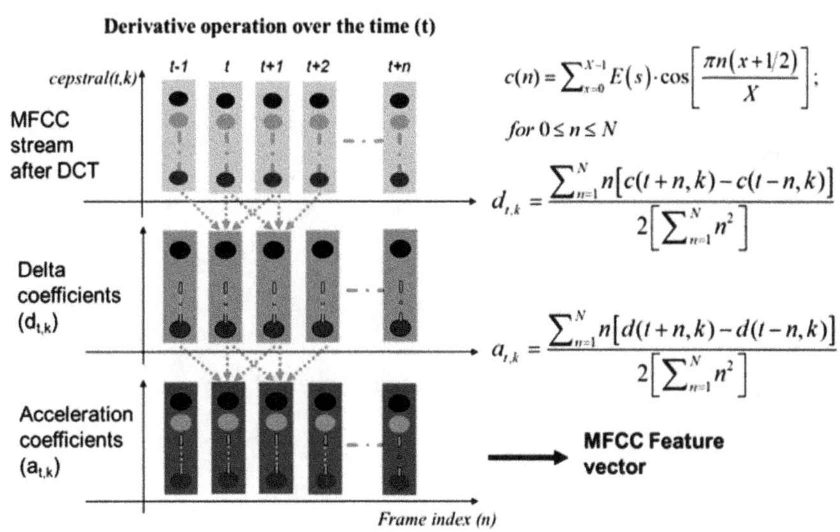

Figure 12. Overall flow of feature extraction

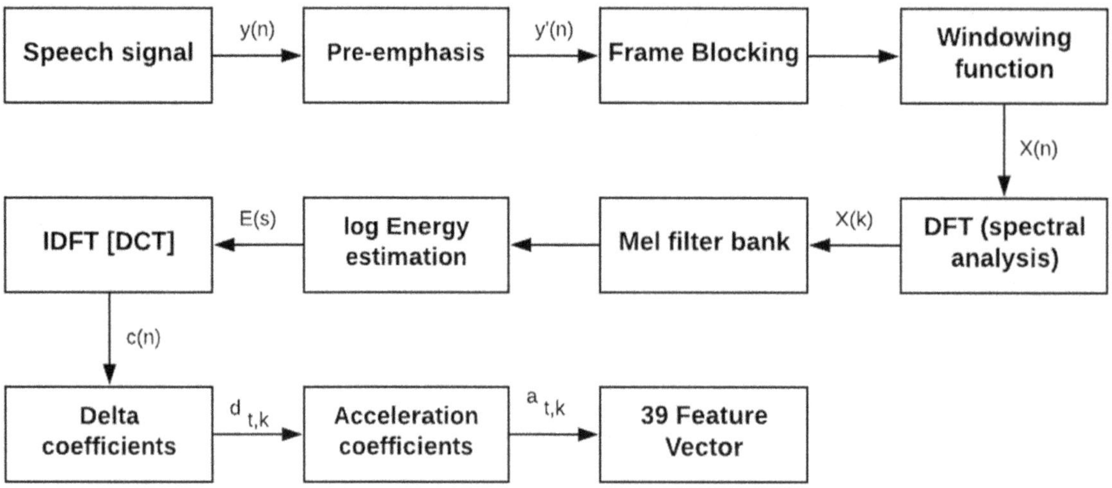

Based on their approach, the classifiers are divided into (i) direct and (2) hierarchical approach classifiers. Direct approach classifiers, classifies the signal/data using all the available features in that instant (of time) step. Whereas, the hierarchical approach classifiers, classifies the signal/data based on the dependency of the features and sub-features suggested by hierarchical scheme. Here, the errors (in hierarchical approach classifiers) usually taken into consideration for modernising of the system regular than that of direct approach classifier but implementation of hierarchical approach classifiers is much more complicated than that of direct approach. A generalized block diagram representation of classification process is shown in the Figure 13.

5.3.1. Fundamental Equation for Model Generation

Likelihood (L) of a word sequence is the combination of the observed acoustic feature vectors (B) and the word sequence (A)

$$L=\arg\max_{A} P\left(B|A\right) \tag{18}$$

Then, by Bayes' Theorem:

$$P\left(A|B\right)=\frac{P\left(B|A\right)P\left(A\right)}{P\left(B\right)} \tag{19}$$

$$P\left(B\right)=\sum_{a} P\left(B|A_a\right)P\left(A_a\right) \text{ [If } A_a \text{ becomes the mutually events]} \tag{20}$$

Figure 13. Generalized block diagram of classifier

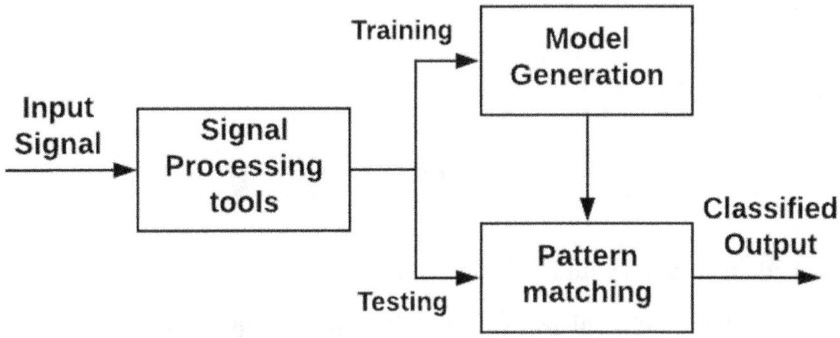

$$P(A|B) = \frac{P(B|A)P(A)}{\sum_a P(B|A_a)P(A_a)} \tag{21}$$

or

$$L = \arg\max_A P(B|A)P(A) \tag{22}$$

Where, $P(B|A)$ represents the Acoustic model and $P(A)$ will be the Language model.

Here in the work, we have used hidden Markov-Gaussian mixture model (HM-GMM) (Povey et al., 2010) and Artificial neural network (ANN) (Liu et al., 2014) as mentioned earlier.

5.3.2. Hidden Markov Model (HMM)

The hidden Markov model (Huang et al., 1990) is a simplest form of dynamic Bayesian network (Rabiner & Juang, 1986). It is used to solve the problem of classifying speech signals or temporal pattern recognition through statistical approach based on modelling of propagative sequences, which is represented by a corresponding observed sequence of that data/signal (Jelinek, 1976). HMM is a stochastic model, where the transition propagative sequence of a state of the system is governed by a *Markov process* and fixed/observable propagative sequence of a state of the system will have a dependency on principal probabilistic information. In short, the HMM will provide us the information about the propagative sequence of a state of an system and since, the Markov process is in hidden state, this model is termed as "Hidden-Markov Model" (Hiroya & Honda, 2004).

The HMM, a probabilistic model of the joint probability of a collection of random variables $\{o_1,\ldots,o_T,q_1,\ldots,q_T\}$. The o_t may be either continuous or discrete observations and the q_t generally "hidden" and they are discrete in nature. There are two conditional independence assumptions (i) the tth hidden variable gives the $(t\text{-}1)^{st}$ hidden variable and it will be independent of previous variables (equation 23), and (ii) the tth observation gives the tth hidden variable and it will be independent of other variables (equation 24)

$$\mathrm{P}\left(q_t \middle| q_{t-1}, o_{t-1}, \ldots, q_1, o_1\right) = \mathrm{P}\left(q_t \middle| q_{t-1}\right) \tag{23}$$

$$\mathrm{P}\left(q_t \middle| q_T, o_T, q_{T-1}, o_{T-1}, \ldots, q_{T+1}, o_{T+1}, q_t, q_{t-1}, o_{t-1}, \ldots, q_1, o_1\right) = \mathrm{P}\left(o_t \middle| q_t\right) \tag{24}$$

If q_t is a discrete random variable with N possible values $\left[1, \ldots, N\right]$. The Hidden-Markov Model (λ) estimates the values of propagative sequence A, B & π through the equation »=$\left[\mathrm{A,B,À}\right]$; where A represents State Transition Matrix, B represents Observation Probability Matrix and π represents Initial state probability distribution and the corresponding model parameter will be:

- State Transition Matrix,

$$A = \left\{a_{i,j}\right\} = \mathrm{P}\left[q_t = j \middle| q_{t-1} = i\right]; \quad 1 \leq i, j \leq N \tag{25}$$

- Observation Probability Matrix $B = \left\{b_j\left(o_t\right)\right\}$, (26)
- For discrete observation:

$$b_j\left(o_t\right) = \mathrm{P}\left[o_t = v_k \mid q_t = j\right]; \quad 1 \leq k \leq M \,\&\, 1 \leq j \leq N \tag{27}$$

- For multivariate Gaussian mixture:

$$b_j\left(o_t\right) = \sum\nolimits_{l=1}^{M} c_{jl} * N\left[o_t \middle| \mu_{jl}, \sum jl\right] = \sum\nolimits_{l=1}^{M} c_{jl} * b_{jl}\left(o_t\right); \\ 1 \leq l \leq M \,\&\, 1 \leq j \leq N \tag{28}$$

- Initial state probability distribution,

$$\pi_i = \mathrm{P}\left[q_1 = i\right]; \quad 1 \leq i \leq N \\ \pi_j = \mathrm{P}\left[q_t = j\right]; \quad 1 \leq j \leq M \tag{29}$$

For the Efficient Calculation of the values of a likelihood model parameters were re-assessed again using Forward Algorithm, Backward Algorithm, Viterbi Algorithm, and Baum-Welch Algorithm.

The maximum Likelihood (ML) hidden-Markov model (ML-HMM), L is given by

$$L = \sum_{i \in \kappa} \alpha_{i,t} \tag{30}$$

Where, the sum of all the possible final states (κ) within the model called emission probabilities, corresponds to the current phonetic transcription of the system. The current phonetic transcription involves *q* states and *t* length of the current observation sequence. Together, *q* and *o* is the implementation of a pronunciation lexicon, an HMM state graph structure for each word that the system is capable of recognizing is shown in Figure 14.

5.3.2.1. Forward Algorithm

The forward variable $\alpha_{i,t} = P\left[o_1, \ldots, o_t, q_t = i \middle| \lambda\right]$ for i^{th} state at t^{th} time can be calculated (equation 33). The $\alpha_{i,t}$ can be defined as

$$a_{i,1} = \pi_i b_i\left(o_1\right); \quad 1 \le i \le N \tag{31}$$

$$\alpha_{j,(t+1)} = \left\{\sum\nolimits_{i=1}^{N} \alpha_{j,t} * \alpha_{i,j}\right\} * b_j\left(o_{t+1}\right); \quad 1 \le t \le T-1 \tag{32}$$

$$P\left(o \middle| \lambda\right) = \sum\nolimits_{i=1}^{N} \alpha_{i,T} \tag{33}$$

where, $\left(\alpha_{j,t+1}\right)$ is the *forward* path probability at time (t+1). $\alpha_{i,j}$ is the transition probability of next state b_j and the current state a_j. $b_j\left(o_t\right)$ is the likelihood state of the observation o_t of the current state.

Figure 14. Graphical representation of the pronunciation lexicon of each word

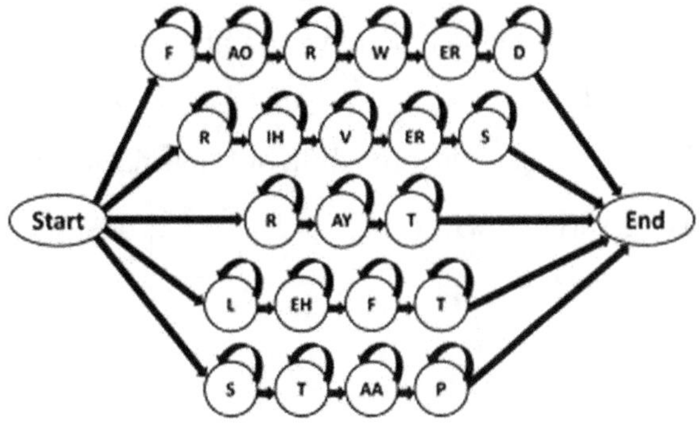

5.3.2.2. Backward Algorithm

The backward variable $\beta_{i,t} = \mathrm{P}\left[o_{t+1},\ldots,o_t \middle| q_t = i,\lambda\right]$ for i^{th} state at t^{th} time can be calculated (equation 36). The $\beta_{i,t}$ can be defined as

$$\beta_{i,T} = 1; \quad 1 \le i \le N \tag{34}$$

$$\beta_{i,t} = \sum\nolimits_{j=1}^{N} \beta_{i,j} * \beta_{j,(t+1)} * b_j\left(o_{t+1}\right); \quad t = T-1, T-2,..,1 \ \& \ 1 \le i \le N \tag{35}$$

$$\mathrm{P}\left(o\middle|\lambda\right) = \sum\nolimits_{i=1}^{N} \beta_{i,1} * \pi_i * \beta_i\left(o_1\right); \quad 1 \le t \le T \tag{36}$$

where, $\left(\beta_{i,t}\right)$ is the backward path probability at time (t) at state (i).when,

$$\delta_{i,t} = \mathrm{P}\left(q_t = i\middle|o,\lambda\right) = \frac{\mathrm{P}\left(o, q_t = i\middle|\lambda\right)}{\mathrm{P}\left(o\middle|\lambda\right)} = \frac{\mathrm{P}\left(o, q_t = i\middle|\lambda\right)}{\sum\nolimits_{j=1}^{N} \mathrm{P}\left(o, q_t = j\middle|\lambda\right)} \tag{37}$$

By combining equation (33, 36 in 37), we get

$$\delta_{i,t} = \frac{\alpha_{i,t} * \beta_{i,t}}{\sum\nolimits_{j=1}^{N} \alpha_{j,t} * \beta_{j,t}}; \quad 1 \le j \le N \tag{38}$$

5.3.2.3. Viterbi Algorithm

The Viterbi algorithm is used to estimate the required optimal or best sequence/path of state for a given observation sequence $\zeta_{t,i} = \max \mathrm{P}\left[p_1, p_2,\ldots,p_{t-1}, p_t = i, o_1, o_2,\ldots,o_t \middle|\lambda\right]$ with the ML estimation (maximum probability) to $\mathrm{P}\left[o,\lambda\right]$. To compute the probability of optimal sequence of state i at given observation o and the model λ using variable will be $\zeta_{t,i} = \mathrm{P}\left[p_t = i\middle|o_t,\lambda\right]$ and using forward & backward variables, it becomes as in equation 39:

$$\zeta_{t,i} = \frac{\alpha_{i,t} * \beta_{i,t}}{\sum\nolimits_{i=1}^{N} \alpha_{i,t} * \beta_{i,t}}; \quad 1 \le i \le N \tag{39}$$

For satisfying the conditional probability (using equation 41), the optimal state i becomes (equation 40)

$$i_t = \arg \max_{1 \le i \le N} \left(\zeta_{t,i}\right); \quad 1 \le t \le T \tag{40}$$

when,

$$\sum_{i=1}^{N} \zeta_{t,i} = 1 \tag{41}$$

Syntax:

1. Initialization:

$$\zeta_{1,i} = \pi_i b_i \left(o_1\right); \quad 1 \le i \le N \tag{42}$$

$$\vartheta_{1,i} = 0 \tag{43}$$

2. Recursion/looping:

$$\zeta_{t,j} = \max_{1 \le i \le N} \left[\zeta_{t-1,i} * \alpha_{i,j}\right] * b_j \left(o_t\right); \quad 1 \le j \le N, 2 \le t \le T \tag{44}$$

$$\vartheta_{t,j} = \arg \max_{1 \le i \le N} \left[\zeta_{t-1,i} * \alpha_{i,j}\right] \tag{45}$$

3. Stop:

$$\bar{P} = \max_{1 \le i \le N} \left[\zeta_{T,i}\right] \tag{46}$$

$$\bar{p}_T = \arg \max_{1 \le i \le N} \left[\zeta_{T,i}\right] \tag{47}$$

4. Optimal Path/sequence using Backtracking:

$$\bar{p}^T = \vartheta_{t+1} * \bar{p}_{t+1}; \quad \left[for\ T-1, T-2, .., 1\right] \tag{48}$$

5.3.2.4. Baum-Welch Algorithm

Till now, the model parameters $»=\left[A,B,À\right]$ were continuously modified to get maximum likelihood variables for the probability $P\left[o,\lambda\right]$. Here, using the variable $\varphi_t\left(i,j\right)$ with the path probability in qi state at time t and estimating the transition probability density of the model, at time t+1 at state qi for a given observational sequence. Then, the variable is defined as (equation 49)

$$\varphi_t(i,j) = \frac{\alpha_{t,i} * a_{i,j} * b_j(o_{t+1}) * \beta_{t+1,j}}{\mathrm{P}(o|\lambda)} \tag{49}$$

As like in equation 41, the variables $\zeta_{t,i}$ & $\varphi_t(i,j)$ are summed over *j* states, to get $\varphi_t(i,j)$

$$\zeta_{t,i} = \sum_{j=1}^{N} \varphi_t(i,j) \tag{50}$$

Similarly, the variables $\zeta_{t,i}$ & $\varphi_t(i,j)$ are summed over time *t*, to get $\varphi_t(i,j)$

$$\sum_{t=1}^{T-1} \zeta_{t,i} = optimal\ number\ of\ transitions\ for\ q_i\ state \tag{51}$$

$$\sum_{t=1}^{T-1} \varphi_t(i,j) = \left[\begin{array}{l} optimal\ number\ of\ transitions \\ due\ to\ the\ transition\ from\ q_i\ to\ q_j\ state \end{array} \right. \tag{52}$$

The Baum-Welch algorithm (equation 53, 54 & 55) is used to re-calculate new parameters for the λ model, using the equation 51 & 52, until an optimal value is convergence to $\lambda_{old} \approx \lambda_{new}$.

$$\pi_i^{new} = \zeta_{1,i};\ 1 \le i \le N \tag{53}$$

$$a_{i,j}^{new} = \frac{\sum_t \varphi_t(i,j)}{\sum_t \zeta_{t,i}};\quad 1 \le t \le T-1 \tag{54}$$

$$b_j^{new}(o_t) = \frac{\sum_t \varphi_t(i,j)}{\sum_t \zeta_{t,i}};\quad 1 \le t \le T-1 \tag{55}$$

Baum-Welch algorithm terminates the iteration, when it observes zero significant changes in the model parameters to build an efficient classification model. Then, the likelihood values of the model parameters using HMM is passed to Gaussian mixture model for further analysis.

5.3.3. Gaussian Mixture Model (GMM)

Gaussian mixture model (Reynolds 1995) is a probabilistic model that segregates the data points into various sub-classes within a (overall) class, if the data points are normally distributed. GMM lies within parametric and non-parametric type density model. i.e., GMM can be used to control the behaviour of the density model in all the possible way (parametric approach) and it can also be modelled arbitrary (non-parametric approach).

The GMM (Reynolds et al., 2000) has two principal components, (i) the mixture or weight component and (ii) the mean (μ) with variances (σ) or covariances (Σ) depending on the model. The mixture or weight component (ϕ) with the constraint $\sum_{n=1}^{N} \phi_n = 1$ for a component (C) to make the total probability distribution function (*pdf*) normalizes to 1 and if the weight component are known then it is a priori distribution or else it is a posteriori distribution. The GMM is nothing but the weighted sum of univariate Gaussian distribution (equation 56).

Gaussian (one dimensional) *pdf* is described by equation 56:

$$a_n(x) = \frac{1}{\sigma_n \sqrt{2\pi}} \exp\left[-\frac{(x-\mu_n)^2}{2\sigma_n^2}\right] \tag{56}$$

Where, 'n' is the Gaussian component [n = 1,...,N] and the mean and variance is shown in equation 57 & 58 at state *i*.

$$\hat{\mu}_i = \frac{1}{T}\sum_{t=1}^{T} x \tag{57}$$

$$\hat{\sigma}_j^2 = \frac{1}{T}\sum_{t=1}^{T}\left[x - \mu_i\right]^2 \tag{58}$$

For a given HMM state, the Gaussian (D-dimensional) *pdf* is described by equation 59:

$$a_i(\vec{x}) = p\left[\vec{x} \middle| \vec{\mu}_i, \Sigma_i\right] = \frac{1}{\sqrt{(2\pi)^D \left|\Sigma_i\right|}} \exp\left(-\frac{1}{2}(\vec{x}-\vec{\mu}_i)^{\mathrm{T}} * \Sigma_i^{-1}(\vec{x}-\vec{\mu}_i)\right) \tag{59}$$

Where, '*n*' is the Gaussian component and N is the D-dimensional *pdf*. If '*D*'-number of components is known, then, the Expectation Maximization or Maximum Likelihood Estimation (MLE) is used to estimate the parameters of the mixture model.

5.3.3.1. Maximum Likelihood Estimation (MLE)

The Expectation Maximization (EM) or Maximum Likelihood Estimation (MLE) (equation 60) is an iterative method to estimate maximum likelihood parameter $a_i(o_t)$ of the k-dimensional feature vector

(o_t) of a given HMM state (j). For estimating the MLE, multivariate Gaussian *pdf* uses diagonal-covariance type equation 61.

$$p\left[x\left|\mu,\Sigma\right.\right]=\sum_{k=1}^{K}\frac{G_k}{\sqrt{2\pi\left|\Sigma_k\right|}}\exp\left(\left(x-\mu_k\right)^{\mathrm{T}}*\Sigma^{-1}\left(x-\mu_k\right)\right) \tag{60}$$

Then, the output of MLE become (equation 61),

$$a_i\left(o_t\right)=\sum_{k=1}^{K}\frac{G_k}{\sqrt{2\pi\left|\Sigma_{ik}\right|}}\exp\left[\left(x-\mu_{ik}\right)^{\mathrm{T}}*\Sigma^{-1}\left(x-\mu_{ik}\right)\right] \tag{61}$$

Where, $\vec{\mu}_j$ represents the mean cepstral vector and σ_j^2 represents the variance cepstral vector.

$$\phi_{tn}\left(i\right)=\frac{\sum_{k=1}\kappa*\alpha_{t-1}\left(i\right)*a_{ik}c_{in}b_{in}\left(o_t\right)\beta_t\left(i\right)}{\alpha_T\left(p\right)} \tag{62}$$

From Baum-Welch algorithm, the previous iteration values ϕ was called and used $\phi_t\left(i\right)$ to calculate the mean $\hat{\mu}_{in}$, weight components $\hat{c}_{in}$, and covariance $\hat{\Sigma}_{in}$ using equations 61 & 62:

$$\hat{\mu}_{in}=\frac{\sum_{t=1}^{T}\phi_{tn}\left(i\right)*o_t}{\sum_{t=1}^{T}\sum_{n=1}^{N}\phi_{tn}\left(i\right)} \tag{63}$$

$$\hat{c}_{in}=\frac{\sum_{t=1}^{T}\phi_{tn}\left(i\right)}{\sum_{t=1}^{T}\sum_{m=1}^{M}\phi_{tn}\left(i\right)} \tag{64}$$

$$\hat{\Sigma}_{in}=\frac{\sum_{t=1}^{T}\phi_{tn}\left(i\right)\left(o_t-\mu_{in}\right)\left(o_t-\mu_{in}\right)^T}{\sum_{t=1}^{T}\sum_{m=1}^{M}\phi_{tn}\left(i\right)} \tag{65}$$

Single K-dimensional diagonal-covariance GMM equation is shown in (equation 66):

$$a_i\left(o_t\right) = \prod_{k=1}^{K} \frac{1}{\sqrt{2\pi\sigma_{ik}^2}} \mathrm{e}\left[-\frac{1}{2}\left(\frac{\left(o_{tk} - \mu_{jk}\right)^2}{\sigma_{jk}^{\ 2}}\right)\right] \tag{66}$$

To avoid the underflow of numeric data, the log of probability of maximum likelihood is calculated using equation 67 and 68

$$\log a_i\left(o_t\right) = -\frac{1}{2}\sum_{k=1}^{K}\left[\log(2\pi) + \sigma_{ik}^2 + \left(\frac{o_{tk} - \mu_{ik}}{\sigma_{ik}^2}\right)^2\right] \tag{67}$$

$$\log a_i\left(o_t\right) = D - \frac{1}{2}\sum_{k=1}^{K}\left(\frac{o_{tk} - \mu_{ik}}{\sigma_{ik}^2}\right)^2 \tag{68}$$

Where, D is a constant term and it can be precomputed using equation (69):

$$D = -\frac{1}{2}\sum_{k=1}^{K}\left[\log(2\pi) + \sigma_{ik}^2\right] \tag{69}$$

Thus, by using the equation (63, 64 & 65) of the EM algorithm, the values of mixture, mean and covariance were estimated.

5.3.3.2. Syntax of EM Algorithm for Performing GMM

1. Initialize, the parameters (mixture/weight, mean and covariance) and find the starting values of log likelihood EM,
2. Find the possible parametric values at time t (step 2 also called as **Expectation step**)

$$\xi_i\left(x_k\right) = \frac{\pi_k * \kappa\left(x_k \middle| \mu_k, \Sigma_k\right)}{\sum_{i=1}^{M} \pi_i * \kappa\left(x_i \middle| \mu_i, \Sigma_i\right)} \tag{70}$$

3. Re-estimate the step 2 for time t+1

$$\pi_i = \frac{1}{K}\sum_{k=1}^{K} \xi_i\left(x_k\right) \tag{71}$$

$$\mu_i = \frac{\sum_{k=1}^{K} \xi_i\left(x_k\right) * x_k}{\sum_{k=1}^{K} \xi_i\left(x_k\right)} \tag{72}$$

$$\Sigma_i = \frac{\sum_{k=1}^{K} \xi_i\left(x_k\right)\left[\left(x_k - \mu_i\right)\left(x_k - \mu_i\right)^T\right]}{\sum_{k=1}^{K} \xi_i\left(x_k\right)} \tag{73}$$

4. Find **log likelihood EM** until the convergence else return to step 2

$$\log \mathrm{P}\left[x \middle| \pi, \mu, \sigma\right] = \sum_{i=1}^{M} \log\left[\sum_{k=1}^{K} \pi_k * \kappa\left(x_i \middle| \mu_k, \Sigma_k\right)\right] \tag{74}$$

5.3.4. Hybrid hM-GM Model

By hybridizing hM-GM model, the ability to find the maximum probability distribution of data (x) jointly among all while in the observation sequence (o_t). All the independent likelihood estimate of GMM & HMM will jointly pass through the decision making block, there the outcome will be only one data $\left[\Psi_M\right]$ [new joint likelihood data] (Povey et al., 2010) equation 75 and Figure 15 shows the process flow of hybrid hM-GM model.

$$\Psi_M(x) = \left[\left(1 - Y\left(x\right)\right) * G_M\right] + \left[Y\left(x\right) * H_M\right] \tag{75}$$

Where, $Y\left(x\right)$ is the weight factor.

5.3.5. Artificial Neural Networks (ANNs)

ANN is an electronic model, which has multiple nodes, having the architecture to mimic the biological neurons of the animal brain. Naturally, the biological neurons are electrically excitable cell that receives an electro-chemical signal from another neuron, process it, and sends the information to the respective place (other neuron, cell, etc.) through a specialized junction called synapses or synaptic junction. The biological neurons are interconnected by this junction to make communication with each other. Artificial Neurons of the Artificial Neural Network imitates four important functions of a biological neuron and that can be mathematical modelled. ANN has nodes to imitate the biological neurons, and it is connected to a links. The links is used to represent the dendrites and synapses of the neurons. Thus, each link has assigned with a particular weight factor. When the node gets an input data, it performs simple operation to define Activation function and adjust the weights of the links, which makes the system to learn. In this work, we have used Feedforward Multi-Layer Perceptron (MLP) and Back propagation algorithm has it is more commonly used in speech processing application (Leung and Haykin 1991).

Figure 15. Hybrid hM-GM block diagram

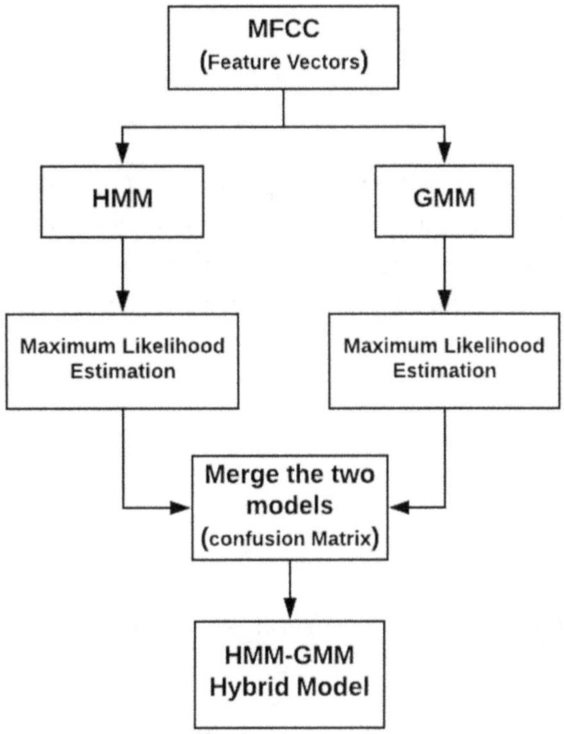

5.3.5.1. Feed-Forward Network

In feed-forward network, the data can only able to flow from input layer to the output layer through the hidden layer unidirectional (only in forward direction), so, called Feed-forward Network and this network doesn't contain any recursive function/process. Simply to say, 1st neuron in 1st layer can only able to transfer data/signal to the 2nd neuron in the 2nd layer if and only if b>a. Multiple layered Feed-forward Network using Back propagation algorithm (Leung and Haykin 1991), can be termed as Multi-Layer Perceptrons (MLP). In generally, The MLP (Bourlard and Morgan 2012) should have at least two layers of perceptrons. Here, It has one input, more than two hidden layers and output layers and it uses a non-linear sigmoid or a radial-basis function to produce complex functions for a given input and this can be expressed as equation 76:

$$Out_i^N = f\left[\sum_{j=1} w_{ji}^{N,N-1} * Out_j^{L-1} + w_{i0}^{N,N-1}\right] \tag{76}$$

Where, Out_i^N is the i node output of layer N, $w_{ji}^{N,N-1}$ is the weight factor present between N-1 and N, $w_{i0}^{N,N-1}$ is the bias term (where w_{i0} =1), and the sigmoid (σ) transfer function (f) is given by equation 77:

$$\sigma(x) = f(x) = \frac{1}{1+e^{-x}} \tag{77}$$

Then, the equation 78 is incorporated with bias term by considering (N-1) = 1, the modified equation is

$$Out_i^N = f\left[\sum_{j=0} w_{ji}^{N,N-1} * Out_j^{L-1}\right] \tag{78}$$

Thus, the MLP's output response is due to the input stream of data given. As, we already know that the ability of MLP depends on weighting factor. So, by continuous tuning of weighting factor is need using training process towards the corresponding targeted output and this can be done by employing Back propagation algorithm by using Least Mean Square Error (LMSR) (equation 79 or 80) (Sohn, Kim et al. 1999)

$$E_{LMS} = \frac{1}{2}\sum_k \sum_i \left|tg_i^k - Out_i^{N,p}\right|^2 \tag{79}$$

Or

$$E_{er} = -\sum_k \sum_i \left\{\left[tg_i^k * \ln\left(Out_i^{N,p}\right)\right] + \left[\left(1 - tg_i^k\right) * \ln\left(1 - Out_i^{N,p}\right)\right]\right\} \tag{80}$$

Using Gradient continuous weight updating, the weighting function becomes equation 81:

$$\Delta w_{ik}^c = -\eta \frac{\partial E\left[w_{ik}^c\right]}{\partial w_{ik}^c} \tag{81}$$

Updating weight Δw_{ik}^c for each weight w_{ik}^c of every training pattern *tp* and each cycle of update is termed as "*epoch training*". Where, w_{ik}^c is the weight factor present between *i* and *k layer*, and η represents learning rate or step length.

5.3.5.2. MLP Classifier

The equation 82 represents a two layer linear network output:

$$Out_c^2 = \sum_b Out_b^1 * w_{bc}^2 = \sum_b f\left[\sum_a in_a * w_{ab}^1\right] * w_{bc}^2 \tag{82}$$

$$\Delta w_{ab}^2 = \eta \sum_c \sum_d \left[tg_d - Out_d^2\right] * Out_a^1 * \delta_{db} = \eta \sum_c \left[tg_b - Out_b^2\right] * Out_a^1 \tag{83}$$

$$\Delta w_{ab}^{1} = \eta \sum_{c} \sum_{d} \left[tg_{d} - Out_{d}^{2} \right] * \overline{f} \left[\sum_{e} in_{e} * w_{eb}^{1} \right] * \left(in_{a} * w_{bd}^{2} \right) \tag{84}$$

Then, the changes due to transfer function

$$\Delta w_{ab}^{2} = \eta \sum_{c} \left[tg_{\tilde{b}} - Out_{b}^{2} \right] * Out_{a}^{1} \tag{85}$$

$$\Delta w_{ab}^{1} = \eta \sum_{c} \sum_{d} \left[tg_{d} - Out_{d}^{2} \right] * w_{bd}^{2} * Out_{b}^{1} \left[1 - Out_{b}^{1} \right] * in_{a} \tag{86}$$

Thus, the equation nfa establishes Back Propagation Learning Algorithm for classification and the probability estimation of MLP using equation gf;

$$\mathrm{P}\left(o \middle| \lambda_{c}\right) = \left[\frac{\mathrm{P}\left(o \middle| \lambda_{c}\right)}{\mathrm{P}\left(\lambda_{c}\right)} \right] * \mathrm{P}\left(o\right) \tag{87}$$

Where, input observed feature vector is o, λ_c represents the true phoneme event, $\mathrm{P}\left(\lambda_c\right)$ represents the priori-likelihood phoneme, and it can be calculated from training dataset, and $\mathrm{P}\left(o\right)$ is the probability of unconditional observation.

Here, in this paper, we used hM-GM and MLPN for classifying the MFCC feature vectors into the Joint Maximum Likelihood Probability for representing the corresponding speech/audio signal. The Phonation model with their corresponding states used in HMM is given in Table 1. The overall function of the various classifiers from MFCC feature vector is given in figure x and the corresponding output of the developed model is check using Five LED indicator system, where each LED represent corresponding signal (Figure 16). The output from classifiers is given to AND Gate Logic with an *if else* condition so, that until the matching the overall system's output remains steady-by mode and the corresponding logic is given in Table 2.

The results of hybrid classifier (hM-GM with ANN) is shown using Phonation model for the commands used to operate wheelchair prototype shown in Table 1 and the corresponding indicator using LED are shown in Figure 16 and Figure 17 shows over all combined process of the developed/proposed Classifier model.

6. FUTURE RESEARCH DIRECTIONS

Current study using Combined, Hybrid HM-GM Classifier and MLPN Classifier with Logic Functions to build an efficient speech recognition system to improve the quality of life of the patients with several level of disabilities. The EM algorithm can able to calculate using the relative frequencies. The EM algorithm is used to re-calculate new parameters for the HMM (λ) model, using the old parameters/data's available. HMM can be modulate and extend, this individuality of HMM maximizes its use in a number of alternative model for developing an automatic speech recognition systems such as Hybridization of HMM- with other classifiers like k-Means, SVM, ANN, Fuzzy c-Mean, Genetic Algorithm, etc. Wavelet (Crouse et al., 1998) based feature extraction methods can also be employed to improve the speech signals feature extraction difference improvement to enhance the probabilities function.

7. CONCLUSION

We observed that introducing if-else with AND Logic as an additional controlling option, the correctness towards the classification gets increased but the overall classification gets decreased by 3-4%. Combining the hybrid hidden Markov-Gaussian mixture model and Multi-layer Perceptron Artificial Neural Network (MLPN), for classifying the human speech/audio signal, the performance (correctness/true value) of system got improved to a larger extent. The Hybrid HM-GM model are purely depend on Maximum Likelihood probability so, the systems reliability was less as it sometimes mislead the command signal to drive the rehabilitative aid (wheelchair). Using these words, a LED system was tested to validate the results and using the words such as Forward, Reverse, Right, Left and Stop, the system to be found working good with an efficiency of about 93%, which was 95% before. To improve the efficiency of the classification, different feature extraction methods need to be used for improving the reliability of the speech signal to be classification. Hence, we propose the model to be good and efficient which in-turn can be used for driving a wheelchair (a rehabilitative aid) for helping the people with differently-disabled, seeking for the help towards the movement/transportation as like in other technics. The movements are pictorially shown in Figure 18.

Table 1. Shows Phonation model of the commands with their corresponding states

Command	Phonation	States
FORWARD	F|AO|R|W|ER|D	6
REVERSE	R|IH|V|ER|S	5
RIGHT	R|AY|T	3
LEFT	L|EH|F|T	4
STOP	S|T|AA|P	4

Figure 16. LED system indication of each command/word

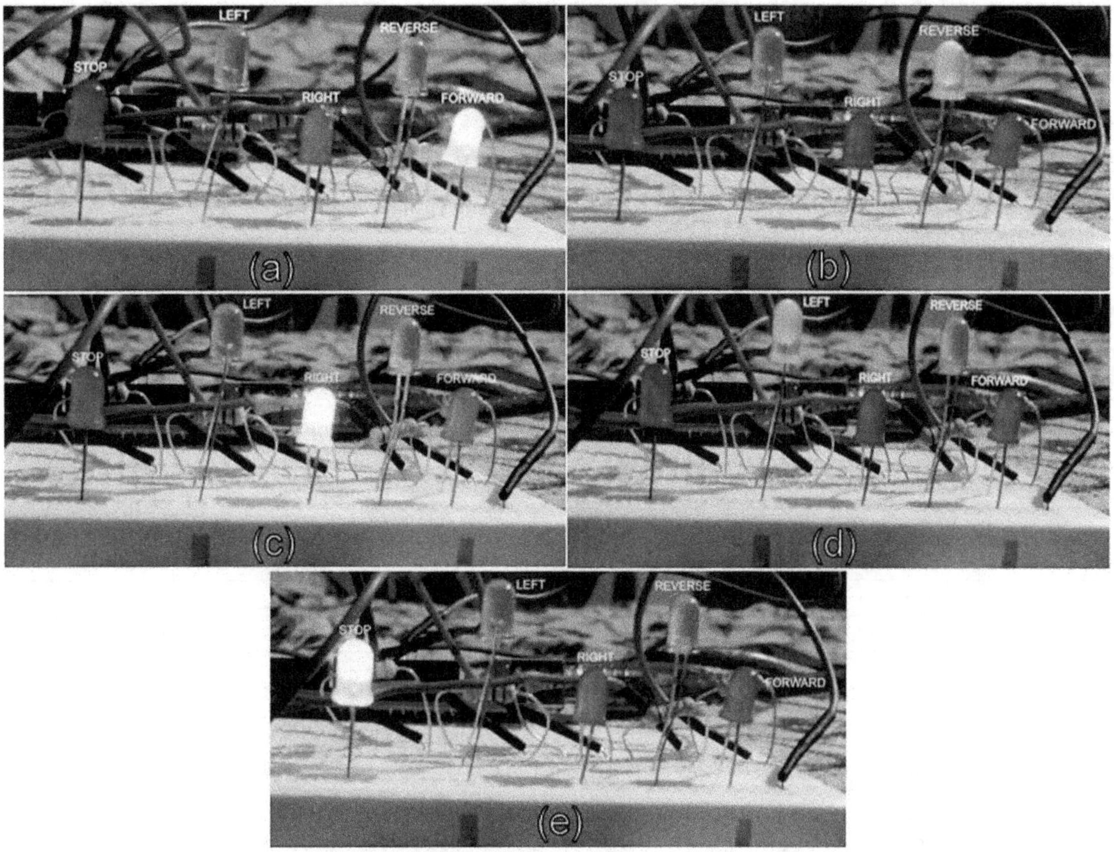

Figure 17. Overall process of combined classifier model
Syntax: conditional if-else logic with AND Gate operation

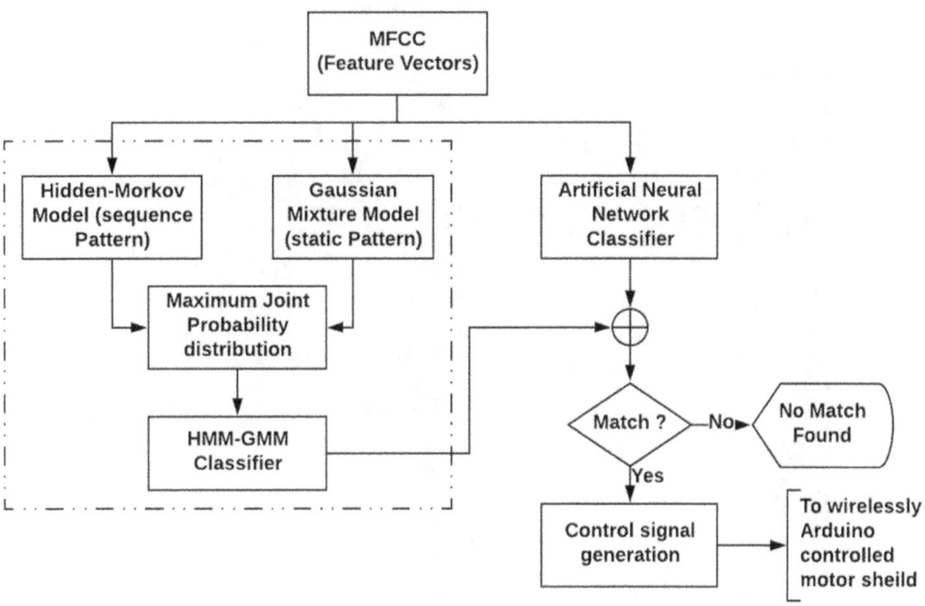

Box 1.

```
If
{
HM-GM = "Forward" && MLPN = "Forward"
Then, print "FORWARD" and send command = 1;
else if
HM-GM = "Reverse" && MLPN = "Reverse"
Then, print "REVERSE" and send command = 2;
else if
HM-GM = "Right" && MLPN = "Right"
Then, print "RIGHT" and send command = 3;
else if
HM-GM = "Left" && MLPN = "Left"
Then, print "LEFT" and send command = 4;
else if
HM-GM = "Stop" && MLPN = "Stop"
Then, print "STOP" and send command = 5;
else
Print "Doesn't Match";
End
```

Table 2. Shows AND Gate logic

HM-GM Classifier	MLPN Classifier	AND Gate Logic
0	0	0
1	0	0
0	1	0
1	1	1

Figure 18. Wheelchair prototype with movement indication

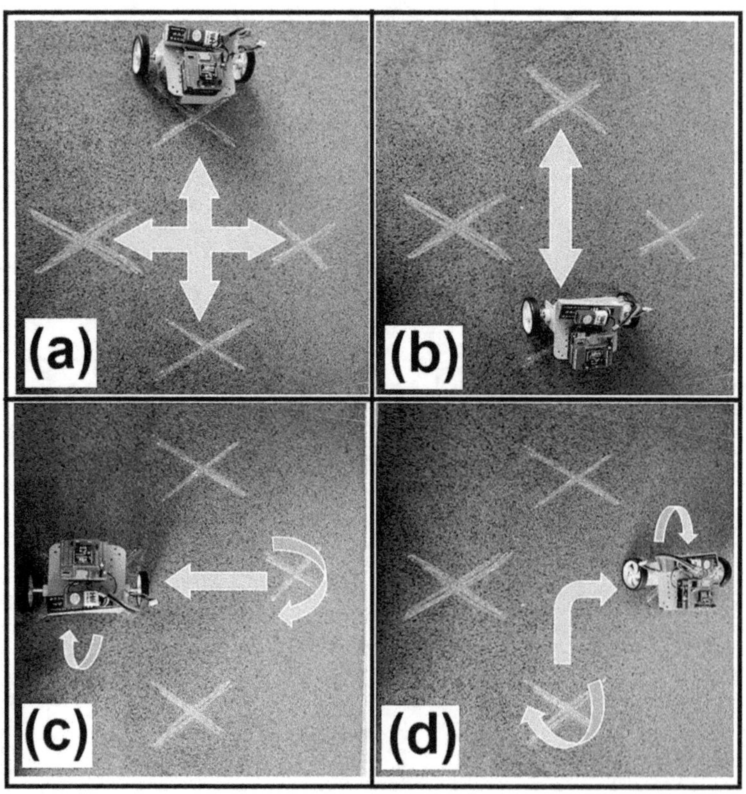

REFERENCES

Ackermann, H. (2008). Cerebellar contributions to speech production and speech perception: Psycholinguistic and neurobiological perspectives. *Trends in Neurosciences*, *31*(6), 265–272. doi:10.1016/j.tins.2008.02.011 PMID:18471906

Ackermann, H., & Riecker, A. (2010). Cerebral control of motor aspects of speech production: neurophysiological and functional imaging data. In *Speech motor control: new developments in basic and applied research* (pp. 117–134). Oxford, UK: Oxford University Press. doi:10.1093/acprof:oso/9780199235797.003.0007

Ahamed, N. U., Sundaraj, K., Ahmad, B., Rahman, M., Ali, A., Islam, A., & Palaniappan, R. (2013). Rehabilitation systems for physically disabled patients: A brief review of sensor-based computerised signal-monitoring systems. *Biomedical Research*, *24*(3).

Ai, O. C., Hariharan, M., Yaacob, S., & Chee, L. S. (2012). Classification of speech dysfluencies with MFCC and LPCC features. *Expert Systems with Applications*, *39*(2), 2157–2165. doi:10.1016/j.eswa.2011.07.065

Ang, K. K., Chua, K. S., Phua, K. S., Wang, C., Chin, Z. Y., Kuah, C. W., ... Guan, C. (2015). A randomized controlled trial of EEG-based motor imagery brain-computer interface robotic rehabilitation for stroke. *Clinical EEG and Neuroscience*, *46*(4), 310–320. doi:10.1177/1550059414522229 PMID:24756025

Atal, B., & Rabiner, L. (1976). A pattern recognition approach to voiced-unvoiced-silence classification with applications to speech recognition. *IEEE Transactions on Acoustics, Speech, and Signal Processing*, *24*(3), 201–212. doi:10.1109/TASSP.1976.1162800

Bahl, L. R., Jelinek, F., & Mercer, R. L. (1990). A maximum likelihood approach to continuous speech recognition. In Readings in Speech Recognition. Elsevier.

Banerjee, A., Datta, S., Das, P., Konar, A., Tibarewala, & Janarthan, R. (2012). Electrooculogram based online control signal generation for wheelchair. In *Electronic System Design (ISED), 2012 International Symposium on*. IEEE.

Barchiesi, D., Giannoulis, D., Stowell, D., & Plumbley, M. D. (2015). Acoustic scene classification: Classifying environments from the sounds they produce. *IEEE Signal Processing Magazine*, *32*(3), 16–34. doi:10.1109/MSP.2014.2326181

Bell-Berti, F., & Harris, K. S. (1981). A temporal model of speech production. *Phonetica*, *38*(1-3), 9–20. doi:10.1159/000260011 PMID:7267724

Bogdashevsky, R., Vladimir, A., Vitaly, Y., George, B., & Harrison, S. (1999). *Speech signal processing for determining psychological or physiological characteristics using a knowledge base*. Google Patents.

Bourlard, H. A., & Morgan, N. (2012). *Connectionist speech recognition: a hybrid approach*. Springer Science & Business Media.

Brandstein, M., & Ward, D. (2013). *Microphone arrays: signal processing techniques and applications*. Springer Science & Business Media.

Crouse, M. S., Nowak, R. D., & Baraniuk, R. G. (1998). Wavelet-based statistical signal processing using hidden Markov models. *IEEE Transactions on Signal Processing*, *46*(4), 886–902. doi:10.1109/78.668544

Deller, J. R. Jr, Proakis, J. G., & Hansen, J. H. (1993). *Discrete time processing of speech signals*. Prentice Hall PTR.

Flanagan, J. L. (2013). *Speech analysis synthesis and perception*. Springer Science & Business Media.

Furui, S. (1981). Cepstral analysis technique for automatic speaker verification. *IEEE Transactions on Acoustics, Speech, and Signal Processing*, *29*(2), 254–272. doi:10.1109/TASSP.1981.1163530

Galas, T., & Rodet, X. (1991). Generalized functional approximation for source-filter system modeling. *Second European Conference on Speech Communication and Technology.*

Gannot, S., Burshtein, D., & Weinstein, E. (2001). Signal enhancement using beamforming and nonstationarity with applications to speech. *IEEE Transactions on Signal Processing*, *49*(8), 1614–1626. doi:10.1109/78.934132

Gay, S. L., & Benesty, J. (2012). *Acoustic signal processing for telecommunication*. Springer Science & Business Media.

Ghoraani, B., & Krishnan, S. (2011). Time–frequency matrix feature extraction and classification of environmental audio signals. *IEEE Transactions on Audio, Speech, and Language Processing*, *19*(7), 2197–2209. doi:10.1109/TASL.2011.2118753

Guenther, F. H. (1994). A neural network model of speech acquisition and motor equivalent speech production. *Biological Cybernetics*, *72*(1), 43–53. doi:10.1007/BF00206237 PMID:7880914

Hagoort, P., Brown, C. M., & Osterhout, L. (1999). The neurocognition of syntactic processing. In The neurocognition of language. Oxford University Press.

Harrington, J. (2010). *Phonetic analysis of speech corpora*. John Wiley & Sons.

Hazan & Baker. (2011). Acoustic-phonetic characteristics of speech produced with communicative intent to counter adverse listening conditions. *The Journal of the Acoustical Society of America, 130*(4), 2139-2152.

Heckmann, M., Domont, X., Joublin, F., & Goerick, C. (2011). A hierarchical framework for spectro-temporal feature extraction. *Speech Communication*, *53*(5), 736–752. doi:10.1016/j.specom.2010.08.006

Hermansky, H. (1990). Perceptual linear predictive (PLP) analysis of speech. *The Journal of the Acoustical Society of America, 87*(4), 1738-1752.

Hiroya, S., & Honda, M. (2004). Estimation of articulatory movements from speech acoustics using an HMM-based speech production model. *IEEE Transactions on Speech and Audio Processing*, *12*(2), 175–185. doi:10.1109/TSA.2003.822636

Hossan, A., Memon, S., & Greggory, M. A. (2010). A novel approach for MFCC feature extraction. In *Signal Processing and Communication Systems (ICSPCS), 2010 4th International Conference on*. IEEE. 10.1109/ICSPCS.2010.5709752

Huang, X., Acero, A., & Hon, H.W. (2001). *Spoken language processing: A guide to theory, algorithm, and system development*. Prentice Hall PTR.

Huang, X. D., Ariki, Y., & Jack, M. (1990). *Hidden Markov models for speech recognition*. New York: Columbia University Press.

Hwang, J.-N., & Hu, Y. H. (2001). *Handbook of neural network signal processing*. CRC Press.

Isshiki, N. (1989). Physiology of speech production. In Phonosurgery. Springer.

Jelinek, F. (1976). Continuous speech recognition by statistical methods. *Proceedings of the IEEE, 64*(4), 532–556. doi:10.1109/PROC.1976.10159

Juang, B.-H., & Rahim, M. G. (1996). Signal bias removal by maximum likelihood estimation for robust telephone speech recognition. *IEEE Transactions on Speech and Audio Processing, 4*(1), 19. doi:10.1109/TSA.1996.481449

Junqua, J.-C. (1996). The influence of acoustics on speech production: A noise-induced stress phenomenon known as the Lombard reflex. *Speech Communication, 20*(1-2), 13–22. doi:10.1016/S0167-6393(96)00041-6

Leung, H., & Haykin, S. (1991). The complex backpropagation algorithm. *IEEE Transactions on Signal Processing, 39*(9), 2101–2104. doi:10.1109/78.134446

Li, Q., & Huang, Y. (2010). Robust speaker identification using an auditory-based feature. In *Acoustics Speech and Signal Processing (ICASSP), 2010 IEEE International Conference on*. IEEE. 10.1109/ICASSP.2010.5495589

Liu, Y., Zhang, P., & Hain, T. (2014). Using neural network front-ends on far field multiple microphones based speech recognition. In *Acoustics, Speech and Signal Processing (ICASSP), 2014 IEEE International Conference on*. IEEE. 10.1109/ICASSP.2014.6854663

Mermelstein, P. (1973). Articulatory model for the study of speech production. *The Journal of the Acoustical Society of America, 53*(4), 1070-1082.

Miller, N. (2013). Measuring up to speech intelligibility. *International Journal of Language & Communication Disorders, 48*(6), 601–612. doi:10.1111/1460-6984.12061 PMID:24119170

Moghimi, S., Kushki, A., Guerguerian, A. M., & Chau, T. (2013). A review of EEG-based brain-computer interfaces as access pathways for individuals with severe disabilities. *Assistive Technology, 25*(2), 99–110. doi:10.1080/10400435.2012.723298 PMID:23923692

Murty, K. S. R., & Yegnanarayana, B. (2006). Combining evidence from residual phase and MFCC features for speaker recognition. *IEEE Signal Processing Letters, 13*(1), 52–55. doi:10.1109/LSP.2005.860538

Nair, A. P., Krishnan, S., & Saquib, Z. (2016). MFCC based noise reduction in ASR using Kalman filtering. In *Advances in Signal Processing (CASP), Conference on*. IEEE. 10.1109/CASP.2016.7746218

Pickett, J. M. (1999). *The acoustics of speech communication: Fundamentals, speech perception theory, and technology*. Allyn & Bacon.

Podder, P., Khan, T. Z., Khan, M. H., & Rahman, M. M. (2014). Comparative performance analysis of hamming, hanning and blackman window. *International Journal of Computers and Applications*, *96*(18).

Povey, D., Burget, L., Agarwal, M., Akyazi, P., Feng, K., Ghoshal, A., … Thomas, S. (2010). Subspace Gaussian mixture models for speech recognition. In *Acoustics Speech and Signal Processing (ICASSP), 2010 IEEE International Conference on*. IEEE.

Rabiner, L. R., & Juang, B.-H. (1993). *Fundamentals of speech recognition*. PTR Prentice Hall.

Rabiner & Juang. (1986). An introduction to hidden Markov models. *IEEE ASSP Magazine, 3*(1), 4-16.

Reynolds, D. A. (1995). Speaker identification and verification using Gaussian mixture speaker models. *Speech Communication*, *17*(1-2), 91–108. doi:10.1016/0167-6393(95)00009-D

Reynolds, D. A., Quatieri, T. F., & Dunn, R. B. (2000). Speaker verification using adapted Gaussian mixture models. *Digital Signal Processing*, *10*(1-3), 19–41. doi:10.1006/dspr.1999.0361

Schultz, T., Wand, M., Hueber, T., & Brumberg, J. S. (2017). Biosignal-based spoken communication: A survey. *IEEE/ACM Transactions on Audio, Speech, and Language Processing*, *25*(12), 2257–2271.

Schwartz, R., Chow, Y., Kimball, O., & Makhoul, J. (1985). Context-dependent modeling for acoustic-phonetic recognition of continuous speech. In *Acoustics, Speech, and Signal Processing, IEEE International Conference on ICASSP'85*. IEEE. 10.1109/ICASSP.1985.1168283

Sohn, J. (1999). A statistical model-based voice activity detection. *IEEE Signal Processing Letters*, *6*(1), 1–3. doi:10.1109/97.736233

Soliman, S. S., & Hsue, S.-Z. (1992). Signal classification using statistical moments. *IEEE Transactions on Communications*, *40*(5), 908–916. doi:10.1109/26.141456

Spencer, L. E. (1988). Speech characteristics of male-to-female transsexuals: A perceptual and acoustic study. *Folia Phoniatrica et Logopaedica*, *40*(1), 31–42. doi:10.1159/000265881 PMID:3384379

Stowell, D., Giannoulis, D., Benetos, E., Lagrange, M., & Plumbey, M. (2015). Detection and classification of acoustic scenes and events. *IEEE Transactions on Multimedia*, *17*(10), 1733–1746. doi:10.1109/TMM.2015.2428998

Sussman, J. E., & Tjaden, K. (2012). Perceptual measures of speech from individuals with Parkinson's disease and multiple sclerosis: Intelligibility and beyond. *Journal of Speech, Language, and Hearing Research*, *55*(4), 1208–1219. doi:10.1044/1092-4388(2011/11-0048) PMID:22232396

Uvanesh, K. (2015). *Linear and non-linear classification of EMG signals for probable applications in designing control system for assistive aids*. Academic Press.

Uvanesh, K., Nayak, S.K., Champaty, S., Thakur, G., Mohapatra, B., Tibarewala, D.N., & Pal, K. (2016). Development of a Surface EMG-Based Control System for Controlling Assistive Devices: A Study on Robotic Vehicle. *Classification and Clustering in Biomedical Signal Processing*, 335.

Veaux, C., Yamagishi, J., & King, S. (2012). Using HMM-based speech synthesis to reconstruct the voice of individuals with degenerative speech disorders. *Thirteenth Annual Conference of the International Speech Communication Association.*

Wang, Y., Ding, N., Ahmar, N., Xiang, J., Poeppel, D., & Simon, J. Z. (2011). Sensitivity to temporal modulation rate and spectral bandwidth in the human auditory system: MEG evidence. *Journal of Neurophysiology*, *107*(8), 2033–2041. doi:10.1152/jn.00310.2011 PMID:21975451

Weismer, G. & Kim, Y. (2010). Classification and taxonomy of motor speech disorders: What are the issues. *Speech motor control: New developments in basic and applied research*, 229-241.

Zhou, X., Garcia-Romero, D., Duraiswami, R., Espy-Wilson, C., & Shamma, S. (2011). Linear versus mel frequency cepstral coefficients for speaker recognition. In *Automatic Speech Recognition and Understanding (ASRU), 2011 IEEE Workshop on*. IEEE. 10.1109/ASRU.2011.6163888

ADDITIONAL READING

Ali, H., Tran, S. N., Benetos, E., & d'Avila Garcez, A. S. (2018). Speaker recognition with hybrid features from a deep belief network. *Neural Computing & Applications*, *29*(6), 13–19. doi:10.100700521-016-2501-7

Mitra, V., Sivaraman, G., Nam, H., Espy-Wilson, C., Saltzman, E., & Tiede, M. (2017). Hybrid convolutional neural networks for articulatory and acoustic information based speech recognition. *Speech Communication*, *89*, 103–112. doi:10.1016/j.specom.2017.03.003

Noda, K., Yamaguchi, Y., Nakadai, K., Okuno, H. G., & Ogata, T. (2015). Audio-visual speech recognition using deep learning. *Applied Intelligence*, *42*(4), 722–737. doi:10.100710489-014-0629-7

Rigoll, G., & Neukirchen, C. (1997). A new approach to hybrid HMM/ANN speech recognition using mutual information neural networks. *Advances in Neural Information Processing Systems.*

Trentin, E., & Gori, M. (2001). A survey of hybrid ANN/HMM models for automatic speech recognition. *Neurocomputing*, *37*(1-4), 91–126. doi:10.1016/S0925-2312(00)00308-8

Uvanesh, K., …. (2016). Classification of Surface Electromyogram Signals Acquired from the Forearm of a Healthy Volunteer. Classification and Clustering in Biomedical Signal Processing, IGI Global: 315-333.

Chapter 3
An Ambient Multi-Agent System for Healthcare Monitoring of Patients With Chronic Diseases

Imane Boussebough
Constantine 2 University, Algeria

Issam Eddine Chaib
Constantine 2 University, Algeria

Billel Boudjit
Paris 13 University, France

ABSTRACT

Chronic diseases are a major cause of death in the world. Thus, many guidelines have been proposed to prevent these diseases. In addition, various systems have been developed to ease health monitoring. However, they are generally behaving as reminders or as anomaly detection systems. After giving an overview of the existed solutions and discussing their drawbacks, the authors present their system which is called ambient healthcare monitoring system (AHMS). It provides a continuous, unobtrusive, and mobile health monitoring of patients with chronic diseases. It is based on the multi-agent paradigm that allows devices to be distributed and autonomous. In addition, it benefits from the characteristics of ambient intelligence (AmI) such as ubiquity and context-awareness. So, AHMS is a promising solution for unobtrusive healthcare monitoring, in which it offers efficient medical services, with less energy consumption, that can significantly reduce the healthcare cost by automating some routine tasks. Consequently, it reduces the latency as well it minimizes the overload on the caregiver.

DOI: 10.4018/978-1-5225-7071-4.ch003

INTRODUCTION

Chronic diseases are among the most widespread diseases in the world. According to the World Health Organization (WHO) (World Health Organization, 2017), in 2015 an estimated 1.6 million deaths were directly caused by diabetes and 17.7 million people died from cardiovascular diseases (CVDs). Thus, healthcare organisations provide various guidelines and recommendations to help patients to deal with these chronic diseases. They recommend respecting diet, controlling vital signs, taking medications and doing physical activities to treat chronic diseases. But, these guidelines limit the patients' lifestyle where a patient should frequently measure his/her physiological parameters and he/she should often visit his/her doctor.

During the past decade, technology had been moving gradually towards Ambient Intelligence (AmI) environments aiming to help inhabitants in everyday life (Hristoskova, Sakkalis, & Zacharioudakis, 2014). AmI tries to adapt the technology to the peoples' needs using omnipresent computing elements, which communicate amongst them in a ubiquitous way (Tapia, Abraham, Corchado, & S.Alonso, 2009). In particular, AmI systems can considerably enhance the healthcare domain (Acampora, Cook, Rashidi, & V.Vasilakos, 2013). Due to the fact that health monitoring of patients within a controlled environment (e.g. hospitals) will disturb them, researchers have proposed to monitor the patients within smart environments, which use AmI technologies. However, previous work has only focused on facilitating the vital sign measuring task, detecting any occurred abnormal situation, and helping caregivers to make suitable decisions. So, these systems can be viewed as reminders (e.g. they remind the patient when the time of taking a drug has arrived) or as anomaly detection systems (e.g. they alert caregivers when a patient is on a critical health situation) or as decision support systems (e.g. they provide to doctors clinical analyses and documentation that assist them to make decisions).

Although the previous solutions are interesting, they don't have mechanisms to apply treatments, in which these systems need for a direct intervention of caregivers. Moreover, patients in critical health situation need for an immediate intervention, where any unnecessary delay can cause the death of the patient. In this purpose, the authors present a multi-agent system named *Ambient Healthcare Monitoring System (AHMS)*, which allows patients to control their health everywhere, at any time, and in an unobtrusive manner without limiting their lifestyle. So, the patient doesn't need to measure his/her vital sign regularly. Instead, the system measures them in a transparent manner using wearable sensors. Also, AHMS helps doctors to remotely monitor the patients' health in real-time by providing a detailed medical information about them. Besides, it uses the guidelines of caregivers (which are saved on the knowledge base) to make instantaneous decisions. These decisions will be directly applied by actuator devices (i.e. it don't need a physical intervention of caregivers). Especially in emergency situations where a delay is not accepted.

The remainder of this chapter is organised as follows: Section 2 presents an overview of the existing systems for health monitoring. Section 3 describes the proposed system, by presenting its objectives, its general architecture, and describes its various agents. An experimental scenario is presented in Section 4, to deepen the understanding of the AHMS operation. Finally, a conclusion and some future works are mentioned in Section 5.

RELATED WORK

In the literature, there are several context-aware systems designed for healthcare monitoring, such as *Ubiquitous Context-aware Healthcare Service System (UCHS)* and *Context-Aware Middleware for Pervasive Homecare (CAMPH)*.

UCHS (Lo, Chen, Cheng, & Kung, 2011) is a decision support system that uses micro sensors to sense user's life vital signal. It is composed of four services, which provide relevant medicine recommendations to its user. It is built upon an integrated service platform, where it uses a semantic network to infer the medical experts and to analyse the influence of the proposed therapy.

CAMPH (Pung, et al., 2009) is a middleware that offers several services are: P2P-based context query processing, context reasoning for activity recognition and context-aware service management. It can be used to develop or deploy home-care services such as patient monitoring, location-based emergency response, and anomalous activity detection. CAMPH provides a continuing-care to elderly with the collaborative interactions of multiple physical spaces (i.e. person, home, office and clinic).

The work in (Kartakis S, 2012) presents the implementation of a smart environment, which uses AmI technologies in a typical hospital room to assist both patients and medical staff. Besides, an oriented interface for clinicians allows vital sign monitoring and access to critical information when they are face to face with a patient.

Additionally, *Philips Healthcare* develops various commercial products for clinical decision support, such as *Philips IntelliVue* (Philips Healthcare, n.d.), and *ProtocolWatch* (Philips Healthcare, n.d.).

Philips IntelliVue (Philips Healthcare, n.d.) offers a unique view of patient's information at his bedside. It incorporates innovations aimed at increasing the utility and value of patient monitor information at the bedside and central station. It gives clinicians immensely powerful tools for real-time clinical analysis by providing context, highlighting patterns, and, for the first time, making deviations instantly recognisable.

ProtocolWatch (Philips Healthcare, n.d.) simplifies the implementation of evidence-based care protocols and sepsis care. It is continually checking monitoring data to provide clarity when it matters most. Whenever criteria for sepsis are met, ProtocolWatch prompts clinicians for tests, observations, or interventions indicated by the care protocol. It also produces a log that can be printed for documentation and quality improvement.

A fundamental problem with much of the previous systems regarding our proposed system is that these systems are not transparent nor pervasive, where it may limit the patient's lifestyle. Moreover, these systems give just medical recommendations to patients without applying any treatment. Thus, add more overload to caregivers that should always make a direct intervention, which might be unhelpful especially in emergency cases.

After discussing the main advantages and shortcomings of the existed systems, we present in the next section the proposed solution to face these drawbacks.

AMBIENT HEALTHCARE MONITORING SYSTEM

Ambient Healthcare Monitoring System (AHMS) is a multi-agent system aimed to transparently and continuously monitor the health of patients with chronic diseases, namely diabetes, hypertension and cardiovascular diseases. Basically, AHMS is responsible for:

- Measuring patient's physiological parameters in real time.
- Taking the appropriate decision according to the current health of patients.
- Allowing doctor to remotely monitor the patients and to get access to their medical data.
- Alerting caregivers (i.e. doctors, family members and ambulance) when a dangerous or critical situation has occurred.
- Applying suitable treatments in an unobtrusive manner using biomedical actuators.
- Offering the longest possible lifetime by reducing battery consumption.

The next subsections will detail the architecture of the system and its components.

General Architecture

In this subsection, the authors describe the general architecture of the proposed system. As illustrated in Figure 1, AHMS is divided into three layers that made it more scalable and consume less battery.

First, health monitoring in ambient environment needs mobile devices to continuously obtain the current context of the patient. Therefore, AHMS has a "*Sensors-actuators layer*", which contains sensors responsible for obtaining physiological data, and actuators charged to inject medications. For instance, the glucometer allows to measure patient's blood glucose, and the insulin pump allows to inject insulin.

However, these devices have a limit resources capacity especially the battery capacity, where communications over long distances consume quickly the devices' battery. Consequently, the authors add a second layer named "*Gateway layer*", which contains relay nodes, such as smartphones, tablets and computers, responsible for collecting physiological data of patients. This layer allows AHMS to respect one of the main requirements of mobility, which is called *Multi-hop wireless communication* mechanism (Karl & Willig, 2005).

Finally, a third layer called "*Processing, storage and communication layer*" is added, which uses a rule-based model that provides a high degree of formality and allows to model and analyse context. In this layer, the *processing unit* analyses and interprets the measured data using deductive rules and infers the knowledge base to obtain suitable decisions; the *storage unit* stores patient's medical data and facilitate a concurrent multiple access of many caregivers; and the *communication unit* allows to send automatic notifications to family members and ambulance using email or SMS in case of critical situations.

In order to monitor patients' health in ambient environments, any proposed systems should use communication technologies that support a low energy consumption, a good transmission rate, a coverage range of few meters and an extensive use in the industrial world. Consequently, the authors choose the following technologies depending on the type of network as follows:

- **In BAN (Body Area Network):** AHMS use *Bluetooth* technology to communicate ambient devices with the gateway. Because it offers a reasonable transmission rate with an average energy consumption and it is integrated into most commercial devices (such as smartphones and biomedical sensors).
- **In PAN/LAN (Personal Area Network/Local Area Network):** the authors prefer the *Wi-Fi* technology to access into LAN and WAN networks. This choice is based on the fact that Wi-Fi technology has a wide range with a very high transmission rate. Although this technology has a very high-energy consumption rate, the batteries used in these networks have an acceptable lifetime and can be recharged easily.

Figure 1. AHMS architecture

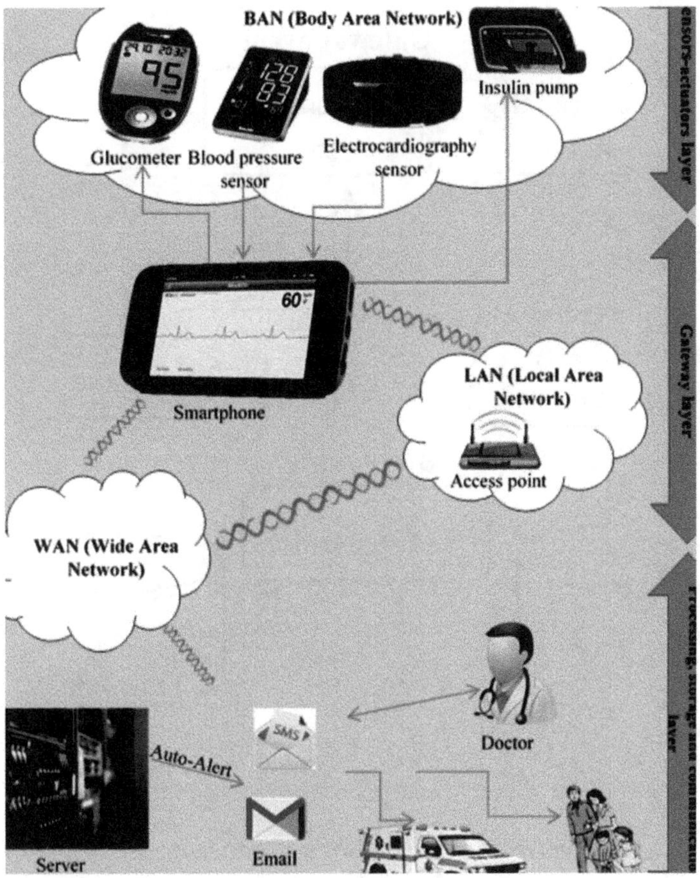

- **In WAN (Wide Area Network):** the authors choose the Wi-Fi and cellular technologies to send decisions, notifications and alerts to users (i.e. patient, doctor, family members and ambulance).

The next section will give more details about the different components of the proposed system.

Detailed Architecture

As mentioned before, AHMS is based on the Multi-agent paradigm, in which it is composed of various agents as follows: *ambient agents, gateway agent, server agent, and doctor agen*t. These agents coordinate between them in order to achieve the objectives of the system as well as possible and to ensure its correct operation, as illustrated in Figure 2.

Ambient Agents

We distinguish two types of ambient agents: *sensor agents* and *actuator agents*. The formers are reactive agents that obtain the physiological parameters of the patient, which are measured by sensors' devices. These agents allow the system to remotely monitor patients' health in transparent, unobtrusive and

Figure 2. The detailed architecture of AHMS

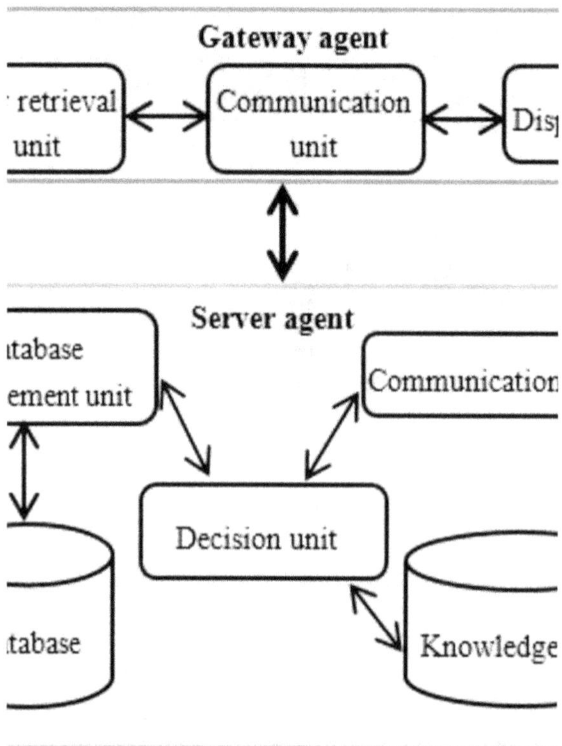

mobile manner. Besides, to perceive current context, sensor agents use a smart technique named *idle listening*, in which devices switch from active state to sleeping state in order to avoid overhearing and increase the energy performance.

The following algorithm summarises the function of the sensor agent:

```
While (true) do
If (a demand of physiological parameters is received or the time of regular
sending is reached) then
1. Obtain measured data from sensors' devices using the acquisition unit.
2. Convert it to a digital value using the analog/digital converter.
3. Send the numerical value to the gateway agent.
4. Put on hold.
End if
End while
```

On the other hand, actuator agents are also reactive agents which apply the necessary treatment by injecting medications using actuators' devices. They also use the idle listening technique, when waiting for a requested action. In addition, the actuator agents allow the system to apply decisions without additional delay and in a transparent way (i.e. without the need for a human intervention).

The following algorithm summarises the function of the sensor agent:

```
While (true) do
If (an injection request is received or the time of regular injection is
reached) then
1. Obtain the medication type and dose using the communication unit.
2. Inject this dose using the corresponding actuator's device.
3. Put on hold.
End if
End while
```

Gateway Agent

It is a reactive agent, which functions in a smartphone, a PDA, a tablet, or a computer. It allows (i) collecting the data measured through sensor agents; (ii) sending these data to the server agent; (iii) sending decisions to actuator agents. This agent represents the interface between patient and server.

The following algorithm summarises the function of the gateway agent:

```
While (true) do
If (any value of a physiological parameter is missed) then
1. Send a demand to the corresponding sensors using the data Recovery unit.
2. Put on hold.
Else
1. Send the values to the Server Agent using the communication unit.
2. Put on hold.
End if
If (new decisions are received) then
3. Send the decisions to actuator agents using the communication unit.
4. Display notifications or alerts, if they exist, using the display unit.
5. Put on hold.
End if
End while
```

Server Agent

It is a cognitive agent, which analyses physiological data sent by the gateway agent and accordingly responds by decisions after inferring the knowledge base using a forward chaining mechanism. The knowledge base contains guidelines for caregivers represented in a formal way as follows: "*if conditions then actions*". Depending on current patient's health, the deductive rules allow deducing suitable actions, which could be a treatment to be performed by actuator agents or a request for data to be measured through sensor agents.

In addition, the server agent can send automatic notifications or alerts, in case of danger or emergency, to doctor, family members and ambulance. It also contains a database that stores patient's medical file and samples history, thus making the decisions take into consideration not only the current measured data values but also previously measured values, personal habits (smoking, physical activities, etc.), current diet, among others.

Briefly, the server agent is decomposed into three different units are *database management unit, communication unit* and *decision-making unit*. It allows to accelerate the decision process and reduce its complexity. The following algorithm summarises the function of the server agent:

```
While (true) do
If (new physiological data values are received from gateway) then
1. Retrieve these values using the communication unit.
2. Get the patient's medical file and samples history using the database man-
agement unit.
3. Infer the knowledge base to determine the suitable decisions (i.e. the
treatments to be applied and notifications or alerts to be sent).
4. Send these treatments to the gateway agent using the communication unit.
5. Send notifications or alerts to the doctor, family members and ambulance
using the communication unit.
6. Store the new physiological data values in the database data using the da-
tabase management unit.
7. Put on hold.
End if
End while
```

Doctor Agent

It is a reactive agent which allows the doctor to create, consult, modify or delete a patient's medical file. Also, it permits to monitor the patient's health remotely, to consult the patient's physiological measurement history, to change the treatment to be used by the patient and to display the received notifications or alerts.

The following algorithm summarises the function of the server agent when interacting with the doctor agent:

```
While (true) do
If (a database access request is received from a doctor) then
1. Retrieve the request using the communication unit.
2. Selecting, modifying or deleting data from patient's medical file, using
the database management unit.
3. Send the retrieved data to the communication unit, in case of a select re-
quest.
4. Put on hold.
End if
End while
```

IMPLEMENTATION AND DISCUSSION

In order to test the good operation of AHMS, the authors use JADE (Java Agent DEvelopment framework) to implement this multi-agent system, then they test it on distinct case scenarios.

For instance, in this section, an experimental scenario of a patient with both *type one diabetes* and *hypertension* is presented. In this scenario, the measured blood glucose value is equal to *1.15 g / l* and the blood pressure value is equal to *90/140 mmHg*, in which in such situation, the patient needs an immediate injection of medications.

As was mentioned before, AHMS use a knowledge base to deduce the suitable actions to be applied by actuator agents. Therefore, the authors implement it using *SWI-Prolog* environment, which is based on *Prolog* language that provides a high level of formality and a multi-threading reasoning process. Figure 3 illustrates an overview of the deductive rules to be inferred in this scenario.

In contrast to the existed solutions in the literature that deal with such scenario by just alerting the patient to take his/her medicament, AHMS inject automatically the medicament in an unobtrusive way using the insulin pump. As well, it alerts the caregivers to ensure that the patient's health had been stable. Figure 4 demonstrates that AHMS has made good decisions and apply the suitable actions without disturbing the patient.

These considerable results had been achieved owing to the scalable architecture of AHMS that adapt to patient's current context (e.g. communication medium availability, gateway capacity). Besides, using knowledge base, database, and multi-unit reasoning agent allow to make decisions in real-time without the need for the physical intervention of caregivers or patients, especially in common situations.

Figure 3. An overview of the knowledge base

```
iventionnelle').
irs monotherapie').


; type 1'); complication('Diabetes

:y('Diabetes'), personalHistory('h
 , PAD>=80.

ise('diabetic hypertension')),valu
iot(personalHistory('coronary insu
 , current_treatment('hypertension

:('hyperglycemia'), complication('
ise('hyperglycemia to alarm'), com
 treatment('Diabetes', 'insulin t
```

Figure 4. The experimental scenario that clarifies AHMS function

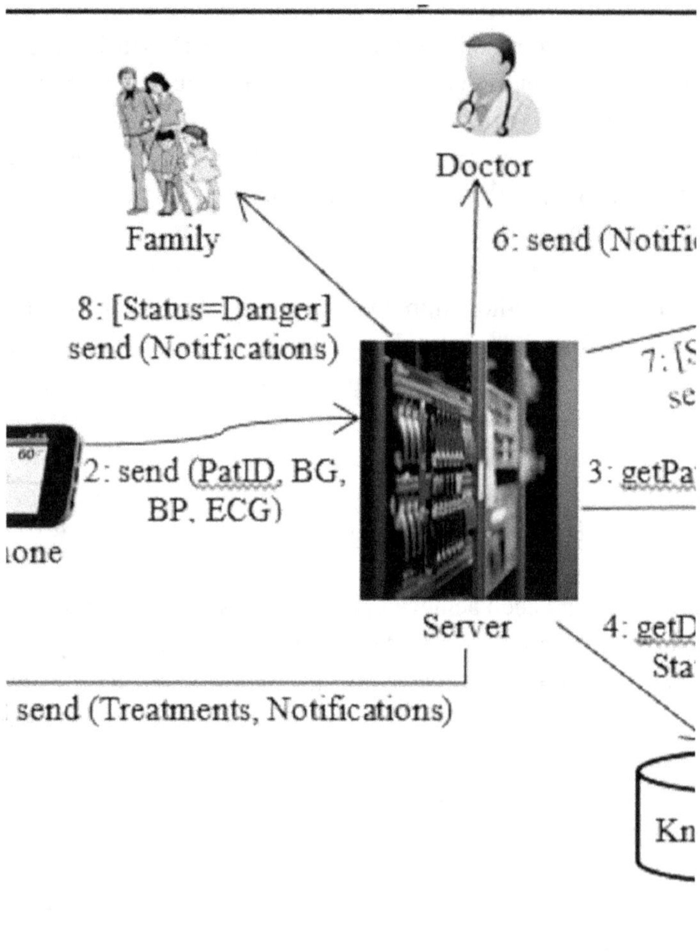

CONCLUSION

In this chapter, the authors present a multi-agent system that can monitor patients at any time. The system consists of sensor agents that measure physiological parameters, actuator agents that inject adequate doses of medicaments, gateway agent playing the role of an intermediary between ambient agents and server agent. The latter contains a decision-making unit responsible for determining, according to the patient's health, the treatment and the persons to be contacted.

By realising AHMS, we want to offer a continuous health monitoring and to minimise the overload on caregivers. Indeed, the use of actuators allows automating the task of injecting medicaments and reduce the delay time between the detection of the anomaly and the applying of treatments.

Essentially, AHMS has confirmed that AmI can efficiently improve the care and life quality of patients with chronic diseases and can offer an easy way for healthcare monitoring at hospitals, medical centres and homes. However, AHMS should face other challenges of ambient environments, namely security and privacy issue.

REFERENCES

Acampora, G., Cook, D. J., Rashidi, P., & Vasilakos, V., A. (2013). A Survey on Ambient Intelligence in Health Care. *Proc IEEE Inst Electr Electron Eng.*

Hristoskova, A., Sakkalis, V., & Zacharioudakis, G. (2014). *Ontology-driven monitoring of patient's vital signs enabling personalized medical detection and alert.* Personalized Medical Detection.

Karl, H., & Willig, A. (2005). *Protocols and architectures for Wireless Sensor Networks.* John Wiley & Sons Ltd. doi:10.1002/0470095121

Kartakis, S. S. V. (2012). *Enhancing Health Care Delivery through Ambient Intelligence Applications.* Academic Press.

Lo, C., Chen, C., Cheng, D., & Kung, H. (2011). Ubiquitous healthcare service system with context-awareness capability: Design and implementation. *Expert Systems with Applications, 38*(4), 4416–4436. doi:10.1016/j.eswa.2010.09.111

Philips Healthcare. (2013). *Neonatal Event Review.* Retrieved from http://www.healthcare.philips.com/main/products/patient_monitoring/

Philips Healthcare. (n.d.a). *Protocol Watch Project.* Retrieved 11 05, 2013, from http://www.healthcare.philips.com/main/products/patient_monitoring/products/protocol_watch/

Philips Healthcare. (n.d.b). *Screen Trends.* Retrieved 08 10, 2015, from http://www.healthcare.philips.com/main/products/patient_monitoring/products/screentrends/index.wpd

Pung, H., Gu, T., Xue, W., Palmes, P., Zhu, J., Ng, W., & Chung, N. (2009). *Context-aware middleware for pervasive elderly home care. IEEE J. Sel. Areas Commun.*

Tapia, D. I., Abraham, A., Corchado, J. M., & Alonso, R. (2009). *Agents and ambient intelligence: case studies.* Academic Press.

World Health Organization. (2017). *Media centre: Facet sheets.* Retrieved 11 25, 2017, from World Health Organization (WHO): http://www.who.int/mediacentre/factsheets/en/

Chapter 4
Healthcare Big Data:
A Comprehensive Overview

Pijush Kanti Dutta Pramanik
National Institute of Technology Durgapur, India

Saurabh Pal
Bengal Institute of Technology, India

Moutan Mukhopadhyay
Bengal Institute of Technology, India

ABSTRACT

Big data has unlocked a new opening in healthcare. Thanks to the considerable benefits and opportunities, it has attracted the momentous attention of all the stakeholders in the healthcare industry. This chapter aims to provide an overall but thorough understanding of healthcare big data. The chapter covers the 10 'V's of healthcare big data as well as different healthcare data analytics including predictive and prescriptive analytics. The obvious advantages of implementing big data technologies in healthcare are meticulously described. The application areas and a good number of practical use cases are also discussed. Handling big data always remains a big challenge. The chapter identifies all the possible challenges in realizing the benefits of healthcare big data. The chapter also presents a brief survey of the tools and platforms, architectures, and commercial infrastructures for healthcare big data.

1. INTRODUCTION

Healthcare industry is going through a trailblazing makeover. Due to the significant advancement in digitised and open and pervasive healthcare systems, it is generating a massive amount of data. This healthcare data is truly comparable to the Big Data both in size and nature, hence termed as healthcare Big Data. Though compared to other industries, the healthcare industry has been lagging behind in the adoption of Big Data technologies, the changed medical and clinical landscape has forced the stakeholders to delve into the development quickly. Suddenly, Big Data has become crucial for almost every operational, clinical, and management task (Bresnick, 2017). The healthcare people are now convinced

DOI: 10.4018/978-1-5225-7071-4.ch004

of the benefits of Big Data and persuading themselves to analyse the data for extracting new insights that have given them the access to promising new threads of knowledge which are being transformed into innovative and purposeful actions (Groves et al., 2013).

Several healthcare use cases are well-suited for incorporating Big Data technologies. The healthcare Big Data analytics has opened up many exciting avenues in different healthcare operations including diagnosis and medical care, clinical decision support, population health management etc. (Bresnick, 2017). The success of healthcare Big Data is mostly dependent on the efficient collection and storage of massive quantities of disparate data acquired from diverse sources and also running it through an in-depth analysis (McDonald, 2017). The effective utilization of healthcare Big Data and obtained knowledge through analytical processes has the potential to save a significant amount of money and most importantly, people's lives (Lebied, 2017).

This chapter provides a preliminary and overall understanding of healthcare Big Data. The rest of the chapter is organised as follows. Section 2 discusses the 'big' aspect of the healthcare data including the ten 'V's of healthcare Big Data. It also covers the basics of healthcare Big Data analytics as well as the present healthcare Big Data market. Section 3 identifies several advantages of Big Data in healthcare. Section 4 mentions some application areas while Section 5 lists some specific examples of healthcare Big Data. The associated challenges are discussed in Section 6. Section 7 provides a brief survey of the different platforms and tools, architectures, and practical infrastructure for healthcare Big Data. Section 8 concludes the chapter.

2. BIG HEALTH DATA

2.1. The Data Overload

Back in 2012, a study estimated that healthcare data boast the largest share (30%) in occupying the overall electronic data storage in the world (Brown, 2015). To make the things graver, healthcare data is growing at a rapid pace, in fact seriously rapid. Among the growing digital universe healthcare is one of the fastest growing sectors. A report from the EMC Corporation along with the research firm IDC suggests that the digital healthcare data is growing at 48% per year whereas the growth rate of the overall digital universe 40% per year for the (IDC, 2014). The report estimates that the size of healthcare data will swell to 2,314 Exabytes by 2020 from a figure of 153 Exabytes in 2013 with an annual growth rate of 48%. The report elaborates that if all the digital healthcare data are stored on a stack of tablet computers, the height of the tower, by the year 2020, would cross 82,000 miles scaling from 5,500 miles in 2013 (Leventhal, 2014). The above statistics are sufficient to get a picture of the growth rate of the healthcare data and if this rate is continued, the healthcare data volume will soon reach the zettabyte and yottabyte scale.

2.2. The 'V's of Healthcare Big Data

2.2.1. Volume

The term 'Big' in healthcare Big Data itself certifying that volume of created and accumulated healthcare data is huge. Over the years, it is expected to grow even further. Clinical notes and trial data, lab results, personal medical records, claims data, FDA submissions, medical device data, human genetics and population data, genomics, radiology images, 3D imaging, and biometric sensor readings are the primary information productive contributors in the exponential growth of healthcare data (Bresnick, 2017) (Raghupathi & Raghupathi, 2014).

2.2.2. Velocity

The healthcare data can be generated either by humans or sensors (Crapo, 2017). Traditional healthcare management systems are typically populated by the human-generated (entered by people) data. In that case, the rate at which the data flows into the system can be manageable. But widespread use of IoT and smart medical devices has led to the generation of real-time health data. Newly accumulated data come in constant and rapid flow which makes collecting and storing really challenging. Also, because of real-time health applications, the unified healthcare system's response time is very crucial. Though trying to react to every health data stream may cause the inefficient and uneconomical use of resources. So, it is important to decide which data require immediate action and which can be deferred.

2.2.3. Variety

Healthcare data come from various sources and, hence, in diverse shapes (e.g. structured, unstructured and semi-structured) formats (e.g. plain text, blobs of text, pictures, video, medical image, etc.) and sizes. Data captured at different estranged locations are typically incompatible because of different data structure and semantics. This requires the development of specialized data structures, communication protocols, and storage systems (Crapo, 2017).

2.2.4. Veracity

Veracity represents the quality of the data. Here, data quality includes integrated, trustworthiness, complete, and bias and noise free. Maintaining these qualities in health data is a serious challenge because of the diversity of sources and channels. Obviously, veracity is, probably, the most sensitive issue among the all 'V's in healthcare Big Data.

2.2.5. Validity

Validity represents the accuracy and correctness of data. The validity of data is also measured by how up to date it is and whether it is generated through standard scientific protocols and methods (Bresnick, 2017).

2.2.6. Viability

From the ocean of healthcare data, it is important to identify the relevant data for each use case (Bresnick, 2017). Relevancy of data is required to maintain for achieving desired and accurate outcome through analytical and predictive measures.

2.2.7. Volatility

As mentioned above, the healthcare data are generated and being changed at a rapid rate. Hence, they tend to live short. But the question is how short? How quickly does the data change? It is important to determine how long the data is relevant, how long to store it and the data of which time period should be considered for analysis (Bresnick, 2017).

2.2.8. Vulnerability

It need not be mentioned explicitly that the privacy and security are of utmost importance for healthcare data especially as data are stored in the cloud and travels to different data junctions (for details, refer Section 6).

2.2.9. Visualization

Healthcare data not only need to be correct and accurate, they have to be presented unambiguously, and attractively to the user. Large and complex clinical reports need to be presented in a way that is meaningful and less time-consuming to understand. Proper visualisation helps in finding valuable insights as it reflects the details in an expressive and usable way.

2.2.10. Value

The ultimate purpose of healthcare Big Data analysis is to gain value in the form of better health services. Better governance, better analytics, and smarter decision making are the core factors for creating maximum value out of healthcare data (Bresnick, 2017). For healthcare organisations, Big Data brings value by shifting profit pools towards the right direction by reducing overall cost.

2.3. Healthcare Big Data vs. Healthcare Smart Data

The healthcare Big Data is basically the data which contains the patient's electronic health records (EHRs) and other related medical information. The objective of this is to provide healthcare services based on the past records. Application of analytics and data science on Big Data gives an opportunity to find the rightful insight. Data analytics instead of trying to combine all the available data, target the right data and thus gives the physician the rightful insights. But still, the gap exists between what is demanded and what is stored in Big Data. But it is not necessary that a voluminous data may always reveal the information which is exactly asked for. Similarly, merely Big Data may not provide valuable and precise insights to the physician.

On the other hand, smart data are data which gives rightful information as per the context. It allows physicians to make smart choices like coordinating the treatment of a patient suffering from multiple illnesses, able to diagnose the diseases better and getting a complete picture of the patient based on the family history. For a particular patient's ailment, based on symptoms smart data accurately advices the right medication and predict any future complications. Smart data is the meaningful data that is extracted from the healthcare Big Data based on the type of data, its volume, and validity. (Bresnick, 2016).

Inferring smart data from Big Data need proper planning and implementation. The focus is what the organization need after Big Data is applied to the system. Based on the system requirement it is wise to enrich the Big Data with the appropriate type of valid data in quality and volume. For example, scanning endless PDF, X-rays of fractures, and blood test data would not necessarily help a physician in diagnosing a patient with stomach ailment or why someone is reacting negatively to a certain medication. To have smart data, the Big Data should be enriched with appropriate and correlated data. It is important to understand that what is being collected is what is being delivered (Bresnick, 2016) (Leventhal, 2014).

2.4. Healthcare Big Data Analytics

Healthcare Big Data analytics is expected to change the face of healthcare. The healthcare sector has been a bit hesitant to embrace the Big Data scenario quickly (TF7 Healthcare subgroup, 2016). With most of the healthcare services now slowly coming to Big Data, a whole new paradigm of services that can be provided to patients can be opened.

Till now the whole treatment and caring of the patient are done by the hospital, but with the advent of Big Data, the treatment has become much easier and more focused (Raghupathi & Raghupathi, 2014). Furthermore, the Big Data analytics will significantly bring down the cost of clinical treatment, administration, medication, etc. The healthcare Big Data will enable the physicians, by providing proper insights, to understand where the attention is needed at any given point of time and take care of the patient accordingly.

The healthcare Big Data, if used properly, has the potential to become the guiding force for the physicians to improve the existing healthcare facilities. It will also help to gain more insight into the health of local population so that the suitable health services can be rendered to them (Crapo, 2017).

2.4.1. Descriptive Analytics

In the descriptive analysis, the various events that have occurred in the past are described. Data mining is performed on the aggregated data to get the details about the event that has happened in the past. The descriptive analysis, in a nutshell, can be summarised by a simple question as "What has happened?" (TF7 Healthcare subgroup, 2016).

Descriptive analytics in healthcare provides insight into the origin and the reason for spreading diseases and how long the quarantine periods might need. It can also shed light on which medicines failed and which combination of drugs succeeded? It can also identify the unhealthy lifestyle that leads to the disease and also the measures taken for its cure.

2.4.2. Diagnostic Analytics

Diagnostic analysis is an analytic technique that uses the descriptive analytics details to identify the reason for an event i.e. it tries to identify the various causes due to which a certain event happened in the past. In a nutshell, diagnostic analytics can be said to ask a simple question "Why did it happen?" (TF7 Healthcare subgroup, 2016).

Diagnostic analytics in healthcare can provide insights into the causes of various disease outbreaks, administrative and patient treatment malpractices, etc. It is also helpful in identifying the reasons - why certain diseases remain dormant and when do they become active i.e. conditions required for the pathogens to germinate. Diagnostic analysis deals with finding out the reason behind an event in the past using techniques of data mining, correlation, and data discovery.

2.4.3. Predictive Analytics

Predictive analytics is an advanced analytics technique which uses data mining, machine learning, artificial intelligence, and statistical modelling to predict future events. Predictive analytics in healthcare empower us to follow the saying "prevention is better than cure" in the true sense.

The predictive analytics in healthcare has a great scope as we can predict diseases that will afflict a person based on his/her habits, genetic makeup or history, or based upon the work environment or home environment (Lebied, 2017). This type of analysis can play its role in a larger scale by helping us in judging the health of the population in the future thus allowing us to take proper precautionary measures. Predictive analytics, if used properly, can prevent many future patients from being in a hospital.

2.4.4. Prescriptive Analytics

Prescriptive analytics deals with finding the best course of action for the predicted scenario derived from the predictive analysis. The prescriptive analysis extends the predictive analysis and descriptive analysis to find out what to do with a predicted event. Based on the available predictions, the predictive analysis provides the answer to the question "What should we do?" (TF7 Healthcare subgroup, 2016). It can suggest possible decision-making options that can lead to mitigating risks.

Prescriptive analytics in healthcare can completely change the face of modern healthcare where not only the diagnosis will be done very quickly but also the treatment will be based on the patients' medical history. This will lead to a better treatment in terms of medicine incompatibilities and side-effects.

2.5. The Healthcare Big Data Market

The healthcare industry has gained a massive business value during the last couple of years. Fuelled by the large-scale adoption of EHR by governments, hospitals, and physicians, it is expected to grow to US$18.7 Billion by 2020 ("Revolutionizing the Healthcare Industry with Big Data, Analytics and Visualization", 2015). Whereas the healthcare and medical analytics are expected to grow at a CAGR of 27.1% to reach US$24.55 Billion by 2021 from US$7.39 Billion in 2016 (marketsandmarkets.com, 2016). The whole healthcare market will be changed due to the transformation of the healthcare data from the normal data to the Big Data. Big Data allows for change of so many things in the health industry, for example, it provides better data storage facilities at a low cost and also allows one to work on the data at a low cost. The Health Big Data market is open to various possibilities such as using the analytics power of the Big Data by the pharmaceutical companies to give better drugs at cheaper costs, reducing the administrative loads on the physicians. The healthcare Big Data will allow organisations to meet the consumer demand for affordable medical care. One of the major contributions of the goodies of using Big Data technologies in healthcare is applied to the unprivileged countries/states where there are inadequate doctors and medical facilities.

3. THE BIG DATA ADVANTAGE IN HEALTHCARE

Digitization of data accumulated from patient records, prescriptions, medical imaging, laboratory, pharmacy and insurance results in an enormous amount of data that is known as healthcare Big Data. This enormous amount of data can lead to knowledge traces that would significantly improve the quality of medical and healthcare services. The Big Data analysis would infer meaningful insights that help in making informed decisions, disease surveillance, and other healthcare and medical services. Patients, physicians, healthcare organization, pharmaceutical companies, policymakers and other stakeholders will be suitably benefited from the knowledge inferred. The applications would be individual and people in mass health surveillance; predicting health issues of individuals like calculating the medical complication and risk associated with a patient, the disease advancement/progression of disease; analysis of the particular kind of treatment suitable for the person; analysis of current treatment strategies to detect whether the diagnosis and applied treatment are correct or not, and thus adjusting the treatment plan accordingly. It may inform the patient about their current and future health state which allows them to make better-informed decision. The projection of Big Data application into the current medical and health service is advantageous in scaling the quality and accountability of health services, some of the advantages are discussed below (Raghupathi & Raghupathi, 2014).

3.1. Reducing Healthcare Cost

Today's healthcare system is a disease centred model where based on the symptoms of disease and lab reports, physicians reccomend the treatment procedure. The treatment procedure is quite centred on clinical expertise and medical evidence, further based on treatment results, other alternative treatment options are suggested. The treatment procedures are recursive, time-consuming and costly. Healthcare Big Data with the enormous amount of data on medical cases, treatment patterns, medicines and their effectiveness, genetic data allows for a patient-centred model of treatment. This information allows analysing and diagnosing the patient correctly and further predicting the correct treatment pattern. In another application, Big Data in genetics ensures personalized profiling and hence personalized medicine for patient allowing accurate treatment. Healthcare Big Data infer knowledge do actually reconcile the redundant costly treatment procedure (Srinivasan & Arunasalam, 2013).

3.2. Reducing Hospital Readmissions

The probability of patient returning back within a month after treatment at the hospital are getting high. This incurs cost and resource to hospital. Big Data analytics applied to the patient medical record, history, chart information, and the patient lifestyle record can identify the patients who are at risk of having medical complications and again readmission. Thus, identifying the patients who need additional care would able to reduce the hospital readmissions ("Seven Big Data Examples That Have Improved Healthcare Operations", 2016).

3.3. Optimized Workforce

Hospitals and other health organizations critically face the classical problem of recruiting staffs and scheduling them. For many staff recruited, there will be a risk of under usage of resources while minimizing the numbers can lead to poor customer services. This problem can be overcome by the application of Big Data. Big Data obtain data from various sources can well predict the number of patients that would come on the daily and hourly basis. Further, hospital admission record analysis over a time series of years can get the future trend on the type and number of patient that would be admitted to the hospital. The application of data science for crunching the raw data delivers information that would allow the organization to optimize its workforce based on the future requirements (Lebied, 2017).

3.4. Real-Time Alerting

One of the biggest functional advantages of Big Data is real-time alerting. Big Data incorporated into services in hospital and clinics would analyse the medical records of patients and thereby in real-time provides advice to a physician for prescriptive decision. Further patient's medical and health data collected by wearable devices (Pramanik et al., 2019) are being analysed in the cloud in association to Big Data to feed real-time information of patient current medical issues, future medical ailment, and preventive measures. The patients' data being collected over time would allow the doctors to see the health status of people in society and thereby taking corrective strategy for any deviation observed. The real-time data is also shared by the health organization to react immediately to any disturbing results found in patient monitoring (Lebied, 2017).

3.5. Analysing Electronic Health Records (EHRs)

Analysing the enormous electronic health record would make a physician comprehend the treatment trends, their effects, and side effects. Moreover, the Big Data allows the updated patient data to be shared among doctors for their treatments and, also, medical cases are exchanged among doctors thus reducing duplicate test and redundant treatment procedure ("7 Big Data Use Cases for Healthcare", 2016).

3.6. Analysing Hospital Networks

Analysing hospital care and management data would be useful in administrating critical medical condition case, strategies for reducing postoperative infection and analysing the medicine (antibiotics) and treatment procedure carried out by doctors which found ineffective in a cure. ("7 Big Data Use Cases for Healthcare", 2016)

3.7. Control Data for Public Health Research

Medical and health organizations, hospitals and small clinics produce huge medical data. This is overwhelming data for medical professionals. As most of the data are raw, unstructured and cluttered, probably these data in their direct form are difficult for medical professional and policymakers to suitably use in public health regulations and decision making. There is a gap between what health professionals want and to what data exists. These data without the application of Big Data is of no use. Application of data analytics can regularize and standardize the public health data, filling the existing gap and thus providing information that can be applied in various regulation and research work for providing better care and health services ("7 Big Data Use Cases for Healthcare", 2016).

3.8. More Efficient Medical Practice

Big Data helps in providing effective treatment for the patient. Big Data analytics gives knowledge about the diseases, their symptoms, treatment pattern, and medicine effectiveness in different stages of illness to the physician that would help them for better-informed healthcare practice while treating a patient.

3.9. Using Health Data for Informed Strategic Planning

On the outbreak of diseases or growth in chronic disease rate among the population, Big Data on public health records like immunizations, distribution, and availability of medical services enables to design strategies for public health. Big Data map the required services over a region in comparison to the available services and thus inferring what necessary steps need to be taken for controlling the public health issues (Eastwood, 2013).

3.10 Optimizing Workflows in Healthcare

Hospitals have multiple departments, limited patient admission capacity, limited doctors and staff with varying schedule and varying flow of incoming patients with different need and treatment make healthcare services in the hospital very dynamic. The patient's health issues span multiple factors like involving treatment from different departments and different physicians at different stages of treatment, laboratory tests, and medication. Further, there are cases of medical complication for inappropriate diagnosis and treatment and hospital readmissions. This volatile state demands completely planned and managed workflow ready for an emergency and changing situations. Healthcare data enriched by multiple sources of data such as real-time patient data (patient health status, location etc.), medical records of patients, nursing information, laboratory data and machine status (available, working etc.) helps to identify the current operational state of hospital and thus allow to take informed decision for better healthcare services by best utilization of resources ("TF7 Healthcare subgroup", 2016).

3.11. Better Safety Practices

The patients who underwent surgery are often suspected of postoperative infections. Big Data analytics of electronic medical record can well inform in previous the susceptibility of patients for getting an infection. This ensures preventive measures like intensive postoperative care, pre- and post-operation preventive medication etc. This predictive analysis promotes better patient safety ("Seven Big Data Examples That Have Improved Healthcare Operations", 2016).

3.12. Patient Engagement

Today's one of the healthcare challenges is patient's engagement leading to patient's awareness, retention and proactive care. A huge spending is done on the healthcare segment though even after that, patients are never properly taken care of resulting in bigger health problems. Patients engagement are found in getting insights, communication, personal wellness tracking, medical management, new disease diagnosis, personal history, immunization, health cost planning, social services research and clinical trial participation etc. Patients want to be engaged so that they are aware, engaged and feel confident (Shah, 2016). This further improves patients' satisfaction and experience leading to the better outcome. Patient interactions with physicians, hospital and clinic staff, pharmacy and pharmaceutical company, laboratory and other counselling staff increases one's engagement. Controlled and updated data about the patient helps the service provider to attune the services to patient's need, helping patients to be more engaged in managing their health issues. To realize the situation Big Data has contributed to a bigger extent. Using Big Data insight, healthcare providers can identify the individuals with critical illness or need support in terms of insurance, medical counselling, care and managing their medical cases. These people are informed regularly. Patients are delivered with a personalized message or called. The personalized messages make people aware of their individual journey as a patient. Utilising Big Data technologies, when the patient makes contact with the clinic or hospital for healthcare service, the physician or the hospital staff may already be aware of patient's history, communication preference and their healthcare journey (Disch, 2016).

3.13. Big Data Is Helping to Prevent Unnecessary ER Visits

Many often patients frequently visit multiple hospitals and clinics for the same or different ailment or disease which causes repetitive treatment procedure, discontinuity in treatment and in the worst case, a wrong treatment that leads to critical health jeopardy and wastage of money and time. In this direction, the application of Big Data would help the patient in reducing unnecessary visits to medical and health agencies, further make sure the treatment is on the right course. Big Data allows the updated medical record of patient to be shared in emergency department so that when patient shifts between hospitals/ clinics or take a new treatment for ailment, the staff will have the knowledge of patient's medical history, treatment procedures carried out, drug administered and the reports of various lab test that are already done. This definitely eases the patient diagnosis, reducing patient overhead and increasing satisfaction (Lebied, 2017).

4. APPLICATIONS OF HEALTHCARE BIG DATA

4.1. Battling the Flu

Flu is an epidemic which may outbreak at any moment of time with potential to spread across in a short period of time. Every year around the world Flu takes millions of lives. Centres for Disease Control and Prevention (CDC), an operating component of the Department of Health and Human Services in the USA is fighting against disease and their control and prevention. The CDC receives 700,000 reports of patients with Flu-like symptoms every week. Doctors, hospitals, and laboratories send a large amount of data to CDC. The reports include the where and what kind of treatment was given by the physician. Big Data analytics has been tremendously useful to get scientific insight from the data stored over time. CDC has made the information public through FluView, an application developed and deployed at CDC (Nambiar et al., 2013). FluView reports in real time how the influenza is spreading across, along to that how vaccines and antivirals can aid patients etc. It gives doctors the answers they need to effectively battle the outbreak, such as knowing which vaccine is effective to which virus strains and whether or not antiviral drugs will be effective in recovery.

Other similar applications where Big Data have been used to capture and analyse the data on the pandemic are FluNearYou[1] and GermTracker[2]. FluNearYou asks the person to input data on their symptoms; based on the symptoms the application generates a map that can allow users to prepare themselves and take preventive measures against infection. GermTracker takes the data from social media posts and analyses them for the disease outbreak. The huge data obtained thus gives a view of a pandemic which doctors might have missed.

4.2. Diabetes and Big Data

Diabetes has become a major health problem in the world. Most of the people are diagnosed with type2 diabetes, a condition where the body cannot use insulin effectively. In these cases, Insulin injections are administered to patients to control sugar level in blood. Diabetes can be controlled by monitoring the patient's sugar levels regularly and further administrating insulin based on the situation.

In managing diabetes and the betterment of patient health, Common sensing has pioneered smart insulin pen cap technology called GoCap[3]. GoCap is a data-driven smart cap that fits over the injection needle of a standard insulin pen and measures the volume of insulin in the pen. GoCap records the time, amount and kind of insulin in the logbook and further sends the data through the Internet to mobile devices of doctors and family members. The information is also displayed and recorded in the mobile device application. The GoCap mobile application helps the patients to enter information about their food intake and glucose levels at the different time of day. These accumulated data on patients helps the doctors to provide personalized treatment to patients.

4.3. Fight Cancer

Big Data on cancer treatment is an accumulation of data collected from cancer patients at different stages of treatment like pre-detection, pre-treatment and end stage. These data can effectively be used in cancer prediction for new cases. Using the historical data of patients, the predictive machine learning algorithm can well identify cancer. Flatironhealth has developed an Oncology cloud service called OncoCloud (Flatiron, 2017) which aims to gather data during diagnosis and treatment and further make it available to the researcher for their advanced study. Another example of Big Data in cancer treatment programme is the Cancer Moonshot Programme (Orcutt, 2016). Cancer is triggered by genetic changes and often genome information is required for therapeutic treatment. In this direction, Big Data as a huge data repository provides enough information about human genomics, patients case reports and their background details. The valuable insight which can be obtained from these data would help to identify the genetic changes which had trigger cancer in a patient and the treatment procedure. Big Data which consist of millions of readable and usable samples would allow scientist all over the world to analyse and work on the data. For widespread and new trends of treatment, sharing of data is essential so that the medical researcher can use a large amount of data on treatment plans and recovery of cancer patients.

4.4. Improved Diagnosis and Treatment

In the healthcare industry, Big Data plays a pivotal role. The application of Big Data includes analysis of the disease pattern and predicts outbreaks. Furthermore, it allows public health monitoring and tracking epidemic and helps doctors and medical health policymakers to prevent future outbreaks. Big Data allows the doctor to keep an efficient record of patient's medical history and thereby enable doctors to provide proper healthcare service for their patients. Further, the data insight allows doctors to carry diagnosis and treatment of patient located remotely connected to the Internet. The patient can contact doctors and get the advice within a minute. The enablement of IoT helps to monitor patient and raise real-time alerts. Big Data helps both sick and healthy patients to connect doctors for improved health and treatment.

4.5. Tackling Opioid Abuse

Opioid abuse is often described as a new "epidemic" in the world. More than 15000 patients die every year on painkiller drug medication and several thousand are killed for the drug overdose or wrong usage. Pain medication is a tricky area for physicians; depending on individual person's capacity doctors prohibit prescribing the opioid use above a certain threshold. Ignoring the prescribed medication and their dosages, patients misuse the drug intakes and often uses them wrongly to what is called as drug abuse. The responsibility of reducing and preventing the drug abuse is split between the patient himself and the healthcare system. In America, to stop this, monitoring programs have started. This includes maintaining a centralized database with data analytics and decision-making system which detect prescription abnormalities, track drug dispensing patterns and preventing the patient from taking dangerous amounts of opioid. Electronic Prescription for Controlled Substances (EPCS) (HealtIT.gov, 2016) - a standard practice which has helped to reduce the opioid epidemic by enabling the practitioners to prescribe medicine electronically which can be shared and monitored everywhere.

4.6. Precision Medicine

The EHR is a major source of Big Data, the EHR contains sociodemographic, medical, and genetics treatment details which allows scientists and clinicians to predict more accurately for a patient's ailment and further reasons for precision medicine. The precision medicine model allows appropriate therapeutic and preventive approaches based on patients' genetic makeup, lifestyle, and environmental factors that work effectively for an individual.

Doctors are often misled in case of instantaneous diagnosis (for emergency) and symptomatic treatments. Applying data science and analytics over Big Data, precise information based on the patient context can be obtained. This information would serve in making precise prescriptive decisions.

4.7. Evidence-Based Medicine

Around the world, evidence-based medicine (EBM) is a standard way of medication. Clinical trial on diseases or ailment treatment methods includes rigorous experiments on patients and involves risk. It is often difficult to generalize the clinical trial methods testing and often the positive test result on a small group of people may not work on the outside world.

Big Data helps in EBM to sort out and identify the effective clinical methods applied to real patients. By data mining over practice-based clinical data of actual patients, it is easy to find out which patient has gone under what treatment, how well the treatment has done or has it any side effects. The data can then be analysed at an individual level to create a patient data model, which can be aggregated across the population to infer wider insights into disease prevalence, treatment pattern etc. Clinicians match the symptoms to a larger patient database and identify the accurate disease in a faster and efficient way (Marr, 2016).

4.8. Genomic Analytics

Researchers are getting a fascinating new perspective on human genome due to advancements made in Big Data analytics. Since genes are all about information, Big Data is a perfect fit for genetics. Researchers are able to look more closely at human genes and they are applying Big Data analytics in this issue. A typical human genome contains more than 20,000 genes, simply mapping a genome requires 100 gigabytes of data. Sequencing multiple genomes and tracking gene interactions, multiples the number by many times. Much of the work done with the human genome and Big Data analytics deals closely with health and medicine. One of the pioneering application of genetics and Big Data is creating personalized medicine and new drugs. One's gene analysis could help in finding the inheritable traits that can be passed to the next generation. This is specifically important for people who are susceptible to passing disease like diabetes, anaemia, heart disease, cancer, obesity etc to their child. Big Data analytics helps the researcher in understanding the human genome and they can get a view of future diseases.

4.9. Clinical Operations

Big Data accumulating a large amount of clinical data from various sources can assist staff in clinical operations. It helps in enhancing the operation of healthcare facilities, the quality of clinical trial and research. Clinicians can do the comparative studies on different patient cases in the different area of treatments. Big Data has changed the mindset of researchers from hypothesis-based treatment to the research-based analysis on a large amount of data resulting in accurate treatment method.

4.10. Patient Monitoring

The wide adoption of EHR in hospitals and clinics has enriched Big Data. Big Data provides a deep Clinical knowledge and understanding of disease and illness. For patient monitoring, various sensors are used to screen for patient's vital statistic like blood pressure, heartbeat, respiratory, oxygen in the blood, and sugar level etc. Any change in the data pattern is analysed along with Big Data and further alerts are raised for preventative measures. Big Data having patient's past medical knowledge, analyses the current statistics to predict the future medical complication and ailments.

4.11. Medical Device and Pharma Supply-Chain Management

Proper functioning of hospitals and clinics availability medical devices and pharmaceutical supplies are proper in quantity is of utmost importance. Many hospitals are not implementing the appropriate supply chain strategies, this cost to hospitals in terms of poor quality services. Nonstandard ordering methods and unnecessary product may cause stockpiling similarly also may cause in supply deficiency. The supply chain is not only about the product but also about the people who buy, move and use them.

Implementing Big Data analytics and automation tool makes supply chain management much easier. Automation allows clinicians to spend more time delivering high-quality care and less time to find for products availability. Technology like RFID (radio frequency identification) has been used for tracking products. The stocking products are fitted with a scannable tag which can provide information about items, manufacturing date, expiry date and shipping date, which allows providers to track the object throughout its life cycle. Predicting the number and type of patient and the supplies required allows maintaining the stock at its optimum level. For the stock, level decreases automatic stock ordering is done (Castle & Szymanski, 2008) (Uzsoy, 2005).

4.12. Drug Discovery and Development Analysis

Drug discovery requires and processing and analysing of unstructured and structured biomedical data obtained from various surveys and experiments. This includes data regarding gene sequencing, protein interaction data, drug data, electronic patient records and clinical trials, self-reporting data etc. These data collected in a huge amount from various sources over time has enriched the medical information base. The pharmaceutical company, while designing a new drug or applying clinical trial, applies analytics to these data to infer knowledge and to build a predictive model for new drug design. This usage of past data has made the drug discovery and development faster in comparison to the traditional method (Jawadekar, 2016).

4.13. Big Data for Personalised Healthcare

There is a rapid advancement in genomic technologies. With large sources of data, it is easier for healthcare professionals to understand the disease mechanisms which leads to better treatment of patients. Many diseases have preventable risk factors. A clear understanding of disease characteristics helps in personalized healthcare and thus reduces the chances of getting the disease. Healthcare professional takes patient's history, do the physical examination and laboratory testing to identify the risk of disease in future. The application of Big Data in this direction makes the process fast and easy. Analytic on patient's health and medical profile gives a personalized medical view which is specific to a patient. The personalized profile for treatment is derived not only from the particular patient's electronic medical report but also from other similar types of patients' case records. Personalized healthcare enables disease risk profiling, disease management plans and wellness plan for an individual patient.

4.14. Infection Prevention, Prediction, and Control

According to the European Centre for disease prevention & control, every year estimated 100,000 patients are infected with hospital-acquired infection (HAI). It is estimated that around 37,000 people died with direct consequences of infections per year. The World Health Organization (WHO) has strict guidelines which can minimize the risk of spreading infections. Some guidelines are easy to follow and some are hard to implement due to limited technology. In this direction, Big Data technology integrates genomics with epidemiology data in order to not just control but also to prevent as well as envisage the possibility of the spread of infections within hospitals and clinics ("TF7 Healthcare subgroup", 2016).

4.15. Health Insurance Fraud Detection

Healthcare fraud is a big problem all over the world. Over the last decade, the healthcare industry had spent billions of dollars on improper claims. More than 1.5 million people have been victimized. These statistics represent avoidable healthcare cost. Healthcare industry is applying analytical controls throughout the treatment process and also incorporating the claims review process. Review process incorporates rule-based data analytics and predictive modelling. The treatment procedure carried and the medicine administrated over the patient is analysed for similar symptom cases to find out whether the treatment and drug used are legitimate as per the context or vague one ("Seven Big Data Examples That Have Improved Healthcare Operations", 2016).

5. USE CASE EXAMPLES

5.1. Asthmapolis

Asthmapolis has launched a GPS enabled tracker called propeller that records the usage of asthma medicine by asthmatics. It helps the medical practitioner to treat asthma more effectively. Propeller[4] uses Bluetooth sensors-based inhaler, mobile application, and advanced analytics. The sensor records information that when and where the patient suffered from an asthma attack and used the inhaler. The information is transferred to a centralized database to be combined with the information at the Center for Disease Control. The combined information identifies the trends and catalyst of asthma attacks in individuals and aggregating the pattern with mass population. This leading information would help the physician to identify when the risk of an asthma attack is higher, and further help them in personalized treatment for asthma patients.

5.2. 23andMe

23andMe[5] is a privately-held personal genomics and biotechnology company. The company is named for 23 pairs of the chromosome in a normal human cell. It is saliva-based direct to consumer genetic testing business. 23andMe extract the genome information from the person saliva for delivering back to the customer. The company has built a huge genetic information bank. The aggregated customer data are available for research team employed by 23andMe and other scientific groups for inherited disorders and other diseases. 23andMe provides raw genetic data which in its original form are not meaningful in different genetic studies. Promethease a personalized online tool for health genetic information processes the raw data from 23andMe and provides personal DNA report (Ramsey, 2015).

5.3. USC Medical Monitor

Parkinson's disease is affecting millions of people today. By 2030 it will be doubled. Since this disease affects a patient's movement, it is important to monitor the patient's mobility condition. In the University of Southern California, computer scientists are teamed up with neurologists, kinesiologist & public health experts to fight against Parkinson's disease (Nambiar et al., 2013). They use different types of devices to monitor patient's movement throughout the day and gather a large amount of data about patient's abnormal movements through 3D sensors, mobile devices and from wearable sensors. The acquired patient data is fitted into algorithms which analyses the kind of changes in movements. The analysed data and reports are sent to researchers and caregivers. Depending on the motion abnormalities alert are sent to the caregiver, depending on which they prescribe appropriate medication and exercises (Nambiar et al., 2013).

5.4. GNS Healthcare and Aetna

Applying Big Data analytics, GNS Healthcare[6] in collaboration with Aetna[7], an insurance-based company aims to treat and prevent metabolic syndrome. The metabolic syndrome can increase the risk of heart disease, strokes and diabetes. GNS uses the claims and health information from Aetna, as a platform called - Reverse Engineering, Forward Simulation (REFS) to create data-driven models. GNS healthcare analyses the risk of getting metabolic syndrome depending on the five conditions i.e. increased waist size, high blood pressure, high triglyceride level, HDL cholesterol and high blood sugar. GNS analysed the data of 37000 Aetna's customers who participated voluntarily in the screening program of metabolic syndrome (Nambiar et al., 2013). The analysed data includes claims, records, pharmacy claims, demographics, laboratory test, biometric screening. GNS & Aetna team uses two analytical models:

1. Claim based model
2. Both claim and biometric data based model

Both analytical models predicted future risk of metabolic syndrome in both population and individual (Nambiar et al., 2013).

5.5. WestMed Medical Group

In the WestMed medical group, as the medical practice growing day by day, the number of physicians grows from 16 to 250. The physicians are seeing 250,000 patients with annual revenue of $255 million ("7 Big Data Use Cases for Healthcare", 2016). Using Big Data, the medical practitioner is now capable of analysing more than 2,200 procedures. The Big Data has helped in streamlining the workflow, shifted clinical work from doctors to nurses, reduced unnecessary testing, and improved patient satisfaction.

5.6. HealthCore (WellPoint)

Healthcore[8] is a clinical outcome research subsidiary of Wellpoint Inc. Healthcore has a team of highly experienced researchers including physicians, pharmacists, epidemiologists, health economists and scientists. They measure safety, efficacy, and effectiveness, compliance of drug, medical devices, and care management interventions in the real-world settings ("Epidomiology and Genomics Research Program", 2018). The Healthcore uses data from different sources like health plan providers, patient's reported information, clinical information from physicians that allows the researchers to answer complex clinical, economic and health policy questions. HealthCore interprets health data and estimates the influence of disease, their treatment and care on the outcome.

5.7. Evolent Health

Evolent Health[9] (previously Valence Health) provides value-based care solutions for health sector like hospitals, health systems and physicians to help them to effectively manage patient populations. Based on each client requirements, customized value-based care model for clinically integrated networks, population health management, health plan administration & TPA, risk adjustment, pharmacy benefit management is designed, built and managed. To handle customer's enormous and heterogeneous data, Evolent Health has adopted Big Data technology. Evolent health has been using MapR for building data repository for storing huge data. MapR offers a distributed data platform to store and analyze Big Data in a distributed fashion which is linearly scalable which can be extended just by adding more machines and/or CPUs, without changing the application code. The MapR platform delivers enterprise-grade security, reliability & real-time performance which lowers both hardware and operational costs of most applications and data. Evolent consumes 3000 inbound data feeds with 45 different types of data. This data includes lab test result, patients' health records, prescriptions, pharmacy records and claims and payment records which are used to make decisions about improving healthcare outcomes & reimbursement. Prior to the MapR, the company takes 20 hours to 22 hours to process millions of data. But MapR cuts the time to 20 minutes, which also requires less hardware.

5.8. United Healthcare

United Healthcare[10] provides health benefits and services to millions of people. Their payment team has the tough task of ensuring the claims are paid correctly and on time and not paying for the fraudulent services. They shifted to a predictive modelling environment based on Hadoop which provides a flexible (seamless integration of new tools and technologies) and cost-effective platform with enterprise-grade features (e.g. high availability and disaster recovery). Bringing the information about claims, prescriptions, plan participants, contracted care providers and associated claim review outcomes to a single framework thus people at United Healthcare are able to identify inaccurate claims in a systematic and repeatable way ("UnitedHealthcare uses Hadoop to Detect Health Care Fraud, Waste and Abuse", 2018). With the help of the data integration from different data silo, it has become easier to find out the fraudulent. United Healthcare also started using NLP to better understand customer satisfaction by converting records of customer's voice (who calls to its call enter) into text and search the indications of customer's dissatisfaction.

5.9. OptumInsight

Optum Labs[11], a collaborative research and development initiative of the Optum Inc of United Health Group and the Mayo Clinic, is pursuing a variety of Big Data analytics projects aiming to improve patient care and costs reduction. It is combining electronic medical record from Mayo & other healthcare organization with claims data from United Healthcare to understand and provide better and more effective health care and also to analyze the total cost of care for specific procedures or diseases (Cambridge & Rochester, 2013).

5.10. Liaison Technologies

Liaison Technology[12] offers a cloud-based solution which provides organizations with the ability to integrate, manage and secure data across the enterprise. They are particularly active in the healthcare industry where a patient's record may be stored in many systems in different formats. The storage is updated in real-time as per the streaming data so that the user always gets the up-to-date view of the data in a single location and in a most suitable format (McDonald, 2017).

5.11. Novartis Genomics

Next Generation Sequencing[13] (NGS), a research initiative carried out at Genomics Institute of the Novartis Research Foundation, is a Big Data application that deals with a huge volume of heterogeneous data. The data includes genome information and other medical data. NGS requires heavy interaction with diverse data from external organizations for experimental and other associated data. The Novartis Genomics suffers from two problems, one integrating heterogeneous datasets and the other in integrating public datasets. To address the problem Big Data technologies like MapReduce and Apache Spark are being used by Novartis. As a result, the combined Spark & MapReduce based workflow and integration layer allow the company's life science researchers to meaningfully take advantage of thousands of experiments that different public organization have conducted (McDonald, 2017) and thus helped in accelerating drug research.

6. CHALLENGES

The major challenges of using the Big Data in healthcare is that health data is completely distributed i.e. one cannot find a complete repository of data related to a patient at one location and in a homogeneous form (Lebied, 2017). The above statement basically points out that we'll need new infrastructure so that data can collaborate together. We have to add other new technologies to the existing older ones like predictive analysis, machine learning and graph analytics (Lebied, 2017). Some important challenges in healthcare Big Data are discussed below.

6.1. Expertise

Whenever a new technology is introduced, expertise on that technology is not achieved overnight. We must understand that most of the hospital IT staffs are not trained to used Big Data. They are familiar with SQL programming. To resolve this knowledge gap quickly and cost-effectively Big Data must allow itself to be extremely user-friendly.

The whole scenario here is that if the expertise of the user is not in the current technology he/she will lose interest in it very quickly and the investment in the technology will be dead. To avoid such mishaps, we the organisations which convert to the Big Data architecture must use various tools which help in bridging the gap between the new technology and the old. The tools must allow for the usage of the languages know previously i.e. the architecture must have backward compatibility. Creating a correct balance of backward compatibility and the new architecture must be balanced for the results.

6.2. Costly Processing and Analysis

The most common challenge in any data processing architecture is that the cost of processing the data. The medical data which comes from various pathological tests itself comes at a huge cost due to the requirement of sophisticated equipment's required to conduct the test. Add to this cost the processing charges for the additional analysis of the data to diagnose a specific disease. To understand the cost and analysis of the medical data, we must come to terms that present-day medical diagnosis and the further prognosis are completely based on the symptoms shown by the patient. These symptoms can be the same for multiple diseases thus leading to a further increase in cost for the diagnosis of the disease. We can very well say that proper handling of the data and its analysis is a very big challenge.

6.3. Security & Privacy

The collection of health data and creating EHR is the way of digitalizing the health data. The major problem with digitalization is the security of the data as well as maintaining the privacy of the patient to whom the data belongs to. The analysis of healthcare data must be done with keeping in mind that under no circumstances the privacy and the personal information of the patient are known anyone including the system i.e. a level of privacy encryption must be imposed on the data that is to be analysed (Patil & Seshadri, 2014). The security architecture of the cloud (or where ever the data is stored) must prevent data breaches and even if breaches cannot be completely avoided try to make sure that data is not traceable to any patient to whom they belong.

6.4. Ransomware Threat

Ransomware is classified as programs that infect the victim's system and prevents the victim from using the system until the ransom is paid. Ransomware basically encrypts the user's files and data and withholds the key to decryption as ransom. Hospitals are particularly vulnerable to this type of attack as the security systems employed by them are not up to the mark thus making the hospitals and medical data repositories as soft targets for such attacks. One can easily understand this as hospitals need their data on a day-to-day basis as the patients' lives depend on the data generated. To process healthcare data, we must up the security from various sources from where the data is collected so that the main systems are not compromised by these attacks.

Ransomware threats can be further reduced by utilising proper antivirus software's as well as having strict monitoring of the data. Also, regular backups of data to places which are completely secure can help from prevention as well as recovery of the valuable data.

6.5. E-Mail Vulnerability in Healthcare

E-mail vulnerability emanates from the various ways in which an email can be used to install a malicious code in the system which in turn can lead to theft of data. As more and more health data are being digitalized, health institutions are falling prey to more and more email-based attacks like phishing, where the people working in those institutions are conned into activating the attack themselves. To remove or to fight against such vulnerabilities, we must follow a three-step approach which includes proactively monitoring the threats to the continuous management of security ("Email Vulnerability in Healthcare", 2017). Also, we must bank for the worst possibility that the data is siphoned off and go for rapid incident response and recovery.

6.6. Data Governance

Data governance is the practice of managing the data assets throughout the lifecycle of the asset so that it meets the organizational needs throughout its lifetime as well as maintains its integrity (Bresnick, 2016). Data governance is required for the health data because as we are digitalizing the data if it is not properly organized, updated and maintained then that data cannot be used for anything other record keeping. We must understand that data governance is important for analytics perspective. To find more from the data we need the data to be organized rather than just being electronic. Some possible solutions to this can be that healthcare institutions hire dedicated data entry operators in their company.

6.7. Data Management

As the digitalization of the healthcare data is done, the need to manage such data also grows. We can't implement traditional methods as our analysis model is based on Big Data architecture. We must manage the data in such a way so that the maximum amount of data is always available for processing. Below are the ways via which data can be managed ("TF7 Healthcare subgroup", 2016):

- **Data Quality:** The quality of data used for processing is important as if we feed low-quality data to the system the analysis of the data will not be worth the effort. We need to focus on data quality as it is the only raw material in the system which will be used to generate valuable results. For every data that is used we must be aware of how the data was collected, conditions under which the observations were made, and how the contents were processed and transformed. This enables reproducibility of experiments as well as the reliability of the data. The quality of the data can significantly influence the conclusion of the whole analysis.

- **Data Quantity:** The quantity of data used for analytics plays a very large role in the healthcare sector. We must understand that this sector is knowledge-intensive and requires data and analytics to improve its practices. The quantity of data used in the analysis, allows us to draw greater insights into the processes. Also, if the quantity of data is less, then the whole analysis can sometimes become questionable as lack of data may not provide proper authenticity to the analysis.
- **Multi-Modal Data:** The healthcare data as mentioned earlier comes from various sources. All these data have various formats used by their respective system. This data can be further classified into structured and unstructured data. The system should accept both the data and try to find synergy among it. This type of integration of data from all sources are helpful in finding new cures for diseases or finding the genomic point of view of disease i.e. can a disease be genetically transferred to the next generation or even if transferred will it remain dormant or not. These types of analysis require data from all the kinds of sources like ancestry of a person, family history of diseases, his/her habits as well as of their family's etc. thus we can say that multi-modal data integration and analysis plays a pivotal role in healthcare analysis.
- **Data Access:** All the analysis of the data and its inference is only possible when and only when access to data is provided. The biggest challenge of today is getting the data i.e. getting access to the data after bypassing the various privacy laws, security barriers etc. and to add hurt to the injury these laws vary from country to country. The health data is highly fragmented i.e. data is distributed among hospitals, pathologies or even specialists whom the patients contact. One of the possible solutions could be that we ask patients to willingly give their data to the analytic system so that all the red tape can be cut easily.
- **Patient-Generated Data:** The patient-generated data (PGD) refers to the data which is generated by the patient's devices and gives us an insight about the patient's habits and can also let us know about the diseases he/she is prone to or maybe suffering from. PGD also provides ways to monitor recently released patients from hospitals and continuously monitor their progress. The major challenge in PGD is that there are various types of devices, a present which is all not compatible with each other as there is no standardization about them. This causes problems and conflicts with the data that is generated.
- **Data Integration:** As it is already known that health data is heterogeneous, so before performing analytics on it we need to integrate the data from all the sources. The data integration in itself is a very big challenge as the data that is provided may be or may not be structurally compatible to each other i.e. they all may exhibit a level of structural heterogeneity if this remains the analysis can be incomplete or inconclusive. To solve this problem, we can use information extraction mechanisms in conjunction with machine learning and semantic web technologies which will help us to get homogeneously integrated data for analysis.

6.8. Fragmented Analytics

As the cost of centralized analytics systems is very high, the industries are now moving towards fragmented analytics model i.e. we analyse the heterogeneous data in fragments and then try to combine the analytics results (Bresnick, 2015). For the healthcare industry, it is assumed that it will not be successful to a very large extent as it is considered to fail at data integration and reporting of states. The Fragmented analytics model is a cheap way of implementing any data analytics system, thus a possible solution can be to maintain tables which show a correlation which previously exists among data and then use that table for data integration and reporting.

6.9. Choosing the Right Healthcare Big Data Analytics Tools

Till now we have seen the various challenges that plague the Big Data applications in healthcare. Adding further to that, we would like to elaborate on how choosing the right Big Data tool also a challenge. We must understand here that the tools must be chosen on the basis of use otherwise we'll end up increasing the cost of the whole architecture, and not even get the proper result. For example, suppose we want to use the Big Data architecture for clinical analysis and not for qualitative benchmarking (Bresnick, 2015). We must understand that the organisations must self-evaluate them and then order better tools which provide better optimisations and digestible reports (Bresnick, 2016).

7. HEALTHCARE BIG DATA IMPLEMENTATION ENVIRONMENTS

7.1. Platforms and Tools

Big Data is implemented in the healthcare domain using various tools. Below some tools and their uses are mentioned:

7.1.1. The Hadoop Distributed File System (HDFS)

The HDFS (Shvachko et al., 2010) is a cluster file system which is used to store structured and unstructured Big Data across multiple systems in a large-scale cluster (Sarkar, 2017). It allows Hadoop to process the massively-scaled volume of data in a fault-tolerant manner. HDFS is used in the healthcare system to collect and aggregate related data while maintaining the data security and privacy in an effectively better way compared to traditional storage systems (Raghupathi & Raghupathi, 2014) (Sarkar, 2017).

7.1.2. MapReduce

MapReduce[14] is a programming model for implementing, analysing and generating Big Data sets. The programming model is composed of the map and reduce methods. The map methods do filtering and data sorting whereas the reduce method summarizes the data. The MapReduce follows the divide-and-conquer approach i.e. it solves by reducing the problem into smaller sub-problems or the input data into independent chunks which are processed completely in parallel, and then the result is combined (Raghupathi & Raghupathi, 2014) (Sarkar, 2017). This algorithm provides a fault-tolerant and flexible way to analyse large data sets over distributed architecture. For large data sets like health data, the data is analysed over a distributed architecture and then the results are collected from different points of processing and combined.

7.1.3. Pig and PigLatin

Pig[15] is a data processing architecture built on top of Hadoop. Pig is designed for making Hadoop simpler to approach and use. The Pig tool can be used for easy and faster cleaning and analyses of big data sets. The pig execution has two modes the Local and Hadoop mode. The PigLatin is a script-based language to express data flow, data input and operation on data to produce the desired output (Hurwitz et al., 2013). The simple and easy to write PigLatin language is used to write programs that bring the structured, unstructured and semi-structured data to the fold which is used to convert and accommodate heterogeneous health data.

7.1.4. Hive

Apache Hive[16] is data warehouse software built over the top of Apache Hadoop. It facilitates data summarization, query writing and processing, and data analysis. Hive helps us easily write queries for getting the results. Hive is a support architecture which supports the structured query language (SQL). It allows the programmers to write queries similar to SQL thus allowing, people to use the Big Data architecture who are unfamiliar with it (Raghupathi & Raghupathi, 2014). Hive helps in maintaining the backward compatibility with the older systems, which worked on SQL, thus allowing for people trained SQL to directly work in the Big Data architecture.

7.1.5. Zookeeper

Apache Zookeeper[17] is a centralized service for distributed systems, it provides maintaining configuration information, registry naming, distributed synchronization and group services. Zookeeper allows synchronization across the resource cluster i.e. it maintains some control regarding which process should use which resource. It helps in parallel computing, by providing centralized resource management services (Raghupathi & Raghupathi, 2014).

7.1.6. HBase

HBase[18] is a Hadoop database which works on non-SQL approach and is easily able to hold all types of data. It is architecturally placed above the HDFS (Hadoop Distributed File System) (Raghupathi & Raghupathi, 2014). It helps in assimilating heterogeneous data and allows reading and writing, randomly in Big Data.

7.1.7. Cassandra

Cassandra[19] is a distributed database system which helps in handling large quantities of data spread across various utility servers (Raghupathi & Raghupathi, 2014). This database helps in health data analysis by allowing us to easily access the data stored on various servers.

7.1.8. Oozie

Oozie[20] is basically used to streamline workflow among tasks (Raghupathi & Raghupathi, 2014). It works by creating synchs among the various parties/processes involved in the system so that conflict does not occur and the workflow moves smoothly.

7.1.9. Mahout

Mahout[21] provides machine learning applications that are helpful in the predictive analysis of healthcare Big Data (Raghupathi & Raghupathi, 2014). It helps in creating applications such that they can learn from past data and able to correlate and analyse similar situations which give results faster, thus making the system more efficient.

7.1.10. Avro

Avro ("Apache Avro™ 1.8.2 Documentation", 2017) provides data serialization services (Raghupathi & Raghupathi, 2014). In healthcare industries, serialization of patients' medical history helps in diagnosing the disease he/she is suffering from or may suffer (observing some pre-symptoms).

7.1.11. Lucene

Apache Lucene[22] is one of the most widely used frameworks for information retrieval. It offers efficient text searching and analysis. It can be used to explore the EMR to satisfy patient-related queries. It can effectively be used in the diagnosis and analysing patient's reports (Raghupathi & Raghupathi, 2014). Also, Lucene can help in analysing the patient's handwriting which can determine his/her psychological state.

7.2. Architectures

7.2.1. Cloud Computing

Cloud architecture provides the most promising architecture for the health industry to switch over to the Big Data platform. Cloud allows the trouble-free and uncomplicated way to collect data in one place and then distribute it among its specialized facilities for further processing thus allowing for a secure way of processing and analysing the data (Pramanik et al., 2018). The cloud architecture provides a centralized data repository from which data is readily accessible for the Big Data analytics. The security of these structures is dependable; also, they allow the usage of the redundancy for reliability. The redundancy in the cloud architecture allows the system to have a protection against possible crashes.

7.2.2. In-Memory Computing

This is a fairly new architecture which provides real-time analysis (Mian et al., 2014). This architecture involves in-memory SQL databases. The basic advantage of in-memory computing is that it is much faster than the traditional systems as disk access time is removed from the equation. This type of architecture is suitable where real-time analysis of data is required (Pramanik & Choudhury, 2018). This architecture can be used even with non-SQL databases. The only drawback of it is that if the system crashes for any reason recovery is near impossible.

7.3. Infrastructure for Big Data in Healthcare

7.3.1. Cisco

Cisco major focus of research is IoT (Internet of Things). For such purpose, Cisco is also working on the processing architecture of IoT data called Fog (Cisco, 2015) (Pramanik et al. 2018). The major application of Fog and IoT is in the healthcare sector. The use of IoT has enabled the health industry, to create a right strategy to deliver the proper healthcare to the patients. Physicians are now able to use the clouds and all the computing powers to securely know about their patient's wellbeing as well as are able to diagnose the disease at an early stage even if the patient is at some distance away from them.

The mobility is the key here which allows the physicians, patients and the administration to be on the same page and provide the best medical care available to the patient.

7.3.2. Watson Health

Watson Health[23] is a complete package developed by IBM, which helps in all aspects of health. It has artificial intelligence as well as machine learning capabilities that help in providing effective diagnosis and medication of the diseases and reduces the job of the hospital staff and people in patient care. Watson can learn about the patient's medical history and is able to provide recommendations to the physician of all the possible new drugs or techniques available in the market, thus saving the time of the physicians to go through all the literature.

7.3.3. Philips HealthSuite

HealthSuite ("About HealthSuite", 2018) is an open cloud-based digital platform designed for the continuous health and personalized care of the user. The suite contains the power of analysing, sharing and orchestrating healthcare services. The analysis part utilizes the machine learning algorithms and various predictive analysis techniques. The sharing features are basically the interoperability of the platform form multiple devices. The orchestrating basically implement the workflow synch, communication like task etc. ("A Cloud-based Platform: Purpose-built for Healthcare", 2018).

8. CONCLUSION

Big Data has influenced almost all the industries in recent years. Healthcare is also no exception. In fact, the healthcare industry is the largest producer of the digital data. Big Data technologies have opened up new opportunities in healthcare. It not only has brought the advantages to the patients but also to the healthcare units and hospitals. To maximise the benefits, careful consideration should be given in adopting the right Big Data tools and the underlying architecture. Though Big Data technology has a significant impact on modern healthcare it needs to progress further to realise its fullest potential. The traditional healthcare system is still lacking in becoming accustomed to the 'big' change. Nevertheless, Big Data has set healthcare industry on the righteous trajectory of rapid transformation and that will surely bring startling benefits to the mankind.

REFERENCES

A Cloud-based Platform: Purpose-built for Healthcare. (2018). Retrieved July 24, 2017, from http://www.usa.philips.com/healthcare/innovation/about-health-suite

About HealthSuite. (2018). Retrieved April 29, 2018, from https://www.philips.co.in/healthcare/innovation/about-health-suite

Apache Avro™ 1.8.2 Documentation. (2017, August 2). Retrieved April 29, 2018, from https://avro.apache.org/docs/current/

7 . Big Data Use Cases for Healthcare. (2016, October 8). Retrieved July 24, 2017, from http://www.ingrammicroadvisor.com/data-center/7-big-data-use-cases-for-healthcare

Bresnick, J. (2015, September 18). *Healthcare Big Data Analytics Suffers from "Fragmented" Approach.* Retrieved May 26, 2017, from http://healthitanalytics.com/news/healthcare-big-data-analytics-suffers-from-fragmented-approach

Bresnick, J. (2015, January 13). *How to Select a Big Data Analytics, Business Intelligence Vendor.* Retrieved July 14, 2017, from https://healthitanalytics.com/news/how-to-select-a-big-data-analytics-business-intelligence-vendor

Bresnick, J. (2016a). *How to Choose the Right Healthcare Big Data Analytics Tools.* Retrieved July 14, 2017, from https://healthitanalytics.com/features/how-to-choose-the-right-healthcare-big-data-analytics-tools

Bresnick, J. (2016b). *The Difference Between Big Data and Smart Data in Healthcare.* Retrieved July 14, 2017, from https://healthitanalytics.com/features/the-difference-between-big-data-and-smart-data-in-healthcare

Bresnick, J. (2016c). *The Role of Healthcare Data Governance in Big Data Analytics.* Retrieved July 14, 2017, from https://healthitanalytics.com/features/the-role-of-healthcare-data-governance-in-big-data-analytics

Bresnick, J. (2017, June 5). *Understanding the Many V's of Healthcare Big Data Analytics.* Retrieved July 20, 2018, from Health IT Analytics: https://healthitanalytics.com/news/understanding-the-many-vs-of-healthcare-big-data-analytics

Brown, N. (2015, September 11). *Healthcare Data Growth: An Exponential Problem.* Retrieved August 8, 2017, from http://www.nextech.com/blog/healthcare-data-growth-an-exponential-problem

Cambridge, Mass & Rochester, Minn. (2013, January 15). *Optum, Mayo Clinic Partner to Launch Optum Labs: An Open, Collaborative Research and Innovation Facility Focused on Better Care for Patients.* Retrieved April 20, 2018, from https://www.optum.com/about/news/optum-labs.html

Castle, B. L., & Szymanski, G. (2008). Supply Chain Management on Clinical Units. In eBusiness in Healthcare (pp. 197-217). London: Springe.

Cisco. (2015). *Fog Computing and the Internet of Things: Extend.* Cisco. Retrieved from https://www.cisco.com/c/dam/en_us/solutions/trends/iot/docs/computing-overview.pdf

Crapo, J. (2017). *Big Data in Healthcare: Separating The Hype From The Reality.* Retrieved July 27, 2017, from https://www.healthcatalyst.com/healthcare-big-data-realities

Disch, W. (2016, August 11). *How to Use Big Data to Improve Patient Engagement.* Retrieved 8 2017, from http://data-informed.com/how-to-use-big-data-to-improve-patient-engagement/

Eastwood, B. (2013, April 23). *6 Big Data Analytics Use Cases for Healthcare IT.* Retrieved July 24, 2017, from http://www.cio.com/article/2386531/healthcare/healthcare-6-big-data-analytics-use-cases-for-healthcare-it.html

Epidomiology and Genomics Research Program. (2018, April 5). Retrieved April 29, 2018, from https://epi.grants.cancer.gov/pharm/pharmacoepi_db/healthcore.html

Evolve, I. P. (2017). *Email Vulnerability in Healthcare.* Retrieved from http://www.evolveip.net/lp/email-vulnerability-healthcare

Flatiron. (2017). *Community Oncology.* Retrieved 8 2017, from https://flatiron.com/community-oncology/

Groves, P., Kayyali, B., Knott, D., & Kuiken, S. V. (2013). *The 'big data' revolution in healthcare.* McKinsey & Company.

HealtIT.gov. (2016, November 4). *Electronic Prescribing of Controlled Substances (EPCS).* Retrieved 8 2017, from https://www.healthit.gov/opioids/epcs

Hurwitz, J., Nugent, A., Halper, F., & Kaufman, M. (2013). *Hadoop Pig and Pig Latin for Big Data.* Wiley.

IDC. (2014). *The Digital Universe Driving Data Growth in Healthcare.* IDC. Retrieved August 7, 2017, from http://www.emc.com/analyst-report/digital-universe-healthcare-vertical-report-ar.pdf

Jawadekar, D. M. (2016, August 4). *Big Data and Pharmaceutical Drug Discovery.* Retrieved August 2017, from https://pharma.elsevier.com/pharma-rd/big-data-and-pharmaceutical-drug-discovery/

Lebied, M. (2017, May 24). *9 Examples of Big Data Analytics in Healthcare That Can Save People.* Retrieved July 26, 2017, from http://www.datapine.com/blog/big-data-examples-in-healthcare/

Leventhal, R. (2014, January 10). *Industry expert: "Big data is closer than it appears".* Retrieved August 2017, from https://www.healthcare-informatics.com/article/how-healthcare-organizations-can-turn-big-data-smart-data

Leventhal, R. (2014, December 4). *Report: Healthcare Data is Growing Exponentially, Needs Protection.* Retrieved August 7, 2017, from https://www.healthcare-informatics.com/news-item/report-healthcare-data-growing-exponentially-needs-protection

marketsandmarkets.com. (2016). *Healthcare Analytics/Medical Analytics Market.* Retrieved August 7, 2017, from http://www.marketsandmarkets.com/Market-Reports/healthcare-data-analytics-market-905.html

Marr, B. (2016, February 16). *How Big Data Is Transforming Medicine.* Retrieved August 2017, from https://www.forbes.com/sites/bernardmarr/2016/02/16/how-big-data-is-transforming-medicine/#244b70277ddc

McDonald, C. (2017, February 27). *5 Big Data Production Examples in Healthcare.* Retrieved July 24, 2017, from https://mapr.com/blog/5-big-data-production-examples-healthcare/

Mian, M., Teredesai, A., Hazel, D., Pokuri, S., & Uppala, K. (2014). In-Memory Analysis for Healthcare Big Data. *IEEE International Congress on Big Data.*

Nambiar, R., Sethi, A., Bhardwaj, R., & Vargheese, R. (2013). A Look at Challenges and Opportunities of Big Data Analytics in Healthcare. *IEEE International Conference on Big Data.* 10.1109/BigData.2013.6691753

Orcutt, M. (2016, June 29). *The Rocket Fuel for Biden's "Cancer Moonshot"? Big Data.* Retrieved April 29, 2018, from https://www.technologyreview.com/s/601784/white-house-cancer-moonshot-data/

Patil, H. K., & Seshadri, R. (2014). Big data security and privacy issues in healthcare. *IEEE International Congress on Big Data.*

Pramanik, P. K. D., & Choudhury, P. (2018). IoT Data Processing: The Different Archetypes and their Security & Privacy Assessments. In *Internet of Things (IoT) Security: Fundamentals, Techniques and Applications.* River Publishers. doi:10.4018/978-1-5225-4044-1.ch007

Pramanik, P. K. D., Pal, S., Brahmachari, A., & Choudhury, P. (2018). Processing IoT Data: From Cloud to Fog. It's Time to be Down-to-Earth. In Applications of Security, Mobile, Analytic and Cloud (SMAC) Technologies for Effective Information Processing and Management. pp. 124-148. IGI Global. doi:10.4018/978-1-5225-4044-1.ch007

Pramanik, P. K. D., Upadhyay, B., Pal, S., & Pal, T. (2018). Internet of Things, Smart Sensors, and Pervasive Systems: Enabling the Connected and Pervasive Health Care. In *Healthcare Data Analytics and Management.* Elsevier.

Raghupathi, W., & Raghupathi, V. (2014). Big data analytics in healthcare: promise and potential. *Health Information Science and Systems, 2*(3).

Ramsey, L. (2015, December 23). *I tried 23andMe's new genetics test - and now I know why the company caused such a stir.* Retrieved August 2017, from http://www.businessinsider.in/I-tried-23andMes-new-genetics-test-and-now-I-know-why-the-company-caused-such-a-stir/articleshow/50302664.cms

Revolutionizing the Healthcare Industry with Big Data, Analytics and Visualization. (2015). Retrieved August 2, 2018, from https://www.einfochips.com/whitepaper/Revolutionizing-the-Healthcare-Industry-with-Big-Data-Analytics-and-Visualization.pdf

Sarkar, B. K. (2017). Big data for secure healthcare system: A conceptual design. *Complex Intelligent Systems, 3*(2), 133–151. doi:10.100740747-017-0040-1

Seven Big Data Examples That Have Improved Healthcare Operations. (2016, April 19). Retrieved July 24, 2017, from Ingram Micro Advisor: http://www.ingrammicroadvisor.com/data-center/seven-big-data-examples-that-have-improved-healthcare-operations

Shah, S. (2016, February 18). *Why patient engagement is so challenging to achieve*. Retrieved August 2, 2018, from http://www.ibmbigdatahub.com/blog/why-patient-engagement-so-challenging-achieve

Shvachko, K., Kuang, H., Radia, S., & Chansler, R. (2010). The Hadoop Distributed File System. In *IEEE 26th Symposium on Mass Storage Systems and Technologies (MSST)*. IEEE.

Srinivasan, U., & Arunasalam, B. (2013). *Leveraging Big Data Analytics to Reduce Healthcare Costs*. IEEE Computer Society.

TF7 Healthcare Subgroup. (2016, December 21). *Big Data Technologies in Healthcare: Needs, opportunities and challenges*. Retrieved July 24, 2017, from http://www.bdva.eu/sites/default/files/Big%20Data%20Technologies%20in%20Healthcare.pdf

United Healthcare uses Hadoop to Detect Health Care Fraud, Waste and Abuse. (2018). Retrieved April 20, 2018, from https://mapr.com/customers/unitedhealthcare/

Uzsoy, R. (2005). *Supply-Chain Management and Health Care Delivery: Pursuing a System-Level Understanding*. Retrieved 2017, from https://www.ncbi.nlm.nih.gov/books/NBK22867/

ENDNOTES

1 https://flunearyou.org/#/
2 https://twitter.com/search?q=%23Germtracker
3 http://www.gocap.me/
4 https://www.propellerhealth.com/
5 https://www.23andme.com/
6 http://www.gnshealthcare.com/
7 https://www.aetna.com/
8 https://www.healthcore.com/
9 https://www.evolenthealth.com/valence-health
10 https://www.uhc.com/
11 https://www.optumlabs.com/
12 https://www.liaison.com/
13 https://www.novartis.com/tags/next-generation-sequencing
14 http://hadoop.apache.org/
15 http://pig.apache.org/
16 https://hive.apache.org/
17 https://zookeeper.apache.org/
18 https://hbase.apache.org/
19 http://cassandra.apache.org/
20 http://oozie.apache.org/
21 https://mahout.apache.org/
22 https://lucene.apache.org/
23 https://www.ibm.com/watson/health/

Chapter 5
Deep Learning and Medical Imaging

Nourhan Zayed
Electronics Research Institute, Egypt

Heba A. Elnemr
Electronics Research Institute, Egypt

ABSTRACT

Deep learning (DL) is a special type of machine learning that attains great potency and flexibility by learning to represent input raw data as a nested hierarchy of essences and representations. DL consists of more layers than conventional machine learning that permit higher levels of abstractions and improved prediction from data. More abstract representations computed in terms of less abstract ones. The goal of this chapter is to present an intensive survey of existing literature on DL techniques over the last years especially in the medical imaging analysis field. All these techniques and algorithms have their points of interest and constraints. Thus, analysis of various techniques and transformations, submitted prior in writing, for plan and utilization of DL methods from medical image analysis prospective will be discussed. The authors provide future research directions in DL area and set trends and identify challenges in the medical imaging field. Furthermore, as quantity of medicinal application demands increase, an extended study and investigation in DL area becomes very significant.

INTRODUCTION

Deep learning (Bengio et al., 2012), is a developed direction in general data analysis, and has been entitled one of the year 2013 ten-breakthrough technologies (Greenspan, Hayit, & Bram van Ginneken, 2016; Wang 2016). It is a significant subfield of Artificial Intelligence (AI) that linked various topics like Machine Learning, Neural Networks, and Classification. Figure 1 represents the connections between the diverse AI fields. This discipline has advanced significantly over the years due to the huge works of scientists like Andrew Ng, Geoff Hinton, Yann LeCun, Adam Gibson, and Andrej Karpathy (Hinton et al., 2015; LeCun et al., 2015; Ng, 2014; Ng et al., 2015).

DOI: 10.4018/978-1-5225-7071-4.ch005

For decades, attaining and extracting the well-founded and distinguishable features is always a pivotal step to complete the task of image recognition and computer vision. Engineering expertise is required in the domain to model a feature extractor that mutated raw data (i.e., such as pixels in the image) into a suitable internal representation or feature vector from which the classical machine learning subsystem could complete its work either classification, prediction, or clustering of the input. An interest and research venture in feature extraction is a key concern in a lot of researches in various applications (Elnemr et al., 2016). Representation learning is a set of procedures that provides a machine to be fed with raw data and to automatically determine the portrayals needed for recognition or grouping (LeCun et al., 2015). Deep learning techniques are representation learning techniques with multiple levels of portrayal, prevailed by composing simple but non-linear modules that each transmuted the representation at one level (starting with the raw input) into a representation at a higher, slightly more abstract level (LeCun et al., 2015). With the composition of enough such transmutations, very complex functions can be learned. Figure 2 demonstrates stream outlines for the disparate parts of an AI system relate to each other within different AI disciplines. Shaded boxes indicate components that are able to learn from data (Bengio et al., 2012; Goodfellow et al., 2016).

A deep learning framework is a multilayer heap of simple modules, all (or most) of which are liable to learning, and many of which calculate non-linear input–yield mappings. Each module in the load transforms its input to elevate both the selectivity and the invariance of the representation. With multiple non-linear layers, a framework can implement extremely sophisticated functions of its inputs that are altogether sensitive to minute details and unkind to large unrelated variations such as the background, pose, lighting and surrounding objects. The hidden layers of a deep multilayer neural network learn to represent the network's inputs in a way that makes it easy to predict the target outputs.

Deep learning is known of sundry hundred years as modern neural networks with multiple hidden layers (Hinton, 2014; Ng et al., 2015; Deeplearning4j Development Team, 2016). Back in the nineteen eightieth, the researchers were excited about the prospect of using neural networks with many layers of hidden neurons, but it was hard to get networks to learn well using standard techniques (i.e. Back-propagation "especially with the problem of gradient descent over the loss function" more details are discussed in sub-section 2.1). Neural nets fell out of favor as other machine learning approaches with comparable better results stemming from statistical machine learning in 1990s and 2000s (Alpaydın, 2012). In the previous couple of years the deep learning has become more useful and gained the attention as the development of the methods of training networks (i.e. good weight regularization/dropout), amount of available training data has increased, its models have grown in size over time as computer hardware (i.e. compute power of the parallel hardware graphical processing units (GPUs), computer clusters) and software infrastructure has improved (Le, 2014; Schmidhuber, 2015).

Recently, There's been vast speculation in the Deep learning and AI research (Examples are Google with DeepMind and its Driverless auto, DeepMind Health to develop compelling healthcare technologies, NVidia with CUDA and GPUs computing, Microsoft InnerEye medical image analysis project, and Toyota with its new plan to devote one billion dollars to AI research) (LeCun et al., 2015; Min et al., 2016), as a lot of the problems that machine learning actually tried to resolve were really resolvable by support vector machines (SVMs) and other models which didn't need such deep networks, but issue like analysis of medical images with the increasing amount of patient data, new challenges and opportunities arise for different phases of the clinical routine, such as diagnosis, treatment and monitoring seem to require much richer representations. Particularly with the fruitful stories, deep learning has solved increasingly complicated medical applications with increasing accuracy over time. Bioinformatics can

Figure 1. The relationship between the different AI fields

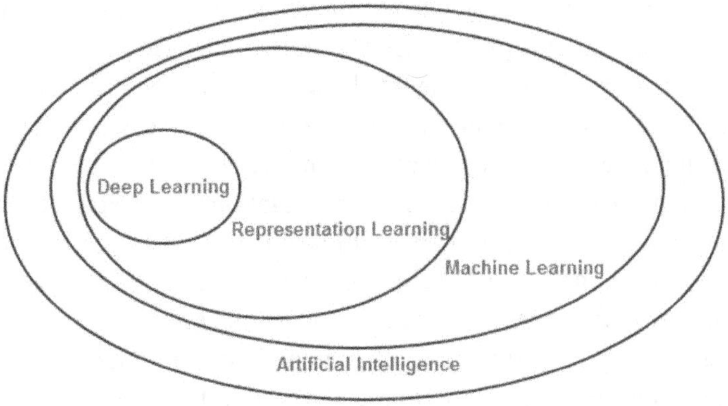

Figure 2. Shows flow charts for the disparate parts of an AI system relate to each other within disparate AI fields; shaded boxes indicate components that are able to learn from data.

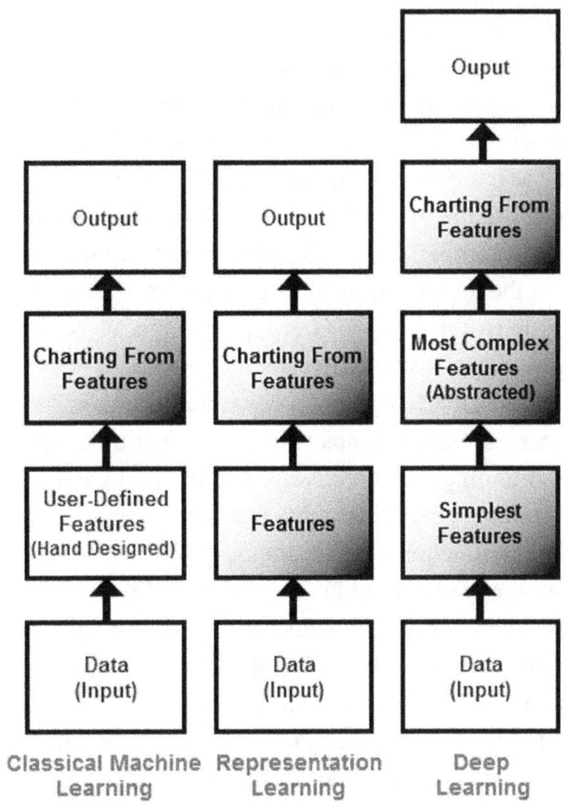

likewise profit by profound from deep learning: splice junctions can be discovered from DNA sequences (Min et al., 2016), finger joints can be recognized from X-ray images (Prasoon, 2014 Anavi et al., 2016), lapses can be detected from electroencephalography (EEG) signals (Turner et al., 2014; Min et al., 2016).

Medical image analysis is essential in today medicine as the medical imaging is a main intrinsic of present-day health care. The skillful diagnosis and/or valuation of a disease depend on the two: image acquisition and image interpretation. Image acquisition has augmented heavily over late years, with gadgets gathering information at fast rates and higher resolution, but evaluating and understanding the emerging different medical modalities (i.e. X-ray, Ultrasound (US), Computed tomography (CT), Magnetic resonance imaging (MRI), and Positron emission tomography (PET)) scans persists a challenging and time monopolizing process. Most interpretations of medical images are executed by radiologists. However, image understanding by individuals is delimited due to its individuality, massive variations across interpreters, and exhaustion. It is robust procedure to find out variations from the norm, and to evaluate estimations and positive or negative disease progress over time (Greenspan, Hayit, & Bram van Ginneken, 2016; Narayan, 2016). This process grasps the attention of the researchers to have new thoughts related to the use of the new era of machine learning in the medical imaging domain as shown in Figure 3. Deep learning is swiftly showing to be the state-of-the-art basis, leading to afflicted accuracy. It has also stimulated new frontiers in medical data analysis with progression not former competent. IEEE Transactions on Medical Imaging produced a special issue in May 2016 focusing in the progress of the deep learning and its progress in medical imaging (Wang, 2016). There were 18 papers in that issue showing a primary impress of deep learning on the medical imaging field. The papers focus on different classical tasks, such as computer aided diagnosis (CAD), lesion detection, image segmentation, image annotation and retrieval, shape modeling, image registration and multimodal analysis, as well as opening up new and novel application domains. Several works that focus on the exploration of the networks and provide insight on the architectures to be chosen for various tasks, parameters, training sets and more (Arel et al., 2010; de Bruijne, 2016; Greenspan, Hayit, & Bram van Ginneken, 2016; Wang, 2016; Deeplearning4j Development Team, 2016) are also included.

Sahiner et al. (1996) were the first to attempt a convolution neural network (CNN) setup for mammography, instead of raw images, texture maps were fed to a simple network with two hidden layers, producing two and three feature images respectively. The method gave acceptable, but not spectacular results. Many things have changed since this publication, however, not only with regard to statistical learning, but also in the context of acquisition techniques. To the best of our knowledge, the exploring beginning of deep learning in the medical field is not before 2012. Ciresan et al. (2012) have focused on the neuronal membrane segmentation in electron microscopy (EM) images problem, which is necessarily to efficiently map 3D brain structure and connectivity.

They used a special type of deep artificial neural network as a pixel classifier followed by a succession of convolutional and max-pooling layers, even without problem-specific post-processing, their approach outperforms all other approaches in the ISBI 2012 EM Segmentation Challenge competition by a large margin in all three considered metrics, i.e. random error, warping error and pixel error. This opens interesting perspectives on applying similar techniques to other biomedical image segmentation tasks (Ciresan et al., 2012) (Brosch et al., 2016). In the last few years, deep learning is making major advances in solving problems that have resisted the best attempts of the AI community for many years.

It has turned out to be very good at discovering intricate structures in high-dimensional data and is therefore applicable to many domains. In addition to beating records in image recognition, predicting the activity of potential drug molecules, analyzing particle accelerator data, reconstructing brain circuits, and predicting the effects of mutations in non-coding DNA on gene expression and disease (Min et al. 2016). It proves its outperforming over other machine-learning techniques at medical images analysis and interpretation application (denoising, heart localization, and parameter estimation) (Rueckert et al., 2016), Computer aided systems for Alzheimer's disease (AD), Mild Cognitive Impairment (MCI) disease diagnosis and prognosis (Suk et al., 2014; Suk & Shen, 2015), lesion detection, semantic imaging, and medical annotation, and the latest breakthrough has been achieved on the neuroimaging multimodality fusion application (Hosseini-Asl et al., 2016).

This state of art chapter, the authors present a survey of the research conducted for deep learning methods over the past years. This chapter is divided into 4 sections. Section 2 depicts a thorough description of different deep learning architectural models. While section 3 the design and the use of deep learning methods in the medical image analysis applications such as computer-aided diagnosis, image segmentation, image annotation and retrieval, image registration, and multimodal image analysis will be surveyed and discussed. Finally, future research directions as well as the challenges exist in the field and conclusions are discussed in section 4, section 5 respectively.

Figure 3. Attention to machine learning has exponentially increased over the past two decades, following a stronger trend than that of medical imaging. The intersection point (in red) indicates that research efforts in medical imaging and deep learning recently became comparable (fifty-fifty), whose combination might boost both.

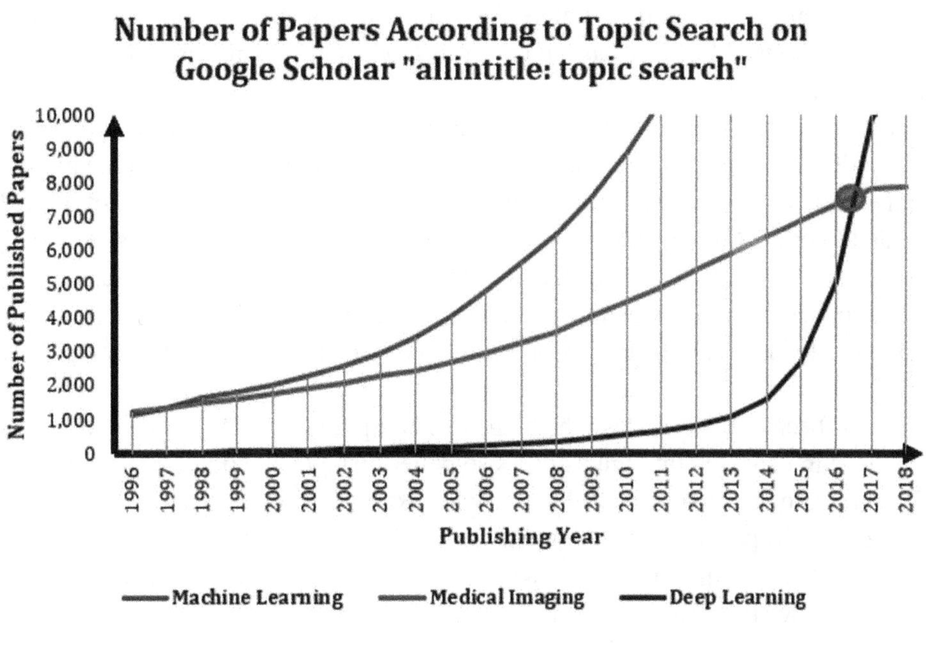

DEEP LEARNING

Deep Learning Key Concepts

Deep learning is in first place about neural networks. Neural networks are a set of algorithms, which are schemed for identifying patterns (Deeplearning4j Development Team, 2016). The patterns they distinguish are vectors having numbers, into which all raw input data must be translated (an appropriate inward representation or feature vector) (Elnemr et al., 2016). Neural networks assist clustering, classifying and predicting. It can be thought as a clustering and classification layer over stored and managed raw data. To be more specific, neural networks educe features that are sustained to other algorithms for clustering and classification; deep neural networks can be thought as components of machine-learning applications involving algorithms for reinforcement learning, classification and regression (Deeplearning4j Development Team 2016; Greenspan et al., 2016). Deep learning maps inputs to outputs. It finds correlations. It is known as a "universal approximator", in light of the fact it can figure out how to approximate the function $f(x) = y$ between any input x and any output y, assuming they are related through correlation or causation at all (Deeplearning4j Development Team, 2016).

Classification encompasses a set of objects and some data features that representing them, and allocating them into categories. Classification tasks depend upon labeled datasets; that is, expertise must relocate their knowledge to the dataset in order for a neural to learn the correlation between labels and data. This is known as supervised learning. Any labels that expertise can generate, any outcomes they care about and which correlate to data can be utilized to train a neural network. The identification of likeness is known as clustering or grouping. Deep learning does not need labels to identify similitudes. Unsupervised learning is learning without labels. The majority of data in the medical world is unlabeled. Precious law of machine learning is: the more data an algorithm can train on, the more precise it will be. Therefore, unsupervised learning has the power to produce highly precise models (Deeplearning4j Development Team, 2016).

Neural nets are robustly structured networks, and contain three kinds of layers - an input, an output, and so called hidden layers, which define any layers between the input and the output layers. Deep learning is the name utilized for "stacked neural networks"; that is, systems composed of a few layers. The layers are made of nodes. A network is an interconnected web of nodes and edges. A node (also called as neuron) is just a spot where input data features processing occurred by a basic calculation with two other numbers, pointed out as the weight and the bias that either enlarge or weaken that input, herewith setting significance to inputs for the task the algorithm is trying to learn. (Deeplearning4j Development Team, 2016)

A classifier has been for each node in the hidden and output layers. These input-weight products are summed and the sum is passed through a node's so-called firing/activation function (fires when it fulfills enough stimuli), to determine whether and to what extent that signal progresses further through the network to affect the ultimate outcome, Figure 4 shows illustration of what node look like components. The activation function (nonlinear transforms) at each node are usually s-shaped functions similar to logistic regression. Logistic regression is a non-linear function that packs input to translate it to a space between 0 and 1 (some sort of sigmoid activation function, "log-sigmoid or the hyperbolic tangent etc."). Pairing adjustable weights with input features is how those features are significantly assigned with regard to how the network classifies/clusters input. (Deeplearning4j Development Team, 2016)

Firstly, the input layer receives the data features. After processing the data, their output will be sent to the first hidden layer. The hidden layer processes this output and sends the results to the next hidden layer. This continues until the data reaches the final output layer, where the output value determines the object's classification (Figure 5). This whole procedure is known as Forward Propagation, or Forward prop. The scores at the output layer determine which class a set of inputs has a place with. A node layer is a line of that neuron like switches that turn on or off as the input is nourished through the net. Each layer's output is all the while the consequent layer's input, starting from an underlying input layer receiving your data. (Deeplearning4j Development Team 2016)

The point of least error as fast as possible is the goal of any neural net (simple multiple layer perceptron (MLP) see Figure 6). The beginning stage is the weights initialization and then updating of those weights and biases continuous repeatedly in a loop till capable of producing accurate classifications and predictions. Every footstep for a neural network encompasses assess, an error mensuration and a small update in its weights, gradual modifications to the coefficients. A collection of weights, whether they are in their start or end state, is also called a model, because it is a trail to model data's relationship to ground-truth labels, to grasp the data's structure. Models regularly begin terrible and wind up less awful, changing over time as the neural network updates its parameters. Neural networks have three key functions: scoring input, calculating loss and applying an update to the model – to begin the three-stage process over once more. A neural network is a corrective feedback loop, remunerating weights that support its right estimates, and rebuffing weights that lead it to error. (Deeplearning4j Development Team 2016)

Deep learning networks are featured from the more conventional single-hidden-layer neural networks, adding multiple hidden layers to the simple MLP, by their depth; that is, the number of node layers through which data pushes through in a multistep process of pattern recognition. Traditional machine learning builds on shallow nets, consisted of one input and one output layer, and at most one hidden layer in between. More than three layers (including input and output) consider as "deep" learning. So deep is a robustly known, technical term that means more than one hidden layer.

In deep networks, each layer of nodes interns on a different group of features resulted from the previous layer's output. The more you go through the neural net, the more abstract (built up) features your nodes can have realized, ever after they gather and fuse features from the previous layer (Figure 7). This is known as feature hierarchy, and it is a hierarchy of increasing complexity and abstraction. Deep learn-

Figure 4. What node look like components; where X0=1, Inputs= Xi, Weights= Wi, and Output=Y

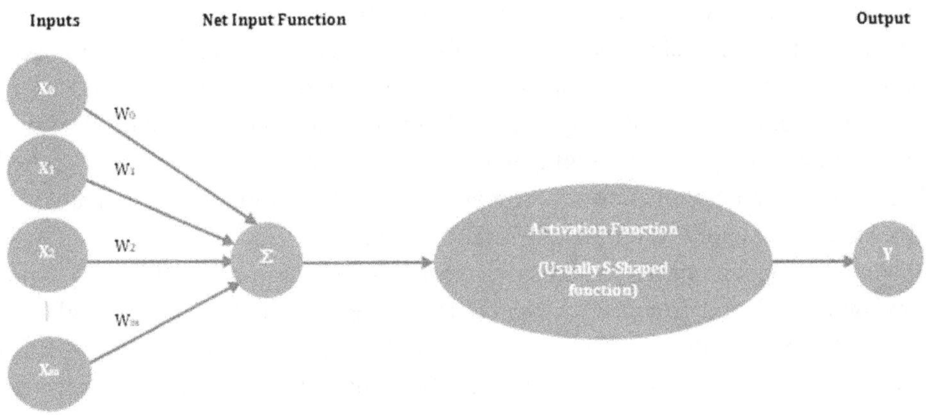

Figure 5. The traditional neural network structure

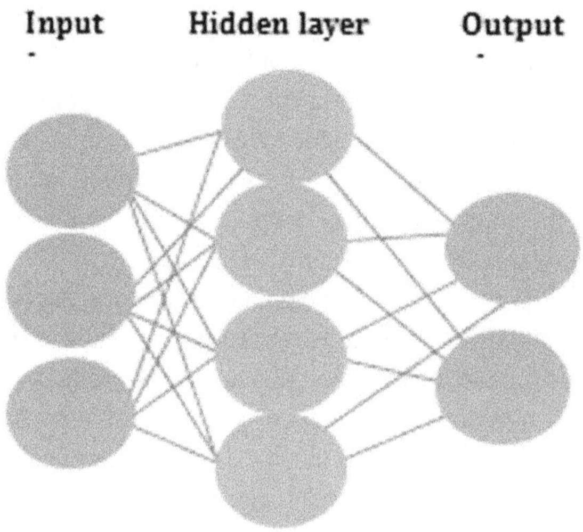

ing networks capability of handling very large, high-dimensional datasets with billions of parameters that pass through nonlinear functions can be made because of this feature hierarchy (Deeplearning4j Development Team, 2016).

The low-layer represents low-level features and the high-layer abstracts those low-level features are one of the key features of the deep learning. First and last, these nets are qualified for disclosing hidden structures within unlabeled, unstructured data, which is the vast plurality of data in the medical field world. Example for unstructured data is raw medical imaging data. Thus, one of the problems deep learning solves best is in processing and clustering unlabeled medical data, perceiving similarities and eccentricity in data that no radiologist/clinical doctor has organized in a relational database or ever put a name to. For example, deep learning can take a million medical images, and cluster them according to their similarities. Deep learning networks do automatic feature extraction without human involvement, unlike most traditional machine-learning algorithms. Given that feature extraction is a task that can consume years of data scientists' teams to achieve, deep learning is a path to take care of the issue of limited experts. It increases the powers of small data science teams, which by their nature do not scale. In the case of neuroimaging and biological data, the deep or hierarchical architecture can be efficiently used to discover latent or hidden representation, inherent in the low-level features from modalities, and ultimately to enhance classification accuracy (Suk et al., 2015).

The issue with such "deep" networks is that it begins to be harder and harder to learn "good" weights for this network. In the beginning of the network training, weights are assigned random initialization values, which can be badly off from the "optimal" solution that targeted to be found. The generally used optimization function that modulates weights with respect to the error they caused is called "gradient descent". The relationship between network error and each of those weights is a derivative, which measures how does the error change as the weight is modulated.

This is the popular Backpropagation algorithm (reverse-mode auto-differentiation) to propagate the "errors" from right to left and calculate the partial derivatives according to each weight to take a step into the opposite direction of the cost (or "error") gradient. Furthermore, due to terrible off beginning, it can become almost impossible to parameterize a "deep" neural network with backpropagation. The

Figure 6. A simple MLP, where y_hat is the final class label that you return as the prediction based on the inputs (x) if this is a classification task. The "a"s are your activated neurons and the "w"s are the weight coefficients.

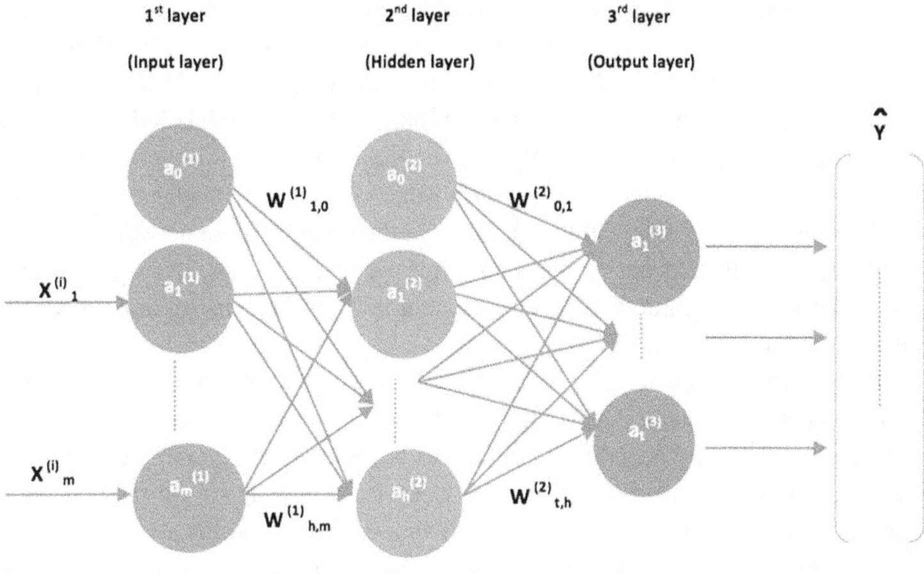

Figure 7. The more you go through the neural net, the more abstract (built up) features your nodes can realize, ever after they gather and fuse features from the previous layer. Successive models layers learn deeper intermediate representations.

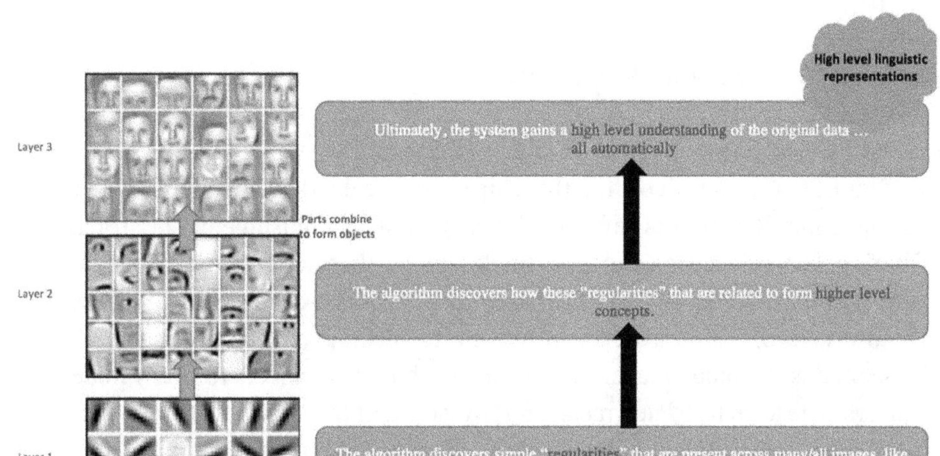

problem is the so-called "vanishing gradient" -- the more layers to be added, the challenging it becomes to "update" the weights because the signal becomes smaller and smaller (Deeplearning4j Development Team 2016).

Hinton, a well-known scientist in the field, was able to innovate a reconstruction method for training deep networks, Restricted Boltzmann machines (RBM) (Arel et al., 2010; Bengio et al., 2012; Deeplearning4j Development Team, 2016) that was a breakthrough that allowed deep nets, to certain limit, to be withstand the vanishing gradient issue. When training on unlabeled data, each node layer in a deep network learns features automatically by over and again endeavoring to reconstruct the input from which it draws its samples, attempting to minimize the difference between the network's guesses and the probability distribution of the input data itself. In the process, these networks learn to recognize correlations between certain relevant features and optimal results – they draw connections between feature signals and what those features represent, whether it is a full reconstruction, or with labeled data (Deeplearning4j Development Team, 2016).

A deep learning network trained on labeled data can then be applied to unstructured data, giving it approach to more input than machine-learning nets. This is a recipe for higher performance: the more data a net can train on, the more accurate it is likely to be. Bad algorithms trained on lots of data can outperform good algorithms trained on very little. Deep learning's ability to process and learn from huge quantities of unlabeled data gives it a distinct advantage over previous algorithms. Deep learning networks end in an output layer: a logistic, or softmax, classifier that assigns likelihood to a particular outcome or label (Deeplearning4j Development Team, 2016). The different models for deep neural network, which differ according to the training method and the architecture, will be discussed in more details in the next subsection.

Deep Learning Models

Restricted Boltzmann Machines (RBMs)

RBM, concocted by Geoff Hinton (Bengio, 2009; Hinton, 2014; Bengio et al., 2012; Deeplearning4j Development Team, 2016), is an algorithm that can automatically detect the inherent patterns in data by reconstructing the input. RBMs are useful for dimensionality diminishment, classification, regression, concurrent filtering, feature learning and topic modeling. Furthermore, it is the basic building blocks for the architecture of deep belief networks (DBN) and autoencoders (AE) deep neural networks algorithms.

Respective to structure, RBMs are shallow two layered neural nets, the first is called visible, or input layer, and the second is the hidden layer. In this net, each node connects to every node in the adjacent layer, across layers. The term restricted means no two nodes of the similar layer are connected, no intra-layer correspondence. RBM can be said to frame a symmetrical bipartite diagram. Symmetrical means that each visible node is connected with each hidden node (Figure 8). Bipartite means it has two parts (layers), and the diagram term is for the web of nodes.

Insomuch as these two layers are part of a deeper neural network, the outputs of the first hidden layer will be passed as inputs (visible layer in that treat) to a second hidden layer, and from there up to the hilt as many hidden layers as exist till they connect to a conclusive classifying layer. (For simple feed-forward movements, the RBM nodes conduct as an AE)

The recreation of the inputs as precisely as likely is the purpose of an RBM. Through a forward path (Figure 9(a)), the inputs are mutated by weights and biases and are hired to activate the hidden layer. In the backward path (Figure 9 (b)), the activations from the hidden layer are mutated by weights and new biases and iterated to the input layer for activation. At the input layer, the adapted activations are inspected as an input reconstruction and emulated to the original input. Kullback-Leibler (KL) divergence, a measure of how one distribution diverges from another one, is utilized to test the accuracy of the net. The training mode employs continuously pinching the weights and biases through both paths till the input is as precise as likely to the reconstruction. Since, RBMs attempt to reconstruct the input in an unsupervised learning way, RBMs should also decipher the structuring blocks and patterns that latent in the data (Deeplearning4j Development Team, 2016). This procedure of provoking consecutive sets of activations by pooling features and then pooling groups of features is the principles of a feature hierarchy, by which neural networks learn more complex and abstract representations of data. Executing these back and forth steps is a process known as Gibbs sampling, and the difference in the correlation of the hidden activations and visible inputs forms the basis for a weight update (Bengio, 2009; Bengio et al., 2012; Hinton, 2014; Deeplearning4j Development Team, 2016).

Existence of two biases is one of the manifestations that distinguish the RBMs from other AE. The hidden bias helps the RBM to produce the initiations and activations on the forward path (since biases impose a floor so that at least some nodes fire no matter how inadequate the data "sparse or dispersed"), while the visible layer's biases help the RBM learn the reconstructions on the retrogressive way (backward path).

RBMs are appealing as a structuring bulk, over more traditional and deeply layered sigmoid belief networks, due to their ease of learning these connection weights. To obtain generative weights, the initial pre-training occurs in an unsupervised insatiable layer-by-layer manner, enabled by what Hinton has termed contrastive divergence (Arel et al., 2010). Although RBM can extract features and reconstruct input data, it still lacks the total ability to combat the vanishing gradient.

Figure 8. The RBMs symmetrical bipartite graph architecture

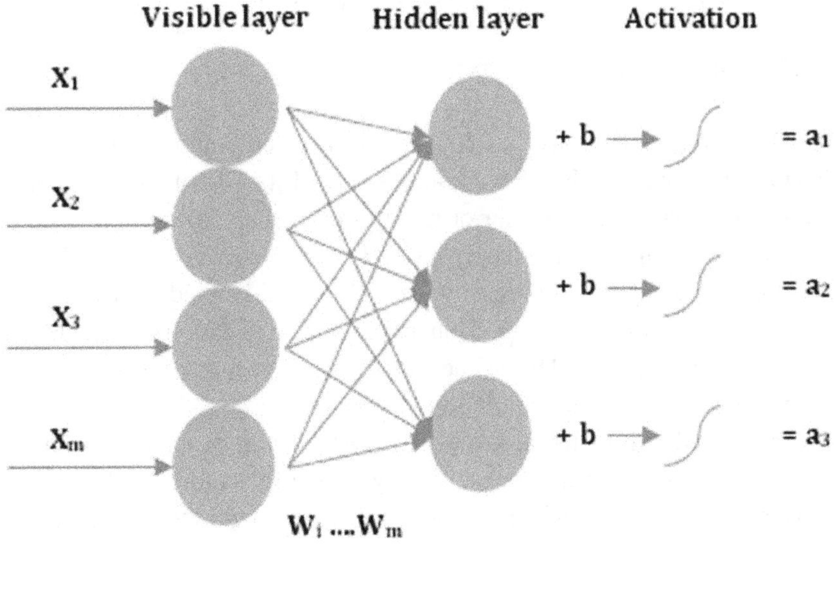

Figure 9. The RBMs in (a) the forward pass, and in (b) the reconstruction on the backward pass

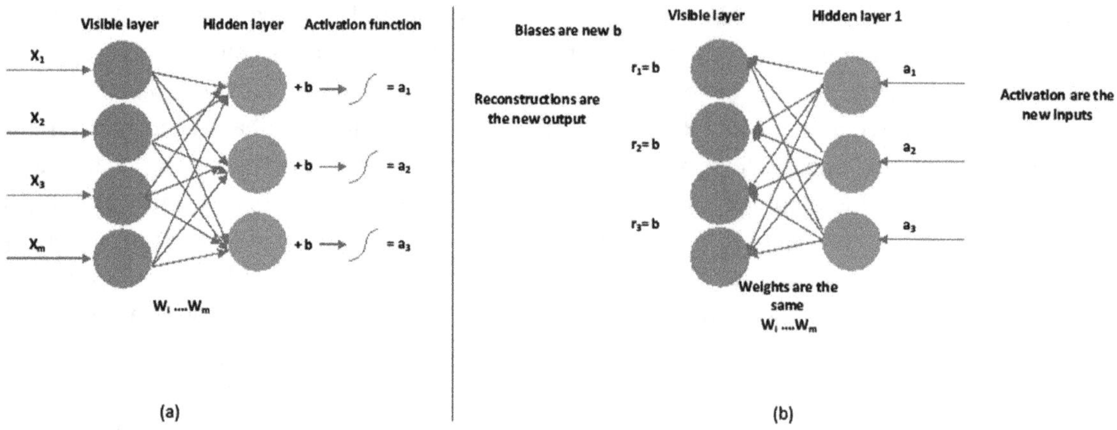

A continuous RBM (CRBM) is a type of RBM that takes continuous input. This endorses the CRBM to handle things like image pixels that are normalized to decimals between zero and one. It should be realized that each layer of a deep learning net needs four components: the input, the coefficients, a bias and the transform (activation function). The input is the numeric information, a vector, bolstered to it from the previous layer (or as the original information). The coefficients are the weights given to various features that pass through each node layer. The bias ensures that at least a few nodes in a layer will be initiated no matter what. The transformation is an additional algorithm that squashes the data after it passes through each layer in a way that makes gradients easier to compute (gradients are necessary for a net to learn). Those transformations and their combinations can be different in each layer. An effective CRBM employs a Gaussian transformation on the visible (or input) layer and a rectified-linear-unit transformation on the hidden layer. That's especially beneficial in facial reconstruction applications. For RBMs handling binary data, simply make both transformations binary ones. Gaussian transformations do not function admirably on RBMs' hidden layers. The rectified-linear-unit transformations utilized for representing more features rather than binary transformations, which employed on DBN (Bengio 2009; Bengio et al., 2012; Hinton 2014; Deeplearning4j Development Team, 2016).

Deep Belief Networks (DBN)

DBN, invented by Geoff Hinton (Hinton et al., 2006) (Mnistdatasetiterator, 2006)(Bengio, 2009), probabilistic generative model, is an algorithm that combines several stacked of RBMs, explained earlier, and end with a softmax layer to create a classifier or it may simply help cluster unlabeled data in an unsupervised learning scenario. Conventional deeply layered neural networks that used backpropagation in their training have three challenges: (1) necessity of a substantial labeled dataset for training, (2) slow learning (i.e. convergence) times, and (3) inadequate parameter selection techniques that lead to poor local optima, which is addressed by the DBN. They are useful for recognizing, clustering and generating images, Furthermore, to video sequences and motion capture data.

In terms of structure, a DBN is identical to a MLP (or RBM), but structure is where their similarities terminate. The existence of the classifier layer leads to give a DBN a radically different training method which allows it to tackle more the vanishing gradient (Deeplearning4j Development Team, 2016).

Figure 10. Illustration of the DBN framework

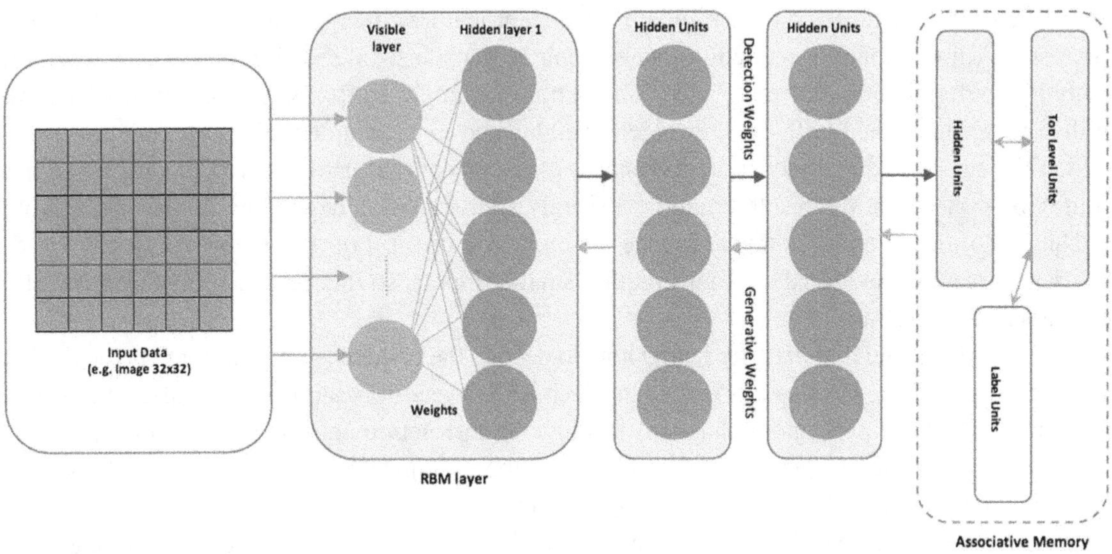

Every RBM layer interacts with both the former and later layers. The nodes of any single layer don't interact with each other laterally. The method is known as layer-wise, unsupervised, voracious pre-training. Basically, the DBN is trained two layers at a time, and these two layers are patronized like an RBM. Excluding the first and final layers, every layer in a deep-belief network has a double function: it turns as the hidden layer to the nodes that come former, and as the input (or "visible") layer to the nodes that come later. Moreover, the first RBM is trained, and its outputs are then used as inputs to the next RBM. This procedure is repeated until the output layer is reached. After this training process, the DBN is competent of identifying the data hidden patterns by having hidden layers that captures higher-order data correlations observed at the visible units. This method is a developed, multilayer feature extractor (Figure 10). Ultimately, a DBN yet demands a set of labels to stratify to the resulting patterns. In such a way, The DBN is adjusted with supervised learning and a small set of labeled examples. In the wake of making minor tweaks to the weights and biases, the net will achieve a slight increase in accuracy.

Thus, the DBN is an effective solution to the vanishing gradient problem (Bengio et al., 2012; Deeplearning4j Development Team, 2016). Furthermore, an extension of a DBN that accepts a continuum of decimals, rather than binary data is called a continuous deep-belief network.

Autoencoders (AE)

AE are group of neural nets that are pretty adequate for unsupervised learning. A deep AE essential motifs are two symmetrical DBNs, usually with an equal number of layers for both encoding and decoding processes. Typically, it has four or five shallow layers, this arrangement of net is speaking to the encoding half, and the second arrangement of four or five layers that make up the decoding half. The layers are RBMs, the building blocks of DBNs. Figure 11 is showing a simplified schema of a deep AE's structure. They are useful for labeling the resulting patterns, dimensionality reduction, image search, image retrieval, denoising, and data reconstruction.

Representation learning core is the AE. They encode input, commonly by insistent large vectors into smaller vectors that grasp their ultimate significant features; that is why, they are useful for data compression (dimensionality reduction), as example it transforms a 256x256 pixel image into a representation with only 30 numbers (Figure 12 illustrates example with 28x28 pixel image). The image can then be reconstructed with the convenient weights and bias; as an addition, random noise can be added at this phase so that to boost the robustness of the discovered patterns. The reconstructed image wouldn't be perfect, but the result would be a seemly approximation depending on the strength of the net. The aim of this compression is to reduce the input size on a set of data before feeding it to a deep classifier. Large computational speedups require smaller inputs, so this preprocessing step is justified regardless of the exertion.

The deep AE second half actually learns how to decode the condensed vector, that one be the input, as it forms its way back. The decoder part of the deep AE is a feed-forward net which also conducts back propagation. The back propagation happens through reconstruction entropy. This part of the network learns to reconstruct the image as shown in Figure 12 the example with layers 100, 250, 500 and 1000 nodes wide, respectively. Those layers initially have the same weights as their counterparts in the pretraining net, except that the weights are transposed; i.e. they are not initialized randomly (Deeplearning4j Development Team 2016).

Binary transformations after each RBM in the deep AE would be used. While Gaussian rectified transformations for the RBMs would be utilized for different sorts of datasets with real-valued data. It ought to be noticed that RBMs do not deliver the most stable, consistent results of all shallow, feedforward networks. By and large, a dense-layer AE works better.

Figure 11. A simplified schema of a deep AE's structure. Input signals are encoded along the path to the hidden layer, and these same signals are decoded along the path to the output layer

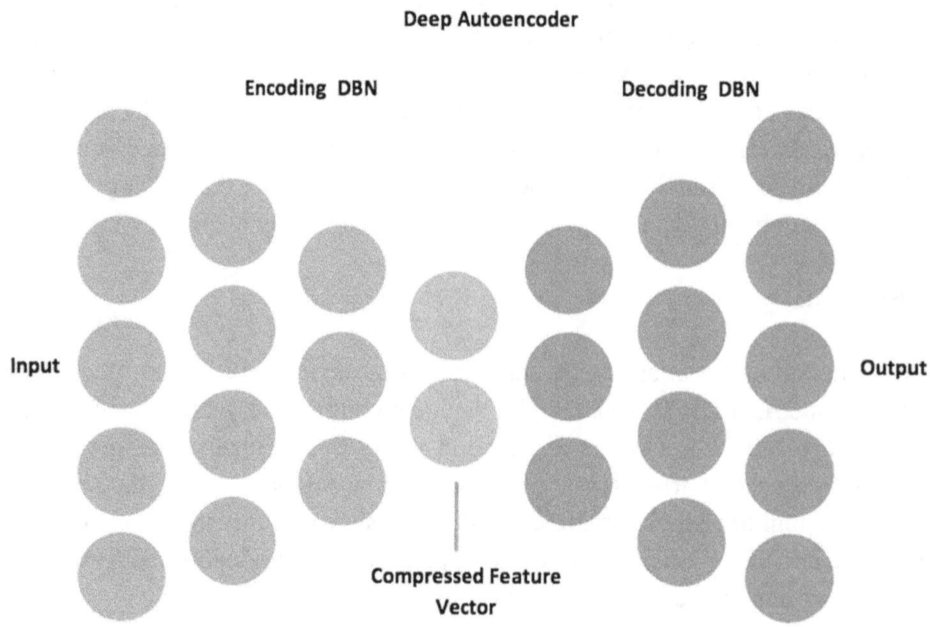

Figure 12. Illustrates example with 28x28 pixel image example passing through the deep AE's structure. Due to the representational capacity of sigmoid-belief units, a form of transformation used with each layer. Sigmoid belief units can't represent as much as information and variance as real-valued data. The expanded first layer is a way of compensating for that. Layers will be 1000, 500, 250, 100 nodes wide, respectively, until the end, where the net produces a vector 30 numbers long. This 30-number vector is the last layer of the first half of the deep AE, the pretraining half, and it is the product of a normal RBM, rather than classification output layer such as softmax or logistic regression, as you would normally see at the end of a deep-belief network.

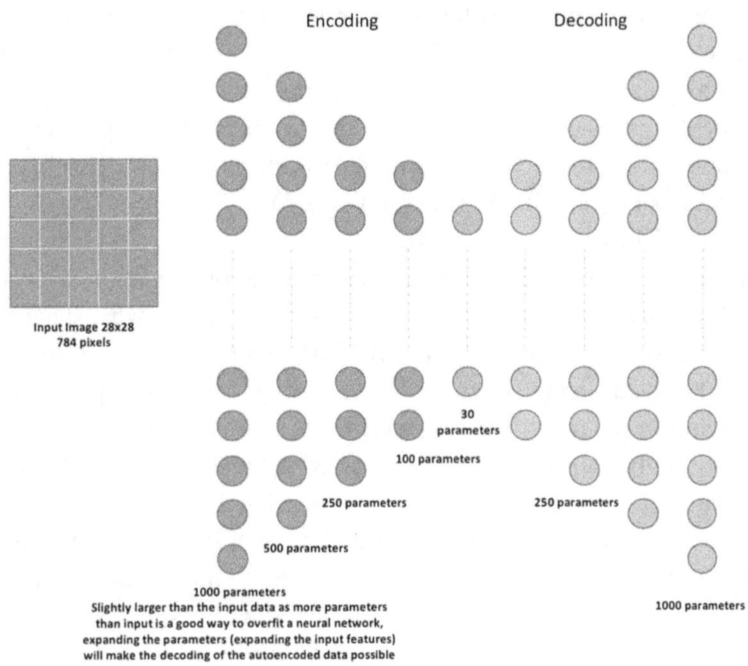

In fact, AE can derive in many aromas including: Variational AE (VAE), Denoising AE (DAE) and Sequence AE. VAEs have subrogated RBMs in many labs because they produce more stable results. DAEs issue a form of regulation by randomly corrupting input (introducing Gaussian noise into the input), which the network learns to ignore in search of the true signal (reconstruct, or denoise). DAEs are an extension of the basic AE, and represent a stochastic version of it (Deeplearning4j Development Team 2016).

A stacked denoising AE (SDA) is to a denoising AE what a deep belief nets is to a RBM. A key capacity of SDAs, and deep learning all the more for the most part, is the unsupervised pre-training, layer by layer, as input is bolstered through. Once each layer is pre-trained to perform feature selection and extraction on the input from the former layer, a second phase of supervised fine-tuning can pursue. A word on stochastic corruption in SDAs: DAEs shuffle data around (rearrange information) and learn about that data by attempting to reconstruct it. The demonstration of rearranging is the noise, and the job of the network is to recognize the features within the noise that will allow it to classify the input. When a network is being trained, it generates a model, and measures the distance between that model and the benchmark through a loss function. Its endeavors to limit and minimize the loss function involve resampling the rearranged inputs and re-reconstructing the data, until it finds those inputs which bring its model closest to what it has been told is true (Deeplearning4j Development Team 2016). Specifically, 'stacked AE' (SAE) is considered to discover latent portrayals from the original neuroimaging and biological features. Noteworthy, the unsupervised characteristic of the pretraining in deep learning, as the SAE model, allows the benefit from the target-unrelated samples to discover general inert feature portrayals, and hence to leverage for further enhancement of the classification accuracy. (Suk et al. 2015)

Convolution Neural Nets (CNNs)

Out of all deep learning architectures, that helped deep learning become one of the hottest topic in AI, are the convolution nets (abbreviated as CNNs, or ConvNets), one of the machine vision applications best tools. CNNs are deep nets that are useful to classify images (name what they see), cluster them by similarity (photo search), and do object recognition (Dmitrievich 2015). They act as local filters of the input space, that are appropriate to discover the strong spatially local correlation in images, this includes 2D and 3D images and videos (Lai 2015) (Emad et al. 2015).

CNNs have multiple of different types of layers as shown in Figure 13: (1) image processing series of layers called convolution filters layers, (2) inlaid with a series of activation layers (tanh or Rectifying Linear Unit (ReLU) functions), and data reduction or pooling layers (known as: maxpooling, downsampling, upsampling), (3) fully connected layers (Lai 2015) (Greenspan, Hayit, Bram van Ginneken 2016).

In the convolution layers, different filters are learned using the back-propagation algorithm in order to extract various features of the input. The low-level features are usually extracted in the first convolution layers, whereas, the higher-level features are extracted in the deep layers. The role of the ReLU is to grow the nonlinear characteristics of the decision function and of the total network without impacting the receptive fields of the convolution layer, in other words the use of ReLU engine reduces the endure from the vanishing gradient problem when backpropagation used for training. The pooling layer has a substantial purpose of diminution the spatial variance (translational and rotational), through computing the max or average value of a particular feature over a region of the image. Most of the precis of representation concepts are usually invariant to most local changes of the input. That makes the representations that seized these concepts as a rule highly non-linear functions of the raw input. This is a substantial process for object classification and detection. The output is then fed to a fully connected layer aiming the classification task, to encode position dependent information and more global patterns (Emad et al. 2015).

From mathematical potential, a convolution is the integral measuring how much two functions overlap as one passes over the other. Think of a convolution as a way of mixing two functions by multiplying them. In the image analysis application, the first static input function is the image being analyzed, the second mobile function is the filter applied to pick up a signal or feature in the image. In the convolutional layers, many filters are passing over a single image, each one picking up different signal (feature). Thus, the first layer of the Deep CNNs consists of "feature maps" which are the results of the convolution processes with an additive bias and possibly compression or normalization of the features as shown in Figure 14. The weights and biases in this layer determine the effectiveness of the filtering process. The former process is pursued by a subsampling (averaging or maximizing) that additionally reduces the dimensionality. The subsampled feature map then receives a weighting and trainable bias and finally propagates through an activation function. The activation function is almost linear and the result is a blurred image when the weighting is small; other weightings can cause the activation output to resemble an AND or OR function. Units in a convolutional layer are organized in feature maps, within which each unit is connected to local patches (kernels) in the feature map of the pervious layer through

Figure 13. The 3 main layers for any CNN

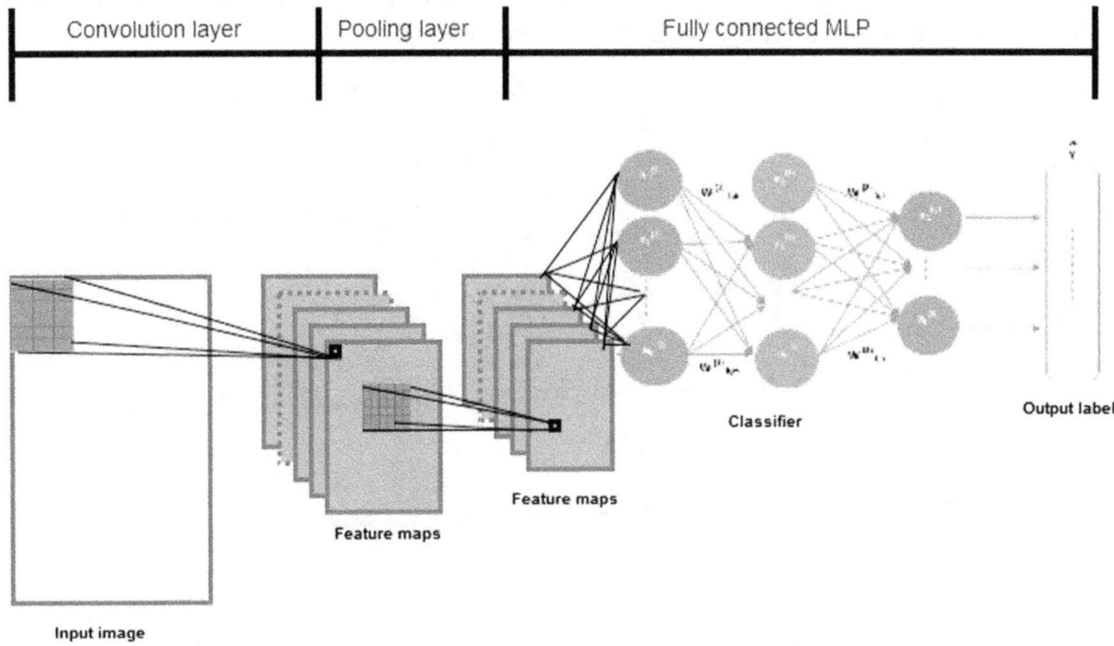

a set of weights called a filter bank. All units in the feature map share the same filter bank. The outputs from a feature map is then passed through another sequence of convolution, subsampling and activation flow as shown in Figure 15. This process can be repeated an arbitrary number of times (Deeplearning4j Development Team 2016).

The convolution filters are learned from training data. This is one of its cons because it reduces the necessity of the time-consuming hand-crafting of features that would otherwise be required to preprocess the images with application-specific filters or by calculating computable features. Nevertheless, applying CNNs have some challenges that need to be eyed such as: Firstly, they demand tens of millions of labelled data points for training. Secondly, they also must be trained with GPUs for the process to be completed in a reasonable amount of time, and finally, training a deep CNN is often complicated by overfitting and convergence issues, which often require repetitive adjustments in the architecture or learning parameters of the network to ensure that all layers are learning with comparable speed (Lai 2015)(Greenspan, Hayit, Bram van Ginneken 2016). The efficient use of GPUs, ReLUs, a new regularization technique called dropout, and techniques to generate more training examples by deforming the existing ones are recommended.

Recurrent Neural Nets (RNN)

In the previous sections of deep network models, they were confined to static patterns, but how can a net decipher and label patterns that change with time. The RNN is a type of artificial neural network that is equipped with recurrent connections, which cement the network to memorize past input patterns and recognize patterns in sequences of data. Though the word sequence usually indicates one dimensional data, it refers here to data paradigms of any dimensionality (Graves et al. 2007). For example, an im-

Figure 14. Illustrates example for the convolution process with different filters applied on the input image (i.e. Different filters, imagine them as passing horizontal line filter, vertical line filter, diagonal line filter each producing a feature map for each convolution process).

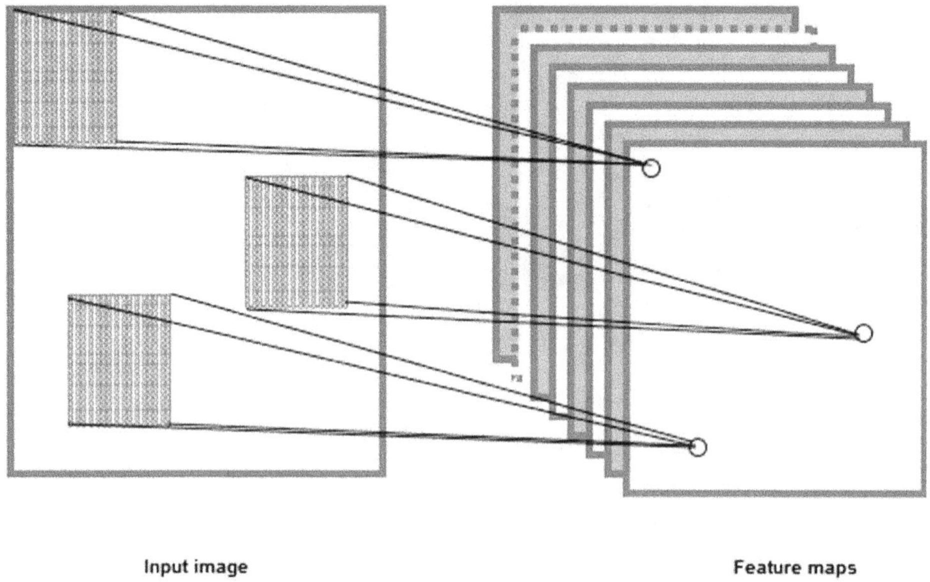

Figure 15. The CNNs complete architecture. From left to right you see: i) The actual input image that is scanned for features. The light rectangle is the filter that passes over it. ii) Activation maps stacked a top one another, one for each filter you employ. The larger rectangle is one patch to be downsampled. iii) The activation maps condensed through downsampling. iv) A new set of activation maps created by passing filters over the first downsampled stack. v) The second downsampling, which condenses the second set of activation maps.vi) A fully connected layer that classifies output with one label per node.

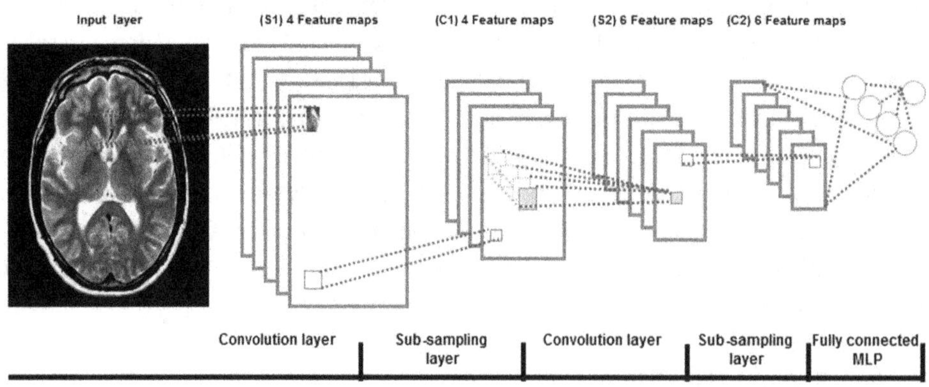

age is a two dimensional sequence, a video is a sequence with three dimension, and a four dimensional sequence as a series of functional magnetic resonance imaging (fMRI) brain scans. A recurrent net has one extra ability – it can forecast the next item in a sequence, essentially acting as an anticipating engine. For the simple RNN at each time step, its current hidden state is a non-linear transformation of the current input and the hidden layer from the last step. RNN is a model that occupies at each time step an input from the outer world and an input from itself (from a previous time step), summarizing all the information it's seen so far (Caswell et al. 2016).

All previous represented deep nets in this state of art article so far are known as feedforward networks since the signal moves in only one direction across the layers. In contrast, RNNs have a feedback loop where the net's yield is sustained once more into the net alongside the next input. Since RNNs have just one layer of neurons, they are structurally one of the simplest types of nets. RNNs, once unfolded in time (Figure 16), can be seen as very deep feedforward networks in which all the layers share the same weights. Like other nets, RNNs receive an input and produce an output. Dissimilar to different nets, the inputs and outputs can arrive in a succession. RNNs are inherently deep in time, since their shrouded state is a component of all previous concealed states (Graves et al. 2013).

RNNs are designed to utilize successive dope of input data with cyclic connections among building blocks like perceptron, long short-term memory units (LSTMs), or gated recurrent units (GRUs) (Min et al. 2016). The feedback loop in the recurrent networks ingesting their own outputs moment after moment as input. RNNs are very robust dynamic systems, but training them has proved to be problematic because the back propagated gradients either enlarge or lessen at each time step, which reintroduces the vanishing gradient problem. In fact, the problem is worse with a RNN in light of the fact that each time step is what might as well be called a layer in a feedforward net. Thus if the net is trained for n time steps, the gradient will vanish exponentially as it would in an n-layer MLP (LeCun et al., 2015).

There are different approaches to take care of this problem, the most widely recognized of which is gating. Gating takes the output of any time step and the next input, and carries out a transmutation before feeding the result back into the RNN. There are several types of gates, the LSTM being the most common, that use special hidden units, the natural behavior of which is to remember inputs for a long time. A special unit called the memory cell acts like an accumulator or a gated broken neuron: it has an association with itself at whenever step that has a weight of one, so it copies its own genuine esteemed state and accumulates the external signal, but this self-connection is multiplicatively gated by another unit that learns to decide when to clear the content of the memory. Other approaches to address this problem include gradient clipping, steeper gates, and better optimizers. GPUs are an essential tool for training an RNN, for increasing the speed of the analysis over central processing unit (CPU) (Deeplearning4j Development Team, 2016).

Nevertheless, RNNs have been inspected less than DBNs and CNNs, they still provide very powerful analysis methods for sequential information. Since most of the biomedical data are typically sequential, the capabilities of RNNs for mapping a variable-length input sequence to another sequence or fixed-size prediction are promising especially for bioinformatics research (Min et al., 2016). Furthermore, Min et al. in their study expected that the RNNs triumphs in natural language processing will lead them to be applied in biomedical text analysis and that employing an attention mechanism will improve performance and extract more relevant information from bioinformatics data (Min et al., 2016). With respect to biomedical imaging, RNNs are currently not the first choice of many researchers. Nevertheless, in our point of view the spread of using dynamic CT and MRI, DTI, fMRI in the medical field would need the incorporation of RNNs and CNNs in the image interpretation/analysis and elevate their importance in the long term.

Figure 16. RNN and the unfolding in time of the computation involved in its forward computation. Updated from (LeCun et al., 2015).

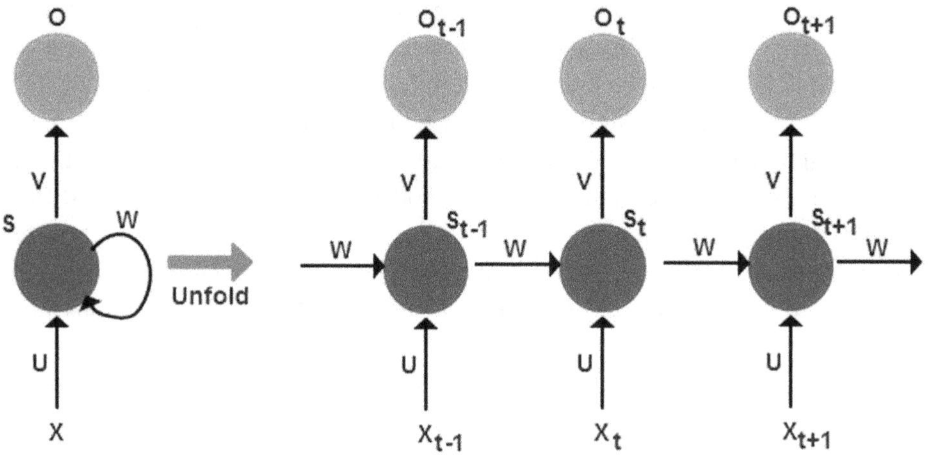

Deep Learning Models Summary and Comparison

To sum up the previous section illustrating the different deep learning architectures check Table 1. There are two main classes of deep learning techniques: purely supervised learning algorithms (e.g., CNNs) and unsupervised and semi-supervised learning algorithms (e.g., DAEs, RBMs, and DBNs).

In brief, while RBMs learn to reconstruct and identify the features of each image as a whole, convolution nets learn images on pieces that the researchers call feature maps. In contrast to RBMs, the approximate inference procedure of DBNs is performed using two-way dependencies, that is, bottom-up and top-down, which allows DBNs to use higher-level information to learn intermediate-level features, thus creating potentially more accurate representations of the data (Salakhutdinov and Hinton, 2012).

Additionally, from table 1 the researchers can deduce that training a deep CNN from scratch (or full training) is a challenge. First, CNNs require a large amount of labeled training data, a requirement that may be difficult to meet in the medical domain where expert annotation is expensive and the diseases (e.g., lesions) are scarce. Second, training a deep CNN requires large computational and memory resources, without which the training process would be extremely time-consuming. Third, training a deep CNN is often complicated by overfitting and convergence issues, which often require repetitive adjustments in the architecture or learning parameters of the network to ensure that all layers are learning with comparable speed. Given these difficulties, several new learning schemes, termed "transfer learning" and "fine-tuning", are shown to provide solutions and are increasingly gaining popularity.

Important to mention, CNN can achieve superior performance on visual object recognition and image classification tasks. However, most of CNNs are designed for 2D natural images. They are not well suited for medical image analysis, since most of medical images are 3D volumetric images, such as MRI, CT and PET. Compared to 2D CNN, 3D CNN can better model the 3D spatial information due to the use of 3D convolution operations. 3D convolution preserves the spatial neighborhood of 3D image. As a result, 3D CNN can solve the discontinuity problem across slices, which are suffered by 2D CNN (Dong Nie et al., 2016).

Furthermore, regarding the biomedical imaging applications, RNNs are currently not the first choice of many researchers. Nevertheless, in my point of view, the long term importance of RNNs and CNNs incorporation in the medical image interpretation/analysis is elevated due to the spread of using dynamic CT and MRI, DTI, fMRI in the medical field. For deep learning to be more useful, many other emergent deep learning architectures have been suggested in the literature, such as deep spatio-temporal neural networks (DST-NNs), multi-dimensional RNN (MD-RNNs), and convolutional AE (CAEs) (Min et al., 2016).

DEEP LEARNING AND MEDICAL IMAGING

Medical image analysis is important in modern medicine. Owing to the huge amount of patients' information, clinical experts, as radiologists and doctors, have to pursue comprehensive analysis, assessments, and interpretation that has become an essential demand. This requires dealing with massive amounts of scans per day, which is a time exhausting task. Furthermore, the different stages of the clinical routine provoked new challenges and prospects, such as diagnosis, detection, monitoring, and treatment. All these expository and motivating reasons and more, elucidate the necessitation to propose new tendencies to incorporate with medical imaging domain (interpretation, registration, fusion, analysis and reconstruction) to produce more precise and generic results.

Rueckert et al. stated in their manuscript that medical image analysis over the former decades has built upon model-based approaches where the underlying image segmentation or multi-modal images registration, has been expressed in terms of a well-defined mathematical model. The main difficulty with this approach is the definition of a suitable model that expressing the prior knowledge about the image analysis problem appropriately and put assumptions and constraints to put the solution space in the model parameters. Over the last years, this attracts significant interest to have data-driven models, since they present the preference that they can model variability of anatomy (both in terms of shape and appearance). They, therefore, represent some of the earliest approaches that use learning in the model construction which can be either statistical (e.g., active shape and appearance models) or probabilistic. The statistical and probabilistic models snag is that they often make simplifying assumptions (i.e. as an example, statistical models are often based on linear models such as principal component analysis while probabilistic models assume that the distributions that are used to model population variability can be sufficiently accurately modelled using Gaussian distributions). This limits the capability to grasp pathologies, and furthermore to model vast variability or heterogeneity in shape or appearance. An alternate, a powerful path is to model the shape and appearance of the anatomy via manifold learning, which is one of the recent trends good example that aim for a close integration of machine learning into the design of image analysis algorithms (Rueckert et al., 2016).

All previously stated algorithms are based on designing the relevant set of features as well as choosing the corresponding learning tool, which is mainly based on the expert knowledge and heuristics (Elnemr et al., 2016). As discussed in the introduction section, instead of trying to designate explicitly a model by hand in order to solve a medical image analysis problem, the idea is to implicitly learn the model directly from data.

Deep learning enables computational models that involve several processing layers to learn data representation with various levels of abstraction (Rueckert et al., 2016) (LeCun et al., 2015). In the coming subsections, this chapter presents how engagement with different deep learning architectural models

Table 1. Different deep learning architectures (summary and comparison)

Deep Network Architecture Name	Unsupervised pre-training	Labeled training data needed	Generative/ Discriminative	Biomedical Imaging Application	Notes, Pros, and Cons
Restricted Boltzmann Machines (RBMs)	Yes	No	Generative	• dimensionality reduction, • classification, • regression, • collaborative filtering, • feature learning and • topic modeling.	• Simplest Deep learning model • The basic building unit for the DBN and AE. • Ease of learning • Lacks total ability to combat the vanishing gradient • Static patterns
Deep belief Networks (DBN)	Helpful	Small Amount	Generative	• recognizing, • clustering • generating images, and • video sequences and motion capture data.	• Multi-layered RPM trained with energy minimizing method • More accurate representations of the data than RBMs. • Existence of classifier layer allows more to tackle the vanishing gradient problem. • Static patterns
Autoencoders (AE)	Helpful	Small Amount	Discriminative (Denoising encoders maps to generative models)	• labeling the resulting patterns, • dimensionality reduction, • image search, • image retrieval, • denoising, and • data reconstruction	• Many types exist SAEs, DAE, etc. • Learn compressed encodings through reconstruction error, minimizing the loss function. • More stable, consistent results • Static patterns
Convolution Neural Networks (CNNs)	No	Large amount	Discriminative	• Anomaly classification • Segmentation • Recognition • Photo search	• Utilize spatial and temporal relationship to reduce learning error • Large computational and memory resources • **Drawbacks of:** Overfitting and convergence issues • **Drawbacks Solved by:** Fine tuning, Regularization, Max-Norm constraints, Dropout (See Glossary) • Static patterns
Recurrent Neural Networks (RNN)	No	Large amount	Discriminative	• Predicting sequence of data, can be forecasting engine • **Future work from my point of view:** • Analysis of FMRI, • Perfusion Data Analysis and • Diffusion Tensor Imaging (DTI) Data Analysis	• Dynamic patterns, recurrent connections(feedback) • Memorizing past inputs • Structurally one of the simplest types of nets • **Drawbacks of:** Training them has proved to be problematic • **Drawbacks Solved by:** Gating, LSTM, gradient clipping, steeper gates, and better optimizers. GPUs are an essential tool for training an RNN to decrease the time of the analysis.

have spectacularly improved the state-of-the-art of medical imaging applications on 3D or 4D image data, etc., as example and not limited to:

- Medical image analysis and interpretation application (medical image denoising, cardiac image analysis for heart localization and parameter measurement, estimations & calculations);
- CAD systems application (computerized prognosis for AD and MCI, organ segmentation, and lesion detection);
- Medical image synthesis application (medical image reconstruction, brain circuits reconstructing, medical semantic imaging, and medical image estimation);
- Medical image labelling, annotation and retrieving application;
- Predicting the disease prognosis and risk assessment, and finally Biometrics.

Deep Learning and Medical Image Interpretation and Analysis

Medical Image Denoising

Different medical imaging modalities including X-rays, MRI, CT, US etc. are susceptible to noise. Recently, for proper image analysis, both manually and automatically, denoising is an essential preprocessing step in the medical imaging field, because of various reasons, different image acquisition techniques, and/or the trend to decrease the patient radiation exposure. As the dose amount of radiation decreases, the noise level increases. It is a challenge then to maintain good image quality while improving patient safety. Agostenelli et al. did experiments with adaptive multi column deep neural networks for image denoising, built using a combination of stacked sparse AE. This system proved to be robust against different types of noise (Agostinelli et al. 2013).

Owing to, the promising results of the models based on deep learning architectures, attraction goes to use these models in the medical image denoising application. Typical of medical image databases, for small sample sizes, (Gondara 2016) presented experimental proof that SDA, constructed using convolutional layers, performed well. Despite the need of very large training datasets for deep architecture models optimum performance. This work illustrated that deep learning techniques succeeded in recovering the signals, even during high levels of noise, at the limit where most triumphant denoising techniques would fail (Figure 17).

Their motivation based on the work proved: the outperforming of the AE in image denoising over the convolutional denoising methods, the less restrictive for specification of noise generative processes, and the performance of DAE constructed using convolutional layers to have a better image with the ability to exploit strong spatial correlations. (Gondara 2016) In their research, for future, they suggest investigating similar architectures on high resolution images and using other image denoising methods such as singular value decomposition (SVD) and median filters for image pre-processing before convolution DAE (CNN DAE), in hope of boosting denoising performance. (Gondara, 2016)

Cardiac Heart Localization and Parameters Measurements, Estimation, and Calculation_

Cardiovascular diseases remain one of the biggest cause of death worldwide. Early detection is the most important step to solve this problem. Firstly, different medical imaging modalities have shown its capa-

Figure 17. Denoising results on different datasets, top row shows real images with second row showing the noisier version ($\mu = 0$, $\sigma = 1$, $p = 0.1$), third row shows images denoised using CNN DAE and fourth row shows results of applying a median filter. Taken from (Gondara 2016).

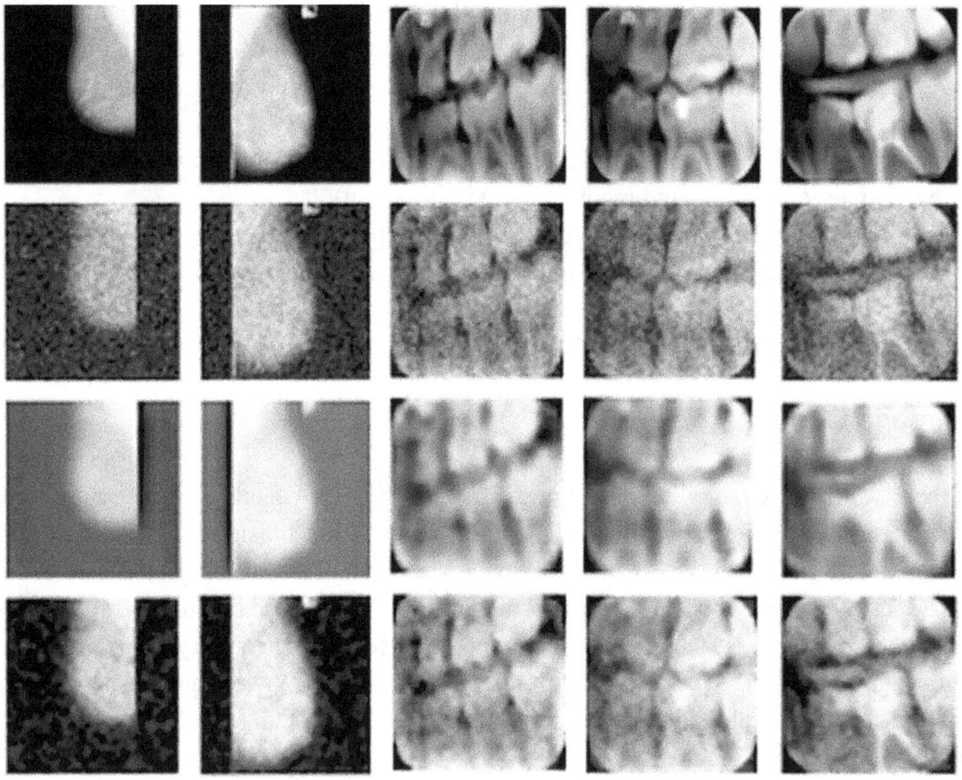

bility of imaging the heart with different parameters in different angles and views. (Shaker et al., 2014) presented a fully automated view classification of cardiac MRI images that uses the deep AE system for automatic feature extraction from a training dataset. This process is very important for medical image analysis, efficient content-based retrieval, as well as CAD systems. The automatic view classification for MRI is very challenging task, as the appearance of the images captured under the same view of the heart for the same patient and among different patients will always be subject to the vast variability in image appearance caused by variation of patient-specific geometry (physical characteristics of the entire body), heart deformations, and disease conditions. The most important task in classifying the images, based on its view application, is to define which features are to be extracted and whether it is based on local or global features or both of them. Major motivation, where the deep learning techniques for feature extraction are very useful to automatically determine a set of most relevant features that can be used in (Shaker et al., 2014).

One more essential step in the early diagnosis is evaluating the cardiac function by calculating many parameters such as ejection fraction (EF), left ventricle (LV) volume, and muscle wall thickness. Unfortunately, determining these volumes can take around 20 minutes for a skilled cardiologist to complete. Automating this process would free the cardiologist for more important tasks. (Hsin & Danner, 2016) proposed automatic method using a deep CNN model to efficiently estimate LV volume from a multiple time series of MRI images taken from different positions and angles through the heart. The best performing algorithms results of another big data challenge project (The Data Science Bowl, 2016), to automatically measure the cardiac function parameters, is dominated by the use of deep CNNs (de Bruijne, 2016). Yaniv Bar et al. applied a deep CNN trained by ImageNet and achieved an area under curve of 0.93, 0.79 and 0.89 for Right Pleural Effusion detection, Enlarged heart detection, and classification between healthy and abnormal chest x-ray, respectively (Bar et al., 2016). This indicates that deep learning techniques pre-trained from wide-ranging non-medical image datasets may provide satisfactory performance for the recognition of medical images. (Wang & Kong, 2016) predicts the end-systolic volume and end-diastolic volume using CNNs to extract features from 2D MRI images time series data and combine information from different axis views (the planes of slice).

Calculation of the heart parameters requires good localization of the whole heart region (ventricles and myocardium) (Mousa et al. 2014), in addition to a good segmentation to muscles and ventricles contours (Mousa et al. 2014) (Mousa et al. 2016). Previously in the literature, segmentation was manually implemented. Manual heart contour is an extremely hard task as it is time-consuming, tedious task, and highly affected by observer variability. Therefore, fully automatic segmentation is an important and challenging task due to the high datasets variability caused by scanners, motion artifacts, different noise sources, and poor contrast between LV and myocardium (Mousa et al. 2016). In the literature of cardiac localization and segmentation, (Carneiro et al. 2010) employs deep neural networks for LV segmentation in US images. (Emad et al. 2015) introduces a new fully automatic approach based on deep CNN to predict and localize the bounding box containing the LV in cardiac MRI in short axis views. In their proposed method they employed a six-layer CNN with different kernel sizes for feature extraction (Figure 18). They based their technique on exhaustive scanning of the input image searching for the LV at four different scales without having any prior knowledge about the position, the shape or the motion profile of the LV. Moreover, need not any prior knowledge or assumptions about neither

Figure 18. The output maps after convolution; First row: the input Image. the second row: The output map of the first convolution layer after applying the 3x3 filters, third row: The output map of second convolutional layer after applying the 6x6 filters on each output map from the previous layers. Taken from (Emad et al. 2015).

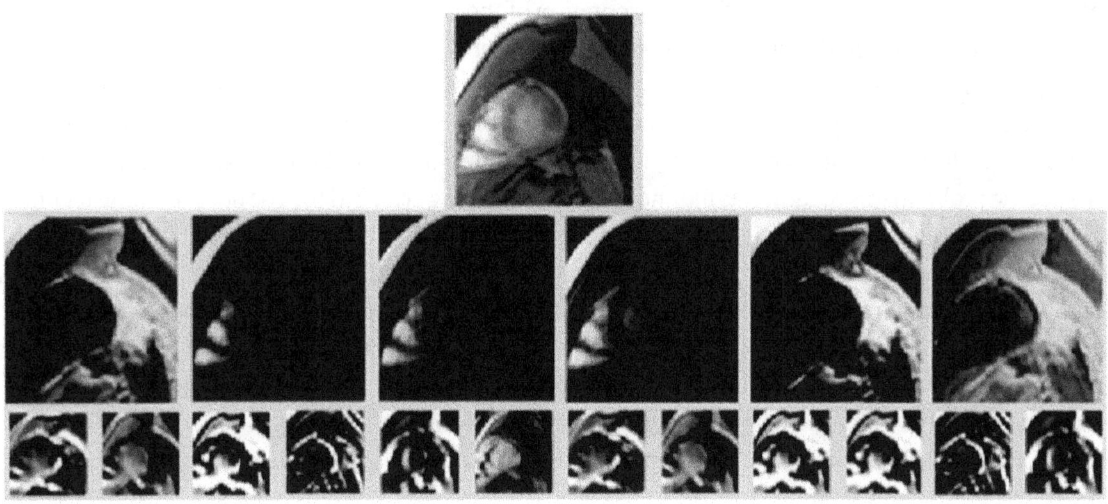

the complete time sequence nor the neighbor slices within the scanned volume. The article presents result with 98.66%, 83.91% and 99.07% for accuracy, sensitivity and specificity respectively, proving robustness of applying the deep learning on localization of the LV to huge variability of the heart shape and size, its positioning within the slice as well as contrast of the images, which are the main problems when applying other conventional (hand crafted) machine learning techniques. One limitation of their algorithm is the computation time (=10 sec/image). Though, they suggest reducing this by employing parallel processing and directed search (Emad et al., 2015).

Recently, (Narayan, 2016) trained a CNN to perform a CNN-based pixel-by-pixel semantic segmentation that combines pooling and upscaling layers on cardiac MRI images to identify the LV and leverage it to compute the volume of the ventricle throughout the course of a heartbeat and compared the results to a set of ground-truth contours. (Ngo et al., 2016) introduces a methodology that engages deep learning and level set for the automated segmentation of the LV of the heart from cardiac cine magnetic resonance (MR) data. In particular, level set methods are based on shape and appearance terms that use small training sets, but present limitations for modelling the visual object variations. Deep learning methods can model such variations using relatively small amounts of annotated training, but they often need to be regularized to produce good generalization. They suggest the combination of these methods in order to bring together the advantages of both approaches, producing a methodology that needs small training sets and produces accurate segmentation results. In (Narayan, 2016), a number of techniques are explored to improve CNN performance on cardiac medical image analysis especially in LV segmentation and cardiac function parameters measure applications. They found substantial improvements in performance at test time when introducing more variety in noisiness, lighting, and contrast to the cardiac MRI images. They presented improved results on both datasets used (The Data Science Bowl, 2016) by adding post-processing technique of taking the largest connected component and filling it in meaningfully to their CNN algorithm. In their article, they raise up a number of broader questions that would benefit from further research related to the use of the deep CNNs in cardiac MRI image analysis application. (Narayan, 2016)

Deep Learning and CAD Systems and Prognosis

CAD is a computerized procedure to provide a second opinion assistance after radiologists of medical image interpretation and diagnosis. The incorporation of the CAD in the diagnosing process can improve the performance of image diagnosis by decreasing inter-observer variation and providing the quantitative support for the clinical decision like biopsy and surgery recommendations, etc. (Cheng et al. 2016).

The conventional design of CAD is often composed of three main steps: feature extraction, feature selection, and classification. In most previous works, engineering on effective feature extraction step for each specific problem was regarded as the one of the most (Cheng et al. 2016). The deep learning techniques could potentially change the design paradigm of the CAD framework for several advantages over the old conventional frameworks. The advantages can be three-fold. First, deep learning can directly uncover features from the training data, and hence the effort of explicit elaboration on feature extraction can be significantly alleviated. The neuron-crafted features may compensate and even surpass the discriminative power of the conventional feature extraction methods. Second, feature interaction and hierarchy can be exploited jointly within the intrinsic deep architecture of a neural network. Consequently, the feature selection process will be significantly simplified. Third, the three steps of feature extraction, selection and supervised classification can be realized within the optimization of the same deep architecture. With such a design, the performance can be tuned more easily in a systematic fashion. (Cheng et al. 2016)

Alzheimer Disease (AD/MCI) CAD Systems and Prognosis

The AD, a progressive brain disorder and the most popular status of dementia in the late life, brings about the death of nerve cells and tissue loss throughout the brain, consequently diminution of the brain volume dramatically through time and affecting most of its functions (i.e. memory, and cognition). Figure 19 (a) shows that AD is sixth cause of death in US in 2015. The percentage changes in selected causes of death (all ages) between 2000 and 2015 Figure 19 (b), authors created this figure based on the data from the National Center of Health Statistics (Murphy et al., 2017). The prodromal stage of the AD is the MCI (Suk et al., 2015). Worldwide, nearly 44 million people are living with the AD. Furthermore, the estimated number of affected people will double for the next two decades, so that one out of 85 persons will have the AD by 2050 (Alzheimer's Association, 2014). There is a lot of neuroimaging modalities for diagnosis structural MRI, functional magnetic resonance imaging (fMRI), and PET. The latter is useful to extract features from, and then classification is done to differentiate between (AD, MCI, and normal control (NC)) groups. MRI images have been known as auspicious indicator for AD progression. Because the expenses of caring for the AD patients is predicted to rise spectacularly, the need of having a (CAD) system for early and precise AD diagnosis becomes crucial (Hosseini-Asl et al., 2016). Previous literature works for CAD systems based on considering simple and low features (i.e. GM tissue volumes from MRI images, the mean signal intensities from PET, the CSF measurement) as AD biomarkers for diagnosis.

Unfortunately, most of these CAD trails in the AD/MCI diagnosis and prognosis are vulnerable to noise and/or artifacts. Furthermore, the necessity for new models capable of discovering the hidden or latent high level information, thus give the attention to the deep architectures to serve efficiently in this application (Suk et al., 2014) (Suk et al., 2015) (Suk & Shen, 2015).

From the state of art, diagnosis of AD proved to be one of the success stories when deep learning is used. In (Gupta et al., 2013), an AE is first used to learn features from 2D patches extracted from either MRI scans for AD or natural images. The parameters of the AE are then used as filters of a convolutional layer for MRI data classification. Sergey and his colleagues work for applying deep neural networks to learn structural and functional brain imaging data and showing that deep learning methods are able to learn physiologically important representations and detect latent relations in neuroimaging data (Plis et al., 2014). In contrary to (Gupta et al., 2013), and to boost the classification performance, (Payan & Montana, 2015) proposed 3D convolutional neural network with softmax function and based on pre-training with SAEs (fine-tuning step). Based on Payan's algorithm, Figure 20 gives a summarization for the architecture of the neural network used for any 3-way classification. Their model proved to be a success in discriminating between healthy and diseased brains. However, their neural network model was too simple and they didn't go on to try more sophisticated neural network models (Hosseini-Asl et al., 2016).

Suk et al. used a three-layer SAE model to separately extract features: Gray matter (GM) tissue volumes from MRI, mean signal intensities from PET, and biological measures from cerebrospinal fluid (CSF) samples; for classifying between AD, MCI, NC with a multi-kernel SVM designed to learn the complementary information from multimodal data. Their results demonstrated accuracy rates of 98.8%, 90.7%, 83.7%, and 83.3% for AD/NC, MCI/NC, AD/MCI, and MCI-C/MCI-NC classification,

Figure 19. a) Top 10 causes of death in 2015, b) Percentage Changes in Selected Causes of Death (All Ages) Between 2000 and 2015. Created from data from the National Center for Health Statistics.

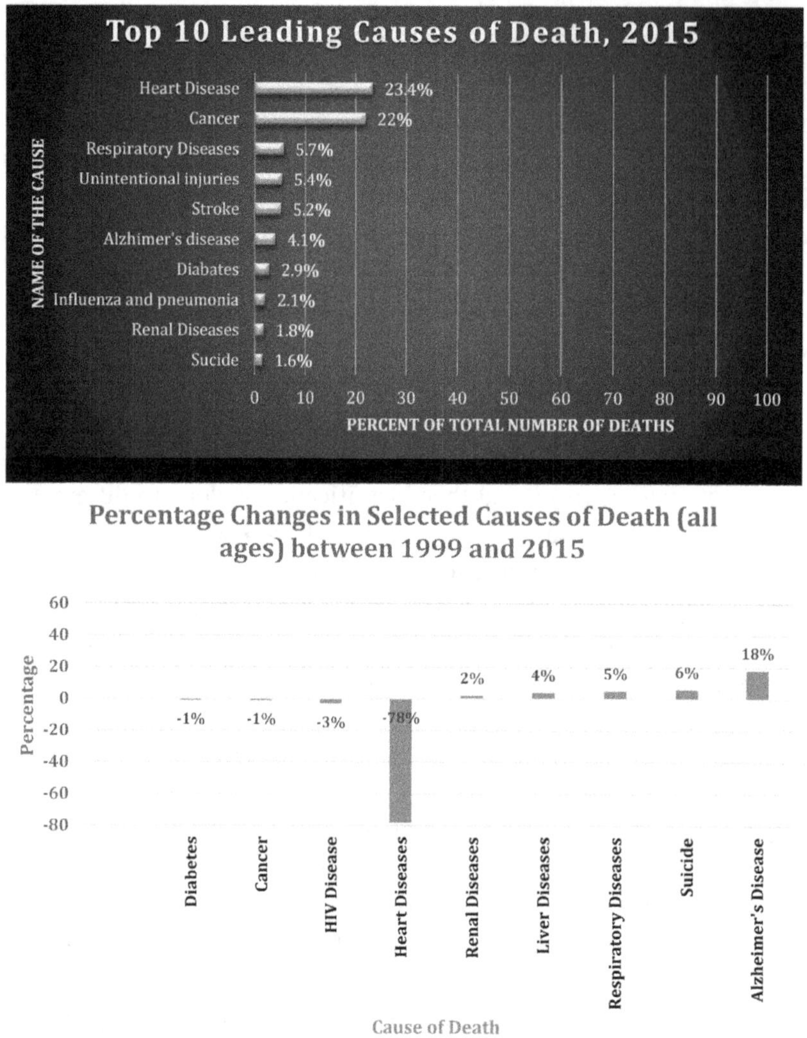

respectively, using the AD Neuroimaging Initiative (ADNI) dataset (Suk et al. 2014) (Suk et al. 2015). One of the cons of this study was that since multiple brain regions may be involved in the structural and functional changes due to AD, and that do not necessarily correspond to the user-defined region of interest (ROIs). Thus, the features extracted from such user-defined ROIs may not be able to reflect small or subtle but potentially important pathological changes. Provoked by this and subsequently (Suk & Shen 2015) joined 3D patches of PET and MRI images, and applied a patch based multimodal deep Boltzmann machine (BM) structure to acquire a common spatial feature characterization from the paired patches. (Brosch et al. 2016) reported accuracy rates of 95.35%, 85.67%, and 74.58% for AD/NC, MCI/NC, and MCI-C/MCI-NC classification, respectively.

Other investigation, Liu and Shen identified the ROI that may be associated with AD by applying deep CNN architecture on the raw MRI images. This preserves the effort spent for manual ROI annota-

Figure 20. Architecture of the neural network used for 3-way classification. V is determined according to the network design you planned, for binary classification, the output layer only will have two units.

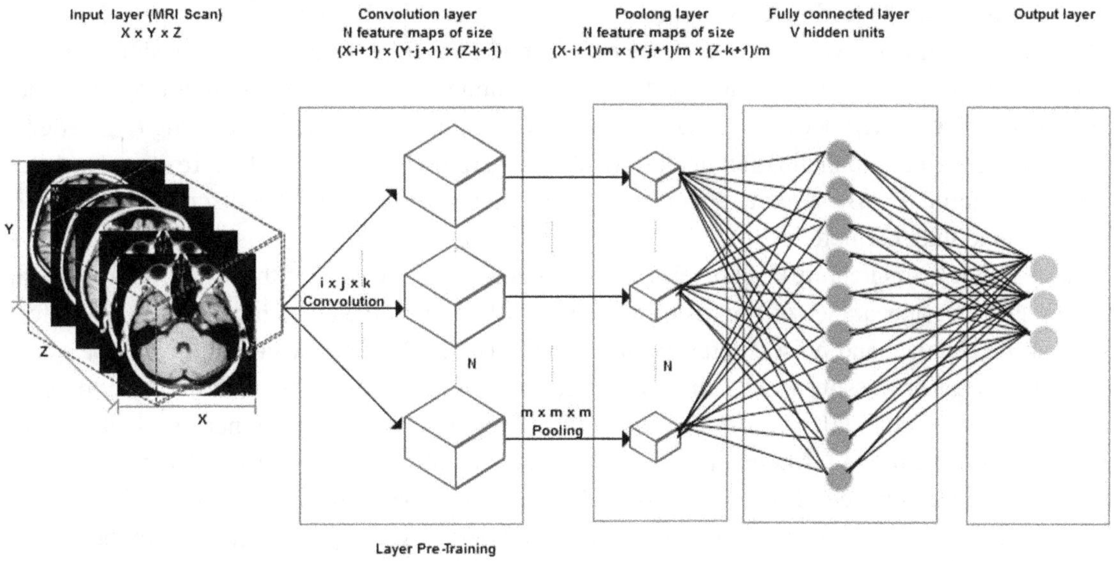

tion (Wang & Kong 2016) (Venugopal & Ramaswamy 2016). Later on, (Liu et al. 2016) investigated a deep learning architecture consisting of a SAE with a softmax output layer for performing four-class classification simultaneously for the following labels: AD, NC, MCI-C, and MCI-NC. They did extract 83 (ROI) from the MRI and PET scans and used multimodal fusion to create a set of features to train stacked layers of DAE. (Liu et al. 2016) (Brosch et al. 2016). Brebisson et al. constructed a deep CNN called SegNet for anatomical brain segmentation (Wang & Kong 2016). Very recently, (Hosseini-Asl et al. 2016) proposed AD diagnostic framework extracts features of a brain MRI with a source-domain-trained 3D-CAE and performs task-specific classification with a deeply supervised target-domain-adaptable 3D-CNN predict the AD on structural (anatomical) brain MRI scans than several other literature predictors.

Lesion Detection and CAD for Lung Nodules and Breast Lesions

The conventional CAD systems exist for the automatic lung nodules detection often produce too many false positives to be of use to oncologists. However, (Ramaswamy & Truong 2016) found that CNNs can successfully be used to classify candidate nodules, with relatively high sensitivity and very high specificity. Their research focused more on the task of lung nodule identification - or, more broadly, being able to classify specific lung scan images as either containing a nodule or not (Ramaswamy & Truong 2016). (Sun et al. 2016) tested the feasibility of using deep learning algorithms for lung cancer diagnosis with the cases from Lung Image Database Consortium (LIDC) database. Three deep learning techniques, CNN, DBN and SDA, were constructed and applied. A structure of 28 image features and an SVM were designed to compare the performance of a conventional CAD system with that of the deep learning techniques. The accuracies of CNN, DBNs, and SDA are 0.7976, 0.8119, and 0.7929, respectively; the accuracy of their designed traditional CAD is 0.7940, which is slightly lower than CNN and DBNs. They also noticed that the mislabeled nodules using DBNs are 4% larger than using traditional CAD and interpreted that as might be resulting from down sampling process losing some size information of the nodules (Sun et al. 2016). The discrimination of malignant/benign for tumors/lesions is considered one of the leading CAD applications. (Cheng et al. 2016) submitted an inclusive study on applying deep learning CAD to differentiate between malignant and benign nodules/lesions. This study illuminates the profits of deep learning methods in shunning the possible errors that may occur due to imprecise errors occurred because of inaccuracy in the results of the image processing (e.g., edge segmentation), as well as the inclination in classification emerging from a feeble feature set, as manifested in a lot of traditional CAD systems. Precisely, they employed the SDA for the discrimination of breast US lesions and lung CT nodules.

The SAE/SDA architectures had potentially the beneficial of addressing the issues of high variation in either shape or appearance of lesions/tumors. Meanwhile, with the advantages of automatic feature extraction mechanism and noise tolerance, the SDA-based CAD scheme can circumvent the potential inaccurate image processing results that could lead to unreliable features in the conventional CAD framework (Cheng et al. 2016). They compared their deep learning algorithm performance with other two popular conventional CAD methods developed specifically for the breast and lung applications, results showed that the deep learning based CAD can achieve better differentiation performance than the comparison methods across different modalities and diseases. The SDA algorithm outperforms the conventional CAD algorithms on both applications in terms of all six assessment used metrics. Additionally, the involvement of more member slices as training data can be very helpful to boost the performance of a deep learning CAD scheme, even if some of the training slices only partially depict the nodules of interest (Cheng et al. 2016).

Very recent accepted research (Kooi et al. 2017), have shown that a deep learning model in the form of a (CNN) trained on a large dataset of mammographic lesions (trained on a large dataset of around 45,000 images) outperforms a state-of-the-art system in (CAD) and therefore has great potential to advance the field of research. They stated a major advantage of the CNN learns from data and does not rely on domain experts, making development easier and faster. On top of this, they have compared the CNN to a group of three experienced readers on a patch level, two of which were certified radiologist and have shown that the human readers and CNN have similar performance (Kooi et al. 2017).

Deep Learning and Medical Images Segmentation Application

Image segmentation is a very important task for medical image analysis. Segmentation applications for medical images include finding important anatomical structures, locating tumors, measuring tissue volume etc. It helps radiologists in visualization and study of the anatomical structures, simulation of the biological processes, localization of pathologies, tracking the diseases, and evaluation of the necessity of radiotherapy or surgeries. Thus, a good segmentation is imperative for accurate quantitative analysis of the medical images and leads to better diagnosis and prognosis (Prasoon 2014) .

Hippocampus Segmentation

Hippocampus is a region in the human brain that is believed to be responsible for memory storage and recall. Damage to the hippocampus by lesions or neurodegenerative diseases such as AD could lead to memory deficits. A reduction in hippocampal volume measurement is a well-known biomarker for AD diagnosis. Several methods have been developed for automatic hippocampus segmentation in MRI images. However, segmentation accuracy is often limited due to the small size of the hippocampus and the complexity of surrounding structures.

Both researches, Wu et al. (2013), and Kim et al. (2013) proposed integrating an unsupervised deep learning architecture into a multi-atlas-based segmentation framework. The authors showed that the deep-learned hierarchical feature representation improved the segmentation accuracy by about 3–4% on overlap metrics over the methods using traditional hand-crafted features in the same segmentation framework (Kim et al. 2013) (Brosch et al. 2016).

(Lai 2015) used the hippocampus segmentation problem (classify each voxel in an MRI Image as non-hippocampus, left hippocampus, or right hippocampus) to evaluate different deep learning techniques for patch-based segmentation uses the ADNI hippocampus MRI dataset as an example. This thesis examined four deep learning approaches: unconventional "stacked 2D", simple 2D patches, "tri-planar", and a full 3D convolutional architecture. Unconventional "stacked 2D" approach offers superior classification results than simple 2D patches without involving considerably additional processing power. The "tri-planar" approach yields a much better classification performance than the 2D approaches, with a reasonable increase in the computational demands. A full 3D convolutional architecture costs a very significant increase in computational power despite the best results. (Lai 2015)

Infant Hippocampus and Brain Segmentation

During the first year of postnatal human brain development, the brain tissues grow quickly, and the cognitive and motor functions undergo a wide range of development. The segmentation of infant brain tissues into white matter (WM), GM, and CSF is of great importance for studying early brain development in health and disease. In addition, the hippocampus segmentation, the part believed to be responsible for human memory and learning function, helps understanding the development of the infant's brain. (Guo et al. 2014) investigated using a two-layer SAE to learn the features for segmenting the hippocampus from infant T1- and T2-weighted (T1w and T2w) brain MRI images (Figure 21). The deep-learned features were used to measure inter-patch similarity for sparse patch matching in a multi-atlas-based segmentation framework, and demonstrated an improvement of 4–8% in Dice similarity over features based on intensity, Haar wavelet, histogram of oriented gradients (HOG) and local gradient patterns (Guo et al. 2014) (Brosch et al. 2016).

Additionally, in studying early brain development in health and disease, segmenting infant brain images is a more challenging task than in the adult brain because infant WM and GM exhibit similar intensity levels in both T1w and T2w MRI images. (Zhang et al. 2015) proposed employing a deep CNN to perform segmentation of brain tissues on T1w, T2w, and fractional anisotropy (FA) DTI images. They trained a three-layer CNN using approximately 10,000 local patches extracted from all voxels in a training set of 10 brain images. The cross-entropy loss functional between the predicted and ground truth labels, and a three-way softmax layer were used to generate a posterior distribution over the three class labels (Brosch et al. 2016). (Zhang et al. 2015) results showed that the proposed model significantly outperformed prior methods on infant brain tissue segmentation. Overall, their experiments demonstrated that CNNs could produce more quantitative and accurate computational modeling and results on infant tissue image segmentation.

Figure 21. Typical hippocampus probability maps and segmentation results for 2-week-old to 9- month-old brain images, produced by three different methods. Red contours indicate the manual ground-truth segmentations, and blue contours indicate the automatic segmentation. Taken from (Guo et al. 2014).

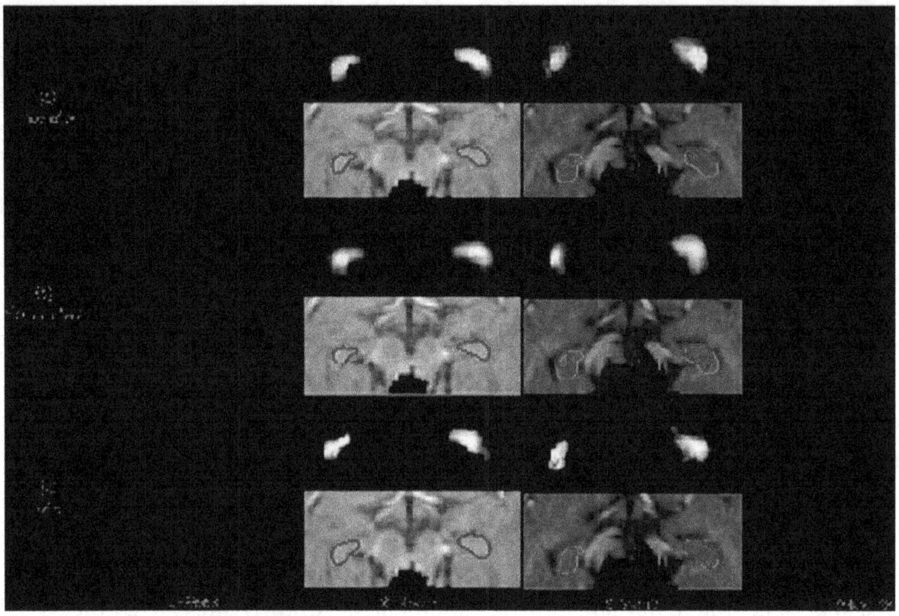

Brain Tumor Segmentation

Automatic segmentation of brain tumors is a challenging problem because the tumors can appear randomly in the brain and have any kind of shape, size, and contrast. Since 2014, there is an increase in the use of neural networks applied to brain tumor and lesion segmentation. Notable mentions are the MICCAI's brain tumor segmentation challenge (BRATS) in 2014 and 2015 and the ISLES challenge in 2015 where the top performing methods were taking use of convolutional neural networks (Havaei, Guizard, et al. 2016). In view of the fact that the input images have high dimensions, the obtainment of a reliable ground truth is very hard (that way the unsupervised learning became more important), and the required high precision for clinical practicality, the brain lesions segmentation became a valuable search application. (Havaei, Davy, et al. 2016) proposed a fully automatic brain tumor segmentation method based on deep CNNs. The proposed method was designed to detect both low-and high-grade glioblastomas (the most common and aggressive cancer that begins within the brain) seen in MRI scans. The proposed deep CNNs learn contextual features at different scales and are fully convolutional, in contrast to traditional CNNs whose final layers are typically fully connected and therefore much more computationally demanding. In brain tumor segmentation, the training samples are highly unbalanced in that the healthy voxels comprise a large percentage of the total brain voxels. The authors tackled this problem by introducing a sequential training procedure in which the model was first trained with unbalanced training data using randomly sampled voxels, and then the top layers of the model were trained with balanced samples that contained the same number of tumor and healthy voxels. (Havaei, Davy, et al. 2016) (Brosch et al. 2016)

(Yoo et al. 2014) were the first to propose an automated feature learning approach for multiple sclerosis lesion segmentation. In this method, uniformly spaced and non-overlapping 3D patches at two scales were extracted from co-registered T2w images and Proton density weighted (PDw) images. Unsupervised feature learning was applied to the T2w and PDw images separately, using a basic architecture of a single RBM for the smaller patches and a two-layer DBN for the larger patches, for each image type. This study established that automatic feature discovery with deep learning is a viable alternative to user preselection of features for WM lesion segmentation (Yoo et al. 2014). The computational demands of deep learning methods have largely restricted the size of the input images, and subdivision into patches has been the most popular workaround for processing larger images such as MRI volumes. For WM lesion segmentation, a patch-based strategy can even have some benefits such as the ability to selectively sample more representative regions (Brosch et al. 2016). However, most patch-based methods are inefficient in that they perform many redundant computations in the overlapping regions of neighboring patches. Some methods have been proposed for speeding up patch-based approaches, (Brosch et al. 2016) presented the convolutional encoder networks, 3D fully convoluted networks (FCN), to process the entire MRI volumes for WM segmentation. By processing entire MRI volumes instead of patches, the algorithm avoids redundant calculations, and therefore could scale up more efficiently with image resolution. Overall, the FCN approach applied to full MRI volumes can be seen as a promising alternative to patch-based methods, especially where computational efficiency is a concern (Brosch et al. 2016).

Deep Learning, Medical Image Synthesis and Registration

Estimating CT Images From MRI Images

CT plays an important role in many clinical applications, e.g., planning for radiotherapy treatment (dose calculation) and correcting the PET attenuation. However, patients are exposed to radiation during the imaging process, this radiation may have harmful effects on the patients. Opposed to CT, MRI is inoffensive and does not comprise any radiation. Therefore, there is a great motivation recently to predict CT image of a particular subject from its MRI, to plan for the radiation treatment. It is technically difficult to directly estimate CT image from MRI image. As displayed in Figure 22, CT and MRI have diverse manifestations. For example, in CT image, the intensity difference between the prostate and bladder is much smaller than that in MRI image. Recently, estimating one model image from other image modality can be done by:

1. The first category is the atlas-based method. However, the performance of these atlas-based methods highly depends on the registration accuracy.
2. The second category is the conventional learning-based method, thus, the performance of these methods is bound to the quality of the feature extraction.
3. The deep learning methods, specifically the CNN becomes popular in both computer vision and medical imaging fields.

As a multilayer and fully trainable model, the CNN is able to capture the complex non-linear mapping from the input space to the output space (Dong Nie et al. 2016) Yet, the direct application of 2D CNN for 3D medical images processing is unconscionable because 2D CNN treats the image aspect slice by slice, hence discontinuous prediction possibly occurs across slices. To tackle this subject, 3D CNNs have been suggested to speculate the absent PET image from the MRI of the same patient in (Liu et al. 2016) research. (Dong Nie et al. 2016)

(Dong Nie et al. 2016) proposed to learn the non-linear mapping from MRI to CT images through a 3D FCN, which is a variation of the conventional CNN. Compared to CNN, FCN generates the structured output, which can better preserve the neighborhood information in the predicted CT image. Specifically, an input MRI image is first partitioned into overlapping patches. For each patch, FCN is used to predict the corresponding CT patch. Finally, all predicted CT patches are merged into a single CT image by averaging the intensities of overlapping CT regions. they evaluated their method on a real pelvic CT/MRI dataset, demonstrating that the FCN deep method can effectively predict CT image from MRI image, and also outperforms three state-of-the-art methods under the comparison as shown in Figure 23. (Dong Nie et al. 2016)

7T MRI Image From 3T MRI Image

The exceptional 7 Tesla (7T) MRI scanners support images that hold anatomy of higher resolution than 3T MRI scanners, hence expediting the diagnostic of brain diseases in early stages. Due to the accessibility of the 3T MRI scanners and the less accessibility of the 7T MRI scanners, (Bahrami et al. 2016)

Figure 22. A pair of corresponding pelvic MR (left) and CT (right) images from the same subject. Taken from (Dong Nie et al. 2016).

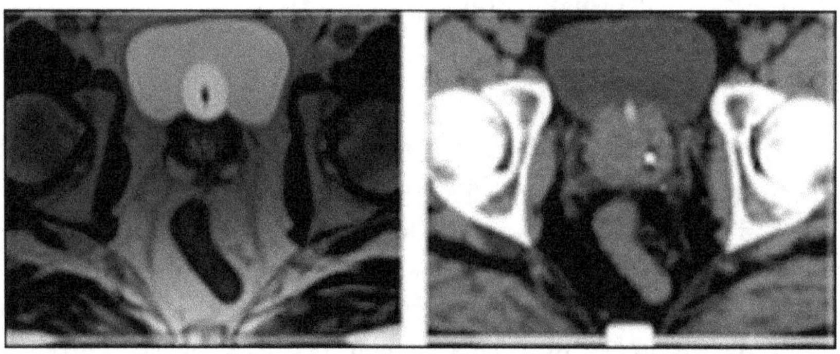

Figure 23. Visual comparison of original MRI images, the estimated CT images by our method and the ground truth CT images on 2 subjects. Taken from (Dong Nie et al. 2016).

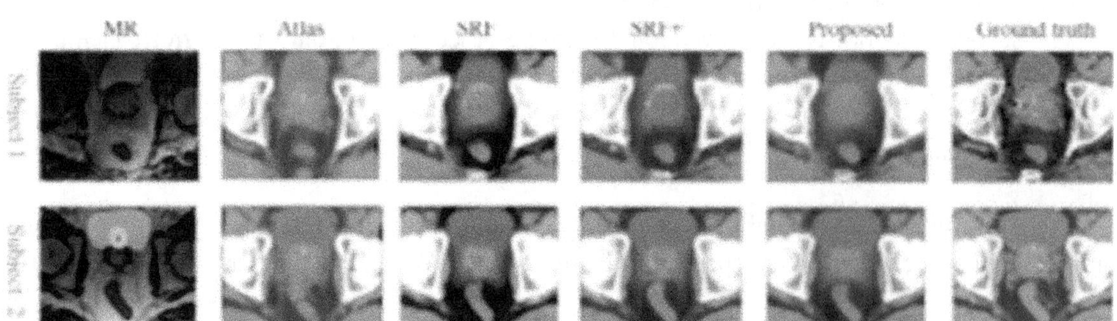

is motivated to utilize 3T MRI to reconstruct 7T-like images. (Bahrami et al. 2016) proposed a deep CNN architecture to reconstruct 7T MRI from 3T MRI using both anatomical and intensity features. The training step is carried out by feeding and training the CNN with the appearance and anatomical characteristics of the 3T patch. This generates the intensity of the center voxel in the equivalent 7T patch. The testing step, on the other hand, aims to map each participant 3T patch to the corresponding 7T-like patch. Their performance is evaluated on 15 subjects, each with both 3T and 7T MRI images. Both visual and numerical results show that the deep CNN method outperforms the comparison methods. (Bahrami et al. 2016)

Registration

The image registration is the process of transforming different sets of data into one coordinate system. Images may be coming from different modalities, or different subjects, different slices or frames. Registration is necessary in order to be able to compare or integrate the data obtained from these different measurements.

Feature selection is a critical step in deformable image registration. Particularly, by selecting the best distinctive features that precisely and succinctly characterize the complex image patches structure, the correspondence detection is improved. This, in turn, enhances the accuracy of the image registration. Moreover, the fast-evolving for imaging modalities, to achieve superior identification for the structural changes in medical imaging, stimulated the development of a method for deformable image registration that scales well to new image modalities or new image applications with little to no human intervention would have a significant impact on the medical image analysis community (Wu et al. 2014)(Wu et al. 2015). To address these concerns, (Wu et al. 2014) (Wu et al. 2015) proposed an unsupervised learning-based image registration framework that uses deep learning trained, using no ground-truth data, to discover compact and highly discriminative features upon observed imaging data. The suggested feature selection technique exploits a convolutional SAE to represent the intrinsic deep features in image patches. Accordingly, the feature representations may be learned directly from the perceived imaging data in a short while. Thus, the feature selection technique becomes more flexible to the incoming imaging modalities. Using two different neuroimaging datasets, they compared their deep learning image registration method demonstrated better dice ratio scores compared to other two existing state-of-the-art deformable image registration methods that use handcrafted features, see Figure 24. (Wu et al. 2014) (Wu et al. 2015).

Deep Learning Medical Image Labelling, Annotation, and Retrieval

Image Retrieval

In a Content-Based Image Retrieval (CBIR) system, learning of effective feature representations and similarity measures is very important for the retrieval performance (Singh 2015). In the recent past, the advancement in medical imaging modalities and technologies has led to the production of digital medical images and cheap large medical image repositories. The size of medical image collections has increased rapidly due to this. To tackle this rapid growth it is required to develop image retrieval systems which operates on a large scale, aiming to build a robust system that creates, manages and queries medical image databases in an accurate manner (Singh 2015). (Zhang & Metaxas 2016) advocates that the scale of image retrieval systems should be significantly increased at which interactive systems can

Figure 24. Typical registration results on 7.0-Tesla MR brain images. Three rows represent three different slices in (a) the template, (b) subject, and (c) Hand-crafted-features registration based results, (d) Deep learning registration based results. Taken from (Wu et al. 2015).

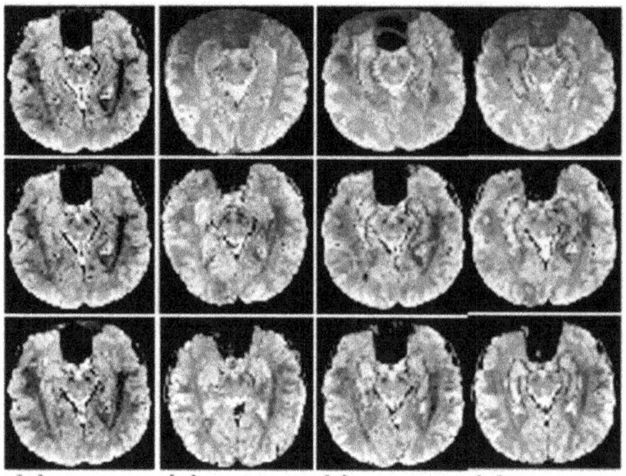

be effective for knowledge discovery in potentially large databases of medical images. Medical image retrieval is one of the few computational components that cover a broad range of tasks, including image manipulation, image management, and image integration. The goal of medical image retrieval is to find the most clinically relevant images in response to specific information needs represented as search queries (Cao et al. 2015).

While substantial amount of research has been conducted in the area of medical image retrieval, real-world tools and applications that can access the medical image data by their content are rare in clinical practice. One of the major barriers (Cao et al. 2015) have identified is that the semantic gap exists between the low-level features (e.g., low-level visual and textual features) and the high-level medical concepts. The key to addressing these issues is to develop new semantic meaningful features from multimodal information to bridge the semantic gap and to enable effective and efficient CBIR. (Cao et al. 2015) developed a new multimodal medical image retrieval approach based on the recent advances in the statistical graphic model and deep learning. They suggest correlating multimodal information (e.g., text and image) or to use the combinations of textual and visual analysis techniques for more effective and efficient CBIR. In addition, they developed a new deep BM based multimodal learning model to learn the joint density model from multimodal information in order to derive the missing modality. This research was tested on a large number of actual medical images. The results indicate that the proposed method is an encouraging solution for indexing and retrieving the new generations of medical imaging technology (Cao et al. 2015).

In other work, (Anavi et al. 2015) utilized the strength of deep learning approaches in a wide range of chest-related diseases and in addition they explored categorization of healthy versus pathology which is an important screening task. Deep learning methods are most effective when applied on large training sets. However, since such large data are generally not available in the medical domain, they explored the feasibility of using a deep learning approach based on non-medical learning (large scale real- life and non-medical image database (ImageNet)). They also applied a feature selection technique to the deep learning representations and show that it can improve the performance of their task (Anavi et al. 2015).

Using deep learning CNN approaches based on non-medical learning, (Bar et al. 2016) illustrated the feasibility of revealing the pathology in chest x-rays by prospecting the extracted features from the CNN layers alongside a set of traditional features, including GIST features descriptor and bag-of-words. The classification results are recorded for each feature set in addition to the fusion of features. Finally, they performed feature selection on the collection of features to show the most informative feature set for the task. Results of 0.78-0.95 accuracy for various pathologies are shown on a dataset of more than 600 radiographs. Owing to the recent progress in feature extraction techniques and classification methods, the CBIR results have been enormously improved. Nevertheless, bearing in mind the growing approachability of imaging for medical big data, decreasing the memory demands along with the computational costs for CBIR systems have become an essential need (Çamlica et al. 2015). In this regard, (Çamlica et al. 2015), proposed a different approach to data reduction. Motivated by the fact that in medical image analysis usually a certain ROI is in focus of user evaluation, they proposed to eliminate some image patches (rectangular blocks) from feature extraction process. This leads to the reduction of both memory requirements and computational expense of the retrieval task.

Deep Learning Disease Prognosis and Risk Assessment (Outcome Prediction)

Brain Tumor Survival Time

High-grade glioma is the most aggressive and severe brain tumor that prompts demise of just about 50% patients in 1–2 years. Thus, the accurate prognosis for glioma patients would provide essential guidelines for their treatment planning. Generally, traditional survival prediction employs clinical information as well as restricted handcrafted features obtained from the MRI images. This task is usually time-consuming, arduous and subjective. (D. Nie et al. 2016) submitted a 3D deep learning framework for predicting the (long or short) overall survival (OS) time for brain gliomas patients, based on automatically extracting deep learned features from multi-modal preoperative brain images (i.e., T1 MRI, fMRI and DTI) of high-grade glioma patients (see Figure 25). The extracted features are then fused together and fed into a binary SVM classifier to predict if the patient has a long or short OS time. Exploratory outcomes demonstrate that their methods can accomplish an accuracy as high as 89.9%, they also find that the learned features from fMRI and DTI play more important roles in anticipating the OS time accurately, which affords valuable deep insights into the functional applications to neuro-oncological. (D. Nie et al. 2016)

Biological Age Estimation

The development of individuals' physical maturation, which is indicated as biological age (BA) estimation in literature, is considered a requisite issue in clinical applications for discovering the endocrinological diseases in adolescents or for optimally planning the time-point for surgical interventions of the pediatrics orthopedic, e.g. for correcting the discrepancy in leg-length. (Stern et al. 2016)

In this work, (Stern et al. 2016) proposed the use of deep CNN for automatic BA estimation from hand MRI volumes comprises of indistinguishable per-bone stage estimation blocks, roused by the way radiologists outwardly perform age estimation using established staging schemes that follow physical maturation. They did fusion of independent age scores from each bone in their CNN by connecting the outputs of all Stage estimation blocks in a fully connected layer in order to achieve a continuous BA prediction (Figure 26). In the results they showed outperforming results the literature automatic BA

Figure 25. The flow chart for their survival prediction system. Updated from (D. Nie et al. 2016)

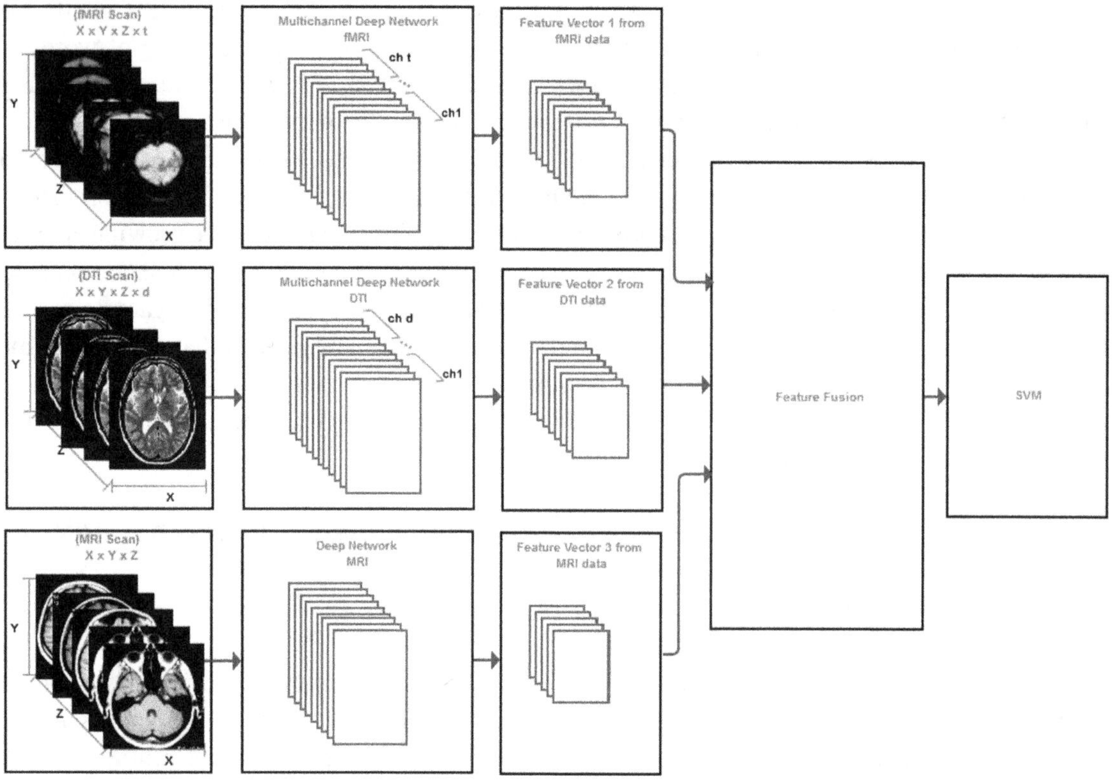

estimation method, achieving a mean error amongst assessed and ground truth BA of 0.36 ± 0.30 years, which is consistent with radiologists performing visual BA speculation.

Deep Learning Hyperspectral Medical Image Analysis

Hyperspectral imaging (HSI), also named imaging spectrometer, stimulated from remote sensing that has been investigated for several applications. HSI is an imaging modality that procures two-dimensional images over numerous electromagnetic spectrum wavelengths generating a hyperspectral image cube (hypercube). Hyperspectral image analysis normally incorporates preprocessing, feature extraction, feature selection, as well as classification or unmixing (Lu and Fei 2014). Notwithstanding that hyperspectral image analysis techniques have been explored exhaustively in remote sensing domain, their application and progression in the medical area still fall behind. The contribution of the spectral features for biomedical applications is not well comprehended and needs more investigations.

Recently, HSI has been auspiciously implemented in medical applications, it provides prominent potency for diagnosing noninvasive disease as well as surgical guidance.

Hypercube that comprises high spectral and spatial resolutions likely hold additional diagnostic information. Nevertheless, the high dimensionality of the spatial and spectral resolutions swells the computational cost for automatic hyperspectral image analysis. Therefore, there is an urge to develop sophisticated hyperspectral image analysis techniques.

Figure 26. Stern et al. CNN architecture. Each stage estimation block performs dimensionality reduction and extracts age relevant features from cropped 3D bone volumes. By feeding feature outputs into a fully connected layer, age estimation is performed. Red arrows indicate weight sharing among SE blocks. Updated from (Stern et al. 2016).

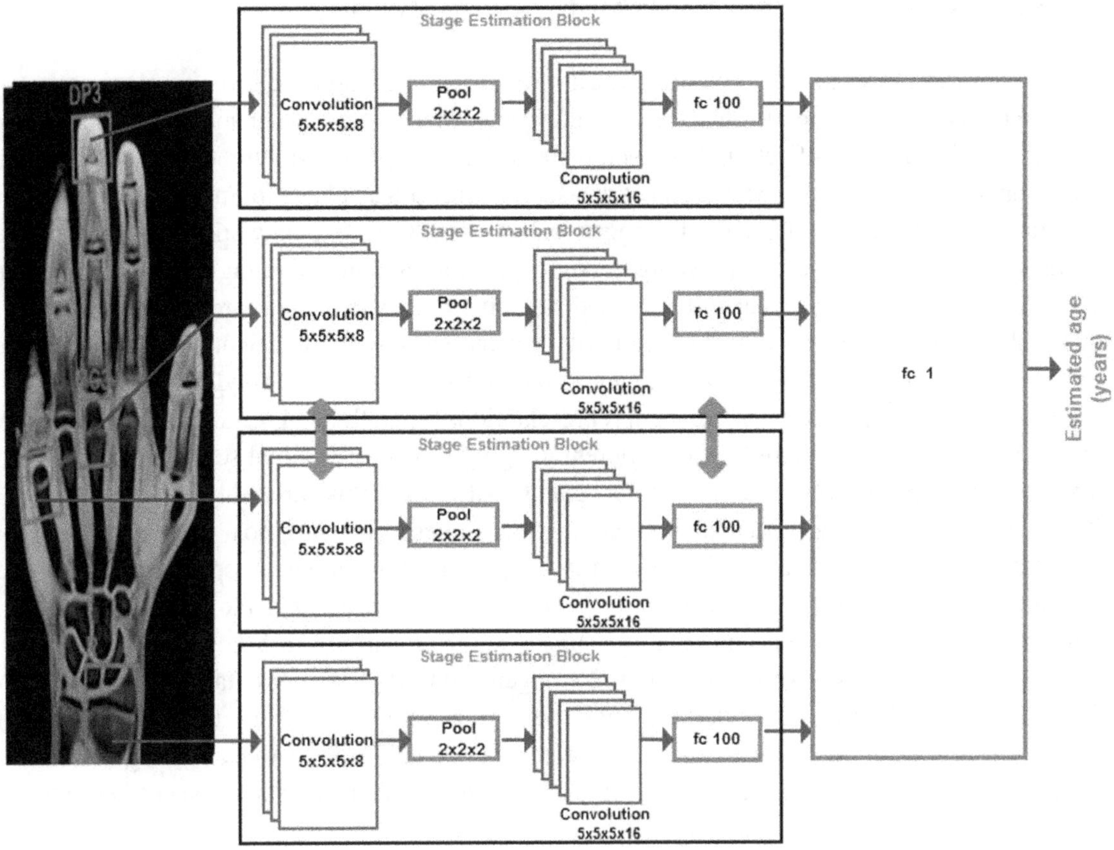

Medical HSI aims to benefit from the fact that biological tissue causes multiple scattering for the delivered light based on its biological structure inhomogeneity, while the absorption mainly occurs in melanin, hemoglobin, and water (Costas et al. 2011). (Costas et al. 2011) presumed that the scattering, fluorescence and absorption characteristics of tissue differ during the evolution of the disease. Accordingly, variations in the disease status should generate corresponding variations in the patterns of the reflected light from the tissue. Since each pixel holds much spectral information, this makes it conceivable to realize the interaction of light with pathology more completely. Furthermore, the spectral signatures of the pixels within the images allows HSI to predict different pathological conditions.

(Halicek et al. 2017) demonstrated that deep learning may be effectively applied for tissue classification after constructing the appropriate architecture. They developed a method to classify normal and cancerous head and neck tissue using deep CNN, which is fully trained on HSI of tissue specimens. The CNN architecture, illustrated in Figure 27, involves six convolutional layers as well as three fully connected layers. The final layer produces a pixel probability to determine its associated class. Several experiments are achieved and validated, the results demonstrate that the proposed deep learning tissue classification framework has a promising performance, near real-time tissue tagging and also outperforms some conventional machine learning techniques.

FUTURE RESEARCH CHALLENGES AND DIRECTIONS

Deep learning works exceptionally well when you have a lot of information and have complex connections that you want to model or approximate. Deep learning is considered as a popular and powerful strategy in pattern recognition and classification. However, there are not many deep structured applications used in medical imaging diagnosis area, because large dataset is not always available for medical images. Therefore, future research faced with major challenges including (a) Can deep networks be used effectively for medical tasks, and are researchers asking the right questions and investigating the right tasks? (b) Is transfer learning from general imagery to the medical domain relevant, do researchers need to work on getting real Big Data for each medical task, or will transfer learning be sufficient? (c) Can researchers rely on learned features alone or may researchers combine them with handcrafted features for the task? (d) Are researchers using strong enough input representations (e.g., 2D vs 3D). Additionally, in practice the available data is often acquired with a different imaging protocol, different scanner model, or from different patient population how can researchers gain benefits from this variability?

There are risks associated with applying learning techniques as a "black box" to perform diagnosis and risk assessment. A flexible learning system in a high-dimensional feature space can carry on out of the blue and this can be hard to distinguish. When derived biomarkers demonstrate great distinctness between disease groups, it is tempting to assume that they must therefore, be good at detecting the underlying signs of disease. Notwithstanding, contingent upon the training data, diagnosis decisions could well be driven not by signs of disease, but by signs of a confounding factor that is correlated with disease status in the training set. Due to these issues, it is not sufficient to know that a given learning approach has excellent performance on a given dataset. The researchers should mean to comprehend

Figure 27. Flowchart of the data processing and deep learning architecture. The spectral signatures from 5×5 blocks extracted from the hypercube are reformatted into 10 × 10 spectral patches. The CNN trained on the spectral patches consisted of six convolutional layers (height, width, and filter numbers are shown) and three fully connected layers (number of neurons in the layer are shown). Taken from (Halicek et al. 2017).

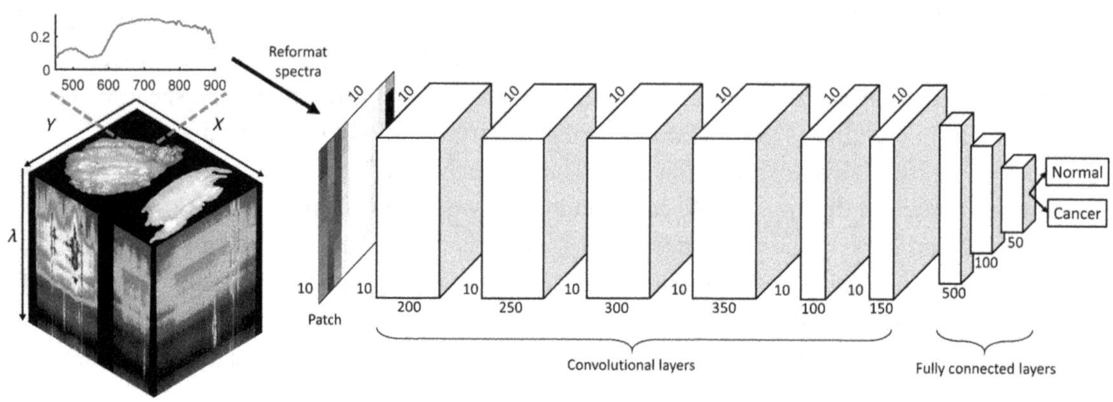

what features drive the decisions and what are the corresponding pitfalls. Generalization performance depends firmly on the size of the training set in relation to the complexity of the representation and learning model, and it is in this way amazing most papers in the field only show a single point on a learning curve when comparing techniques. It would be more informative to show not just average performance on a specific training set, yet in addition, learning curves visualizing performance as a function of the amount of training data as well as examples of cases in which the algorithm fails. (de Bruijne 2016)

Additionally, the main challenge of the HSI field is the high-dimensionality, the significant increase in the spectral bands may cause the curse of dimensionality, which may lead to decrease in classification performance. Furthermore, the HSI is particularly complex in two aspects: high level of data redundancy because of the high correlation between adjacent spectral bands, and the disparities of the hyperspectral signatures.

The suggested future work is directed for four scopes. Enhancing the deep learning techniques regarding learning structures, accuracy and speed, as well as increasing their capabilities and applications. The following points of research are suggested for future work in order to face many existing challenges in the medical field:

- Breakthrough results in using deep learning on computer vision were obtained on the ImageNet Large Scale Visual Recognition Challenge (ILSVRC) based on the ImageNET dataset (http://www.image-net.org/). This dataset is very large compared to most of the training and test datasets used in the medical papers (millions versus 100's or 1000's). From the literature review, the chapter authors can conclude that the medical image analysis community could likely benefit strongly if similarly, large publicly available medical image datasets were constructed. This is a challenging task for many reasons: Firstly, it is difficult to obtain funding for the construction of such datasets. Secondly, scarce and expensive medical expertise is needed for high quality annotation of medical imaging data. Thirdly, privacy issues make it more difficult to share medical data than natural images. Fourthly, the breadth of applications in medical imaging requires that many different datasets need to be collected.
- A portion of the representations are inspired by progresses in neuroscience and are loosely based on interpretation of information processing and communication patterns in the nervous system such as neural coding which attempts to define the relationship between various stimuli and associated neuronal responses in the brain. More understanding, as well as with continued and determined research efforts to develop new learning algorithms and architectures for deep neural networks, would enrich the medical imaging analysis field.
- Fusing different hybrid deep learning architectures, as well as the combination of the learned features with the handcrafted features for the task is shown to be beneficial, but need more investigation, optimization, and development of techniques to limit the calculation time provide valuable research topics.
- Mining of multimodal medical data (X-ray, MRI, CT, echo videos, time series data, text) would be useful, this state of art paper suggests a future direction to Multimodal fusion deep learning, Multiprotocol fusion deep learning, Multi-Data fusion deep learning.
- HSI is an arising technology that needs further extensive studies and investigations, which necessitate consolidating more HSI data for patients, analyzing the influence of dimensionality reduction, and exploring more network models structures and weights initialization methods to optimize the classification performance and enhance the generalizability.

CONCLUSION

For Several medical imaging analysis applications, extracting robust and discriminative features from medical image is the most difficult yet the most critical step. Feature extraction procedures are broadly employed in many areas such as pattern recognition, machine learning and data mining. Features should be easily computed, robust, rotationally invariant, and obtuse to different contortions and variations in the images. Most existing machine learning techniques are using handcraft features that need expert engineering to extract. Deep learning is the new trend to extract and abstract these features from the unsupervised data automatically. This manuscript provides a comprehensive survey on the state of art on various deep learning architectural models. Several typical and advanced approaches of deep learning application on medical images are explored, discussed and evaluated. It is worth be noted that deep learning can have a large impact on medical image analysis applications such as computer diagnosis, image segmentation, image reconstruction, image annotation and retrieval, image registration and multimodal image analysis.

REFERENCES

Agostinelli, F., Anderson, M. R., & Lee, H. (2013). *Adaptive Multi-Column Deep Neural Networks with Application to Robust Image Denoising*. NIPS. Available at http://papers.nips.cc/paper/5030-adaptive-multi-column-deep-neural-networks-with-application-to-robust-image-denoising.pdf

Alpaydın, E. (2012). *Introduction to machine learning.* The MIT Press.

Alzheimer's Association. (2014). Alzheimer's Disease Facts and Figures. *Alzheimer's & Dementia, 10*(2), 1–80. PMID:23871765

Anavi, Y. (2015). A Comparative Study for Chest Radiograph Image Retrieval Using Binary, Texture and Deep Learning Classification. *Proceedings of the 37th Annual International Conference of the IEEE Engineering in Medicine and Biology Society*, 2940–2943. 10.1109/EMBC.2015.7319008

Anavi, Y. (2016). *Visualizing and enhancing a deep learning framework using patients age and gender for chest x-ray image retrieval.* Available at: http://proceedings.spiedigitallibrary.org/proceeding.aspx?doi=10.1117/12.2217587

Arel, I., Rose, D. C., & Karnowski, T. P. (2010). Deep Machine Learning - A New Frontier in Artificial Intelligence Research. *IEEE Computational Intelligence Magazine, 5*(4), 13–18. doi:10.1109/MCI.2010.938364

Bahrami, K. (2016). Convolutional Neural Network for Reconstruction of 7T-like Images from 3T MRI Using Appearance and Anatomical Features. In *Deep Learning and Data Labeling for Medical Applications: First International Workshop, LABELS 2016, and Second International Workshop, DLMIA 2016, Held in Conjunction with MICCAI 2016, Athens, Greece, October 21, 2016, Proceedings*. Cham: Springer International Publishing. 10.1007/978-3-319-46976-8_5

Bar, Y. (2016). Chest pathology identification using deep feature selection with non-medical training. *Computer Methods in Biomechanics and Biomedical Engineering. Imaging & Visualization*, 1–5. Available at http://www.tandfonline.com/doi/full/10.1080/21681163.2016.1138324

Bengio, Y., Courville, A., & Vincent, P. (2009). *Learning Deep Architectures for AI*, Bengio, Y., Courville, A. & Vincent, P., 2012. Representation Learning: A Review and New Perspectives. *IEEE Transactions on Pattern Analysis and Machine Intelligence*, *35*(8), 1798–1828. doi:10.1109/TPAMI.2013.50 PMID:23787338

Brosch, T. (2016). Deep learning of brain images and its application to multiple sclerosis. In G. Wu, D. Shen, & M. R. Sabuncu (Eds.), *Machine Learning and Medical Imaging* (pp. 69–96). Elsevier. doi:10.1016/B978-0-12-804076-8.00003-7

Çamlica, Z., Tizhoosh, H. R., & Khalvati, F. (2015). Autoencoding the retrieval relevance of medical images. *5th International Conference on Image Processing, Theory, Tools and Applications 2015, IPTA 2015*, 550–555. 10.1109/IPTA.2015.7367208

Cao, Y. (2015). Medical Image Retrieval: A Multimodal Approach. *Computational Advances in Cancer Informatics*, *13*(S3), 125–136. PMID:26309389

Carneiro, G., Nascimento, J. C., & Freitas, A. (2010). *Robust left ventricle segmentation from ultrasound data using deep neu- ral networks and efficient search methods*. Isbi. Available at http://ieeexplore.ieee.org/xpls/abs_all.jsp?arnumber=5490181

Caswell, I., Shen, C., & Wang, L. (2016). *Loopy Neural Nets: Imitating Feedback Loops in the Human Brain*. Stanford.

Cheng, J.-Z. (2016). *Computer-Aided Diagnosis with Deep Learning Architecture: Applications to Breast Lesions in US Images and Pulmonary Nodules in CT Scans*. Nature Publishing Group. Available at: http://www.pubmedcentral.nih.gov/articlerender.fcgi?artid=4832199&tool=pmcentrez&rendertype=abstract

Ciresan, D. (2012). *Deep Neural Networks Segment Neuronal Membranes in Electron Microscopy Images*. Nips. Available at https://papers.nips.cc/paper/4741-deep-neural-networks-segment-neuronal-membranes-in-electron-microscopy-images.pdf

de Bruijne, M. (2016). Machine learning approaches in medical image analysis: From detection to diagnosis. *Medical Image Analysis*, *33*, 94–97. doi:10.1016/j.media.2016.06.032 PMID:27481324

Deeplearning4j Development Team. (2016). *Deeplearning4j: Open-source distributed deep learning for the JVM*. Apache Software Foundation License 2.0. Available at: http://deeplearning4j.org

Dmitrievich, I. A. (2015). *Deep Learning in information analysis of electrocardiogram signals for disease diagnostics* (Diss.). Moscow Institute of Physics and Technology.

Elnemr, H. A., Zayed, N. M., & Fakhreldein, M. A. (2016). Feature Extraction Techniques: Fundamental Concepts and Survey. Handbook of Research on Emerging Perspectives in Intelligent Pattern Recognition, Analysis, and Image Processing, 264–294.

Emad, O., Yassine, I. A., & Fahmy, A. S. (2015). Automatic Localization of the Left Ventricle in Cardiac MRI Images Using Deep Learning. *37th Annual International Conference of the IEEE Engineering in Medicine & Biology Society (EMBC)*, 683–686. 10.1109/EMBC.2015.7318454

Gondara, L. (2016). *Medical image denoising using convolutional denoising autoencoders*. Available at: http://arxiv.org/abs/1608.04667

Goodfellow, I., Bengio, Y., & Courville, A. (2016). *Deep Learning*. Available at: http://www.deeplearningbook.org

Graves, A., Fernandez, S., & Schmidhuber, J. (2007). *Multi-Dimensional Recurrent Neural Networks*. Available at: http://arxiv.org/abs/0705.2011

Graves, A., Mohamed, A., & Hinton, G. (2013). Speech Recognition with Deep Recurrent Neural Networks. *IEEE International Conference on acoustics, speech and signal processing*, 3, 6645–6649. 10.1109/ICASSP.2013.6638947

Greenspan, H. (2016). *Special Section on Deep Learning in Medical Applications*. Available at: http://www.ieee-tmi.org/deep-learning-in-medical-applications.pdf

Greenspan, H., van Ginneken, B., & Summers, R. M. (2016). Guest Editorial Deep Learning in Medical Imaging : Overview and Future Promise of an Exciting New Technique. *IEEE Transactions on Medical Imaging*, *35*(5), 1153–1159. doi:10.1109/TMI.2016.2553401

Guo, Y. (2014). Segmenting Hippocampus from Infant Brains by Sparse Patch Matching with Deep-Learned Features. *Medical Image Computing and Computer-Assisted Intervention. MICCAI 2014: 17th International Conference, Boston, MA, USA, September 14-18, 2014, Proceedings*, 308–315. 10.1007/978-3-319-10470-6_39

Gupta, A., Ayhan, M. S., & Maida, A. S. (2013). Natural Image Bases to Represent Neuroimaging Data. *Journal of Machine Learning Research: Workshop and Conference Proceedings*, *28*(3), 977–984.

Havaei, M., Davy, A., Warde-Farley, D., Biard, A., Courville, A., Bengio, Y., ... Larochelle, H. (2016). Brain tumor segmentation with Deep Neural Networks. *Medical Image Analysis*, *35*, 18–31. doi:10.1016/j.media.2016.05.004 PMID:27310171

Havaei, M., & Guizard, N. (2016). *Deep learning trends for focal brain pathology segmentation in MRI*. Available at: http://arxiv.org/abs/1607.05258

Hinton, G. (2014). Where do features come from? *Cognitive Science*, *38*(6), 1078–1101. doi:10.1111/cogs.12049 PMID:23800216

Hinton, G., Bengio, Y., & Lecun, Y. (2015). *Deep Learning tutorial*. Nips.

Hinton, G. E., Osindero, S., & Teh, Y.-W. W. (2006). A Fast Learning Algorithm for Deep Belief Nets. *Neural Computation*, *18*(7), 1527–1554. doi:10.1162/neco.2006.18.7.1527 PMID:16764513

Hosseini-Asl, E., Keynto, R., & El-Baz, A. (2016). *Alzheimer's Disease Diagnostics by Adaptation of 3D Convolutional Network*. Available at: http://arxiv.org/abs/1607.00455

Hsin, C., & Danner, C. (2016). *Convolutional Neural Networks for Left Ventricle Volume Estimation*. Academic Press.

Kim, M., Wu, G., & Shen, D. (2013). Unsupervised deep learning for hippocampus segmentation in 7.0 Tesla MR images. *Lecture Notes in Computer Science*, *8184*, 1–8.

Kooi, T., Litjens, G., van Ginneken, B., Gubern-Mérida, A., Sánchez, C. I., Mann, R., ... Karssemeijer, N. (2017). Large scale deep learning for computer aided detection of mammographic lesions. *Medical Image Analysis*, *35*, 303–312. doi:10.1016/j.media.2016.07.007 PMID:27497072

Lai, M. (2015). *Deep Learning for Medical Image Segmentation*. Available at: http://arxiv.org/abs/1505.02000

Le, Q. V. (2014). *A Tutorial on Deep Learning Part 1: Nonlinear Classifiers and The Backpropagation Algorithm*. Tutorial.

LeCun, Y., Bengio, Y., & Hinton, G. (2015). Deep learning. *Nature*, *521*(7553), 436–444. doi:10.1038/nature14539 PMID:26017442

Liu, W., Zheng, W.-L., & Lu, B.-L. (2016). *Multimodal Emotion Recognition Using Multimodal Deep Learning*. Available at: http://arxiv.org/abs/1602.08225

Min, S., Lee, B., & Yoon, S. (2016). Deep learning in bioinformatics. *Briefings in Bioinformatics*. doi:10.1093/bib/bbw068 PMID:27473064

Mnistdatasetiterator, A. (2006). *Tutorial : Deep-Belief Networks*. Academic Press.

Mousa, D., Zayed, N., & Yassine, I. A. (2014). Automatic cardiac MRI localization method. *Proceedings of the 7th Cairo International Biomedical Engineering Conference, CIBEC 2014*, 153–157. 10.1109/CIBEC.2014.7020942

Mousa, D., Zayed, N., & Yassine, I. A. (2016). Factors Affecting the Segmentation of the Heart Ventricles in Short Axis Cardiac Perfusion MRI Images. *International Journal of Computers and Technology*, *15*(11), 7218–7226. doi:10.24297/ijct.v15i11.4376

Murphy, S.L. (2017). National Vital Statistics Reports - Deaths: Final Data for 2007. *National Vital Statistics Reports - Deaths: Final Data for 2015*, *66*(6).

Narayan, T. (2016). *Automated Left Ventricle Segmentation in Cardiac MRIs using Convolutional Neural Networks*. Deep Learning.

Ng, A. (2015). *Deep Learning Tutorial.* University of Stanford. Available at: http://ufldl.stanford.edu/tutorial/supervised/ConvolutionalNeuralNetwork/

Ngo, T. A., Lu, Z., & Carneiro, G. (2016). Combining deep learning and level set for the automated segmentation of the left ventricle of the heart from cardiac cine magnetic resonance. *Medical Image Analysis*, *35*, 159–171. doi:10.1016/j.media.2016.05.009 PMID:27423113

Nie, D. (2016). 3D Deep Learning for Multi-modal Imaging-guided Survival Time Prediction of Brain Tumor Patients. In *Medical Image Computing and Computer-Assisted Intervention MICCAI'2016* (pp. 212–220). Springer. doi:10.1007/978-3-319-46723-8_25

Nie, D. (2016). Estimating CT Image from MRI Data Using 3D Fully Convolutional Networks. In *Deep Learning and Data Labeling for Medical Applications: First International Workshop, LABELS 2016, and Second International Workshop, DLMIA 2016, Held in Conjunction with MICCAI 2016, Athens, Greece, October 21, 2016, Proceedings*. Cham: Springer International Publishing. 10.1007/978-3-319-46976-8_18

Payan, A., & Montana, G. (2015). *Predicting Alzheimer's disease: a neuroimaging study with 3D convolutional neural networks*. Miccai.

Plis, S.M. (2014). Deep learning for neuroimaging: A validation study. *Frontiers in Neuroscience*, *8*, 1–11.

Prasoon, A. (2014). *Deep Feature Learning and Cascaded Classifier for Large Scale Data Segmenting Cartilage in Knee MRIs*. University of Copenhagen.

Ramaswamy, S., & Truong, K. (2016). *Pulmonary Nodule Classification with Convolutional Neural Networks*. Academic Press.

Rueckert, D., Glocker, B., & Kainz, B. (2016). Learning clinically useful information from images: Past, present and future. *Medical Image Analysis*, *33*, 1339–1351.

Sahiner, B., Heang-Ping Chan, Petrick, N., Datong Wei, Helvie, M. A., Adler, D. D., & Goodsitt, M. M. (1996). Classification of mass and normal breast tissue: A convolution neural network classifier with spatial domain and texture images. *IEEE Transactions on Medical Imaging*, *15*(5), 598–610. doi:10.1109/42.538937 PMID:18215941

Schmidhuber, J. (2015). Deep Learning in neural networks: An overview. *Neural Networks*, *61*, 85–117. doi:10.1016/j.neunet.2014.09.003 PMID:25462637

Shaker, M. S. (2014). Cardiac MRI View Classification using Autoencoder. *7th Cairo International Biomedical Engineering Conference*, 125–128.

Singh, A. V. (2015). *Content-Based Image Retrieval using Deep Learning*. New York: B. Thomas Golisano College of Computing and Information Sciences Rochester Institute of Technology Rochester.

Stern, D. (2016). *Medical Image Computing and Computer-Assisted Intervention – MICCAI 2016*. Cham: Springer International Publishing. Available at http://link.springer.com/10.1007/978-3-319-46723-8

Suk, H. & Shen, D. (2015). Learning in Diagnosis of Brain Disorders. In S.-W. Lee, H. H. Bülthoff, & K.-R. Müller (Eds.), *Recent Progress in Brain and Cognitive Engineering*. Springer. Available at: http://link.springer.com/10.1007/978-94-017-7239-6

Suk, H., Lee, S.-W., & Shen, D. (2015). Latent feature representation with stacked auto-encoder for AD/MCI diagnosis. *Brain Structure & Function*, *220*(2), 841–859. doi:10.100700429-013-0687-3 PMID:24363140

Suk, H.-I. I., Lee, S.-W., & Shen, D. (2014). Hierarchical Feature Representation and Multimodal Fusion with Deep Learning for AD/MCI Diagnosis. *NeuroImage*, *101*(2), 569–582. doi:10.1016/j.neuroimage.2014.06.077 PMID:25042445

Sun, W., Zheng, B., & Qian, W. (2016). Computer aided lung cancer diagnosis with deep learning algorithms. In *SPIE Medical Imaging* (pp. 1–8). SPIE. Available at http://proceedings.spiedigitallibrary.org/proceeding.aspx?doi=10.1117/12.2216307

The Data Science Bowl. (2016). *Transforming How We Diagnose Heart Disease*. Available at: https://www.kaggle.com/c/second-annual-data-science-bowl

Turner, J. T. (2014). *Deep Belief Networks used on High Resolution Multichannel Electroencephalography Data for Seizure Detection. In AAAI Spring Symposium Series* (pp. 75–81). Bengio. Available at http://www.aaai.org/ocs/index.php/SSS/SSS14/paper/viewPDFInterstitial/7747/7787

Venugopal, V. & Ramaswamy, S. (2016). *DeepMD: Transforming How We Diagnose Heart Disease Using Convolutional Neural Networks*. Academic Press.

Wang, K., & Kong, Y. (2016). *Diagnosis of Heart Disease via CNNs*. Available at: https://books.google.de/books?id=ms2oBgAAQBAJ

Wu, G., Kim, M. W., Qian, G., Yaozong, L. S., & Shen, D. (2014). *Unsupervised Deep Feature Learning for Deformable Registration of MR Brain Images*. Academic Press.

Wu, G., Kim, M., Wang, Q., Munsell, B. C., & Shen, D. (2015). Scalable High-Performance Image Registration Framework by Unsupervised Deep Feature Representations Learning. *IEEE Transactions on Biomedical Engineering*, *63*(7), 1505–1516. doi:10.1109/TBME.2015.2496253 PMID:26552069

Yoo, Y. (2014). *Deep Learning of Image Features from Unlabeled Data for Multiple Sclerosis Lesion Segmentation*. Mlmi. doi:10.1007/978-3-319-10581-9_15

Zhang, S., & Metaxas, D. (2016). Large-Scale medical image analytics: Recent methodologies, applications and Future directions. *Medical Image Analysis*, *33*, 98–101. doi:10.1016/j.media.2016.06.010 PMID:27503077

Zhang, W., Li, R., Deng, H., Wang, L., Lin, W., Ji, S., & Shen, D. (2015). Deep convolutional neural networks for multi-modality isointense infant brain image segmentation. *NeuroImage*, *108*, 214–224. doi:10.1016/j.neuroimage.2014.12.061 PMID:25562829

Chapter 6
Medi-Rings for Senior Citizens:
Distributed EMR System

Siva Sankar Yellampalli
UTL Technologies Ltd., India

N. Ravi Kiran
UTL Technologies Ltd., India

Ishwar Malapur
UTL Technologies Ltd., India

ABSTRACT

In this chapter, the authors propose Medi-Ring, a compact system to carry all the medical records for senior citizens to avoid improper medication, delay in treatment in emergency situation. The three main aspects of Medi-Ring are NFC technology, system memory, and a controller. NFC technology is used for transferring the data, the system memory is used to store the medical records which includes patient's details, doctor's prescription, and all other medical details. A controller is used to control the whole system. As the proposed Medi-Ring is wearable, compact, and flexible, it can be used as a medical companion for senior citizens.

INTRODUCTION

Mostly in medical emergency, a patient can be treated with a proper medication if and only if the previous medical records of the patient are available. In developing countries such as India such records are not accessible during medical emergency because of the lack of infrastructure. In western countries, several Electronic Medical Record [EMR] options such as object storage systems, compliance WORM storage, IBM's Hippocratic databases etc [Hasan R.,2007] are available to maintain the medical records where the data is loaded into a centralized network. EMR is a real time transaction processing database for clinical patient information [Hasan R.,2007]. EMR is a record in digital format which requires resources such as internet to synchronize with central network and needs technical persons to maintain it. In developing countries such as India, medical records are mostly handwritten. Handwritten paper medical

DOI: 10.4018/978-1-5225-7071-4.ch006

records have their own set of advantages and disadvantages. The main advantages are that they are very cost effective, gives more leeway for the doctor to represent the symptoms in form of diagrams etc for easy understanding, to increase speed of diagnosis common elements can be typed and can have boxes for selecting etc [Hasan R.,2007]. Along with the advantages they have disadvantages such as storage problems, accessibility issues, fragmentation of manual medical records if the patient visits different Doctors for multiple aliments, difficulty in transfer of medical records from one hospital to another and also manual records can be associated with poor legibility which can contribute medical errors [Boumstein, J. 2013]. In India medical records in most of the hospitals are manual in nature. 50% of medical records in India are unusable or partly usable as they are not properly stored or the handwriting of the medical practitioner is not legible. As mentioned in article of Times of India, World Health Organization lists India among the top 10 killers in the world due to medical errors. While a British National Health system survey in 2009 reported that 15% of its patients were misdiagnosed [Malatha Iyer, 2011].

Due to the manual medical records, during medical emergency, patients in India have to be taken to the same hospital for treatment. If patient is taken to another hospital, physician or doctor will have no access to patient's previous medical records leading to re-simulate all the treatments which consumes lifesaving minutes. To overcome the problems associated with manual medical records, some hospitals have migrated to electronic medical records to serve patients better. Some of the challenges faced by the hospitals in India due to electronic medical records are high installation cost, need for reliable internet facility, and need for uninterrupted power supply [Hasan R.,2007]. Due to high patient to doctor ration in India EMR implementation which requires a centralized network, becomes very expensive in terms of cost of installation. In addition to this EMR are associated with another problem –data security. An article from NDTV gadgets beta, "Your medical Record is worth more to hackers than your credit card", The FBI warned health care providers to guard against cyber-attacks after one of largest U.S hospital operators, community Health system Inc., said Chinese Hackers had broken into its computer network and Stolen the personal information of 4.5 million patients[Reuters,2014]. This article clearly states that the centralized networks are more prone to security threats and very expensive for implementation. To address the problems discussed, the medical records can be stored locally than global, which can be accomplished with a wearable gadget "Medi-Ring". As every person in his life has to visit the hospital for a regular check-up, each time it is required to carry necessary report or previous check-up report. There may be chance that some patients may forget to carry reports and some may have lost the report. In such case the patient as well as doctor will face a problem, and this may insist them to take another check-up which will be burden to the patient. So in order to avoid such problems, proposed medi-ring, which can store the file and transfer the files to other system.

BACKGROUND

In historical convention, keeping medical files and medical prescriptions throughout the India was manual and medical records in papers and some books. There are many disadvantages of keeping the records in manual format- large storage area, maintenance, retrieval, legibility of practitioner's hand writing etc. The retrieval system is complex as the index has to be maintained separately for ease of access. Maintenance is difficulty as the records have to be regularly inspected and protected from termites, moisture, water seepage etc. To overcome these problems many hospitals are converting their manual records into computerized patient records and storing them in the digital form. The records are stored according to the patient ID. Depending on the ID of the patient they will retrieve the data or medical files from the computer. The main disadvantage is anyone with patient ID can retrieve the information and modify the doctor's prescription or the data can be stolen and used for illegal activities. To secure computerized medical records additional security features have to be incorporated in the system such as access by only authorized personal, have a closed loop system so that external hacks can be stopped etc. In legal proceedings, it is doctor's duty to produce documents and prove the documents are not altered. For computerized records if they are not maintained with sufficient security measures it would be difficult to ascertain in the court of any proceeding that the records are not tampered with. The confidentiality of the documents should not be broken by doctor or any hospital personal as important documents or medical records of the patient such as endoscopic video, Electro cardio gram data, EEG data, etc are stored in the online system. The documents can be secured in computer and it should not share without patient biometric, even though doctor should not see documents without the patient. This can be done implementing biometric for security.

There are many court decision results are available in India, for sharing the patient details those are

1. National commission has told that if there any negligence in the submitting the patient details and medical records to the court, action to be taken on the on the hospital. [Kanaiyalal Ramanlal,1996]
2. If any patient or relatives of the patient asks for the report, the doctor should not give the report if any case held on the patient. The Bombay high court verdict. [Raghunath Raheja,1996], if any case is not there on patient, doctor has to give the patient details.
3. Hospitals and doctors are guilty if they are not produced the patient records and details to the court. [Kanaiyalal Ramanlal,1996]
4. It is the duty of the doctor to keep the record until the patient case id is disposed. [Thomas, J. 2009]

The Figure 1 shows the Medical record room in various Indian hospitals, in some hospitals they will not maintain the record room all the records are given to patient itself.

Due to the various security concerns related to Electronic Medical Records and the effort that should go into safeguarding the records which are stored in a centralized location as shown in Figure 2, we are proposing a Medi-ring where the data would be personalized and the data can be accessed only in the presence of the patient. This technique will also help in avoiding the complex infrastructure set up that is needed to store all the medical records at a centralized location. Medi-ring also addresses the concern of availability of medical records at the time of emergency as the records would be carried by the patient in person. It is very helpful in emergency and doctor can check the previous medical reports using a Medi-ring read out device. The proposed solution, Medi-ring is suitable in India as the hospitals are still in the process of setting up EMR solutions. Medi-ring solution would save investment to the hospitals for setting up a centralized data storage system and in a developing country that money can be used for providing better medical facilities to the patients. The schematic of the proposed Medi-ring is shown in figure 3

Our proposed system contains memory, communication device and controller to control whole system.

Figure 1. Medical record room

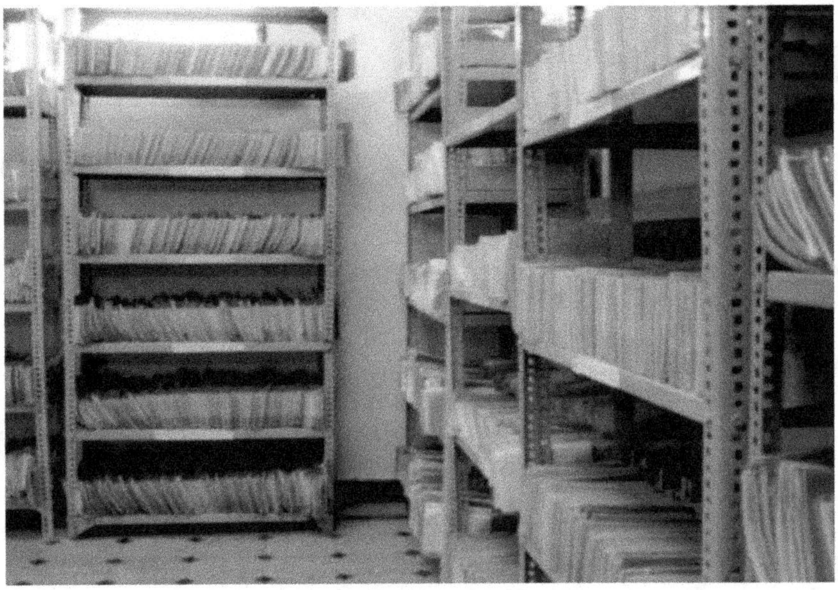

Figure 2. Digital-centralized medical reports accessing from server

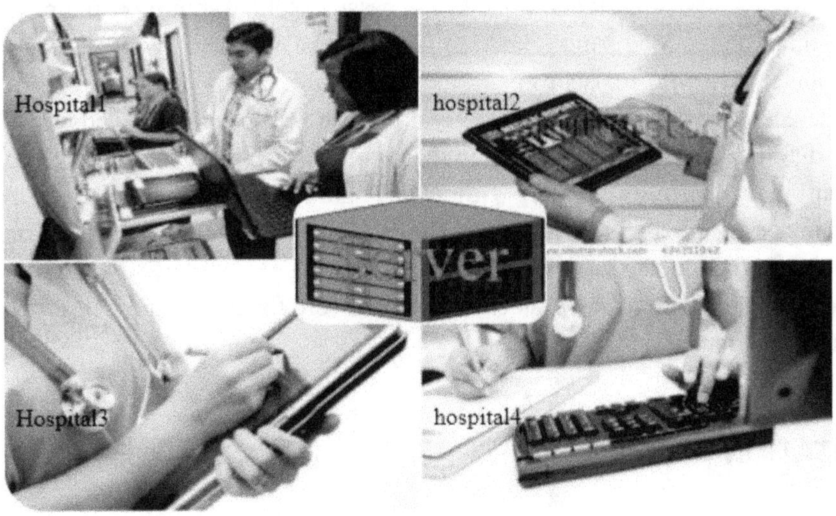

WORKING PRINCIPAL AND OPERATION

The NFC based Medi-ring consist of NFC Transceiver, SD card or Flash memory and controller. The prescriptions and other medical records such as BP reports, CT scan, blood reports etc given by the physician are loaded into this system with peer to peer communication through the SPI interface [SPI Block Guide v3.06, 2003]. The various reports are classified based on date and type of report for easy accessibility. The patient can have separate passwords for access to different folders so unauthorized access can be minimize, for example pharmacist can only look at the prescription and not at other medi-

Figure 3. Shows the proposed system

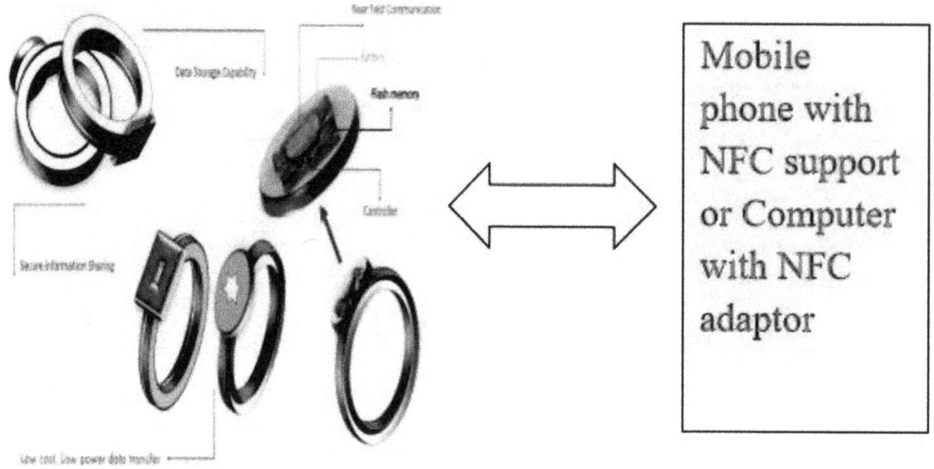

cal reports. The data can be transferred from any android application based system or desktop system. The data (text file or any other compatible formats) is loaded into flash memory via SPI interface. The conceptual diagram of a physician accessing previous records and loading the new record is shown in figure 4. The loaded data is stored in flash memory until the next data loaded with authenticated password. The Medi-ring has been designed to be in the passive state to minimize the power consumption and to avoid a battery in the Medi-ring. The Medi-ring will be activated by magnetic induction when it is brought in contact with NFC transceiver.

When this device power ups, the data stored inside flash memory is retrieved back. Figure 5 shows the conceptual diagram of Pharmacist receiving the records from an NFC receiver. The patient can get the exact precautionary pharmacy and drug without any hard copy or any centralized networks even during the emergency condition. Figure 6 illustrates the concept of a patient with medi-rings in emergency condition where data is extracted via NFC receiver.

The date stored in mediring can be protected with password for access and it is not prone for hacking as it is not connected to internet.

IMPLEMENTATION

The goal of the project is to prototype the proposed medi-ring system, which is used for a medical purpose. The system can be easily justified with the transfer of data through NFC between the smartphones.

More number of options are available to design a ring, in this project we have to transfer a file, receive a file, from & to memory. Three components are required to build this model as shown in block diagram of medi-ring in Figure 7.

1. Transceiver module to transmit and to receive the data.
2. SD (secured digital) card to store the data.
3. A controller to control whole operation.

Figure 4. The conceptual diagram of a physician accessing previous records and loading new record

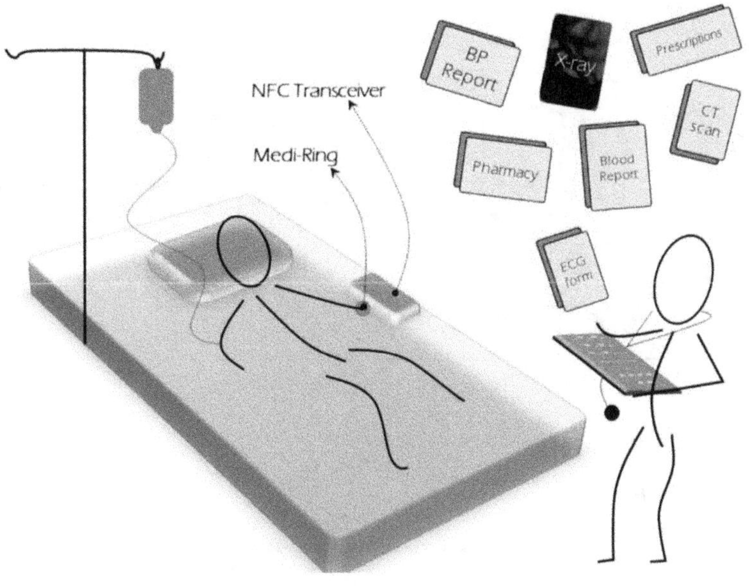

Figure 5. The conceptual diagram of pharmacist receiving the records from an NFC receiver

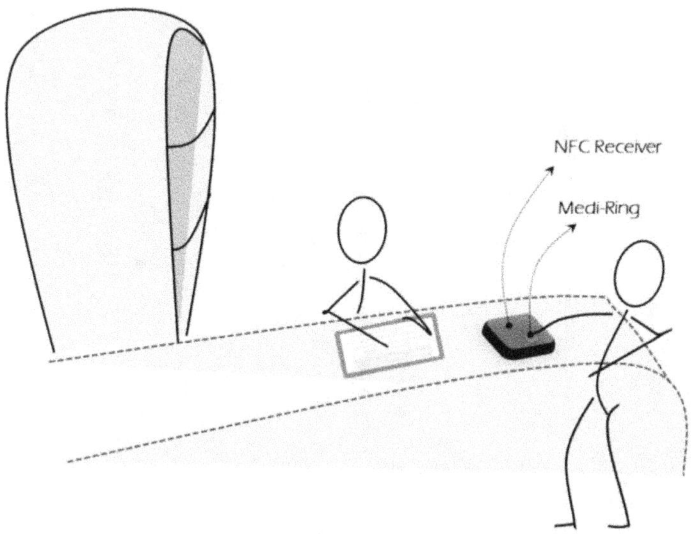

Choosing transceiver model we have two mediums, wired and wireless [Kasper, T., 2007]. Wired is not preferred because of its high cost and circuit complexity. Due to the advantage of wireless transceivers such as low cost and less area overhead we have adopted wireless transceivers. In wireless transceiver there are multiple option like WIFI, Zigbee, Bluetooth, NRF, RF, NFC, etc . In this work, NFC transceivers is used due to following requirement and advantage. Requirements is that the patients have to transfer his report only in front of doctor avoiding long distance data communication. This will be possible only by adopting NFC, because NFC communicate within the range of 10cm [Louliej,2012]

Figure 6.

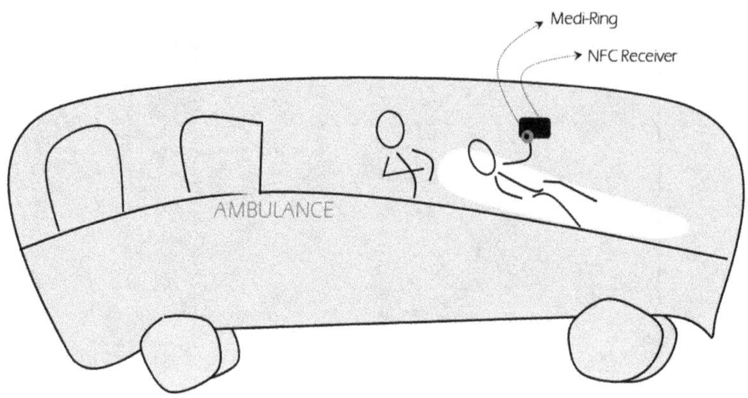

Figure 7. The Block diagram of a medi-ring

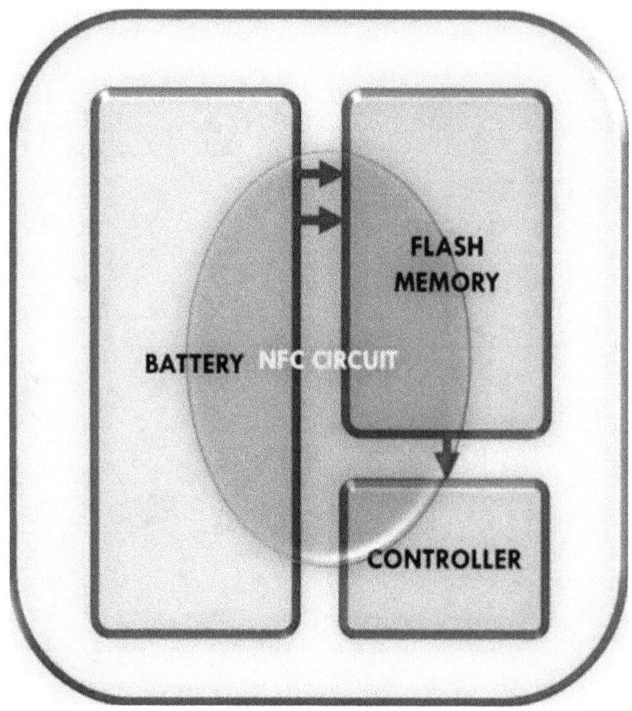

[Zou, J. 2010]. Advantage of NFC [ECMA International. 2013] is that it is user friendly, secured data transmission, small in size and compared to other transceivers it is low cost. In this project TRF7970A NFC model from Texas Instruments as shown in figure 8 is used. It works at 13.56 Mhz, supports all standards of NFC, it is a low power device, operate at 2.7 to 5.5 VDC and it is easily available and easy to interface with the controller. So for prototyping we used this model. It is having SPI protocol to communicate with other devices. In this project it is needed to have memory to store file/ data. SD card is highly preferred due to high availability, low cost, easy interfacing with controller and it can be made

Figure 8. TRF7970A NFC model from Texas Instruments

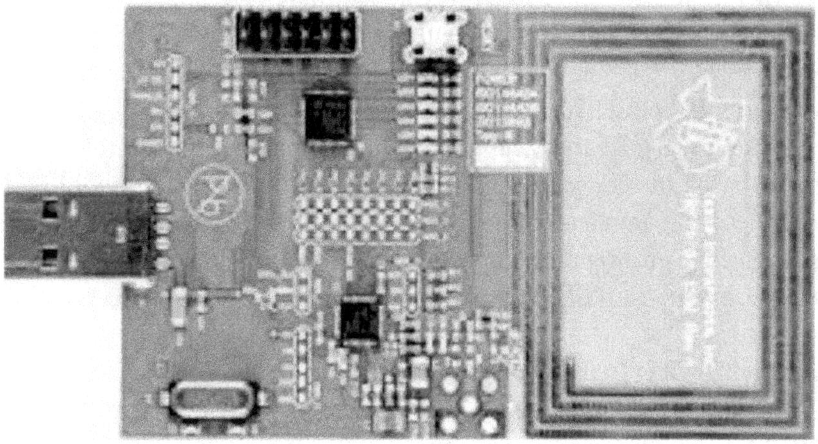

communicate with SPI protocol. In this system we do not need a high-end controller for the operation since this project includes only file transferring and receiving. This can be done by using basic controller. The project requires two SPI devices which is used to transfer data between NFC to controller and from controller to SD card or vice versa.

DESIGN OF THE PROPOSED SYSTEM

The proposed hardware system consists of three components. Mainly controller, NFC module, and flash memory/memory card/pen drive. In any embedded product controller is the heart of the system, here also need the controller for controlling the whole operation will discuss the in detail in next topic. For NFC module is used for transmitting and receiving data, it is wireless protocol less with data rate min 102kbps and max 424kbps.For storing the data or medical files require a memory device, here Pen drive is used as a memory device for prototyping.

1. **Controller:** Controller is a system which contains the CPU, memory, I/O ports and Interrupts. The controllers are classified according to the number of ports available – 8 bit, 16bit and 32 bit controllers. In this work a 32 bit controller is used as it has a very high speed controller and also have more RAM, ROM, I/O ports/peripherals. To design the Medi-ring we require a controller with SPI and USB protocol support is needed as USB drive (USB Protocol) and NFC Module (SPI protocol) has to be interfacing with controller. For prototyping here an ARM_cortex_m3- LPC 1768, 32-bit controller has been used.
    a. **ARM Cortex-M3 LPC1768:** Figure 9 shows the ARM cortex-m3 LPC1768 board with NXP IC. The IC having 100 pin packages. It contains almost all peripherals.

ARM Cortex-M3 based smaller scale controller for implanted applications for LPC1768 that require an abnormal state of coordination and it's devour low power. The fringe supplement of the LPC1768 have up to 512 kilo bytes of glimmer memory and up to 64KB of information memory furthermore its comprises of Ethernet MAC, USB interface that can be arranged as either Host, Device, or OTG likewise working 8 channel broadly useful DMA controller, 4 UARTs, 2 CAN channels(CAN 2.0B), 3 SSP controllers, SPI interface, 3 I2C interfaces, 2-information and 2-yield I2S interface, 8 channel 12-bit ADC, 10-bit DAC, engine control PWM, 4 universally useful clocks, 6yield broadly useful PWM, ultra-low power clock with segregated battery supply, and up to 70 universally useful inputs and yields pins.

ARM Cortex-M3 based smaller scale controller for implanted applications for LPC1768 that require an abnormal state of coordination and it's devour low power. The LPC1768 ARM expands framework helps, for example, effective investigating components and its abnormal state of bolster piece coordinated. Its devoured recurrence of up to 100MHz.

2. **Communication Device:** In this project, the patient has to transfer the medical report or medical files from MediRing to target device and also from target device to Medi-Ring. In our project we can use any of this, but our main concentration of the project it should be wearable and compact system, for this reason we are not going to use wired communication and also it will increase the complexity of the design. So now our main concentration on wireless communication. For our project we don't need long distance communication because patient has to transfer medical report or medical prescription only in front of the doctor for this we are going to use NFC, i.e. Near Field Communication.

DESIGN OF NFC

NFC is a wireless technology; it operates in the range of 10cm or less. NFC operates at 13.56 MHz frequency and it is standard ISO/IEC18000-3 wireless interface with data rates of 106kbps to 424 kbps. Compared to the conventional contactless technology in this frequency range which supports only active-passive communications, communications between NFC-capable devices can be active-active (peer-to-peer) as well as active-passive. This feature of NFC therefore makes NFC technology a link to the RFID world. NFC technology is backwards compatible with the widely used Smart Card infra-

Figure 9. LPC1768 ARM Cortex_m3 Controller

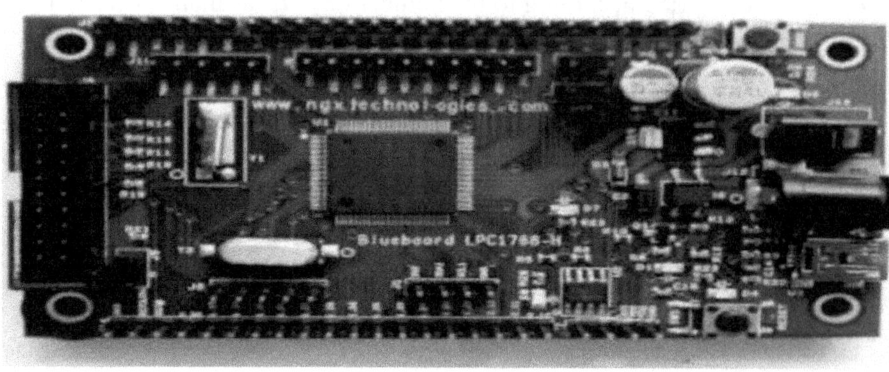

structure based on ISO/IEC 14443 A (e. g. NXP's MIFARE technology) and ISO/IEC 14443 B as well as with the Sony FeliCa card (JIS X 6319-4) []. In NFC communication the device that initiates the communication is called the initiator and the device that responds is called the target. For NFC communication it should have both an initiator and a target. The initiator generates RF field that can used to power the passive target. This is how the NFC device operates on passive devices like smart poster, tags, stickers and cards. NFC is designed using loop antennae by creating electromagnetic induction between the coils. Initiator will generate the electromagnetic field, this field is used for communication between the initiator and the target. The target in NFC technology are also called as NFC tags. NFC tags can be classified as read-only or read & write tags. If the tags have prewritten data and they allow Initiators to read the data but not alter it, tags are called read only tags. If the NFC tags allow the initiator to rewrite the data, they are classified as read & write tags. In addition to this classification NFC forum specified/ Classified the tags into four different categories depending on the communication speed, security, read and write options. Table 1 lists the different types of Tags available in market.

WORKING OF NFC

Near field communication is based on inductive-coupling. Like the RFID Standards 14443 and FeliCa NFC uses an inductive coupling [International Organization for Standardization, 2013, ECMA International, 2013]. Similar to the transformer principle, the magnetic near-field of two conductor coils is used to couple the polling device (initiator) and listening device (target). NFC works using magnetic induction between two antennas located within each other's 'near field'. Modulation schemes are amplitude on/ off keying (OOK) with different modulation depth (100% or 10%) and BPSK.

Figure 10 illustrates the communication in an NFC device where one side is passive device/tag other side is active device/initiator. In NFC communication between tag and initiator happens due to electromagnetic Coupling.

There are two modes of operation in NFC - Active Mode and Passive Mode [Information Technology-Telecommunication and Information Exchange between Systems—Near Field Communication—Internface and Protocol (NFCIP-1),2013]. In Active mode, both devices with NFC chip generate an electromagnetic field and exchange data. In Passive mode, only one active device generates the necessary electromagnetic field and the other device uses the electromagnetic field generated by the active device to exchange in-

Table 1. Types of tags

Tag Types	Standard	Read/Rewrite Capability	Memory	Speed	Data Collision Protection
Type1	ISO 14443A	Read Re-write Read only	96 bytes to 2KB	106Kbps	No
Type2	ISO 14443A	Read Re-write Read only	96 bytes to 2KB	106Kbps	Yes
Type3	Japanese JIS X 6319-4	Preconfigured Read Re-write Read only	Variable up to 1MB per service	212 Kbps to 424 Kbps	Sony Felica
Type4	ISO 14443A	Preconfigured Read Re-write Read only	32Kb per service	All speed	Yes

Figure 10. Communication using inductive coupling

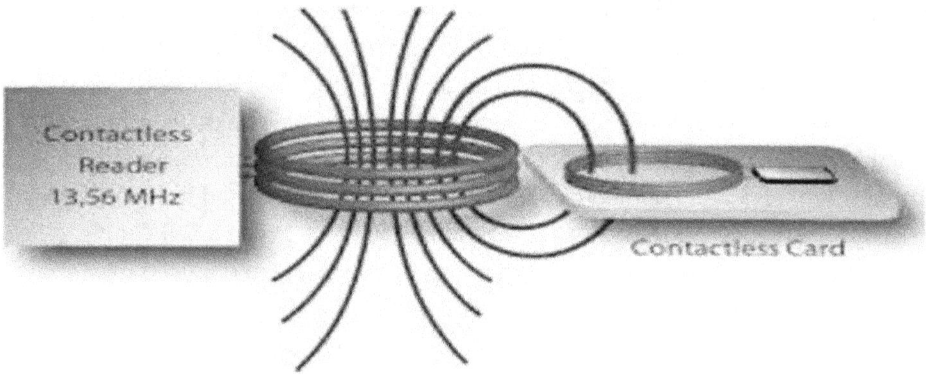

formation. In passive transmission mode NFC devicesuses13.56 MHz carrier signal of the active device as the energy source. Modulation scheme of the active/polling device is ASK. In passive transmission mode, data transmission from a passive/listening device to the active device due to the coupling of the coils of a polling and a listening device affects the impedance of the active polling device. A variation in the impedance of the listening device causes amplitude or phase changes to the antenna voltage of the polling device which is detected by the polling device. This technique is called load modulation. Load modulation is carried out in listening mode (as with ISO/IEC 14443) using an auxiliary carrier at 848 kHz which is modulated by the baseband and varies the impedance of the listening device. The modulation scheme is ASK (as with ISO/IEC 14443 A PICC's) or BPSK as with 14443 B PICC's). There is a third passive mode which is compatible to FeliCa where the load modulation is without an auxiliary carrier directly as ASK on the 13.56 MHz carrier. For NFC peer-to-peer mode where both the devices are active NFC devices, signal in both the directions are modulated and coded like a polling device. In active mode the energy consumed during transmission is less compared to passive mode as each NFC devices use their own power supply and the carrier signal is switched off after end of transmission. In this work we have made the NFC on the Medi-ring passive mode.

In modes of operation of NFC can be further classified into three modes depending on whether information is read from the listing device or if read & write operations are happening. The three modes of operation are:

- **Card Emulation Mode (Passive Mode):** The NFC device behaves like an existing contactless card conforming to one of the legacy standards
- **Peer-to-Peer Mode**: two NFC devices exchange information. The initiator device (polling device) requires less power compared to the reader/writer mode because the target (listener) uses its own power supply.
- **Reader/Writer Mode (Active Mode):** The NFC device is active and reads or writes to a passive legacy RFID tag.

Every mode (card emulation, peer-to-peer, reader/writer mode) can be combined with one of the following transmission technologies: NFC-A (backward compatible to ISO/IEC 14443 A) NFC-B (backward compatible to ISO/IEC 14443 B) NFC-F (backward compatible to JIS X 6319-4). To support all the different technologies, an NFC device in polling mode first attempts to get responses from NFC-A, NFC-B and NFC-F tags with the according request signals. When NFC polling device receives a response from an compatible device, the NFC device sets up the corresponding communication mode (NFC-A, NFC-B or NFC-F mode). Coding and modulation varies depending on active or passive communication mode, NFC-A, -B, -F communication, and bitrate. Table 2 shows the coding, modulation and data rates for NFC-A, NFC-B and NFC-F modes.

b. **TRF7970ATB NFC Module:** The selected TRF7970ATB NFC MODULE supports Near Field Communication (NFC) Standards NFCIP-1 (ISO/IEC 18092) and NFCIP-2 (ISO/IEC 21481). The module has Integrated Encoders, Decoders, and Data Framing Crystal or Oscillator. For NFC Initiator, Active and Passive Target Operation for All Three Bit Rates (106 kbps, System Components (MCU, Peripherals, 212 kbps, 424 kbps) is available and Card Emulation is also possible. The input Voltage Range is 2.7 VDC to 5.5 VDC. It has a Programmable I/O Voltage Levels from 1.8 VDC to 5.5 VDC. The Programmable System Clock Frequency Output (RF, RF/2, RF/4) from 13.56-MHz or 27.12-MHz. Programmable Power Modes for Ultra Low-Power System Design (Power Down < 1 µA). Parallel or SPI Interface (With 127-Byte FIFO). Temperature Range: –40°C to 110°C. It supports all three types of modes. figure 11 shows the TRF7970ATB module

3. **Semiconductor Memory:** In this project we require the memory device for storing medical files and prescription history. Semiconductor memories can be broadly classified based on their characteristics such as capacity, access time and organization. The memories directly connected to CPU are called primary memory.

There are two types of semiconductor memory

Table 2. Coding, modulation and data rates for NFC-A, -B or -F modes

NFC-Forum Standard	Polling / Listening	Coding	Modulation	Data Rate	Carrier frequency
NFC-A	Polling	Modified Miller	ASK 100%	106 kb/s	13.56 MHz
	Listening	Manchester	Load modulation (ASK)	106 kb/s	13.56 MHz +- 848 kHz subcarrier
NFC-B	Polling	NRZ-L	ASK 10%	106 kb/s	13.56 MHz
	Listening	NRZ-L	Load modulation (BPSK)	106 kb/s	13.56 MHz +- 848 kHz subcarrier
NFC-F	Polling	Manchester	ASK 10%	212 / 424 kb/s	13.56 MHz
	Listening	Manchester	Load modulation (ASK)	212 / 424 kb/s	13.56 MHz (without subcarrier)

Figure 11. TRF7970ATB module

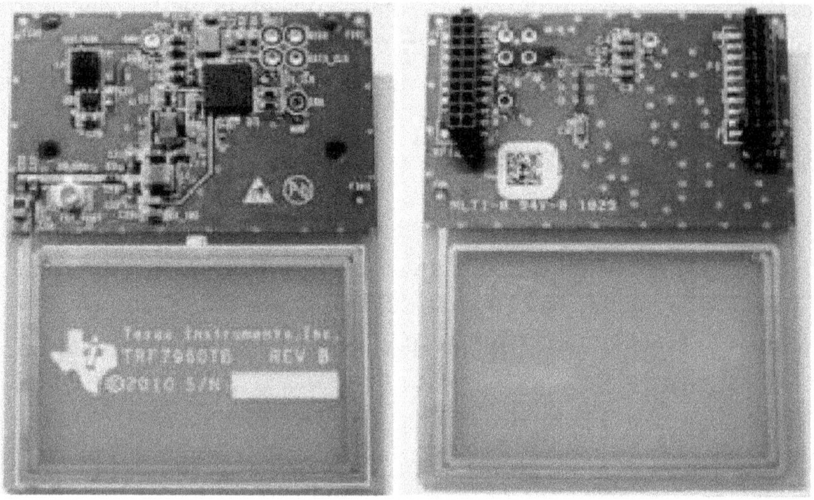

1. **Volatile Memory:** It is the type of memory, when there is no power it will lost the data. This type of memory is used as a primary memory in computer. Like RAM, Cache Memory.
2. **Non-Volatile Memory:** It is the type of memory, even there is no power the data will retain. This type of memory is used as a secondary memory of computer. Like Hard disk, memory sticks.

For this project prototyping non-volatile memory is used, because patient data of files should not be erased when power off and it should be permanent memory. So when comes to Non-volatile memory there are many types,

1. ROM 2. PROM 3. EPROM 4. EEPROM 5. Flash EPROM 6. Mask ROM

ROM: It means Read-only memory, this is non-volatile memory, it does not lose it data when no power.

PROM: It means Programmable ROM, this is also a type of ROM, in this internally have fuses in every bit, you want store any data by burn the fuses, if the data is wrong total memory will be discarded, and this is also called one time programmable ROM.

EPROM: It is the higher version of PROM, in this VU radiation is used to erase the memory and again it can be programmed. For erasing data it takes around 20-25 minutes.

EEPROM: It means electrically erasable programmable ROM. This is also a type of nonvolatile memory, in this drawback of EPROM is of erasable time is reduced totally by using electrical signals to erase the ROM.

Flash EPROM: It is very advanced type of non-volatile memory, the entire chip can be erased within half second, so that the name is called Flash memory.

Mask ROM: It is the type of ROM, its contents are programmed in manufacturing process only and not user programmable memory.

Figure 12. USB memory stick/USB pendrive

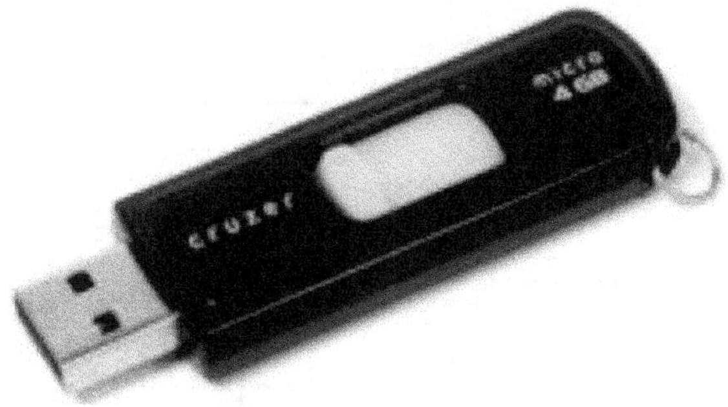

Now for project Flash Memory/Flash EPROM is used for prototyping.

There are many flash memories devices are available in market, so as availability and learning purpose there have two option for us, one is SD card, other is USB memory stick/USB Pendrive. Figure 12 show the USB memory stick used in the project.

This type of memory sticks are used for portability, also we need to test our system is writing and reading data from the USB stick, by connecting to computer.

4. **LCD:** In this work we used LCD for testing purpose. LCD is a Liquid crystal device which is used for display here the LCD is using as output device, LCD displays all the monitoring 1parameters of the vehicle in 16x2 display

Figure 13 shows the Liquid Crystal Display is used to display the information or result from the microcontroller. It's one of the most common devices that are used to interface with microcontroller. 16x2 and 20x2 are two types of LCD displays that are used in common where, the first number indicates the number of characters fit in a line and the latter is the number of rows.

IMPLEMENTATION AND TESTING OF THE SYSTEM

The block diagram of the system prototype is shown in figure 14. As seen in the block diagram the final system will not need an LCD display. LCD is used in the prototype to help in debugging. As seen

Figure 13. Liquid crystal device

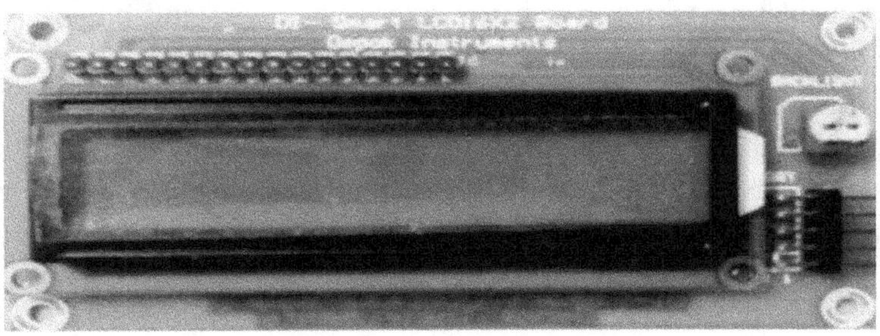

Figure 14. Block diagram of the proposed Medi-ring system

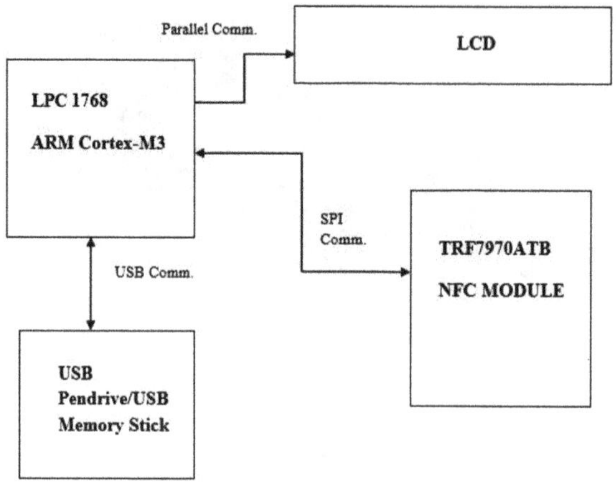

in Figure 14 The important part of the system is the interface of the controller with NFC module and interface of the controller with USB memory stick. In the next subsection we will be looking at the technique to interface NFC module and USB memory stick to the controller.

INTERFACING USB PEN DRIVE WITH LPC1768 CONTROLLER

In LPC_1768 controller will support USB2.0 [USB Implementers Forum. 2005] with full speed. The controller has a total of 32 endpoints (16 physical and 16 logical) and supports all data transfer types. LPC 1768 controller allows us to scale endpoints in runtime. The packet size can be modified using software based on endpoint. LPC 1768 support soft-connect and has good-link feature. It allows dynamically switch b/w CPU controlled mode and DMA mode. It supports direct memory access transfer on non-controlled endpoints. It has two buffers in Bulk and Isochronous endpoints. The Data transmission supported by LPC 1768 is divided into four types depending on the type of data it copes with.

1. Control Transfer
2. Isochronous transfer
3. Interrupt Transfer
4. Bulk transfer

Control Transfer: In this type of transfer a device will send the request to the host, and appropriate data will find the particular pipe for data transfer. After some time status bit will return to the host, so that data might be bidirectional, it uses same endpoint for each direction. Figure 15 shows the control transfer in USB

Isochronous transfer: This type of communication the data accuracy is not critical, for transmission it will uses timing mechanism. In this type constant data transfer rate can be maintained. In this type request will send to Device, depending on the response it will transfer data. Figure 16 shows the isochronous transactions.

Figure 15. Control transfer with ACK without ACK

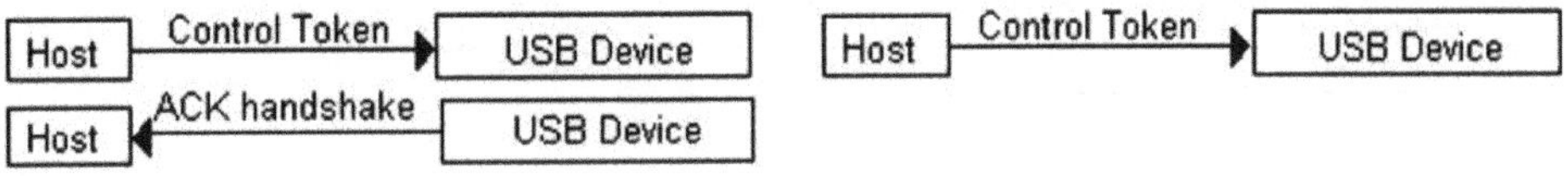

Figure 16. Isochronous transactions communication sequence

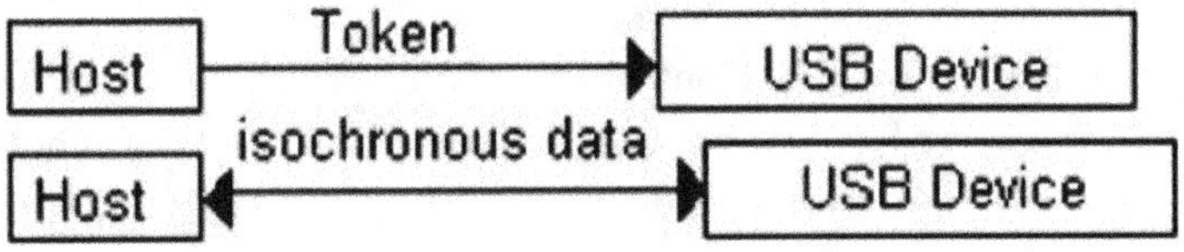

Interrupt Transfer: As the name tells that it uses interrupt routine for transferring small and high priority data. Figure 17 show that Interrupt transfer communication sequence, if data is not waiting it will send NAC data.

Bulk transfer: the name suggests it is made for large amount of data handling. It means transfer large amount of data at a time. If host wants to transfer bulk data it will send the token to the other USB device depending on the input or output it will response and transfer occurs. Figure 18 shows the bulk transactions

The USB protocol frame format is shown in Figure 19. The frame format consists of an 8 bit Sync field called synchronous field. As the name suggests it is used for timing correction of the data. An 8 bit PID field follows the Sync field. The PID field four bits are used for identifying the data type and packet format data, and remaining four bits which are once complemented are now used as check bits. The PID field determines to which group the data belongs to and also decide the input or output device. PID field is followed by Address field. Address field gives the address of a function used in the end of the pipe. Endpoint field as seen if Figure 19 is of 4-bit. Endpoint field is used for sending or receiving of the packet. Data field is 0-1023 bytes which used to transfer the data bits in the USB.

Figure 17. Interrupt transaction communication sequence

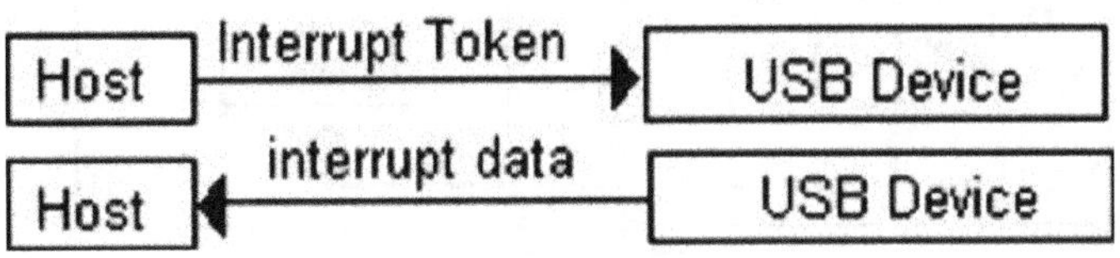

Figure 18. Bulk transfer communication sequence

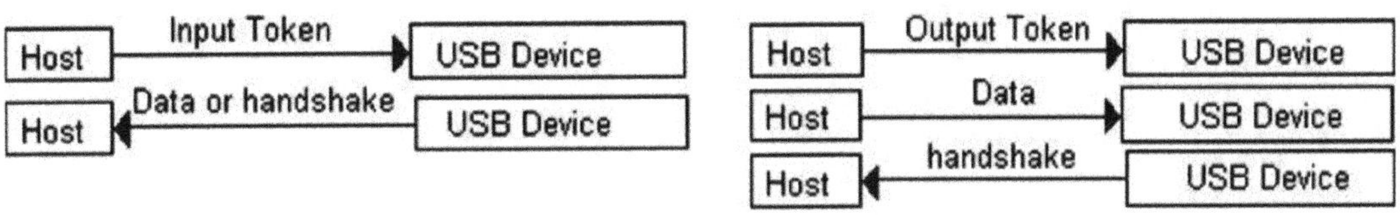

Figure 19. Typical data packet of USB protocol

Sync (8)	PID (8)	Address	Endpoint (4)	Data (0-1023 bytes)

Architecture of USB Device Controller

Figure 20 shows the architecture of USB Controller in LPC1768. USB controller consists of analog transceiver. The analog transceiver has two bidirectional pins D+ and D- as shown in Fig. 20. As seen in the architecture there is a serial interface engine for full speed USB implementation, Endpoint is implemented using SRAM FIFO ant it is interfaced with AHB bus.

In our project USB acts as a host, the architecture of host controller as shown figure 21.

This device has support fully open host controller interface .it supports the USB-operation, USB_suspend, USB_reset, USB_resum operations.

Algorithm of USB Interfacing With LPC1768 Controller

Figure 22 shows the communication between controller and USB Pendrive.

Figure 23 shows the final interfacing of USB flash drive to controller and testing

Figure 20. Architecture of USB controller

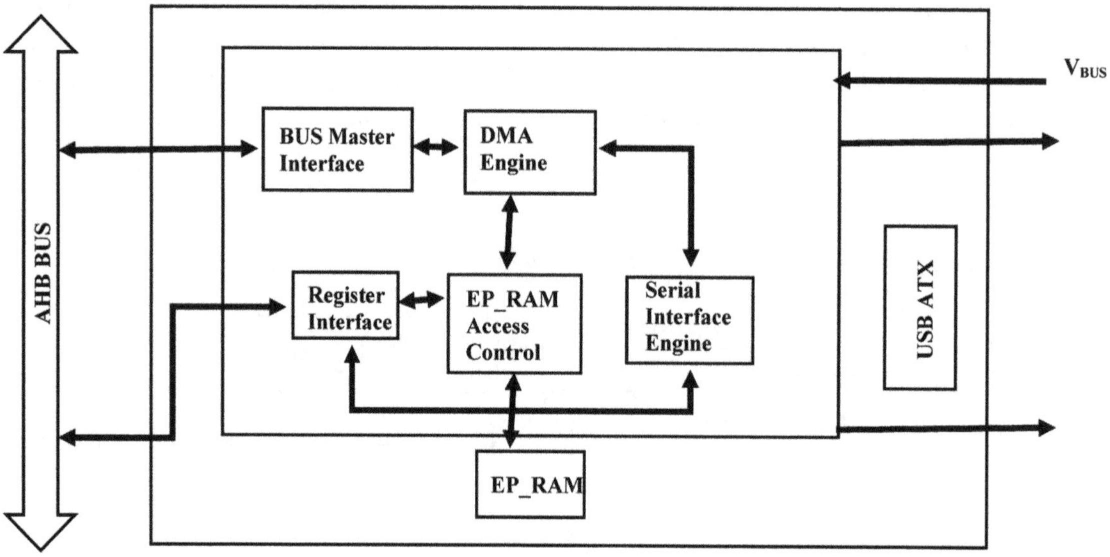

Figure 21. Architecture of USB host controller

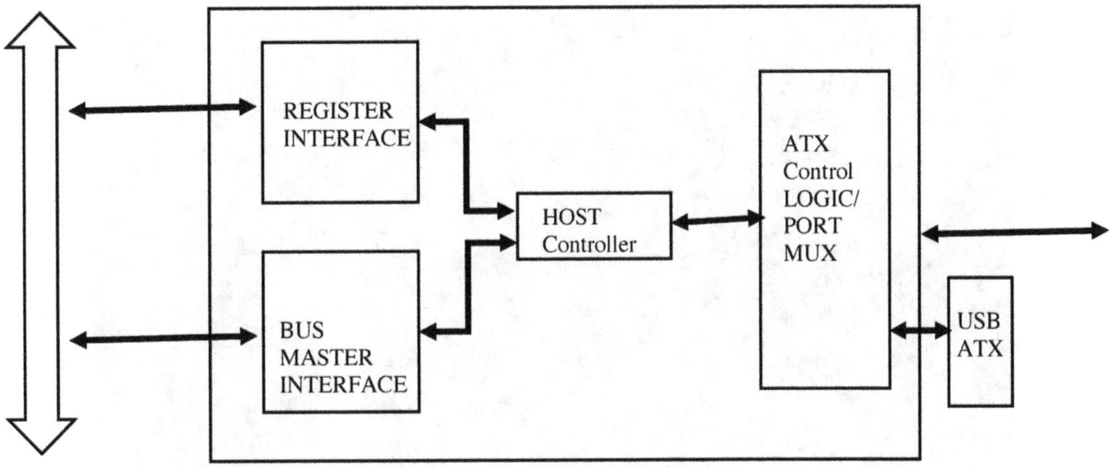

Figure 22. Flow chart of USB communication with controller

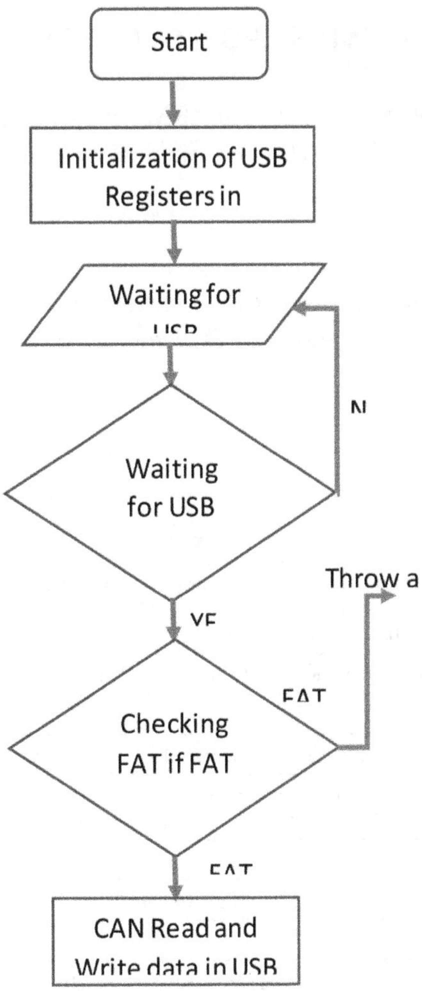

Figure 23. Hardware interfacing and testing of usb flash drive with controller

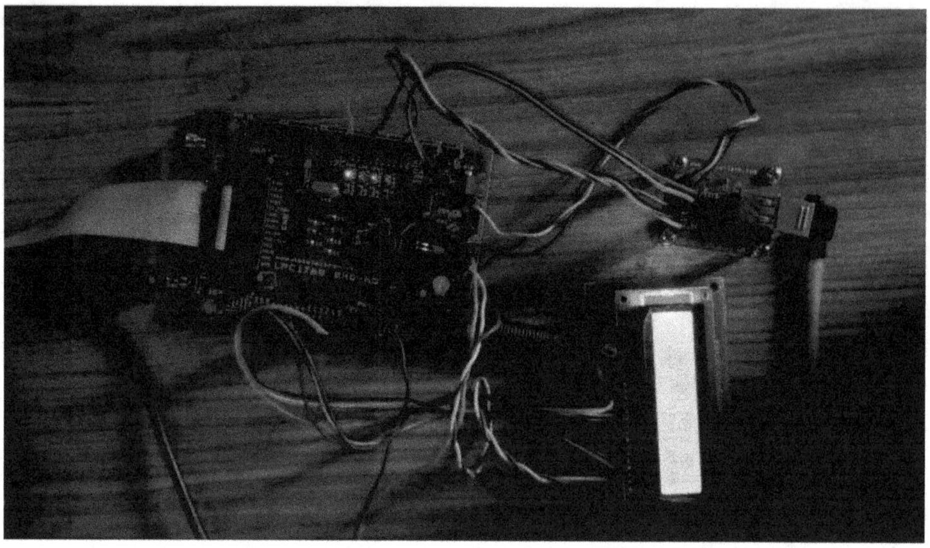

TRF7970ATB INTERFACING WITH LPC1768 CONTROLLER

As in the Figure 23 shows the interfacing between ARM cortex m3 and TRF7970ATB. Here the interfacing protocol is SPI, because TRF7970ATB NFC module has only support of SPI communication.

SPI Registers in LPC 1768

There are four register in SPI protocol 1. SPCR-SPI control register. It is used to configure the SPI and it is the 32-bit register. Below table 3 shows the SPCR register description of all 32 bits and functions

Table 3. SPCR resister

31:12	RESERVED
11:8	BITS When bit 2 (BIT ENABLE) of this register is 1, this field controls the number of bits per transfer: 1000 -- 8 Bits per transfer 1001 -- 9 Bits per transfer 1010 -- 10 Bits per transfer 1011 -- 11 Bits per transfer 1100 -- 12 Bits per transfer 1101 -- 13 Bits per transfer 1110 -- 14 Bits per transfer 1111 -- 15 Bits per transfer 0000 -- 16 Bits per transfer
7	SPIE This bit is used to enable SPI interrupt.(0 OR 1)
6	LSBF (0 or 1)
5	MSTR This bit is used for Master mode select. 0 -- Slave Mode. 1 -- Master Mode.
4	CPOL This is used for controlling clock polarity. 0 -- SCK is active high. 1 -- SCK is active low.
3	CPHA(0 OR 1)
2	BIT ENABLE This is used to clear the 16-byte Rx FIFO
1:0	RESERVED

SPSR: SPI status Register, it is also 32 bit register, below table 4shows the register description of SPSR.

Table 4. SPSR register

31:8	7	6	5	4	3	2:0
RESERVED	SPIF	WCOL	ROVR	MODF	ABTR	RESERVED

SPDR:SPI data register, it is 32 bit register,so 0:7 bit is data low bits,8:15 data high bits,16:31 are Reserved. This register contains data to be transmit and received data.

SPCCR: SPI Clock control register, it is also 32 bit register, it used for controlling of SCK in master. In this register 0:7 bits for counter, 8:31 bits are reserved.

Algorithm of SPI Communication With TRF7970ATB

Figure 24 shows the communication between controller and mobile

In the figure 24 shows the how we are communication with the NFC and other NFC module, If the there is no response from NFC module, it will wait, again it will send the command, if get the response it will communicate with other mobile or any NFC active device, to transfer and receive data.

Figure 25 Shows the Final interfacing controller with NFC module

Figure 24. Communication between controller and TRF7970ATB NFC module

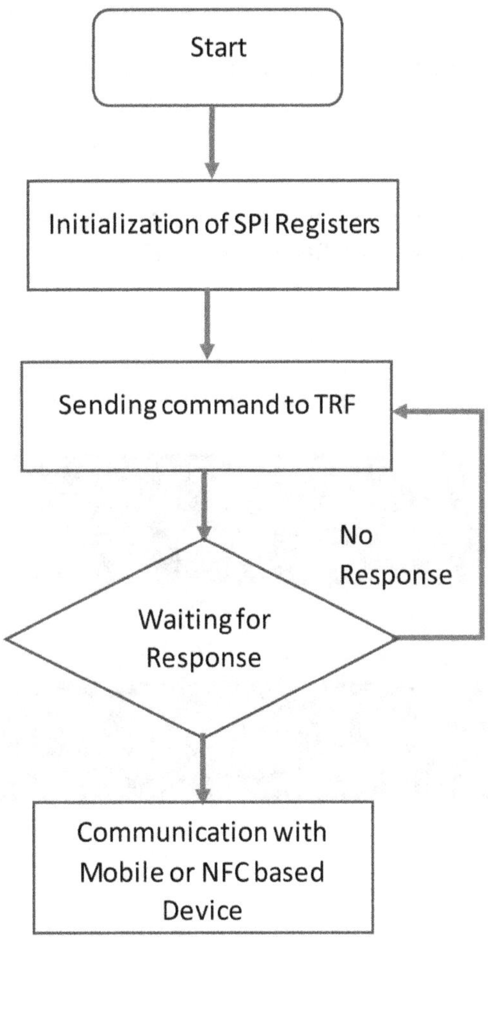

Figure 25. Hardware interfacing b/w controller and TRF7970ATB NFC module

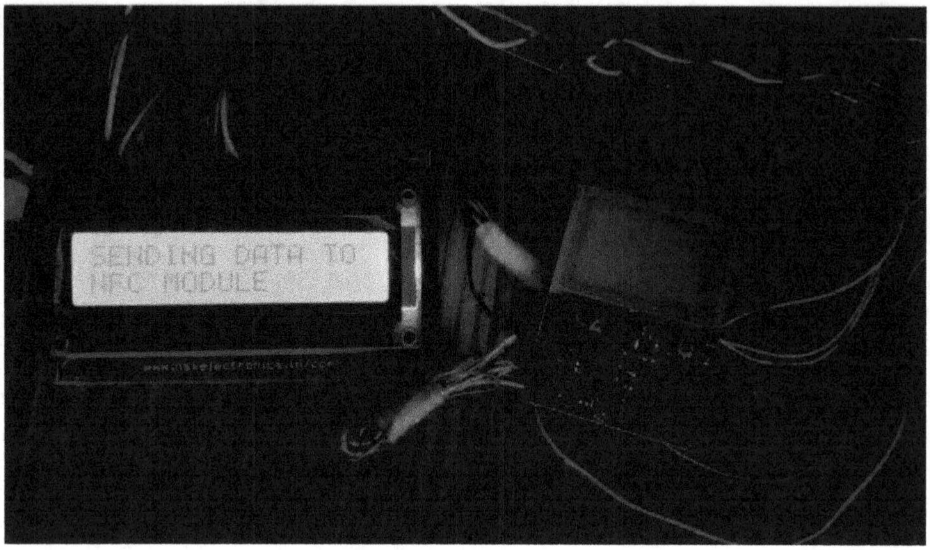

Results

The photo of initial LCD was shown below. The display indicates the main purpose of this project.

USB Host Initialization

Figure 27, Figure 28, Figure 29 and Figure 30 show the USB host initialization process; if USB Drive is not plugged to controller it will ask for USB plug in, if it's done its go for Host initialization.

Figure 26. Indication of project name Medi-ring in LCD

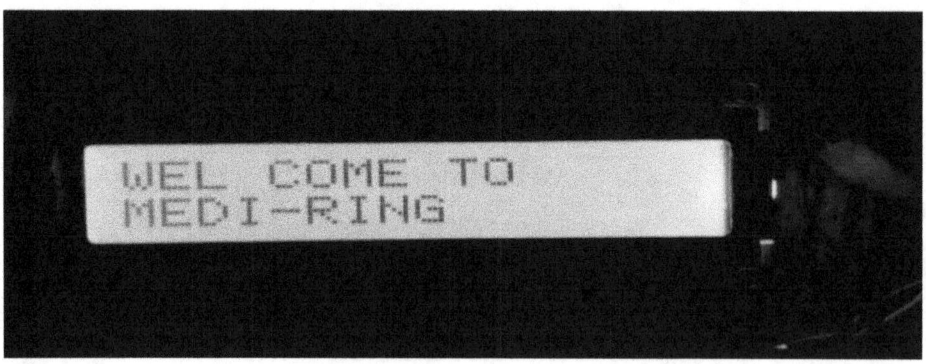

Figure 27. USB host initialization

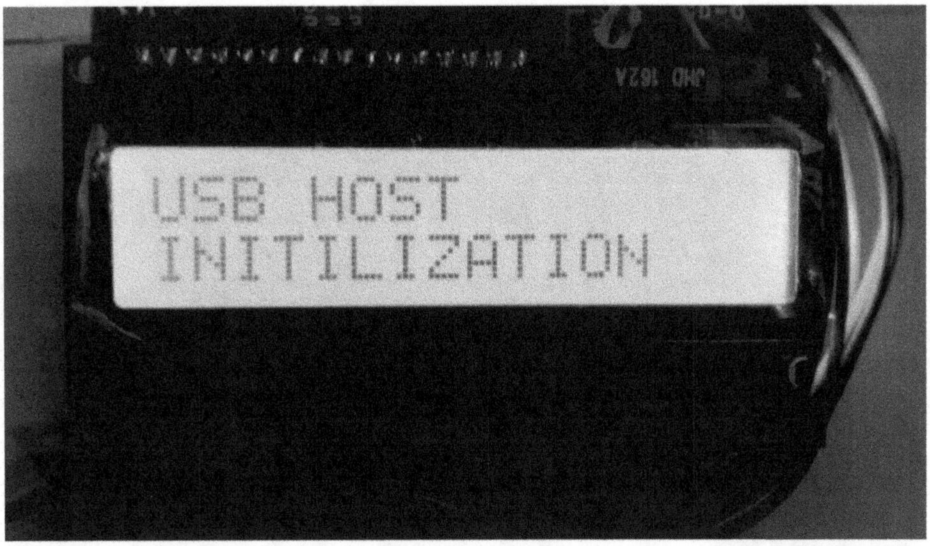

Figure 28. Waiting for USB flash drive plug in

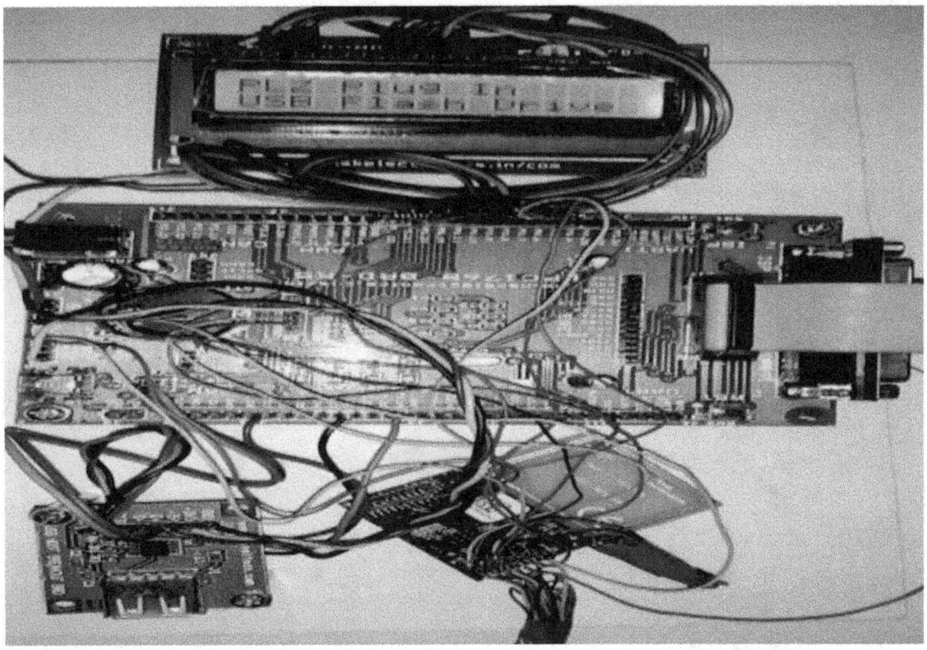

SPI INTERFACING

Figure 31 show the initialization of SPI is done and Figure 32 shows the NFC module interfacing with controller using SPI protocol. And also seen wired connections

Figure 29. USB flash drive plugged in

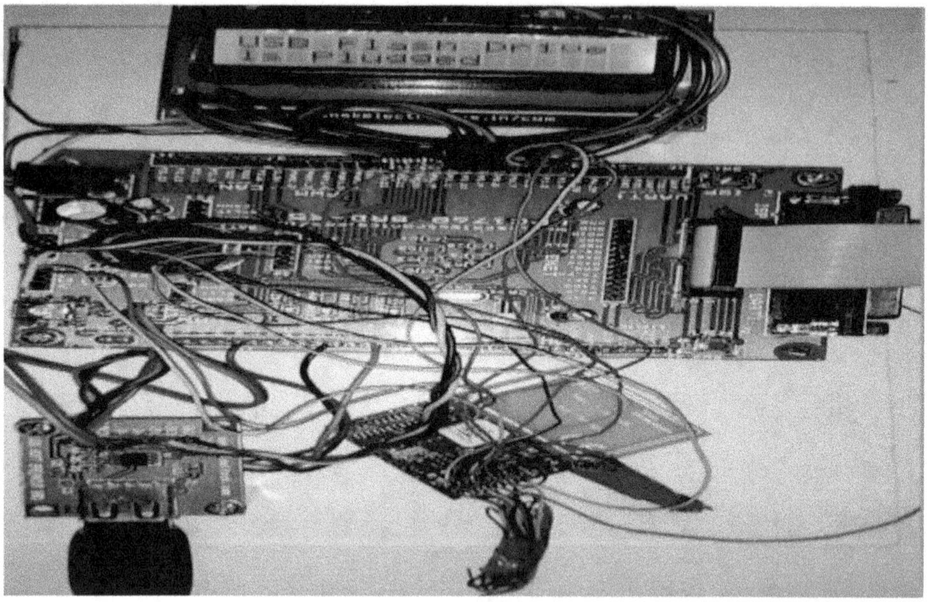

Figure 30. USB HOST is initialization completed

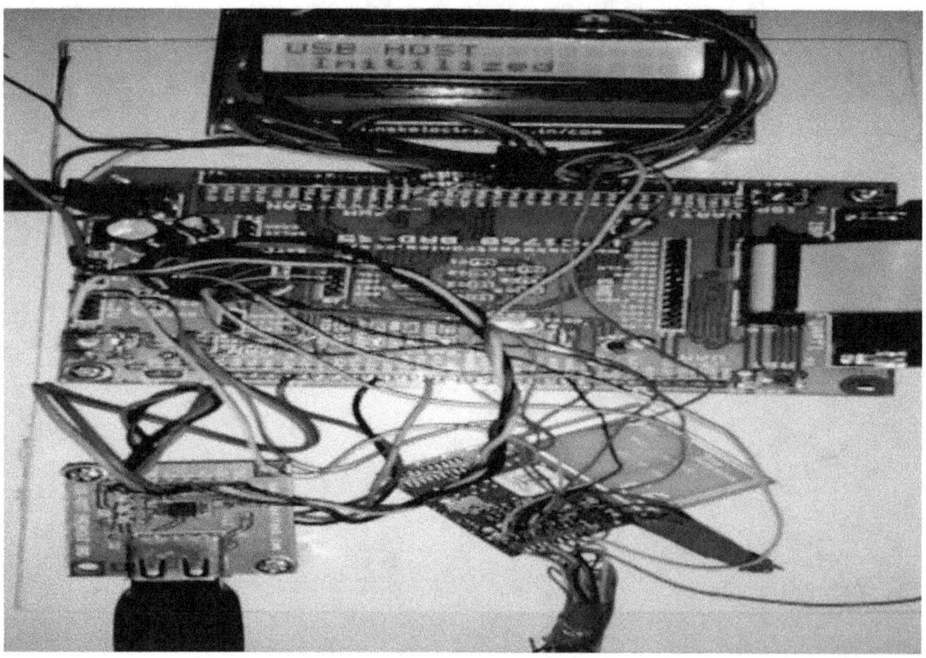

Figure 31. Initialization of SPI registers in LPC1768

Figure 32. NFC TRF7970ATB interfacing with controller

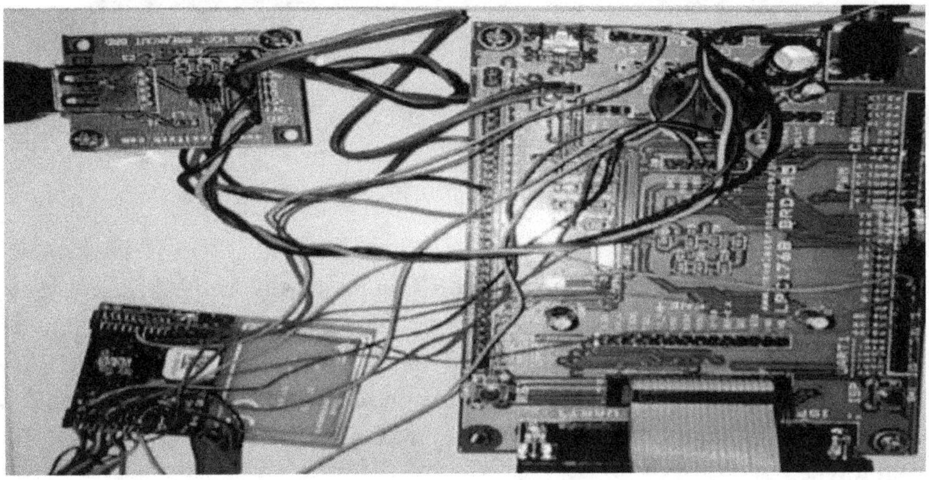

As seen all the figures and hardware implementation is programming Keil software, tested in simulation and also testing of hardware is done. Final module interfacing that is interfacing NFC module and flash drive to single controller Below Figure 33, show the final project hardware of MEDI-RING.

Figure 33. Final hardware of the Medi-Ring

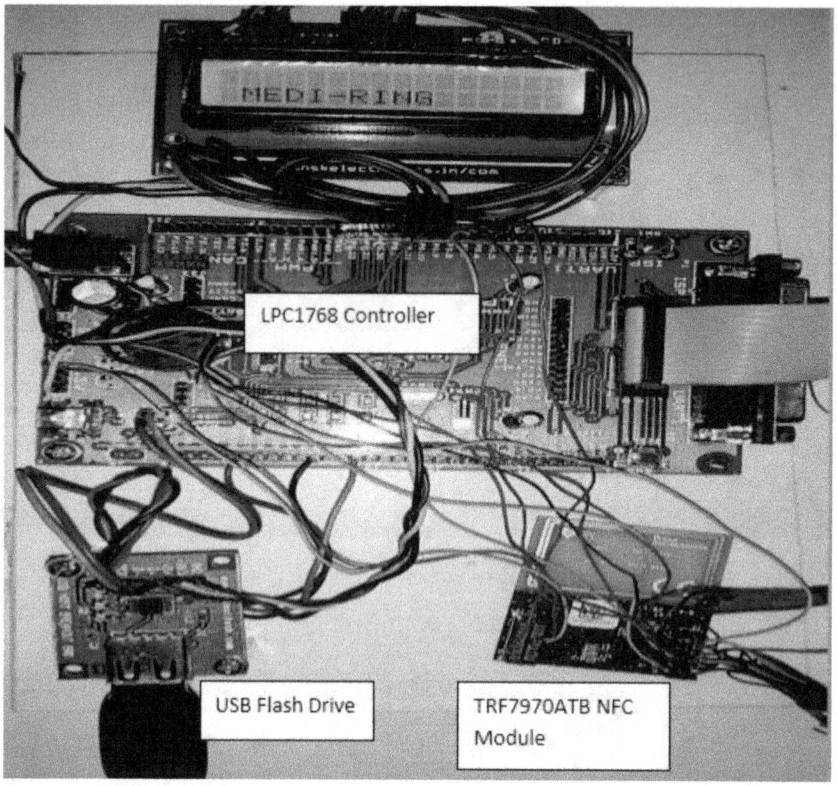

CONCLUSION

This chapter concentrates on implementation of Medi-Ring for storing medical files or prescriptions of a patient. This includes interfacing of USB flash drive with controller and NFC module with controller. And here completed programming of USB host and SPI communication in LPC1768 controller and interfaced both USB drive and NFC module with controller. And also tested the data writing into the USB drive and reading from USB drive. The system is developed on this embedded firmware is a satisfactory prototype.

REFERENCES

Boumstein, J. (2013). *The case for Outsourced Invoice Scanning and data Capture*. Academic Press.

Burkland, S. (2005). *Near Field Communication in Smartphones (Unpublished work)*. Berlin Institute of Technology. Retrieved from http://citeseerx.ist.psu.edu/viewdoc/versions?doi=10.1.1.455.3514

Dr. Shyam Kumar v Rameshbhai, Harmanbhai Kachiya, 2002 (1) CPR 320, I (2006) CPJ 16 (NC)

ECMA International. (2013). *Near Field Communication-Interface and Protocol (NFCIP-1)*. Retrieved from https://www.ecma-international.org/publications/files/ECMA-ST/Ecma-340.pdf

ECMA International. (2013). *Near Field Communication-Interface and Protocol (NFCIP-2)*. Retrieved from https://www.ecma-international.org/publications/standards/Ecma-352.htm

Force v. M Ganeswara Rao. 1998 (3) CPR 251; 1998 (1) CPJ 413 (AP SCDRC).

Hasan, R., Winslett, M., & Sion, R. (2007). Requirements of Secure Storage Systems for Healthcare Records. In W. Jonker & M. Petković (Eds.), Lecture Notes in Computer Science: Vol. 4721. *Secure Data Management. SDM 2007*. Berlin: Springer. doi:10.1007/978-3-540-75248-6_12

Implementers Forum, U. S. B. (2005). *USB 'A' Plug Form Factor (Revision 1.0)*. Retrieved from http://www.usb.org/developers/docs/devclass_docs/CCWG_A_Plug_Form_Factor_Guideline_Revision_1.0_.pdf

International Organization for Standardization. (2013). *Information Technology-Telecommunication and Information Exchange between Systems—Near Field Communication—Internface and Protocol (NFCIP-1)*. Retrieved from https://www.iso.org/standard/56692.html

International Organization for Standardization. (2016). *Identification Cards-Contactless Integrated Circuit Cards-Proximity Cards-Part 2: Radio Frequency Power and Signal Interface (ISO/IEC 14443-2:2016)*. Retrieved from https://www.iso.org/standard/66288.html

Iyer, M. (2011, April 20). Medical errors in top 10 Killers: WHO. *Times of India*.

Kanaiyalal Ramanlal Trivedi v Dr. Satyanarayan Vishwakarma 1996 (3) CPR 24 (Guj); I (1997) CPJ 332 (Guj); 1998 CCJ 690 (Guj)

Kasper, T., Carluccio, D., & Paar, C. (2007). An Embedded System for Practical Security Analysis of Contactless Smartcards. Information Security Theory and Practices. Smart Cards, Mobile and Ubiquitous Computing Systems Lecture Notes in Computer Science, 150-160. doi:10.1007/978-3-540-72354-7_13

Louliej, A., Jabrane, Y., Said, B. A., & Ouahman, A. A. (2012). Reduction of power envelope fluctuations in ECMA-368 ultra wideband communication system. *2012 International Conference on Multimedia Computing and Systems*. 10.1109/ICMCS.2012.6320132

Motorola. (2003). *SPI Block Guide v3.06 (S12SPIV3/D)*. Retrieved from https://opencores.org/usercontent,doc,1499360489

Raghunath Raheja v The Maharashtra Medical Council and Ors AIR 1996 Bombay 198

Reuters. (2014, September 25). *Your Medical Record Is worth More to Hackers than Your Credit card.* NDTV.

Thomas, J. (2009). Medical records and issues in negligence. *Indian Journal of Urology, 25*(3), 384. doi:10.4103/0970-1591.56208 PMID:19881136

Zou, J., Zhang, C., Dong, C., Fan, C., & Wen, Z. (2010). Mobile payment based on RFID-SIM Card. *2010 10th IEEE International Conference on Computer and Information Technology*.

Chapter 7
Edge Detection on Light Field Images:
Evaluation of Retinal Blood Vessels Detection on a Simulated Light Field Fundus Photography

Yessaadi Sabrina
Badji Mokhtar University, Algeria

Laskri Mohamed Tayeb
Badji Mokhtar University, Algeria

ABSTRACT

Digital fundus imaging is becoming an important task in computer-aided diagnosis and has gained an important position in the digital medical imaging domain. One of its applications is the retinal blood vessels extracting. Object detection in machine vision and image processing has gained increasing interest due to its social and security potential. Plenoptic imaging is a promising optical technique. This technique computes the location and the propagation direction information of the object light, which are used as efficient descriptors to detect and track the object displacement. In this chapter, the authors use an edge detection technique to extract and segment blood vessels in the retinal image. They propose a novel approach to detect vessels in a simulated light fields fundus image, based on the image representation with the first and the second order derivative, well known as gradient and Laplacian image descriptors. Since the difficulties to get a light field image of a fundus in the retinal image, the authors test their model in the image provided by Sha Tong et al.

DOI: 10.4018/978-1-5225-7071-4.ch007

INTRODUCTION

As a crucial technique in computer vision and image processing, object detection has often been used for object segmentation and tracking for computer vision systems (Belongie, Malik, & Puzicha, 2002). It is based on the detection of instant objects like the human body, face, car, bicycles, or buildings. This approach plays an important role in visual surveillance applications, pedestrian detection and tracking, image retrieval, and face recognition (Moeslund, 2012; Tekalp, 2015).

Different techniques and methods have been proposed to yield an efficient solution, as we can cite the background subtraction, the saliency detection, and many other ones. Earlier measurement methods suffer from drawbacks due to complexes scene properties (geometrics, illumination, ..., etc.). (Tekalp, 2015; McAndrew, 2015).

To improve these limits, new optical methods for describing objects are efficiently and largely invaded in computer vision and machine learning (Cristóbal, Schelkens, & Thienpont, 2013). Quite recently, considerable attention has been paid to plenoptic imaging, this approach captures information on the three-dimensional light field of appropriate scene and records, simultaneously, the location information and the propagation direction of the object light plane (Levoy, & Hanrahan, 1996; Levoy, 2006; Xu, & Lam, 2017). These computed measures are used as efficient descriptors to detect and track moving objects (Zobel, Fritz, & Scholz, 2002).

In this chapter, we propose a new sensing strategy for blood-retinal vessels detection and extraction based on, first, the extraction of visual information of a frame image such as a discrete object, specifically: edges. At this level, we focus on the description of light field images based on the detection and the localization of significant intensity variation, or what it is called: edge.

First and the second derivative, well known as Gradient and Laplacian, will be used to compute the edge image, that we will use to extract retinal blood vessels in retinal images.

RELATED WORK

The extraction of visual information of a frame image, such as a discrete object, specifically: edges, was an important issue to accomplish the object detection task. This technique is called the edge detection.

Edge detection is a long-standing problem in computer vision. It is an important phase for several computer vision and image processing techniques, as pattern recognition, image segmentation, image matching, object detection and tracking. This method aims to locate pixels of high variation in intensity from the other neighbor's pixels (Canny, 1983; Ziou, & Tabbone, 1998).

In the graphics community, successful approaches have been proposed to perform the object detection process, based on edge detection, under a variety of condition scene and camera constraints. See Ziou and Tabbone (1998) for an interesting overview of researches in this field. Certain of these methods proved very good model accuracy in the two-dimension image plane, therefore they suffer from object moving and background changes.

However, existing solutions suffer from many underlying assumptions, due to complexes scene properties (geometrics, illumination, ..., etc.). Recently, the computer vision community has converged in using light field imaging as a new representation of the image scene. The light field imaging, or, as Gortler, Grzeszczuk., Szeliski, and Cohen (1996), called "The Lumigraph", are 4-dimensional images containing both, orientation, and position information of each point of the object. Effectively, Light field imaging record the 3D Information of the scene in the image plane, this information is represented by the location of the individual light rays, that is defined by the position coordinates and the propagation direction of the incoming light, defined by the incidence angles (Adelson, & Bergen, 1991; Levoy, & Hanrahan, 1996; Levoy, 2006).

As a new technique, the light field was largely used for several technologies of computer vision and image processing, object detection was one of these techniques (Dansereau, 2013). Although, few works were presented for object detection, using the light field image. Efficient but few techniques were proposed, in literature.

In their work, Dansereau, Williams, and Corke, (2016), proposed a framework to detect changes in mobile light field cameras. Shimada, Nagahara, and Taniguchi, (2013) used the light field for object detection, their method generates an arbitrary in-focus plan and an out-focus one that filled the background region. The object detection is used for video surveillance, too, and performed by computing the viewpoint of spatial-temporal light field consistency in processing the light rays.

In a second work, Shimada., Nagahara., and Taniguchi, (2015), presented a new change detection strategy using light rays, they determine in-focus and an out-focus area, by generating an active surveillance field. Light rays source is defined by the evaluating of the focusses. The temporal changes are captured by the update of the light rays background.

Depth estimation technique for the 4D plenoptic function, using light field image was used to provide a metric to the foreground and background separation models, as the work of Boyle, (2016). Or to construct a depth map databases, as we can find in the work of Raj, Lowney, and Shah, (2016). For more work, readers can see the work of Hansen, and Holk (2011), and Liu, Hou, Sun, and Tan, (2017).

By far, nearly all existing edge detection algorithms used images provided by a regular camera.

High image quality is the more challenging requirement for medical imaging systems. Medical diagnosis task is generally based on image analysis, it requires more details in images to deal with difficult analysis and avoid the wrong diagnosis.

Due to its capabilities to perform image quality, light field camera has a potential to manipulate single one and computationally extract important features as position, orientation, and depth information. This new technology may have an important use in some medical imaging systems. Plenoptic imaging flexibly manipulates the image as it can adjust the focus plain doc a digital focusing/refocusing and changing the viewpoint. In medical imaging, the analysis task will be a simple task as the viewer interacts with image and explore object image anatomy by a simple operation of focusing/refocusing feature of interest through multiple viewpoints in different depth levels (Turola, & Gruppetta, 2013).

As it is a new technology a few medical applications are following this new trend. In DERMOPLENO project of the Multimedia Signal Processing-LP Groups of the superior thechnico institute (Instituto Superior Técnico), researchers aim to develop new methods and tool using the Plenoptic function for medical imaging tasks, as we can cite: acquisition, computational analysis, and coding. Their work was about the skin cancer analysis, known as Melanoma. To get Melanoma Plenoptic high-resolution images. The images contain rich visual information of both spatial and orientation ones, as for example the RGB intensity and angles of orientation of light rays. The project aims to get compressive databases of high-resolution images. it aims to explore the efficiency of the light field in data representation to reduce the amount of data by their capabilities to perform compression methods by expanding the capacity of storage and the rapidity of databases access.

In neurosurgery, Brian. R Chen and al had explored the light field technology to get more information from a single image using its different views, and getting the organ anatomy at different depth levels, by refusing/ focusing on any object of interest.

As one of interesting use of light field: The Light Field Speckle (LFLS) belonging to the MSP-Leiria group. This project uses the dynamic speckle to extract Dynamic Patterns and combining it with light field images to get more optical proprieties to create more significant rich image descriptions: texture and pattern images concerns.

In 2012, Tumlinson, and Everett, (2015), from Carl Zeiss Meditec Corporation, proposed a light field camera from fundus photography. They managed to define and remove aberrations, in addition to reducing the glare effects in fundus images.

The other study made by Turola, and Gruppetta, (2013), on the application of 4D light field technology to retinal imaging. They performed some numerical simulations in Matlab.

Hence, in literature, there are few works based on LF imaging for retinal imaging specifically retinal blood vessels detection and extraction. This kind of image application had a great impact on the human health as it helps to control and surveil the whole-body health through the state of retinal blood vessels.

Situated in the posterior of the eye, this makes retina not directly accessible with present a major difficulty to explore and to analysis it. Researchers are exposed to a relevant challenge due to several reasons (Tong, & Melanson, 2017):

- Noisy fundus images: as the retina is low reflective a highly sensitive to the light, imaging it is difficult as it requires to both illuminate and photograph it simultaneously. This produces a low ratio of signal to noise. And the appearance of ghost reflection due to the scalping surface of the retina and parasite light that must be eliminated.
- Another relevant is about the variation of the intensity and color of the retinal image views, depending on the changing of image sequences. This influences the depth map and as result will create difficulties to reconstruct 3D images through 2D images series.
- The difference between the spherical form of the retina and the planar one of the camera restricts the field of view area, that can cause the loose of important information on the retinal image, and false diagnosis may be concluded.

In general, light field imaging still is in its infancy in the medical imaging domain, and limited research where leading this way.

In our work, we expose the feasibility of using the light field imaging technology in the fundus photography as a revolutionary solution of the limited exposed above. In our proposed method we use a different kind of image fundus representation: the simulated fundus light field image, which provides high-quality 2D retinal images, that will be used to perform edge position pixel. The edge detection task is performed by the computing of the first and the second derivative as known as the Gradient and the Laplacian operators, respectively.

THE FOCUS OF THE CHAPTER

This chapter will be divided into two parts:

- The first part we will talk about the light field imaging, as a new method for image acquisition and representation. Where we give the theoretical definition of the light field notion and the plenoptic function of light. Finally, we will give a brief description of the main tools, sensors, and databases.
- In the second part, we will expose, in details our model for edge and blood vessels detection.
  - First, we construct the edge image, based on the definition of the first, (Gradient), and the second derivative, (Laplacian), operators. As we give their theoretical aspects and the adaptation for image and edge detection.
  - Second, the application of the above theoretical formulas to detect and extract blood vessels in the retinal image.
- The end of this chapter is about a conclusion and future researches.

FIRST PART: LIGHT FIELDS IMAGING

In his notebook, Leonardo Davinci described the body of the air "as a set of full of an infinite number of radiant pyramids caused by the objects located in it" (Adelson, & Bergen, 1991). The radiant pyramids referee above is what we called the light field. The light field is described as: "a set of rays passing through any point in space", these rays are different in sense of orientation and intensity (Adelson, & Bergen, 1991; Levoy, 2006).

In "Thoughts on Ray Vibrations", Michael Faraday proposes to interpret light as a field. The term of the light field was, firstly introduced and defined, in 1936, by Gershun in his book: The Light Field, Translated into English by Parry Moon and Gregory Timoshenko (Gershun, 1939).

Light fields imaging is a technique that is widely used in recent research. As it used, both, orientation and position of each light provided by the object to describe it. It offers a new image formation, based on multiple view representation approach for images in the real scene (Levoy, 2006; Xu, & Lam, 2017).

Light field object models are used to capture and store the appearance of an object from different points of view. They represent objects using their different views and render a photo-realistic view of different kind object shape. A simple interpolation technique can achieve the rendering phase (Levoy, & Hanrahan, 1996).

Definitions

- In literature, the light field is defined as a description of the radiance of light rays in 4D space. It describes the image as a field of rays, according to their orientation and their position (Levoy, 2006).
- The light field is a vector function that describes the amount of light flowing in every direction through every point in space. The direction of each ray is given by the 5D plenoptic function, and the magnitude of each ray is given by the radiance (Adelson, & Bergen, 1991).

Light Field in 4D

The light field in 4D is defined, using two distant planes: *UV* and *ST*, intersecting the optical axis. The amount of coming light ray at the plane *UV*, through the plane *ST*, is defined by the 4-Dimensional plenoptic function $LF(u, v, s, t)$ (Levoy, 2006).

Where: *(u, v)* and *(s, t)* denote, respectively, the distance between the two planes *UV* and *ST* from the optical axis.

The Light Field in 2D

The light field in 2D is defined, using two distant planes: U and S, intersecting the optical axis.

The amount of coming light ray at the plane U, through the plane S, is defined by the 2-Dimensional plenoptic function LF *(u, s)*.

Where *u* and *s* denote, respectively, the distance between the two planes *U* and *S* from the optical axis.

In our work, we will use the light field in 2D space, as a basic definition to perform our experiment phase (Levoy, 2006).

Light Fields Characteristics

The light field has caused an important stir in recent years. They are characterized by:

- Light field represents 3D objects with their different views and render a photo-realistic image of that object by view interpolation method.
- They offer a new representation of the image, so the post-processing phase is more flexible and efficient. This due to the high quality of the 2D image produced with new modern cameras, known as Lytro camera and plenoptic camera (Levoy, 2006).

The Plenoptic Function

The 5D plenoptic function describing 'everything that can be seen' with references to psychophysical and physiological literature on vision. It was called the "photic field" by Party moon, pat Hanraha and Levoy, give it the name of the 4D light field (Levoy, & Hanrahan, 1996).

Figure 1. Light filed two planes parametrization

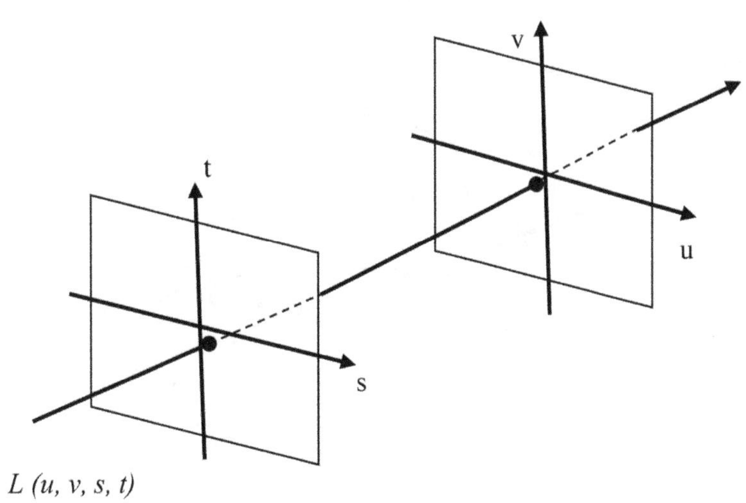

Definition

The plenoptic function is the dubbed name of the radiance along unchanging light rays arrangement in a 3D space. As a function it describes the cats light coordinates: x, y, z, and the angles ɵ and ϕ. if we assume that radiance is constant along an empty space, the Plenoptic function will be defined as a 4-D function.

Light Field Parametrization

The parametrization of a 4D set of rays has three different descriptions. The light rays see Figure 2, two planes, that is illustrated in Figure 1 and the spherical representation, Figure 3. The most used is based on the definition of ray's coordinates using 2 planes in a random position (Levoy, 2006).

That parametrization made a special definition of the light field: as a collection of perspective images positioned on the first plane, let it be *ST*, and projected into the second plane, the *UV* plane. Each perspective is taken from the well-defined position of the observer (Levoy, 2006).

Figure 2. Light rays parametrization

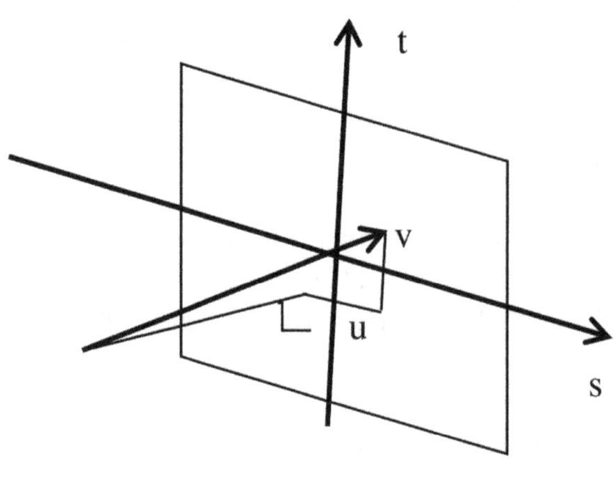

Figure 3. The spherical parametrization

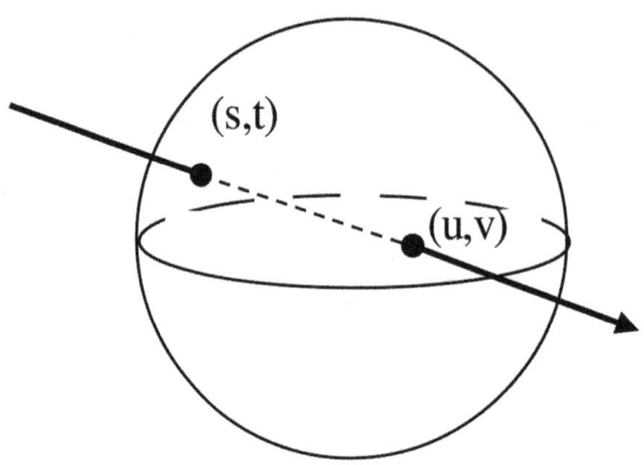

The 4-D Light Field Sampling

Image rendering conveying an object's shape on a computer display, using, previously, captured rays sampling. The number and the arrangement of images and the resolution of each image are together called the sampling of the 4D light field (Levoy, 2006).

Light Fields Database

To deal with the wide increase of research in computational photography, specifically, the large use of Light field imaging, large and colossal databases were created to evaluate and test the researcher's works. The reader can get a good reference for benchmarking light field datasets in the work of Wanner, Meister, and Goldluecke, 2013, and Honauer, Johannsen, Kondermann, and Goldluecke, 2016). Several, and important databases were built for different sort of Light Field images, as we can cite:

- **Stanford Light Field Archive:** This database is constructed using a different type of light field sensor, as a camera array, gantry, and a light field microscope. It provides an Archive with 20 light fields sampled
- **UCSD/MERL Light Field Repository:** This database contains both video and static light fields. Sampled light fields are represented in one dimension of viewpoints.
- **Synthetic Light Field Archive:** Many artificial light fields construct this repository, with some specificities like including some nice challenges like reflections, transparencies, and occlusions.
- **Middlebury Stereo Datasets:** The Middlebury Stereo Dataset provides a single 4D light field and additional 3D light fields. Fortunately, this database contains the ground truth data, as well as some corresponded depth information.

Light Field Data Acquisition

In computer vision, data acquisition is a very important task, and require more sophisticated sensors to perform it and to get high image quality. However, conventional cameras, lose most image information specifically those about light distribution. That significantly decreases the efficiency of the vision system.

To perform the light field vision application variant system acquisition were created. As we can cite:

Gantry Camera

A simple camera placed on a moving gantry, see, Figure 4. It was used to acquire the light field data by three important universities, as Stanford University, Cornell University, and Virginia University. Due to the expensive cost of such sensors, researchers used the Lego Mindstorms Gantry to capture the Light field data. It is based on just moving the camera through the four sides of the Lego gantry. MIT graphics group had built a simple vertical XY-table for Light field acquisition.

Camera Array

As the Light Filed data was largely used, many vision systems work with dynamic scenes. Camera Array system, in Figure 5, performs this kind of acquisition. Researchers at the Stanford University built

Figure 4. Planar Gantry Camera. Lego Mindstorms gantry.

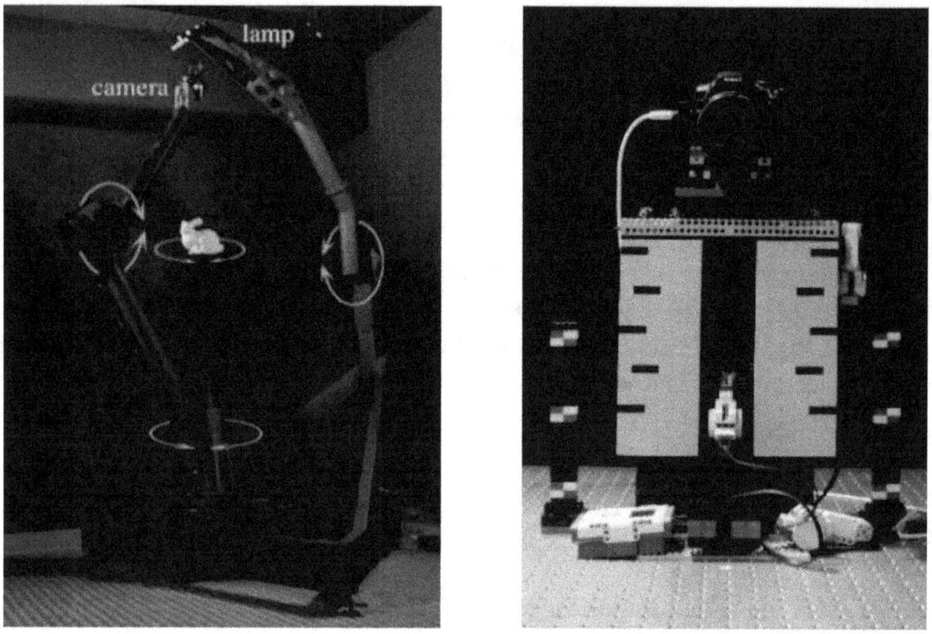

several camera arrays to perform application in computational photography. Since that, camera array systems were significantly developed, and becoming more compact and efficient. Cameras array are commercialized in the market and are available for personal use.

ViewPLUS, designed and manufactured the world's first camera with PCI Express external: The ProFUSION 25, a 5x5 camera array system with 25 VGA resolution, and high-quality senses.

Another type of camera well known for its very small size, smaller than a coin: the PiCam (Pelican Imaging Camera-Array), a passive camera that can acquire both stills and video. This camera is outfitted with an ultra-thin high-performance monolithic camera array, that enables the acquisition of a high-quality image with a super-resolution. Since this camera is small enough, smartphones and other mobile advice will be equipped with.

Coded Aperture Camera

Programmable Aperture Camera is used for captured different aperture shape by blocking undesirable light rays and keep useful ones. To overcome the low quantity of light caused by the small aperture size, researchers can use computational methods, to recover the whole light field. MIT Media Lab proposes The Aperture camera as a coded aperture camera, illustrated in Figure 6.

Lenslet Camera

The first generation of the lenslet camera was first proposed by Ng et al, this is a hand-held camera that captures whole light field by placing the Lenslet in front of the image sensor. Lenslet camera can capture both static and dynamic scenes. The light field camera Lytro is the commercial camera of this type of

Figure 5. Camera array systems. a. Profusion25. b. PiCam. c. Camera array on a smartphone.

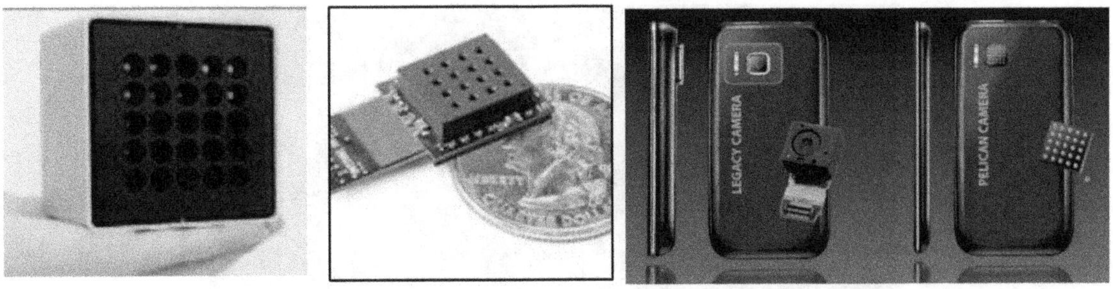

Figure 6. The coded Aperture camera: The aperture MIT

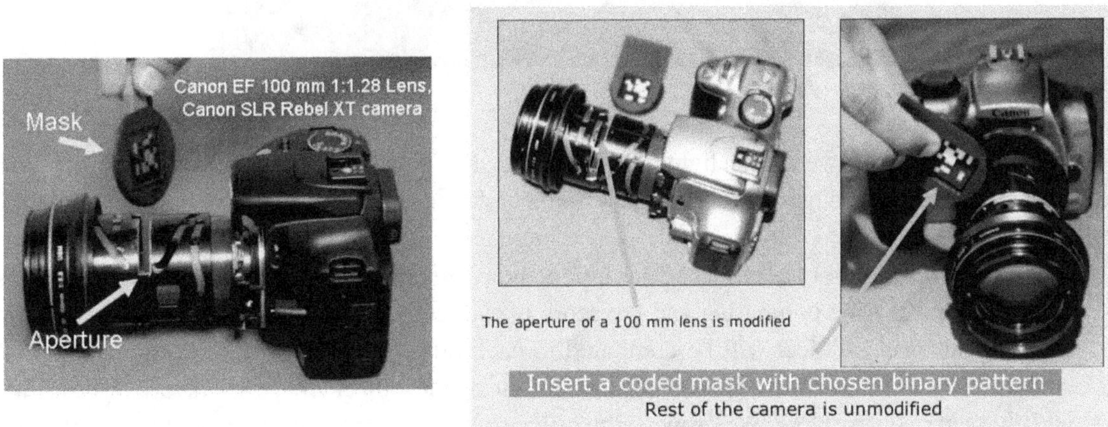

camera. The second generation was developed by Georgiev et al, called the focused plenoptic camera, well known for their high image resolution. Figure 7 illustrates an example of the lenslet camera: The Lytro Illum.

SECOND PART: EDGE AND OBJECT DETECTION MODEL

Overview of the Proposed Idea

Object recognition and tracking are basically based on two crucial tasks:

- The first is the data acquisition: at this level, we have work, as possible, on high-quality images, this can influence the efficiency and the time answer of the recognition or detection model. So, an efficient data acquisition sensor or large databases of high-quality image perform significantly the data acquisition task. Preprocessing phase will be neglected as we can get high-quality images, with only special sophisticated cameras.

Figure 7. Lenslet Camera: The Lytro Illum

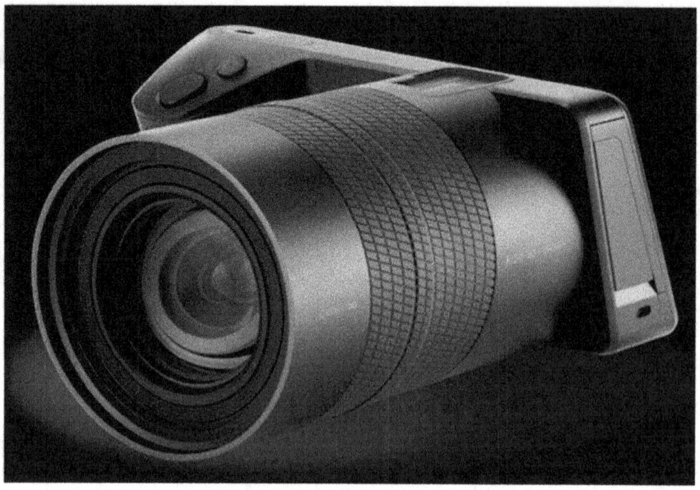

In our proposed model, we use the light field image. As they have the characteristics to describe object and scene in high-quality image resolution, with efficient information about pixel position and orientation.

- The second task is about the object description and representation. This is an important task, as it influences in the time computing and the score of the recognition process. In image recognition, images and images-object will be compared to each other to make a recognition decision. The comparison is computed using a good description of the object image by invariant descriptors and characteristics vectors. We propose the utilization of the image gradient and the Laplacian of the object image, well known in arithmetic as the first and the second derivative function, respectively. These descriptors will be used to create edge images.

Experimental Setup

Our work is divided into two main experiments:

- The edge detection and image edge representation: in this first experiments we use the theoretical and arithmetical definition of derivative to create gradient and Laplacian images. as we consider the use of the intensity image, the gradient is defined by the computing of the first derivative, and the Laplacian as the second derivative, using the 3*3 Sobel operator.
  - Both gradient and Laplacian image is used to describe the edge image and the edge image object for the second experiment of the object detection.
- The blood vessels detection: in this level, the application of the gradient and Laplacian formulas to detect and extract blood vessels in the retinal image.

A discussion about these results and a conclusion for future works will be presented at the end of this chapter.

Dataset

Our model was tested using the fundus image proposed by Tong and Melanson, (2017). In their work, the image is the result of the simulation of the light field fundus photography using a Zemax tool. The quality of the image of the simulated light field fundus is better than this representing the simple retina image. This high quality used to detect vessel in retinal images. All light fields are rendered as .png images.

Experiment Tools

All experiments are achieved on a PC with an Intel Core i7, with a windows 64 bits operating system. The computing is performed in Matlab 2017a.

Edge Detection and Derivative Functions

Edge detection is one of the major steps in image processing: image segmentation, tracking, detection of defects in industrial products and so on.

In a neighborhood of pixels, the discontinuity in the intensity values is a discriminant characteristic, which makes it possible to determine the different regions in an image (edges). Based on the discontinuity property in the image intensity, the edge can describe the line as an edge segment, which the intensity value of their pixels is lower or higher than the one at the background, on each side (Gonzalez, & Woods,2002; McAndrew, 2015).

Differentiation is an appropriate way to determine this discontinuity in an image. It can be expressed by the calculation of partial derivatives of the discrete function representing the image intensity. The definition of the image by the first derivative (the gradient) or the second derivative (the Laplacian) has been widely used, to describe the image in terms of its outlines. This representation is efficient, as it is an optimal representation of the image basing, only, on its significant descriptors (Gonzalez, & Woods, 2002; McAndrew, 2015).

First Derivative and the Gradient of an Intensity Image

To enable edge detection, the Gradient vector is frequently used. The gradient vector of an image at any given pixel position is orthogonal to the direction of edges in this image, and its magnitude is maximal in this direction. Using these geometrical properties, we will use gradient magnitude and direction image for computing a non-maximum suppressed image. This image will be called the edge image (McAndrew, 2015).

Mathematical Definition

For a function of intensity values, I (x, y), the gradient, at (x, y) position, is defined as the two-dimensioned column vector ∇ I, where:

$$\nabla I \equiv Grad\left(I\right) \equiv \begin{pmatrix} G_x \\ G_y \end{pmatrix} \tag{1}$$

where

$$G_x \equiv \frac{\delta I(x,y)}{\delta x} \tag{2}$$

$$G_y \equiv \frac{\delta I(x,y)}{\delta y} \tag{3}$$

Geometrical Properties of the Gradient

The gradient of an image has a very important property, it always points in the direction of the greatest rate of change of I at the location (x, y). As a vector, two parameters may describe the gradient, these two descriptors are the magnitude and the direction (Gonzalez, & Woods,2002; McAndrew, 2015).

The Gradient Magnitude

The gradient magnitude denotes the rate of change in the direction of the gradient vector, at a given location. this magnitude computes a length of the gradient vector (Gonzalez, & Woods,2002):

$$Mag(x,y) = Mag(\nabla I) = \sqrt{G_x^2 + G_y^2} \tag{4}$$

For more suitable computation, the magnitude in equation (4), can be approximated by absolute values of G_x and G_y, as followed:

$$Mag(x,y) \approx |G_x| + |G_y| \tag{5}$$

The Gradient Orientation

The computing of the angle gives the gradient vector orientation as followed:

$$\theta = tan^{-1}\left({G_x}/{G_y} \right) \tag{6}$$

In case of G_y is equal to zero at the (x, y) position, the angle θ is equal to Π/2 if G_x is positive or -Π/2 else.

Gradient and First Order Derivatives

The local change in intensity value of an image can be detected using derivative functions (first or second derivative) at the pixel position of an image.

Using the notation in Table 1, the image I (x, y) denotes the 3x3 image pixel, p_5 is pixel with (x, y) location. p_1 denotes the location x-1, y-1, and so on.

The approximation of the first derivative can be computed using a different kind of masks, the major characteristics of these masks are that the sum of their coefficients is always equal to zero, which means, in constant intensities, the mask will give a response of zero. this corresponds to the definition of derivatives (Gonzalez, & Woods, 2002).

The first order directional derivatives in x and y-direction are defined by:

$$I_x\left(x,y\right) = p_6 - p_5 \tag{7}$$

$$I_y\left(x,y\right) = p_8 - p_5 \tag{8}$$

In 1965, Roberts proposed a mask of 2x2 of cross gradient operators, defined by, see Table 2 (Gonzalez, & Woods,2002).

The Roberts mask operators don't have a center of symmetry, they are of even size, so they will be awkward to implement.

Table 1. The region neighborhood

P_1	P_2	P_3
P_4	P_5	P_6
P_7	P_8	P_9

Table 2. Roberts cross gradient operators

-1	0
0	1

(a)

0	-1
1	0

(b)

The filters in which we are interested are the Sobel mask operators, masks of 3x3 size, that presented in Table 3. At each (x, y) position of pixel *p*, the approximation in the x-direction is obtained by the sum of the third and the first row of the 3x3 image region neighborhood, implemented by the mask of Table 3 (a), and the approximation in the y-direction is obtained by the sum of the third and the first column of the 3x3 image region implemented by the mask of Table 3(b).

Using the 3x3 neighborhood of p_5 center, the approximations of G_x (x, y) and G_y (x, y) is obtained are as follow:

$$G_x(x,y) = (p_7 + 2 * p_8 + p_9) - (p_1 + 2 * p_2 + p_3) \tag{9}$$

$$G_y(x,y) = (p_3 + 2 * p_6 + p_9) - (p_1 + 2 * p_4 + p_7) \tag{10}$$

Table 3 illustrates the G_x and G_y filter operators, obtained from the equation (9) and (10).

Gradient Vector Properties

The gradient magnitude and orientation can be computed using the substitution of G_x (x, y) and G_y (x, y) of the equation 9 and 10 in the equation 5. The magnitude and the orientation image, at each point of (x, y) position are computed as below (Gonzalez, & Woods,2002):

$$Mag(x,y) \approx |(p_7 + 2 * p_8 + p_9) - (p_1 + 2 * p_2 + p_3)| +$$

$$|(p_3 + 2 * p_6 + p_9) - (p_1 + 2 * p_4 + p_7)| \tag{11}$$

And the orientation, defined by the angle θ is computed using the followed equation:

Table 3. The Sobel mask operators

-1	-2	-1
0	0	0
1	2	1

(a)

-1	0	1
-2	0	2
-1	0	1

(b)

$$\theta = tan^{-1}\left(\frac{\left(p_7 + 2 * p_8 + p_9\right) - \left(p_1 + 2 * p_2 + p_3\right)}{\left(p_3 + 2 * p_6 + p_9\right) - \left(p_1 + 2 * p_4 + p_7\right)}\right) \tag{12}$$

Figures 8, Figure 9, and Figure 10 show the original, the magnitude and the orientation gradient images obtained using the equations 11 and 12.

Figure 8. The original Light field image

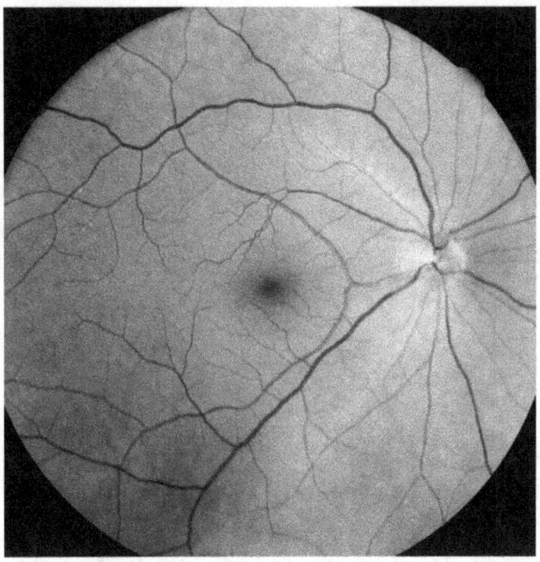

Figure 9. The magnitude image

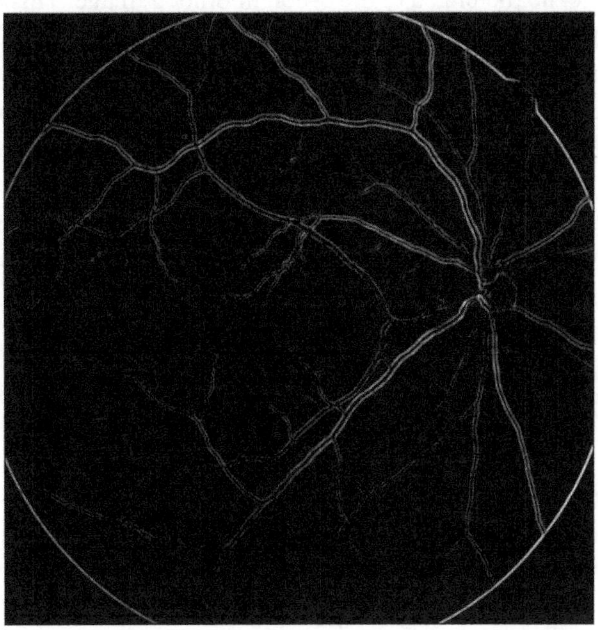

Figure 10. The orientation image

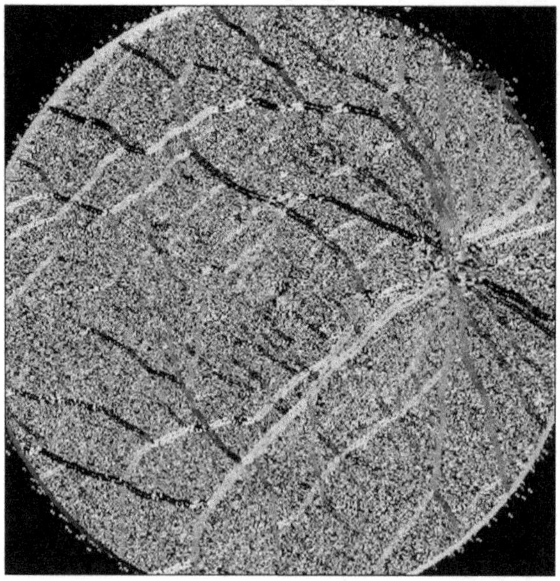

Non-Maxima Suppression Algorithm

Optimal edge operator would have marked points belonged to the edge line as a maximum. To find these point positions, we have to non-maximum suppress the magnitude gradient image, through the gradient direction of each of their points.

The Non-maxima suppression algorithm is based on the definition of the nine-pixel neighborhoods, by taking the pixel p (x, y) at the position (x, y), as an image region center of the amplitude image. Since the pixel of maximum amplitude value in the direction of the gradient will be chosen, as pixel edges, we can have an unreal pixel i.e. not belonged to the 3-neighborhood image. This means that it's magnitude value is unknown and must be estimated. The estimation of the magnitude value will be done by using the interpolation algorithm (Canny, 1983).

Let p (x, y) be the accurate pixel at the (x, y) position, we will define two other unreal points, in and at the opposite side of the gradient direction. Gradient magnitude values at these new points can be estimated using those of the two pixels in the neighborhood image, lying in the same line.

In equation 13 and 14, we estimate, as an example, the value of the magnitude of a point situated between p (x, y+1) and p (x+1, y+1). The value of interpolated magnitude gradient is computed using these following two equations:

$$G_1 = \frac{G_x}{G_y} * G\left(x+1, y+1\right) + \left(1 - \frac{G_x}{G_y}\right) * G\left(x, y+1\right) \tag{13}$$

$$G_2 = \frac{G_x}{G_y} * G(x-1, y-1) + \left(1 - \frac{G_x}{G_y}\right) * G(x, y-1) \tag{14}$$

We mark the point p (x, y) as maximum if G (x, y) > G_1 and G (x, y) > $G_{2,}$ and its magnitude value will be equal to 255 (white pixel) else, it's value will be zero (black pixel).

The values of the orientation angle belong to the interval value of [-π/2, π/2[.

Images, below, show the obtained edge detector image, Figure 11 (a) before the thresholding phase, and Figure 11 (b) after the thresholding algorithm.

Second Derivative for Image Representation

In what follows, we will use the representation of the image by the Laplacian operator.

Laplacian and the Second Derivative of an Image

The Laplacian is an isotopic derivation operator (invariant to the rotation of the image), and linear (calculated from the derivation which is a linear operation) (Gonzalez, & Woods,2002; McAndrew, 2015).

The Laplacian of a function f is calculated as follows:

$$\nabla^2 f = \frac{\partial^2 f}{\partial x^2} + \frac{\partial^2 f}{\partial y^2} \tag{15}$$

In image processing, the expression (15) is expressed in a discrete form, using pixel intensity values, in a well-defined neighborhood in the picture.

The definition of the second, partial and directional derivatives according to x and y are expressed by the following equations:

Figure 11. The edge image using gradient operator

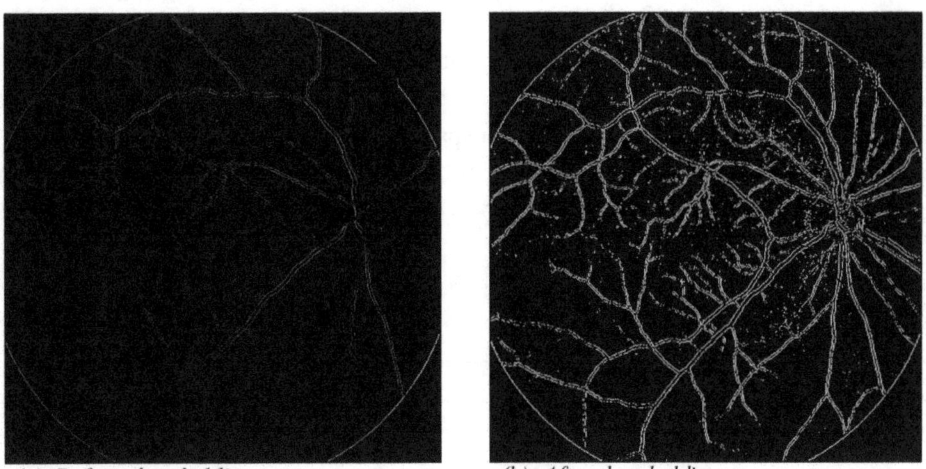

(a). Before thresholding *(b). After thresholding*

$$\frac{\partial^2 f}{\partial x^2} = f\left(x+1,y\right)+f\left(x-1,y\right)-2*f\left(x,y\right) \tag{16}$$

$$\frac{\partial^2 f}{\partial y^2} = f\left(x,y+1\right)+f\left(x,y-1\right)-2*f\left(x,y\right) \tag{17}$$

And so, the Laplacian is obtained by summing equations (16) and (17), as follows:

$$\nabla^2 f = f\left(x+1,y\right)+f\left(x-1,y\right)+f\left(x,y+1\right)+f\left(x,y-1\right)-4*f\left(x,y\right) \tag{18}$$

Several masks can be used to calculate the Laplacian of a picture. In the following examples, we will use the representation in 8-neighbors for the Laplacian definition see Table 4 (Gonzalez, & Woods, 2002).

In correspondence with the definition of the derivation, we note well that the sum of the values of all the mask is equal to zero, so if there is no change in intensity, the sum of the product of pixels with this mask is well equal to zero (Gonzalez, & Woods, 2002).

Experimental Results

Computing using the equations 18, Figure 12 (a) and Figure 12 (b) show, respectively, the obtained Laplacian image before and after thresholding.

FUTURE RESEARCH DIRECTIONS

As an additional material test, we propose to use different image representation, the histogram of oriented gradients (*HOG*), Laplacian of Gaussian (LoG), or an eigenvalues images to perform the edge detection task.

To deal with space color definition. An additional comparison of edge detecting in a light field image represented in the three coordinates L*, a*, and b* with the whole image in the L*a*b* CIE 1976 color space domain. The difference in results was very significant.

Edges obtained with the image represented in L* and b* coordinates are more significative than those obtained with a* and L*a*b* CIE 1976 color space. different Gradient edge images represented in: Figure 14 (a): L*, Figure 14 (b): a*, Figure 14 (c): b*, Figure 14 (d): L*a*b* color space, and images of Laplacian edge are in: Figure 15 (a): L*, Figure 15 (b): a*, Figure 15(c): b*, Figure 15 (d): L*a*b* color

Table 4. The Laplacian mask operator

0	1	0
1	-4	1
0	1	0

Figure 12. The edge image using Laplacian operator

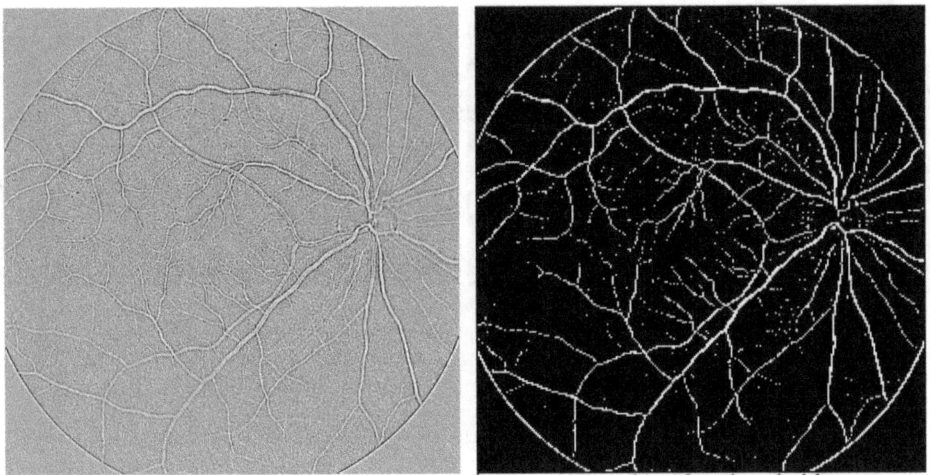

(a). Before thresholding (b). After thresholding

space, demonstrate the influence of color space color for the blood vessels detection process of simple images of: Figure 13 (a): L*, Figure 13 (b): a*, Figure 13 (c): b*, Figure 13 (d): L*a*b* color space.

Based on these obtained results, we invite researchers to use, other color space representation, following the image type and application, to perform, as possible, the edge detection process.

CONCLUSION

In this chapter, we proposed a new sensing strategy for blood-retinal vessels detection and extraction based on, first, the extraction of visual information of a frame image such as a discrete object, specifically: edges. we have presented a new object detection technique on simulated light fields fundus images. Our technique is based on the blood vessels detection of the retinal image, using the differentiation method.

Throw multiple experiences, we have shown that working on light field images deal, efficiently, with the object detection process drawbacks.

Figure 13. Images using L(a), a*(b), b*(c), and (d) L*a*b* color space*

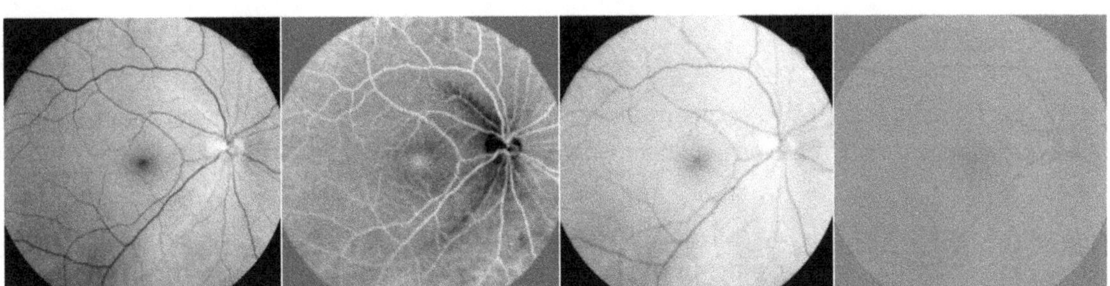

(a) (b) (c) (d)

Figure 14. Gradient edge image using L(a), a*(b), b*(c), and (d) L*a*b* color space*

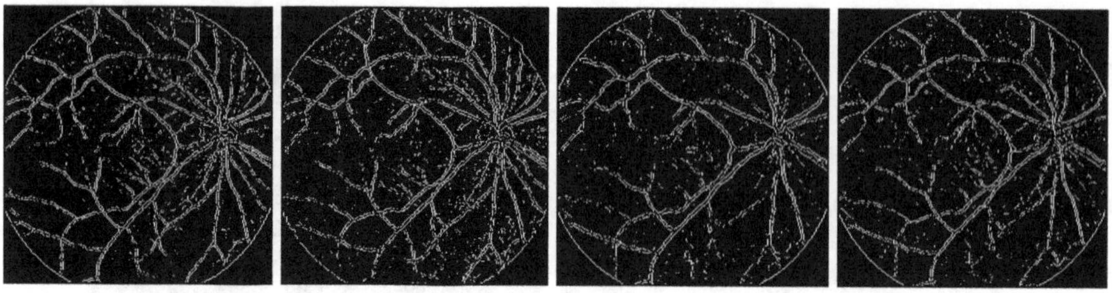

(a) (b) (c) (d)

Figure 15. Laplacian edge image using L(a), a*(b), b*(c), and L*a*b* color space (d)*

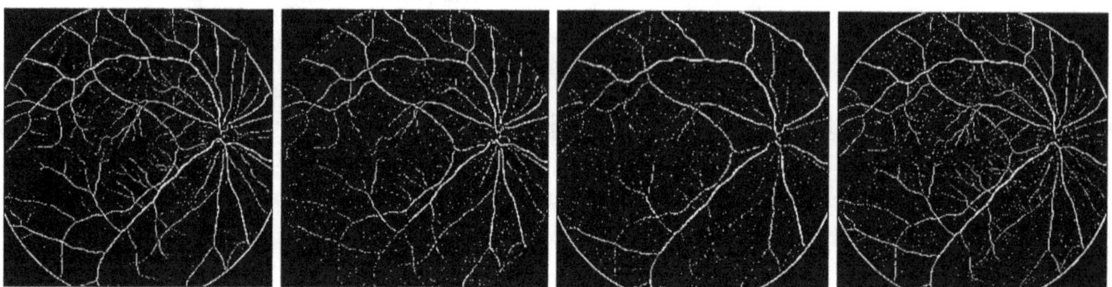

(a) (b) (c) (d)

We have proved, during experiments and test that the use of the derivative method of edge detection had performed the blood vessels detection task in terms of optimality representation and efficiency results.

The proposed method can be readily used in the medical imaging field, the vessel detection in retinal light field image.

Since the difficulties to get a light field image of a fundus in the retinal image. The retinal image can be simulated using powerful optical design tools, like Zemax and Oslo. These tools are very efficient and have been tested for such a task.

In conclusion, the study has shown the importance of the image color representation in an image processing or a computer vision system. And its influences on the time computing and result quality.

REFERENCES

Achanta, R., Estrada, F., Wils, P., & Süsstrunk, S. (2008, May). Salient region detection and segmentation. In *International conference on computer vision systems* (pp. 66-75). Springer. 10.1007/978-3-540-79547-6_7

Adelson, E. H., & Bergen, J. R. (1991). *The plenoptic function and the elements of early vision*. Academic Press.

Belongie, S., Malik, J., & Puzicha, J. (2001). Matching shapes. In *Computer Vision, 2001. ICCV 2001. Proceedings. Eighth IEEE International Conference on* (Vol. 1, pp. 454-461). IEEE. 10.1109/ICCV.2001.937552

Belongie, S., Malik, J., & Puzicha, J. (2001). Shape context: A new descriptor for shape matching and object recognition. In Advances in neural information processing systems (pp. 831-837). Academic Press.

Belongie, S., Malik, J., & Puzicha, J. (2002). Shape matching and object recognition using shape contexts. *IEEE Transactions on Pattern Analysis and Machine Intelligence*, *24*(4), 509–522. doi:10.1109/34.993558

Boyle, K. C. (2016). *Occluded Edge Detection in Light Field Images for Background Removal*. Academic Press.

Canny, J. F. (1983). *Finding edges and lines in images*. Academic Press.

Cristóbal, G., Schelkens, P., & Thienpont, H. (Eds.). (2013). *Optical and digital image processing: fundamentals and applications*. John Wiley & Sons.

Dansereau, D. (2016). *Light field toolbox v. 0.4*. Available at: http://www.mathworks.com/matlabcentral/fileexchange/49683-lightfield-toolboxv0-4

Dansereau, D. G. (2015). Light field toolbox for matlab. *Software Manual*.

Dansereau, D. G., Pizarro, O., & Williams, S. B. (2013, June). Decoding, calibration and rectification for lenselet-based plenoptic cameras. In *Computer Vision and Pattern Recognition (CVPR), 2013 IEEE Conference on* (pp. 1027-1034). IEEE. 10.1109/CVPR.2013.137

Gershun, A. (1939). The light field. *Studies in Applied Mathematics*, *18*(1-4), 51–151.

Gonzalez, R. C., & Woods, R. E. (2002). *Digital image processing*. Academic Press.

Gonzalez, R. C., Woods, R. E., & Eddins, S. L. (2009). *Digital Image Processing Using MATLAB*. Gatesmark Publishing.

Gortler, S. J., Grzeszczuk, R., Szeliski, R., & Cohen, M. F. (1996, August). The lumigraph. In *Proceedings of the 23rd annual conference on Computer graphics and interactive techniques* (pp. 43-54). ACM.

Hansen, M., & Holk, E. (2011). *Depth map estimation for plenoptic images*. Academic Press.

Hazirbas, C., Leal-Taixé, L., & Cremers, D. (2017). *Deep Depth from Focus*. arXiv preprint arXiv:1704.01085

Honauer, K., Johannsen, O., Kondermann, D., & Goldluecke, B. (2016). A dataset and evaluation methodology for depth estimation on 4d light fields. In *Asian Conference on Computer Vision* (pp. 19-34). Springer.

Levoy, M. (2006). Light fields and computational imaging. *Computer*, *39*(8), 46–55. doi:10.1109/MC.2006.270

Levoy, M., & Hanrahan, P. (1996, August). Light field rendering. In *Proceedings of the 23rd annual conference on Computer graphics and interactive techniques* (pp. 31-42). ACM.

McAndrew, A. (2015). *A computational introduction to digital image processing*. Chapman and Hall/CRC.

Moeslund, T. B. (2012). *Introduction to video and image processing: Building real systems and applications*. Springer Science & Business Media. doi:10.1007/978-1-4471-2503-7

Murphy, K. P. (2012). *Machine Learning: A Probabilistic Perspective*. Academic Press.

Myung, I. J. (2003). Tutorial on maximum likelihood estimation. *Journal of Mathematical Psychology*, *47*(1), 90–100. doi:10.1016/S0022-2496(02)00028-7

Ng, R., Levoy, M., Brédif, M., Duval, G., Horowitz, M., & Hanrahan, P. (2005). Light field photography with a hand-held plenoptic camera. *Computer Science Technical Report CSTR*, *2*(11), 1–11.

Raj, A. S., Lowney, M., & Shah, R. (2016). *Light-field database creation and depth estimation*. Dept. Computer Science, Stanford University, Technical Report.

Shimada, A., Nagahara, H., & Taniguchi, R. I. (2013). Object detection based on spatiotemporal light field sensing. *Information and Media Technologies*, *8*(4), 1115–1119.

Shimada, A., Nagahara, H., & Taniguchi, R. I. (2015, August). Change detection on light field for active video surveillance. In *Advanced Video and Signal Based Surveillance (AVSS), 2015 12th IEEE International Conference on* (pp. 1-6). IEEE. 10.1109/AVSS.2015.7301785

Tekalp, A. M. (2015). *Digital video processing*. Prentice Hall Press.

Tumlinson, A. R., & Everett, M. J. (2015). *U.S. Patent No. 8,998,411*. Washington, DC: U.S. Patent and Trademark Office.

Turola, M., & Gruppetta, S. (2013, October). 4D light field ophthalmoscope: a study of plenoptic imaging of the human retina. In *Frontiers in Optics* (pp. JW3A–36). Optical Society of America. doi:10.1364/FIO.2013.JW3A.36

Umbaugh, S. E. (2017). *Digital Image Processing and Analysis with MATLAB and CVIPtools: Applications with MATLAB® and CVIPtools*. CRC Press.

Venkataraman, K., Lelescu, D., Duparré, J., McMahon, A., Molina, G., Chatterjee, P., ... Nayar, S. (2013). Picam: An ultra-thin high-performance monolithic camera array. *ACM Transactions on Graphics*, *32*(6), 166. doi:10.1145/2508363.2508390

Wanner, S., Meister, S., & Goldluecke, B. (2013, September). *Datasets and benchmarks for densely sampled 4d light fields*. VMV.

Xu, Y., & Lam, M. L. (2017). Light Field Vision for Artificial Intelligence. In *Artificial Intelligence and Computer Vision* (pp. 189–209). Cham: Springer. doi:10.1007/978-3-319-46245-5_11

Yücer, K., Sorkine-Hornung, A., Wang, O., & Sorkine-Hornung, O. (2016). Efficient 3D object segmentation from densely sampled light fields with applications to 3D reconstruction. *ACM Transactions on Graphics*, *35*(3), 22. doi:10.1145/2876504

Ziou, D., & Tabbone, S. (1998). Edge detection techniques-an overview. *Pattern Recognition and Image Analysis C/C of Raspoznavaniye Obrazov I Analiz Izobrazhenii, 8*, 537-559.

Zobel, M., Fritz, M., & Scholz, I. (2002, November). *Object Tracking and Pose Estimation Using Light-Field Object Models* (pp. 371–378). VMV.

ADDITIONAL READING

Bolan, J., Hall, E., Clifford, C., & Thurow, B. (2016). Light-field imaging toolkit. *SoftwareX*, *5*, 101–106. doi:10.1016/j.softx.2016.05.004

Deschenes, F., Ziou, D., & Auclair-Fortier, M. F. (2004). Detection of lines, line junctions and line terminations. *International Journal of Remote Sensing*, *25*(3), 511–535. doi:10.1080/0143116031000139845

Gortler, S. J., Grzeszczuk, R., Szeliski, R., & Cohen, M. F. (1996, August). The lumigraph. In *Proceedings of the 23rd annual conference on Computer graphics and interactive techniques* (pp. 43-54). ACM.

Hainich, R. R., & Bimber, O. (2016). *Displays: fundamentals & applications*. CRC press. doi:10.1201/9781315367408

Ihrke, I., Restrepo, J., & Mignard-Debise, L. (2016). Principles of Light Field Imaging: Briefly revisiting 25 years of research. *IEEE Signal Processing Magazine*, *33*(5), 59–69. doi:10.1109/MSP.2016.2582220

KEY TERMS AND DEFINITIONS

Depth Map: Represents an image that contains distance information, this information describes the relation between object surfaces and a viewpoint.

Gradient: Known in arithmetic as the first derivative function, is a vector describing the position and the orientation of a variation. this variation is a function defined by the variation of its various parameters. The symbol ∇ denotes it.

Laplacian: Usually denoted by the symbols $\nabla\cdot\nabla$, ∇^2 or Δ, Laplacian operator, or a second-order derivative operator, it is defined on Euclidean space by the divergence of the gradient of a function.

Lumigraph: Dubbed name of the 4D plenoptic function that describes all upcoming light rays at all positions and directions.

Oslo'Edu: Optics software for layout and optimization for the educative task, it is an optical design tool to perform the optical design researches.

Plenoptic Function: Represents the intensity of observed light by a five-dimensional function, light is described in 3-dimensional space, at every position and direction.

Radiance (*L*)**:** Measured in watts (*W*) per steradian (*sr*) per meter squared (*m*2), the radiance represents the amount of light flux living a surface.

Rendering: The process of extracting 2D projected images from the radiance equation.

Zemax: Is an optical design program, it offers the possibility to design and analyze both imaging and illumination systems. Zemax is sold American company, Zemax LLC, and manly used by Microsoft Windows.

Chapter 8
Telemonitoring Healthcare System-Based Mobile Agent Technology

Nardjes Bouchemal
University Center of Mila, Algeria

Ramdane Maamri
Constantine 2 University, Algeria

Naila Bouchemal
Altran Technology, Algeria

ABSTRACT

Generally, distributed computing through a handheld/mobile device has to be considered with care because of the limited capabilities on these devices. Especially in ubiquitous telemonitoring healthcare, which refers to the disposition of any type of health services, such that medical staff members (physicians, emergency workers, other healthcare providers, etc.) through mobile computing devices can access them and expect data to be made available. In this chapter, the authors present a new system based on ubiquitous agents to assist telemonitoring employees, not only anytime and anywhere but also on any device.

INTRODUCTION

Patients, in Ubiquitous telemonitoring healthcare systems, will be monitored at long distance, and medical control support devices may be embedded in devices collecting vital-sign information from sensors (blood pressure, temperature, etc), (Koehler, 2011).

These new systems must have special characteristics such as permanent connection, storage capability for patient's healthcare information and intelligence.

That requires the introduction of new technologies such as cloud computing for the storage and accessibility and intelligent agent for the assistance and decisions.

DOI: 10.4018/978-1-5225-7071-4.ch008

Telemonitoring healthcare systems work with two important components; the system itself and network construction. The systems have the following important goals (Miller, 2009; Qinghua, 2010)

- Provides an electronic healthcare record for the patient conditions in the past and in the present time.
- Issues and alarm if there is anything wrong with the patient's vital signs or if one of his/her family member's see something is wrong.
- Sends a report, to include general information about the patient's health status.
- Presents the patient's health status such as temperature and other vital signs to the medical experts to analyze and they can offer advice.
- Offers support service in emergency situations (first-aid).

It is clear that telemonitoring healthcare systems must be permanently connected with the medical staff, which is not evident in the context of ubiquitous environments where devices have reduced energy autonomy and can be off-line at any time.

It is not enough to gather information about the context, but that information must be processed by self-adaptable and dynamic mechanisms and methods that can react independently of each particular situation that arises.

In this sense, agents and Multi-Agent Systems comprise one of the areas that can contribute expanding the possibilities of ubiquitous healthcare systems and telemonitoring systems. An agent can be defined as a computational system situated in an environment and is able to act autonomously in this environment to achieve its design goals (Wooldridge, 2002).

On the other hand, such as many other users, physicians are surrounded by many mobile and ubiquitous devices. We want to take advantage of this diversity to let them always connected.

For that, we propose in this chapter an approach based on Ubiquitous Mobile Agent System.

Its goal is to recognize physician devices; with the ability to migrate from one device to another.

The rest of the chapter is organized as follow: section 2 summarizes some works based on the use of agents in telemonitoring systems. We present in section three our contribution, the implementation and experimentations on JADE-LEAP. Finally, some conclusions are drawn.

RELATED WORK

Intelligent agents have the ability to make decisions defined by their inherent properties, such as: reactivity, pro-activity and sociability. These properties are intended to enable the agent to meet the objectives for which they were designed, following rules of behavior that enable them to communicate with their environment (Wooldridge, 2002). Recent research has discussed the benefits of using agent technology and applications in the health care and telemonitoring domain (Isern, 2010).

De Paz et al. presented a project: Autonomous aGent for monitoring ALZheimer's patients (AGALZ), which facilitates the monitoring and tracking of patients with Alzheimer's (De Paz, 2015).

A telemonitoring system aimed at enhancing remote healthcare of dependent people at their homes has also been developed. The main contribution is the use of an experimental architecture that allows the interconnection of heterogeneous Wireless Sensor Networks (Tapia, 2010).

De Meo et al. presented multi-agent system that supports personalized patient access to health care services. The proposed system combines submitted queries with the corresponding patient profiles to identify services likely to satisfy patient needs and desires, (De Meo, 2011).

Vaidehi et al. presented a design for a health care monitoring system based on multi-agent and wireless sensor networks which can collect, retrieve, store and analyze patient vital signs. The multi-agent system is applied to manage these sensors and to collect and store data in a database, (Vaidehi, 2013).

Camarinha-Matos and Vieira presented an MA-based architecture for health care centers to remotely observe and help elderly people living alone at home, (Camarinha, 1999).

Wu et al. proposed a multi-agent web service framework based on a service-oriented architecture to support qualified and optimized medical data translation in an e-healthcare information system, (Wu, 2012).

Su and Wu designed a highly distributed information infrastructure—MADIP—by using the multi-agent and MA paradigm, which can automatically notify the responsible care-provider of abnormalities, offer remote medical advice and perform continuous health monitoring as needed, (Su, 2011).

Kim proposed a methodology for the design and implementation of u-healthcare, linking distributed mobile agents with medical entities into a collaborative environment (Kim, 2013).

Authors in (Su, 2014) presents the design and development of a mobile multi-agent platform based open information systems (IMAIS)with an automated diagnosis engine to support intensive and distributed ubiquitous fetal monitoring.

In most of presented systems, permanent connection is needed with healthcare staff. It is easy when using traditional wire-based communication systems, where users are connected to their desk PC.

But nowadays, users (including healthcare staff) need to have information anywhere and anytime to monitor patients and disabled persons.

For this, most of existing systems introduce ubiquitous devices and agents concept, but the problem is when these devices are offline (ex. problem of connection or insufficient battery), not available or does not have enough resources, Table.1.

CONTRIBUTION: UBIQUITOUS MOBILE AGENT SYSTEM

Physicians, such as most of today's users, have many handheld devices (smart phones, laptops, tablet, smart swatch, etc.) that provide them access to patient information.

The process may operate even if devices have limited energy capabilities or have no connectivity.

The idea is to connect monitor physician with his patient anywhere and anytime, through Ubiquitous Mobile Agent (UMA) that can migrate from one device to another and takes advantages from all of them especially in case of energy insufficiency, limited storage space or failure connectivity.

UMA System Architecture

The system is composed essentially of Ubiquitous Mobile Agent (*UMA*) to assist monitor physician and Device Agents (*DevA*) embedded in each device.

In patient side, we proposed Patient Agent (*PatA*) to assist patient, collect information from sensors and assure communication with the monitor physician (Figure 1). Below, we detail each agent.

Table 1. Presented systems analysis

Systems	Domain	Type of Agents	Ubiquitous Devices	Devices Problems Considered	
				Autonomy energy	Connection Quality
De Meo*et al.*	Personalized e-Health service access	Stationary	Yes	No	No
Wu *et al.*	Medical data transmission	Stationary	Yes	No	No
Vaidehi	In-home monitoring	Stationary	Yes	No	No
De Paz et al.	In-home monitoring	Mobile	Yes	No	Yes
Su and Wu,	Health care monitoring	Mobile	Yes	No	No
Alonso, *et al.*,	Health care monitoring	Stationary	Yes	No	No
Kim	Ubiquitous health care systems	Mobile	Yes	No	No
Su and Chu	Ubiquitous fetal monitoring	Mobile	Yes	No	No

Table 2. Example of StatusDevice of four devices

Device	StatusDevice		
	Energy Capacity	Connected	Storage Capacity
Lap Top	Low	Yes	Low
Smart Phone	Low	No	High
Tablet	Medium	Yes	Medium
Smart Swatch	Medium	No	Low

- *Ubiquitous Mobile Agent*
    - UMA is a Mobile agent, having the list of monitor physician devices: *ListDevice*= {*D1, D2,..,Dn*}. It is initially embedded on one of them (ex. smart phone).
    - UMA establishes a wireless network including all *ListDevice* devices.
    - UMA must have a permanent communication with the patient through Patient Agent (*PatA*) and with devices through Device Agent (*DevA*).
    - UMA has a detailed status of each device *StatusDevice* including: *EnergyCapacity* (time of battery), *Connected* (yes or no), *StorageCapacity*.
    - *StatusDevice* is collected from Device Agents. Table.2 summarizes example of status devices of laptop, smart phone and a tablet.
- *Device Agent.* DeviceAgent (*DevA*) is a stationary agent embedded in each device. Its role is to collect and transmit *StatusDevice* to UMA.
- *Patient Agent.* At the patient level, we planned to install PatientAgent (*PatA*) to communicate with UMA. It transmits health status information or alerts in emergency situations.

Process Description

- Initially, we suppose that UMA is embedded in *Di* from *ListDevice*.
- When UMA receives information from PatA (Health Status or Alert Messages), it verifies capabilities of its actual device.
- If *StatusDevice* is weak (*EnergyCapacity =low, Connected= No* or *StorageCapacity = low*), UMA requests *StatusDevice* from all devices by contacting *DevA* of each one.
- UMA evaluates the most powerful device, migrates and concludes its task (alert message or ordinary health status information).

IMPLEMENTATION AND EXPERIMENTATION

Implementation Using JADE-Leap

JADE is a set of Java classes that allow a developer to build a FIPA-compliant multi-agent system quite easily, (Bellifemine, 2007; FIPA, 2013). An add-on to JADE, called LEAP, was released. It replaces some parts of the JADE kernel, creating a modified environment called JADE-LEAP (Jade, 2013; Jade Leap, 2013), which allows the implementation of agents in mobile devices with limited resources.

In this example there is a multi-agent system with six agents. Two of them are running on the main container of the platform, which is connected through Internet with a container on a PC that holds another two agents.

These four agents communicate wirelessly with two agents running in mobile devices (one on a tablet and one on a smart phone).

Note that in JADE-LEAP each agent is represented by a container. The rest of programming (behaviors, messages, etc.) is identical to JADE.

Experimentation Scenario

- We propose three devices to Dr. Reda (the monitor physician) and we create three agents: *DevA1for* smartphone, *DevA2* for tablet and *DevA3*for *laptop*.
- Anissa is an elderly woman with heart failure, she lives alone and she is telemonitored by Dr. Reda.

Figure 1. Components of UMA System

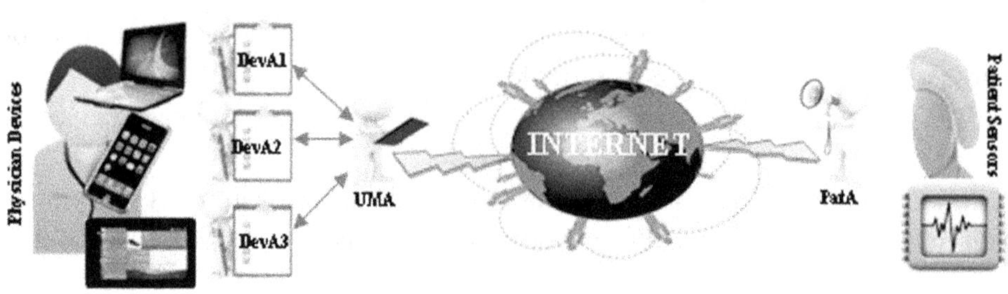

- She has sensors to collect her health status and to alert Dr. Reda in emergency situation.
- We create *PatA*, an agent installed on a laptop. Its aim is to alert Dr. Reda in case of heart crisis and to transmit Anissa's health status.
- Tonight, Anissa has heart attack symptoms; her agent: *PatA*sends an alert message to UMA.
- Dr. Reda was sleeping and his phone and laptop were on offline mode. UMA looks for available devices (tablet), migrates and makes alerts to Dr. Reda.

Figure 2 presents proposed agents communication using dummy agent. We can see UMA migration from Main-container to Container2.

Experimentation Results

We have done experiments according to the power of smartphone battery and its storage capability. We propose smartphone because it is the most used device.

For this, we increase the power, we send alerts from PatA and we calculate the response time in two cases:

- When using UMA system, UMA migrates to another device in order to alert Dr. Reda.
- The second case without UMA system: when Dr. Reda does not respond, PatA resends the alert to another device.

In the second experiment, we calculate the response time according to the memory storage capability. We established graphs in figure 3.

We can see that the response time of the monitor physician is lesser, even if the battery energy or the memory storage capability is low. This is due to the migration of UMA to alert Dr. Reda.

Figure 2. Interactions of system agents using dummy agent of JADE

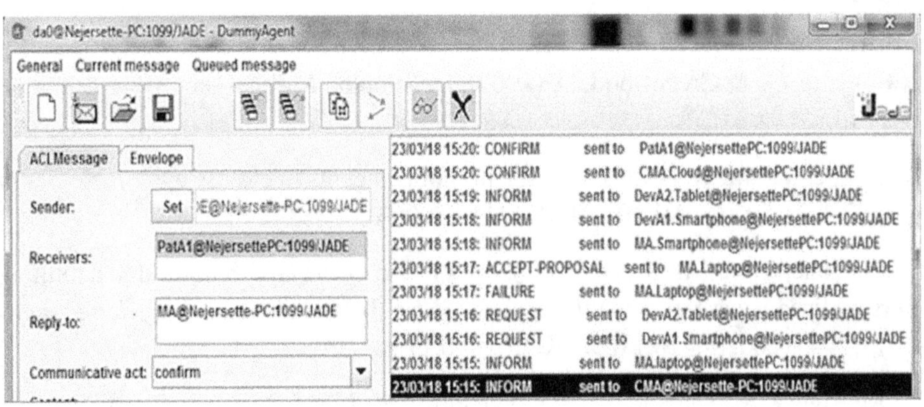

Figure 3. Response time using UMA system (according to battery and memory capacity)

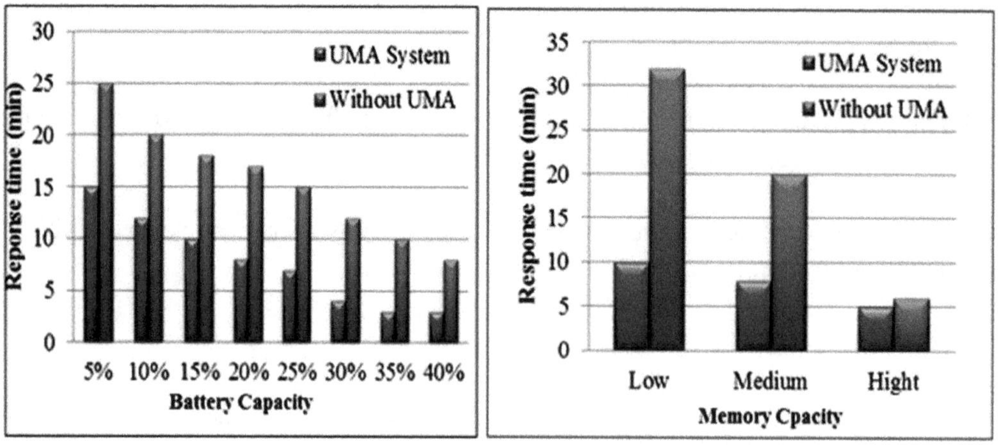

CONCLUSION

We proposed in this chapter an approach based on ubiquitous mobile agents in order to assist monitor physician to telemonitor his patient.

The monitor physician hands several mobile, ubiquitous and restricted devices.

Our proposal is to take advantage from all devices surrounding him; by allowing the ubiquitous mobile agent to migrate on, in order to complete its task (alerting the physician or just receiving health status information).

Also, at patient level we designed patient agent. Its role is to have permanent communication with UMA. We have done the implementation of our proposal using JADE-LEAP framework.

In future works, we would like to detail patient level and to consider more than one patient.

REFERENCES

Bellifemine, F., Caire, G., & Greenwood, D. (2007). Developing Multi-Agent Systems with JADE. John Wiley & Sons Ltd.

Camarinha, L. M., & Vieira, W. (1999). Intelligent mobile agents in elderly care. *Robotics and Autonomous Systems*, *27*(1-2), 59–75. doi:10.1016/S0921-8890(98)00083-9

De Meo, P., Quattrone, G., & Ursino, D. (2011). Integration of the HL7 Standard in a multiagent system to support personalized access to e-health services. *IEEE Transactions on Knowledge and Data Engineering*, *23*(8), 1244–1260. doi:10.1109/TKDE.2010.174

De Paz, J. F., Rodríguez, S., Zatoand, C., & Corchado, J. M. (2015). An Integrated System for Helping Disabled and Dependent People: AGALZ, AZTECA, and MOVI-MAS Projects. Springer International Publishing.

FIPA ACL Message Structure Specification. (2013). Retrieved from http://www.fipa.org/specs/fipa00061/SC00061G.pdf

Isern, D., Sánchez, D., & Moreno, A. (2010). Agents applied in health care: A review. *International Journal of Medical Informatics*, *79*(3), 145–166. doi:10.1016/j.ijmedinf.2010.01.003 PMID:20129820

JADE-LEAP. (n.d.). Retrieved from http://sharon.cslet.it/project/jade

Java Agent Development Framework (JADE). (n.d.). Available online: http://jade.tilab.com

Kim, H.-K. (2013). Convergence agent model for developing u-healthcare systems. *Future Generation Computer Systems*.

Koehler, F., Winkler, S., Schieber, M., Sechtem, U., Stangl, K., Bohm, M., ... Anker, S. D. (2011). Impact of Remote Telemedical Management on Mortality and Hospitalizations in Ambulatory Patients With Chronic Heart Failure: The Telemedical Interventional Monitoring in Heart Failure Study. On behalf of the Telemedical Interventional Monitoring in Heart failure. *Circulation*, *123*(17), 1873–1880. doi:10.1161/CIRCULATIONAHA.111.018473 PMID:21444883

Miller, A. B., & Pina, I. L. (2009). Understanding heart failure with preserved ejection fraction: Clinical importance and future outlook. *Congestive Heart Failure (Greenwich, Conn.)*, *15*(4), 186–192. doi:10.1111/j.1751-7133.2009.00063.x PMID:19627293

Qinghua, Z., Guoquan, C., Zhuan, W. T., Hongyu, S., & Ningning, X., (2010). Research on home health care telemedicine service system concerned with the improvement of medical resources utilization rate and medical conditions. *The 12th International Conference on Advanced Communication Technology (ICACT)*, *2*, 1555-1559.

Su, C. J., & Chu, T. W. (2014). A Mobile Multi-Agent Information System for UbiquitousFetal Monitoring. *International Journal of Environmental Research and Public Health*, *11*(1), 600–625. doi:10.3390/ijerph110100600 PMID:24452256

Su, C.-J., & Wu, C.-Y. (2011). JADE implemented mobile multi-agent based, distributed information-platform for pervasive health care monitoring. *Applied Soft Computing*, *11*(1), 315–325. doi:10.1016/j.asoc.2009.11.022

Tapia, D. I., Alonso, R. S., De la Prieta, F., Zato, C., Rodríguez, S., Corchado, E., ... Corchado, J. M. (2010). SYLPH: An Ambient intelligence based platform for integrating heterogeneous wireless sensor networks. *IEEE International Conference on Fuzzy Systems (FUZZ)*, 1–8. 10.1109/FUZZY.2010.5584145

Vaidehi, V., Vardhini, M., Yogeshwaran, H., Inbasagar, G., Bhargavi, R., & Hemalatha, C. S. (2013). Agent based health monitoring of elderly people in indoor environments using wireless sensornetworks. *Procedia Computer Science*, *19*, 64–71. doi:10.1016/j.procs.2013.06.014

Wooldridge, M. (2002). *An introduction to multi agents systems*. Sussex, UK: John Wiley & Sons Ltd.

Wu, C.-S., Khoury, I., & Shah, H. (2012). Optimizing medical data quality based on multiagent web serviceframework. *IEEE Transactions on Information Technology in Biomedicine*, *16*(4), 745–757. doi:10.1109/TITB.2012.2195498 PMID:22614723

Chapter 9
Research Investigation and Analysis on Behavioral Analytics, Neuro Imaging, and Pervasive Sensory Algorithms and Techniques for Autism Diagnosis

Sasikala R.
VIT University, India

Sureshkumar N.
VIT University, India

ABSTRACT

Interdisciplinary research on autism diagnosis and training for the autistic children are current requirements. Behavioral analytics are the techniques followed by pediatricians for identifying ASD in children. However, the techniques successfully accepted by the pediatricians worldwide would be useful for the parents and pediatricians only for the elementary school-aged children, and the system is not helping for early diagnose among children of age 2. Machine learning, image processing, and pervasive techniques are trending for early diagnosis of ASD. Hence, the chapter has done a research-based survey and detailed analysis on behavioral analytics algorithms, neuro imaging, and eye tracking techniques for early diagnosis. The behavioral analytics survey mainly focuses on social and meta-cognitive skills, and the input dataset has been taken from parents, trainers, teachers, and peer groups. The chapter also identifies that computing technologies with neuro-imaging and pervasive techniques are better than the behavioral skill analysis for early diagnosis.

DOI: 10.4018/978-1-5225-7071-4.ch009

INTRODUCTION

Scientific report says early diagnosis and identifying level of autism in early stage helps the therapist to start treatment in initial stage which improves learning, communication and social skills of young children with autism. Dr. Arora, a paediatrician who has worked in AIIMS says "The autistic children numbers are alarming and calls for policy-making and interventions to bring these children into mainstream society," and he also says "Autism warrants immediate attention,". Most of the time, children are diagnosed much later but when proper techniques used, it can be diagnosed at the age of 24 months. The paediatricians,, Geneticists, molecular biologists and biochemists are working together to understand and treat how brain cells talk and how it is to be treated(Kulage KM 2014).

A specialized paediatric care must be required globally which makes the system for children from receiving care that could improve their wellbeing. The cloud based medical assistance technologies greatly expand the reach of paediatric specialists, increase collaboration among clinicians and researchers, and make quality healthcare available to more children worldwide. The physical or occasional system based behaviour analytics (Bauer O et al 2017) are the mechanisms which usually doctors follow for identifying Autism(Zheng Z et al 2016, 2017). In addition to IOT based and pervasive devices(Tentori M 2017) (Cabielles-Hernández et al 2017), an eye-tracking device based research study found that differences in gaze preference can be detected in infants as young as two months. The research work showed that the infants watching videos, mostly look at mouths more than eyes and also infants look at objects more than people are diagnosed as autism. The infants with autism usually experienced a decline in attention to other people's eyes. The eye tracking devices are easy to handle and portable and it can be fixed away from infants. The other research study on autism diagnosis is based on electroencephalography(EEG) signals(Auzias et al). The feature extraction and classification techniques assist the diagnosis process of Autism. Hence, the research study on EEG and eye tracking devices(Liu W et al 2016) supports the paediatricians to start treatment before mature brain circuitry is established (i.e., between ages 1 and 3 years). It helps the paediatricians to start treatment early and efforts provide best chance of promoting effective and positive connections between brain cells. Hence stimulation and treatment will be easily happening while brain connections are actively being created. In contrast, Identifying autism among kids in elementary school aged can start treatment later in brain development (i.e., at age 4 or later), which leads to more challenging job of trying to change brain cell connections in the later stage. Screening process for autism among 1 year old children using a broad band screen allows scientists with the opportunity to study the disorder during the first year or two of life(Wedyan 2016, Cheung SC 2015).

. A strong preference for moving geometric images over social images was highly specific to this ASD subtype compared with toddlers with typical development, language delay, and global developmental delay as well as unaffected siblings of toddlers with ASD. In conclusion, although it is unclear what the future will hold, it is possible that diagnosis may move away from a purely clinical judgment approach to a more objective research domain approach that instead focuses on the combined techniques such as cloud based pervasive Image processing and analytics to help the biomarkers. From various study, we identified that still more computing techniques of research analysis required in Autism diagnosis. The objective of the paper is to analyse the possibilities of autism diagnosis in various levels, Video Analytics, sensor based pervasive eye tracking device and behaviour analytics. Hence, an integrated early diagnosis and treatment system can be developed for the global attention and the centralized database would be useful for making further research on this area(Fischer S 2017, Chandler DL 2016, Camada MY 2017).

LITERATURE REVIEW ON DIAGNOSIS OF AUTISM

From the survey of various diagnosis techniques, it is identified that most of the hardware based technologies are latest and more research works are in the last 3 to 4 years. Hence, the analysis is concentrating the latest techniques.

Behavoural Analytics

Food Selectivity and Refusal

Children with ASD have a common problem of food refusal, food selectivity and unusual behaviour in mealtime. In (Bandini, L.G et al 2017), research addressed food selectivity in childhood persist into adolescence. The study analysed the following behaviours in the mean age of 6.8 and 13.2:

- Food Selectivity (FFQ and YAQ)
- Food refusal
- Food repertoire (showing interests in unique food)
- Problematic Meal Time Behaviour (MIOH)

The statistical analysis showed that food refusal improved and food repertoire increased from childhood into adolescent. Hence introducing variety of food and healthy diet from childhood age is very necessary for ASD children

Social Functioning

(Freeman et al 2017) examined Executive and Social Functioning in Elementary-Aged Children with Autism and study report done survey on elementary school aged children with ASD. Executive functioning is a set of process helps to analyse neurologically based skills which involves mental control and self-regulation. It depends on three types of brain functions: self control, mental flexibility and working memory. The following measures are taken for Executive and social functioning analysis:

- NEPSY-II - Performance-Based for metacognitive and Behaviour analysis
- DAS-II (Performance-Based) for metacognitive
- BRIEF – Teacher Ratings for meta cognitive and Behaviour Analysis

The results and Statistical analysis proved that executive functioning performances are associated with social functioning. Also the executive and social functioning analyses are significant measures for ASD analysis. Various Techniques used by Clinics for screening ASD suspected children and its inputs from Paediatricians and analysis techniques are given in Figure 1.

Social Functioning With Machine Learning Techniques

Chawarska and Volkmar (2005) summarized the findings of these studies to include:

- Vocalizations
- Eye gaze patterns
- Not showing interest to play with peers and interactive games
- Inconsistency in responding when we call by name
- Limited non-verbal communications
- Limited social referencing

A comparison of Machine Learning techniques(Short E et al 2011) for modelling Human Robot interaction(Peca A 2016) with children with autism has done research on 18 different features including the main behaviour of Autism Kids: child vocalizations. The research developed machine learning based model for vocalization behaviour of children with ASD.

Neuro Imaging Based Diagnosis

(Katuwal, Cahill, Baum, & Michael, 2015) discussed about the morphometric features of brain were derived by the FreeSurfer and the classification can be performed by using three different classifiers: Support Vector Machines (SVM), Random Forest and the Gradient Boosting Machine. Features are analysed based on the classification on the frontal and temporal regions and based on this information the prediction is done diagnosis can be made.

(Zhao, Qiao, Shi, Yap, & Shen, 2017) discussed about a neuro-imaging based diagnosis of the ASD and suggested a framework that integrates canonical correlation analysis and the Fisher discriminant criterion. They performed feature weightage analysis evaluating certain brain regions that play vital role in the diagnosis which includes the precuneus, orbito-frontal cortex and putamen. They are extremely allied with the human emotional modulation and memory.

Table 1. Machine learning based model for vocalization behaviour of children

<table>
<tr><td>Technique</td><td colspan="5">Machine Learning</td></tr>
<tr><td>Dataset</td><td colspan="5">Children interaction with Robot</td></tr>
<tr><td>Concept</td><td colspan="5">Behavioural analysis</td></tr>
<tr><td>Hypothesis</td><td colspan="5">1. Conditional Random fields (CRF)
2. Outperforms Decision Tree in recognition of Child vocalizations
3. Recognition using the full multi-modal feature set will outperform recognition using only audio features.</td></tr>
<tr><td>Results</td><td colspan="5">Total feature set had 241 features validation method: Leave 1 out
Testing: 64 additional features with information gain as parameter on CRF</td></tr>
<tr><td rowspan="3">Multimodal data</td><td></td><td>Mean F1</td><td>Variance</td><td>Error Rate</td><td>Variance%</td></tr>
<tr><td>CRF</td><td>0.0889</td><td>0.0156</td><td>26.35%</td><td>1.62%</td></tr>
<tr><td>DT</td><td>0.1181</td><td>0.0017</td><td>28.19%</td><td>1.74%</td></tr>
<tr><td rowspan="3">Audio only data</td><td></td><td>Mean F1</td><td>Variance</td><td>Error Rate</td><td>Variance%</td></tr>
<tr><td>CRF</td><td>0.1784</td><td>0.0035</td><td>21.48%</td><td>3.22%</td></tr>
<tr><td>DT</td><td>0.0714</td><td>0.0021</td><td>20.02%</td><td>2.51%</td></tr>
<tr><td rowspan="2">Best features testing</td><td></td><td>F1</td><td>Variance</td><td>Error Rate</td><td>Variance%</td></tr>
<tr><td>CRF</td><td>0.2281</td><td>0.0700</td><td>19.81%</td><td>1.61%</td></tr>
</table>

Figure 1. Developmental screen process steps

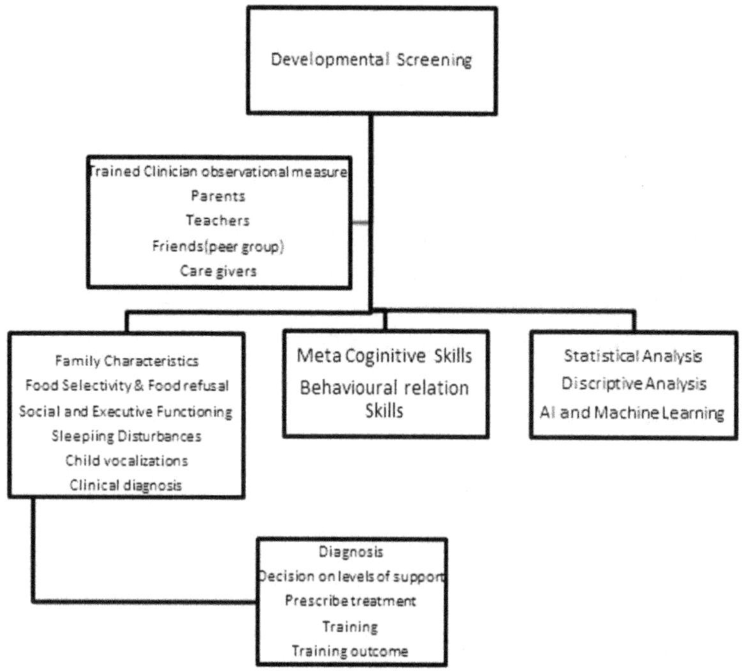

Figure 2. Eye tracking and neuro imaging process

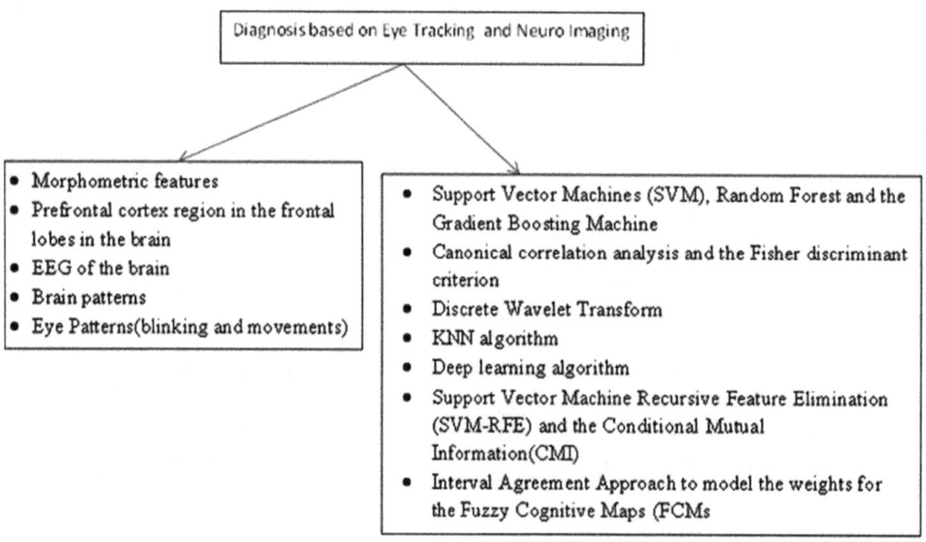

(Ibrahim, Djemal, & Alsuwailem, 2017) used the feature extraction and classification techniques for the diagnosis of autism. First for the pre-processing of the EEG signal is done in order to remove the major artifacts prior to the decomposition into various EEG sub-bands, by using the discrete-wavelet-transform (DWT). Shannon entropy and the largest lyapunov exponent non linear methods were studied. It measures the chaoticity and complexity in the EEG recording as well as with the two conventional methods that includes standard deviation and the band power. The KNN algorithm is used for classification and it yields better performance in terms of speed and accuracy with the large EEG dataset.

(Heinsfeld, Franco, Craddock, Buchweitz, & Meneguzzi, 2017) suggested that the deep learning algorithms to be applied with large brain imaging datasets, by studying the patterns of the patient's brain. The pattern of functional connectivity is evaluated to reveal the neural pattern that helps with the classification for the disease diagnosis. Thus a deeper study is made using the deep learning model.

(Alzubi, Ramzan, & Alzoubi, n.d.) proposed a hybrid feature selection approach for the Single Nucleotide Polymorphisms (SNPs) said to be a fusion of both filter and wrapper method Support Vector Machine Recursive Feature Elimination (SVM-RFE) and the Conditional Mutual Information(CMI) methods. This approach is performed and compared with the traditional classifiers like SVM, Naive Bayes, Linear Discriminant Analysis and k-nearest neighbourhood algorithms. The accuracy of this approach is 89%.

(Farsi, Doctor, Petrovic, Chandran, & Karyotis, 2017) introduced the Interval Agreement Approach to model the weights for the Fuzzy Cognitive Maps (FCMs) to understand and identify the uncertainty with the imprecise data. This approach is used in the classification for the diagnosis of autism providing an effective decision support system to enhance the medical modelling and reasoning.

A consolidated report of Various Eye tracking and Neuro imaging inputs and techniques are given in Figure 2.

Pervasive Computing for ASD

(Kashanian H, Ajami NB and Deghati M) used wearable sensors and cloud computing technology for emotional interaction with autism Patients and the components used are smart clothes, Emotion Analysis with multimodal Data and Control Emotional interaction.

(Torii, Ohtani, & Ishii, 2017)discussed about the image processing techniques by after image used in the blink determination to capture the eye movement and to understand the degree to which the eye ball run off the track based on the image. Also the change that occurred in the right and left eyes is also determined. Initially the pixel indicating the eyes of the subject is selected from the captured frame of the image. Then a reference image called as an afterimage is set, from the pixel showing the subject's pupil. In the acquired image, from the center of the subject's pupil is divided into four. Then the number of pixels of the overlapping part is counted from each divided part based on the obtained afterimage. This image is then processed with precision in 30-40 fps from a camera and then the amount of change detected in the pixels of the movement of the right and left eyeballs is converted to numbers. After this the sequence of eyeball movement is converted into graphs for further diagnosis. This method was found to be effective to determine the non-autistic and autistic people more precisely in the early stage.

(Subrahmaniam, 2013) discussed about the animation, computer graphics and the eye tracking techniques with respect to the human psychological conditions not only as a technology but also as a diagnostic approach and instrument in the diagnosis of autism. In this approach certain analysis can be made with the video and pre-defined set of events and responses can be made and interpreted out of it.

(Thabtah, 2017) with machine learning, classification models can be built which can be used as the screening tool in many decision making processes. An effective study is made on this research. The process reduced the screening time for diagnosis and improving the sensitivity and specificity and as a result simplifies the overall processing.

(Jameson, Lorence, & Lee, 2012) discussed about making interactive data capture from the digital video for the diagnosis. This paper explains about how the models are developed and automated for use. The integration and computerization of various models and techniques helps in the recognition of the primitives and the annotations from the videos. This approach is discussed with the large scale autism dataset.

(Patnam VS, George FT, George K, Verma A, 2017) is applied the concept of Predict meltdown in Kids and alert parents and the Recurrent Convolutional Neural Network (Deep Learning Model) algorithm implemented on dataset of images and videos of Kids and 93% of accuracy is attained.

(Alwakeel SS et al. 2015) proposed wearable sensor devices for identifying distraction. The machine algorithm embedded with sensors for taking decision (table 2).

(Atyabi A et al 2017) described the targeting diagnosis and classification of ASD children by using data mining and speech generating devices. The details are given in table 3.

(Zhang L et al 2017 and Kuriakose S) projected VR based devices for adolescent autism kids. The core arguments of research are revealed in Table 4.

Analysis on Various Parameters of Autistic Diagnosis and Datasets

Table 5 shows various possibilities of Autistic Diagnosis datasets and Analysis parameters and its concluding points are given.

RESEARCH DISCUSSION AND CONCLUSION

- From the survey it is identified that Social skills, meta cognitive skills analysis assist the Doctors and Parents to diagnose autism in Elementary school aged children.
- Neuro Imaging and Eye tracking diagnosing systems assist the doctors to detect the autism early stage such as less than 24 months.
- Research on Machine learning algorithms and Image processing techniques for autism diagnose creates great impact in identifying autism kids.

Table 2.

Technique	Machine Learning for Wireless sensor network
Concept	Activity recognition and alert system with wearable sensor devices. ACSA (Autistic Child sensor and assistant System)
System Architecture and Operation (3 components)	1. ACSA Wearable sensor 2. ACSA parent application 3. Machine learning and query processing
Proposed solution	ACSA wearable device should be worn anywhere on body based on the need. The device is connected to Home automation system. Distraction of the child can be prevented.
Components of ACSA Sensor	GSM Module, GPS Sensor, Temperature Sensor, Heart beat sensor, Repetitive and undesired movement sensor with accelerometer, Gyroscope and magnetometer, sound sensor, Real-time OS, ambient control, Intelligent battery control
Future Work	Implementation of the work Online Machine Learning Framework

Table 3. Diagnosis and classification of ASD children by using data mining

Technique/Approach	Ensemble classification AAC- Augmentative and Alternative Communication		
Concept	Pattern Recognition and datamining on massive streaming data from speech generating devices. Classify patients as ASD and Non-ASD based on temporal Behavioural and frequency profiles.		
Algorithm	Support Vector machine and Ensemble learning Unsupervised class labelling with bootstrapped ensembles		
Problem Statement	No existing study to utilize patterns of AAC apps to classify AD and Non-ASD		
Methodology	AAC app-> freespeech -> platform(ipad)		
Experiment	**Step 1:** Data Cleaning **Step 2:** Feature Engineering (outlier detection, missing value imputation, selection, extraction) **Dataset:** 1. Freespeech app data released in January 2012.Among 6033 users, the dataset contains 5372 user data. Attributes: Keypress, on-screen events, backend events 2. 214 user surveys (180 disclosed) 81-ASD and 99 Non-ASD patients **Step 3:** Machine Learning (Clustering and Regression analysis) Parameter setup: CV- Leave one Out Validation 100 iterations and 100 bootstraps		
Results		ASD Error Rate	Non-ASD Error rate
	Class label Prediction using 20 Key press Samples		
	SOM(SVM)	21.8129%	53.3854%
	K-Means	21.8245%	53.3854%
	Class label prediction using only 1st 20 Key press of 1st Session of each participant		
	SOM (SVM)	39.1304%	58.9744%
	K-Means	39.1304%	58.97744%
	Logistic Regression produces accuracy of 70%		

Table 4. VR based devices for adolescents autism kids

Concept	VR based driving system to teach driving for adolescent autism kids. Estimation of Cognitive load measurement from Multimodal data collected from VR.
Block Diagram Proposed in the system	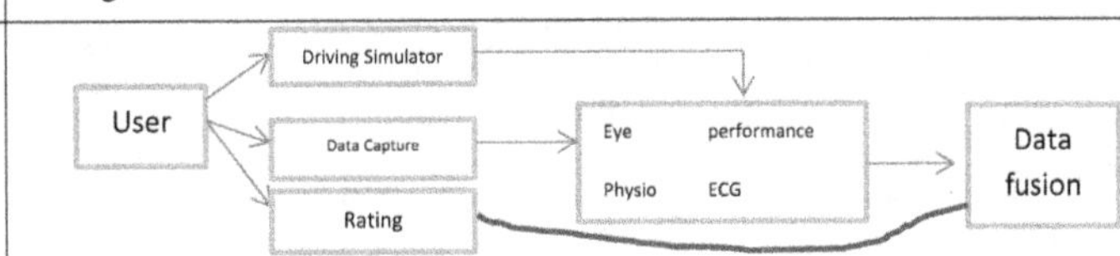
Dataset	20 Adolescents (13-18 years) 6 sessions 19 Male and 1 Female 1. Eye Features: Blink, Pupil Diameter, fixation, Saccade. 2. Other: EEG Signals 3. Peripheral Physical features 4. Performance features
Classification Algorithms	SVM, KNN, Decision Tree, Discriminant analysis and Artificial Neural Networks
Results	84.43% - Feature Level Fusion 81.48% - Decision Level Fusion 83.42% - Hybrid Level Fusion

Table 5. Autistic diagnosis datasets, algorithms and result analysis

Year	Title	Technique	Concept Algorithm	Dataset Parameters	Result
2017	Feature fusion via hierarchical supervised local CCA for diagnosis of autism spectrum disorder	Machine learning	Behavioural phenotype of ASD. hierarchical supervised local CCA(canonical correlation analysis) and Fisher discriminant criterion	Neuro Images(MRI) Feature weightage	Improves the discriminative power of the extracted features and to reduce the sensitivity
2017	Electroencephalography (EEG) signal processing for epilepsy and autism spectrum disorder diagnosis	Machine learning	reveal abnormality in communication between brain regions. discrete-wavelet-transform (DWT), kNN algorithm	Brain signals Chaoticity and complexity in EEG signals. Shannon entropy	Feature extraction and classification techniques improving the performance in terms of accuracy and speed.
2017	Identification of autism spectrum disorder using deep learning and the ABIDE dataset	Deep learning	pattern of functional connectivity is evaluated to reveal the neural pattern Deep Neural Network (DNN)	brain imaging datasets (ABIDE data) Accuracy Sensitivity Specificity Time	70% accuracy Identify the areas of the brain that contributed most to differentiating ASD from typically developing controls as per the deep learning model.
2017	Hybrid Feature Selection Method for Autism Spectrum Disorder SNPs	Machine learning	separate the affected samples from the normal ones(genes) Support Vector Machine Recursive Feature Elimination (SVM-RFE) and the Conditional Mutual Information(CMI)	Autism Spectrum Disorder(ASD) SNP dataset Accuracy Sensitivity Specificity Time	Classification Accuracy 89%
2017	Measurement of Ocular Movement Abnormality in Pursuit Eye Movement (PEM) of Autism Spectrum Children with Disability	Image processing	Behavioural analysis Gaze direction, blink Image processing	Image data Density function distribution, cumulative frequency function, and ROC curve	Eye movements to be used for the diagnosis of children who has autism spectrum.
2015	The predictive power of structural MRI in Autism diagnosis	Machine learning	Brain morphometric feature analysis Support Vector Machines (SVM), Random Forest and the Gradient Boosting Machine	ABIDE data Accuracy Sensitivity Specificity	67% accuracy. Classification on the frontal and temporal regions and based on this information the prediction is done.
2013	CG&A with Eye Tracking for Cognitive Behavior Analysis and Psychoanalysis	Computer graphics and animation	Tools: OpenGL, Microsoft DirectX Gaze Time, Area of Interest (or) Region of Interest, fixation, Index of Cognitive Activity Animation, computer graphics and the eye tracking techniques	Video Real-time Rendering, Cut scenes	Pre-defined set of events and responses can be made and interpreted out of it.

continued on following page

Table 5. Continued

Year	Title	Technique	Concept Algorithm	Dataset Parameters	Result
2012	Integrating Computerized Primitives and Annotated Video Patterns: A Proposed Model for Autism Diagnosis and Research	Data mining	Gesture, recognition, and annotated video Gaussian mixture models	Digital video Event inference from the video	Recognition of the primitives and the annotations from the videos.
2011	A comparison of machine learning techniques for modelling Human-Robot interaction with Children with autism	Machine Learning	Behavioural analysis Conditional Random fields	Children Interaction with Robot Error rate, variance, mean F1 measure	CRF outperforms DT and Multi-modal feature set is efficient than only audio dataset
2015	A machine learning based WSN system for Autism activity recognition	Machine Learning with WSN	Architecture ACSA nil	Nil 3 components	1.ACSA wearable device 2. Parent application 3. Query Processing
2017	An exploratory analysis targeting diagnostic classification of AAC app usage pattern	Ensemble Learning	Classify ASD and Non-ASD SVM, Ensemble learning and boot-strapped Ensembles	Freespeech app user dataset 2012 Error rate	70% accuracy with Logistic Regression
2017	Cognitive load measurement in a virtual reality based reality based driving system for Autism intervention	Machine learning	VR based driving system for autism kids SVM, KNN, DT, DA, ANN	20 Adolescent ASD patients Feature level fusion, Decision level fusion and Hybrid level fusion	84.43% on Feature level fusion
2017	Communication with Autistic people through wearable sensors and cloud technology	Emotion analysis	WSN and cloud based architecture for emotional interaction with Autism kids nil	Architecture 3 components Smart clothes, Emotion analysis and control interaction	Architecture – 3 layer 1.User Terminal 2.Communication layer 3. Cloud based service layer
2017	Deep learning based Recognition of meltdown in Autistic Kids	Deep Learning	Predict meltdown in kids and alert parents RCNN	Images and Videos of kids Accuracy and Loss	93% on complete samples and 92% on 5 Samples
2017	Design of a physiology-sensitive VR based social communication platform for children with Autism	Machine learning	VR based anxiety sensitive device Fuzzy Logic	9 ASD patients and care givers feedback Social responsiveness scale cutoff T-score, Social Communication Questionnaire, Spence Children Anxiety Scale	

- Food selection and Food refusal is one of the major characteristic of autism toddlers in early stage and research on this area assists the parents in later stage.
- Wearable technologies, Deep learning, Cloud computing, Eye tracking and sensory processing are the recent research trends in autism spectrum disorders diagnosis.
- Early diagnosis aids Doctors and Parents to provide more training in the initial stage and reduce the impact of autism issues in later stage.

The significance of the above approaches is to expand knowledge and collaboration between physicians and organizations, connect teams to research, diagnose, treat rare and complex cases and advance capacity for children's healthcare on a global scale.

ACKNOWLEDGMENT

The authors thank VIT University for providing 'VIT SEED GRANT' for carrying out this research work.

REFERENCES

Alwakeel, S. S., Alhalabi, B., Aggoune, H., & Alwakeel, M. (2015). A Machine Learning Based WSN System for Autism Activity Recognition. In *Machine Learning and Applications (ICMLA), 2015 IEEE 14th International Conference* (pp. 771-776). IEEE. 10.1109/ICMLA.2015.46

Alzubi, R., Ramzan, N., & Alzoubi, H. (n.d.). *Hybrid Feature Selection Method for Autism Spectrum Disorder SNPs.*

Atyabi, A., Li, B., Ahn, Y. A., Kim, M., Barney, E., & Shic, F. (2017). An exploratory analysis targeting diagnostic classification of AAC app usage patterns. In *Neural Networks (IJCNN), 2017 International Joint Conference* (pp. 1633-1640). IEEE. 10.1109/IJCNN.2017.7966047

Auzias, G., Takerkart, S., & Deruelle, C. (2016). On the Influence of Confounding Factors in Multisite Brain Morphometry Studies of Developmental Pathologies: Application to Autism Spectrum Disorder. *IEEE Journal of Biomedical and Health Informatics, 20*(3), 810–817. doi:10.1109/JBHI.2015.2460012 PMID:26208373

Bandini, L. G., Curtin, C., Phillips, S., Anderson, S. E., Maslin, M., & Must, A. (2017). Changes in food selectivity in children with autism spectrum disorder. *Journal of Autism and Developmental Disorders, 47*(2), 439–446. doi:10.100710803-016-2963-6 PMID:27866350

Bauer, O., Le Sourd, A. M., Nardi, G., Bourgeron, T., Olivo-Marin, J. C., Ey, E., & de Chaumont, F. (2017). Unbiased analysis of mouse social behaviour using unsupervised machine learning. In *Biomedical Imaging (ISBI 2017), 2017 IEEE 14th International Symposium* (pp. 878-881). IEEE. 10.1109/ISBI.2017.7950656

Cabielles-Hernández, D., Pérez-Pérez, J. R., Paule-Ruiz, M., & Fernández-Fernández, S. (2017, April 1). Specialized Intervention Using Tablet Devices for Communication Deficits in Children with Autism Spectrum Disorders. *IEEE Transactions on Learning Technologies*, *10*(2), 182–193. doi:10.1109/TLT.2016.2559482

Camada, M. Y., Cerqueira, J. J., & Lima, A. M. Stereotyped gesture recognition: An analysis between HMM and SVM. In *Innovations in Intelligent Systems and Applications (INISTA), 2017 IEEE International Conference* (pp. 328-333). IEEE.

Chandler, D. L. (2016). Opening New Worlds for Those with Autism: Technology Is Creating Great New Possibilities for Those on Every Part of the Spectrum. *IEEE Pulse*, *7*(4), 43–46. doi:10.1109/MPUL.2016.2563819 PMID:27414634

Cheung, S. C. (2015). Integrating multimedia into autism intervention. *IEEE MultiMedia*, *22*(4), 4–10. doi:10.1109/MMUL.2015.86

Farsi, A. Al, Doctor, F., Petrovic, D., Chandran, S., & Karyotis, C. (2017). *Interval Valued Data Enhanced Fuzzy Cognitive Maps: Towards an Approach for Autism Deduction in Toddlers*. doi:10.1109/FUZZ-IEEE.2017.8015702

Fischer, S. (2017). Minibrain Storm: Cerebral Organoids Aren't Real Brains? But They Provide a Powerful Platform for Modeling Brain Diseases Like Zika Infection, Alzheimer's, and Even Autism. *IEEE Pulse*, *8*(3), 31–34. doi:10.1109/MPUL.2017.2680360 PMID:28534760

Freeman, L. M., Locke, J., Rotheram-Fuller, E., & Mandell, D. (2017). Brief Report: Examining Executive and Social Functioning in Elementary-Aged Children with Autism. *Journal of Autism and Developmental Disorders*, *47*(6), 1890–1895. doi:10.100710803-017-3079-3 PMID:28260182

Heinsfeld, A. S., Franco, A. R., Craddock, R. C., Buchweitz, A., & Meneguzzi, F. (2017, August). Identification of autism spectrum disorder using deep learning and the ABIDE dataset. *NeuroImage. Clinical*, *17*, 16–23. doi:10.1016/j.nicl.2017.08.017 PMID:29034163

Ibrahim, S., Djemal, R., & Alsuwailem, A. (2017). Electroencephalography (EEG) signal processing for epilepsy and autism spectrum disorder diagnosis. *Biocybernetics and Biomedical Engineering*, 1–11. doi:10.1016/J.BBE.2017.08.006

Jameson, R., Lorence, D., & Lee, J. (2012). Integrating computerized primitives and annotated video patterns: A proposed model for autism diagnosis and research. *Journal of Medical Systems*, *36*(3), 2037–2045. doi:10.100710916-011-9666-5 PMID:21537855

Kashanian, H., Ajami, N. B., & Deghati, M. Communication with autistic people through wearable sensors and cloud technology. In *Fuzzy and Intelligent Systems (CFIS), 2017 5th Iranian Joint Congress* (pp. 139-143). IEEE. 10.1109/CFIS.2017.8003672

Katuwal, G. J., Cahill, N. D., Baum, S. A., & Michael, A. M. (2015). The predictive power of structural MRI in Autism diagnosis. *Proceedings of the Annual International Conference of the IEEE Engineering in Medicine and Biology Society*, 4270–4273. 10.1109/EMBC.2015.7319338

Kulage, K. M., Smaldone, A. M., & Cohn, E. G. (2014). How will DSM-5 affect autism diagnosis? A systematic literature review and meta-analysis. *Journal of Autism and Developmental Disorders*, *44*(8), 1918–1932. doi:10.100710803-014-2065-2 PMID:24531932

Kuriakose, S., & Lahiri, U. (2017). Design of a Physiology-Sensitive VR-Based Social Communication Platform for Children with Autism. *IEEE Transactions on Neural Systems and Rehabilitation Engineering*, *25*(8), 1180–1191. doi:10.1109/TNSRE.2016.2613879 PMID:28114071

Liu, W., Yu, X., Raj, B., Yi, L., Zou, X., & Li, M. (2015). Efficient autism spectrum disorder prediction with eye movement: A machine learning framework. In *Affective Computing and Intelligent Interaction (ACII), 2015 International Conference* (pp. 649-655). IEEE. 10.1109/ACII.2015.7344638

Patnam, V. S., George, F. T., George, K., & Verma, A. Deep Learning Based Recognition of Meltdown in Autistic Kids. In *Healthcare Informatics (ICHI), 2017 IEEE International Conference* (pp. 391-396). IEEE. 10.1109/ICHI.2017.35

Peca, A. (2016). Robot enhanced therapy for children with autism disorders: Measuring ethical acceptability. *IEEE Technology and Society Magazine*, *35*(2), 54–66. doi:10.1109/MTS.2016.2554701

Rothkoff, G., Reisman, M., Tal, N., Shani, O., Nissim-Rafinia, M., Meshorer, E., & Shifman, S. (2017). Isoform Dependent Functions of AUTS2 During Neuronal Differentiation. *European Neuropsychopharmacology*, *27*, S372–S373. doi:10.1016/j.euroneuro.2016.09.401

Short, E., Feil-Seifer, D., & Matarić, M. (2011). A comparison of machine learning techniques for modeling human-robot interaction with children with autism. In *Proceedings of the 6th international conference on Human-robot interaction* (pp. 251-252). ACM. 10.1145/1957656.1957756

Tentori, M., Escobedo, L., Hernandez, C., Matic, A., & Hayes, G. R. (2016). Pervasive Displays in Classrooms of Children with Severe Autism. *IEEE Pervasive Computing*, *15*(3), 48–57. doi:10.1109/MPRV.2016.49

Thabtah, F. (2017). *Autism Spectrum Disorder Screening : Machine Learning Adaptation and DSM-5 Fulfillment*. Academic Press.

Torii, I., Ohtani, K., & Ishii, N. (2016). Measurement of Ocular Movement Abnormality in Pursuit Eye Movement (PEM) of Autism Spectrum Children with Disability. In *Applied Computing and Information Technology/3rd Intl Conf on Computational Science/Intelligence and Applied Informatics/1st Intl Conf on Big Data, Cloud Computing, Data Science & Engineering (ACIT-CSII-BCD), 2016 4th Intl Conf* (pp. 235-240). IEEE.

Volkmar, F., Chawarska, K., & Klin, A. (2005). Autism in infancy and early childhood. *Annual Review of Psychology*, *56*(1), 315–336. doi:10.1146/annurev.psych.56.091103.070159 PMID:15709938

Wedyan, M., & Al-Jumaily, A. (2016). Upper limb motor coordination based early diagnosis in high risk subjects for Autism. In *Computational Intelligence (SSCI), 2016 IEEE Symposium Series* (pp. 1-8). IEEE. 10.1109/IRIS.2016.8066059

Zhang, L., Wade, J., Bian, D., Fan, J., Swanson, A., Weitlauf, A., ... Sarkar, N. (2017). Cognitive load measurement in a virtual reality-based driving system for autism intervention. *IEEE Transactions on Affective Computing.*, *8*(2), 176–189. doi:10.1109/TAFFC.2016.2582490 PMID:28966730

Zhao, F., Qiao, L., Shi, F., Yap, P. T., & Shen, D. (2017). Feature fusion via hierarchical supervised local CCA for diagnosis of autism spectrum disorder. *Brain Imaging and Behavior*, *11*(4), 1050–1060. doi:10.100711682-016-9587-5 PMID:27535871

Zheng, Z., Fu, Q., Zhao, H., Swanson, A. R., Weitlauf, A. S., Warren, Z. E., & Sarkar, N. (2017). Design of an Autonomous Social Orienting Training System (ASOTS) for Young Children With Autism. *IEEE Transactions on Neural Systems and Rehabilitation Engineering*, *25*(6), 668–678. doi:10.1109/TNSRE.2016.2598727 PMID:28644796

Zheng, Z., Young, E. M., Swanson, A. R., Weitlauf, A. S., Warren, Z. E., & Sarkar, N. (2016). Robot-Mediated Imitation Skill Training for Children With Autism. *IEEE Transactions on Neural Systems and Rehabilitation Engineering*, *24*(6), 682–691. doi:10.1109/TNSRE.2015.2475724 PMID:26353376

Chapter 10
Data Analysis and Integration in Healthcare

Kara S. Evans
Waynesburg University, USA

Elizabeth Baoying Wang
Waynesburg University, USA

ABSTRACT

Healthcare providers treat a plethora of conditions associated with the human body for a patient to achieve optimal healthiness. However, aspects of a patients' entire wellbeing can often be overlooked, which leads to issues such as drug interactions, missed diagnoses, and other gaps in care. Healthcare can benefit from implementing better data management and integration to improve data analysis, which could bridge gaps in care. This chapter will explain data analysis and data integration, why they are pertinent in the healthcare system, and their associated rewards and challenges. After analyzing these healthcare facets, this chapter will conclude with a proposal for healthcare providers to leverage technology for patients' general wellbeing and a healthier population.

INTRODUCTION

There has been ample research about the influence and role of information technology in medical systems. Technology is increasingly used in pertinent roles, such as acquiring data, processing data, communicating collaborative data to caregivers, as in nurses and doctors, and administering treatment to patients. The increase in the use of technology is accounted for by various reasons, as Payne et.al. states, "The reported benefits of Health Information Technology (HIT) include improved healthcare quality and safety, decreased costs, and an enhanced ability to conduct research" (Payne, 2016). These rewards have motivated hospital systems to increase their technological prowess. However, while the available technological aspects of healthcare advance in some hospital systems, others have been left in an antiquated state, which could be detrimental as information technology continues its rapid improvements. Many medical systems continue using relational databases for both patient information and general business information, while higher end medical systems are migrating to much more fluid forms of data manage-

DOI: 10.4018/978-1-5225-7071-4.ch010

ment. However, both types of systems need to continue or begin to apply data analysis and data integration to truly make the most of the vast amounts of data collected by medical practitioners. As Brumen states, "Medical data stored in online systems are true goldmines. However, if they are not analyzed, they are useless" (Brumen, 2013). Herein will serve as an encouragement for healthcare providers to continue their pursuit of new technologies for both caregivers and patients, primarily by recognizing the importance of data analysis and integration in modern medical systems. As Payne et.al. aptly explains, "technology assumes a primary role in delivering high quality, safe, and cost effective clinical care and wellness promotion, and is thus worthy of further pursuit, energy, and effort" (Payne, 2016).

Herein, the current uses and possibilities of data integration will be explored in medical fields, specifically with federal initiatives to incorporate data analysis in the healthcare system. The chapter will divulge several benefits and challenges associated with incorporating data analysis and integration in healthcare systems. Benefits include: improved diagnosis, preventative diagnoses, accurate records of prior and current treatment, protection from drug interactions, overdoses, and allergies, real time diagnoses and treatment, a more cost effective system, and enhanced research for future improvements. Some challenges include: data security, patients' privacy concerns, the learning curve for clinicians, incentives for data integration, analysis, and sharing, implementing a standard for integration and sharing, and maintaining a patient-centric practice. This chapter will end with a proposal for healthcare providers to collaborate on medical analysis and integration across health professions, and the associated risks and rewards with an application on that scale.

BACKGROUND

Without practices that involve data analysis and integration, healthcare providers fall into possible mishaps with fatal drug interactions, missed diagnoses, and other deadly accidents that could happen without the preemption of information technology and analytics. Also, analytics preempts issues like later cancer stages and heart problems in at risk patients, which would be left out if no data analysis or data integration was used in hospital systems. Additionally, without Electronic Medical Records (EMRs) or other networked sharing of patient data, doctors in the same hospital systems could find inconsistencies or mistakes within a patient's Personal Health Record (PHR). In traditional databases, only one person or computer can access a patient's data to change it to avoid race conditions. A race condition happens when two different people or processes are accessing a piece of data to change it and something gets left out by accident. There would be no inclusive way to share patients' data with all of his or her caregivers, especially in large healthcare systems. Using different analysis systems could allow different caregivers to simultaneously access data and change it, or even allow machines to automatically put data into the patient's record.

As well, currently, patients are primarily responsible for their own information, which can lead to issues with misremembrance and confusion, especially with older patients or patients experiencing trauma. To elaborate, a patient must tell their physician every medication they are taking, with no possible way to accurately verify all their medications. Or, a patient who had an emergency and was admitted into another hospital may not remember what treatment was given to them, which could cause issues for the primary care physician. In addition, data analysis and integration is imperative when considering research. Without data analysis and integration, research cannot be comprehensive, encompassing all possible patients across spans of age, race, socioeconomic backgrounds, and genetic profiles. Especially in population health research, this information is invaluable. Therefore, these issues and more unmentioned create the need for the preemption given through comprehensive data analysis and data integration.

Data analysis relies heavily on the use of statistics from known patient information. This analysis phase is best as an automated background function connected to all devices on the hospital's network. Once the data has been collected and analyzed, data integration is the practical application of that information. Once the data has been collected and analyzed, data integration is the practical application of that information. For example, if an analysis of the medical system's patients reveals a high population of obesity in adults, the hospital can use that information to effect change. Perhaps the hospital would then begin a test group involving adults to monitor the population's health, or maybe the nurses would advise more heavily on the subjects of exercise and healthy eating. Likewise, analysis may reveal an individual has a high risk for heart problems later in life. Being able to automate analysis processes can catch high risk patients before they begin to experience symptoms of heart failure or some other issue. In finding one issue, that issue's symptoms or signs can be added into tests so that the issue can be found earlier in patients. Both data analysis and data integration have become and will continue to be invaluable in improving the quality and quantity of healthcare for the general population

DATA ANALYSIS AND INTEGRATION IN MEDICAL FIELDS

Data analysis and integration has been implemented in a few areas by some medical providers. Data analysis is the systematic use of data to drive fact-based decision making for measurement, planning, learning, and management (Wills, 2014). Data integration is defined as the implementation of data analysis into various applications. Data analysis and integration is based on collection and protection of medical data and records.

Medical Data and Records

In recent years, the federal government of the United States, through The Centers for Medicare and Medicaid Services (CMS) and the Office of the National Coordinator for Health Information Technology (ONC), has created several initiatives to aid medical systems as they transfer to actively using data analysis and data integration.

Initiatives and Programs

The ONC's mission is to support the adoption of health information technology and promote information sharing across the nation (HealthIT, 2017). The ONC is under the Department of Health and Human Services (HHS), which was created in 2004. The ONC and CMS both strive to uphold and enforce all Health Insurance Portability and Accountability Act (HIPAA) regulations in order to promote privacy and security (HealthIT, 2017). In the medical profession, the HIPAA regulations are of special, immediate importance to uphold patient privacy as well as prevent medical systems from violating doctor and patient confidentiality. Likewise, several ONC initiatives specifically affect Electronic Medical Records (EMRs), such as the Health Information Technology for Economic and Clinical Health (HITECH) Act of 2009 and the ONC2015 initiative, which provide incentives to adopt Electronic Medical Records into healthcare systems, both large and small practices (HealthIT, 2017). In addition to these initiatives, "CMS initiated the Medicare and Medicaid EHR Incentive Programs. The programs are referred to as 'EHR Incentive Programs' or 'Meaningful Use' programs", which lay out EHR adoption via a staged approach with requirements providers should meet at each stage (HealthIT, 2017). Another initiative by CMS is the electronic Clinical Quality Measures (eCQMs), which utilize information technology to measure health care quality within a system. According to the eCQM Resource Center, eCQMs provide a variety of quality reporting and incentive programs for clinics that participate (ECQMs, 2015). From these various incentive programs, data analysis and integration are becoming more feasible for healthcare systems.

Electronic Medical Records

Numerous systems are moving to enhance and innovate medical procedures using information technology. Medical records are experiencing the greatest change. Presently, writing records solely on paper is an antiquated process, but most medical providers have moved to traditional relational databases. However, as technology advances, so ought the systems which are used to house important data. The newest innovation is big data, which is defined as large data sets that can be analyzed via computers to reveal trends, patterns, and associations, and is made up of five key parts to be effective and useful for data managers: volume, variety, velocity, veracity, and value. For medical systems, the technology that uses big data is Electronic Medical Records (EMRs). Electronic Medical Records, sometimes called Electronic Health Records (EHRs), which are electronic records, with consolidated diagnosis and treatment activities of a patient (Kohli, 2016). In these EMRs, many aspects of a patient's medical history can reside, such as dietary history, family medical history, and Personal Health Records (PHRs). EMRs were provided specifically by the initiatives mentioned in the previous section. McDonald asserts that EMRs would "then encourage the sharing of patient information by clinicians everywhere in an attempt to lower costs, speed diagnosis, and improve patient outcomes," and "predictive modeling over data derived from EMRs is being used for early diagnosis and is reducing mortality rates" (McDonald, 2017). Wills provides an example of successful EMRs: "Kaiser Permanente, headquartered in Oakland, California, has shown the way forward through its implementation of HealthConnect, which allows for data exchange and integration of electronic health records (EHRs)" (Wills, 2014). From using their system, HealthConnect, Kaiser has saved approximately 1 billion dollars as of 2013 and have improved their disease management of cardiovascular diseases (Wills, 2014). EMRs have begun to show their effectiveness in the medical sphere and will continue to be implemented by hospital systems in order to effect the benefits associated with electronic record keeping.

Biometric Wearables and Microsensors

In addition to EMRs, research and implementation are being accomplished by a few in more groundbreaking innovations, such as microsensors, which can monitor blood-flow in a patient, biometric wearables, which monitor a patient for various purposes, and detector monitoring, which provides real-time monitoring for system parameters and events (Nelson, 2017). Micro-technology has continually shown promise in revolutionizing medical procedures. One way is through micro-cameras, which can be swallowed by the patient in order to navigate the patient's gastrovascular system and locate issues without or before surgery. Hopefully, doctors will be able to use more micro-cameras in the future to minimize risk to patients and locate issues more quickly. Micro-technology could also be used instead of certain surgery procedures sometime in the near future. In addition, some monitors have real-time alerts over the hospital's network, which enables doctors and nurses to receive notifications wherever they are in the hospital. This would help with emergencies that require timely action as well as let the attending doctors and nurses continually view a patient's vitals without being in the room. As well, there is increased interest in using technology to monitor patients at all times, even when they are at home. For instance, patients with diabetes could have biometric wearables that monitor and assist with their glucose levels. Using technology like this, those patients would not have to worry about their glucose levels, and if a drop happened, a doctor could be notified and treatment administered before the patient even realizes they have a problem. From these innovations and more, data analysis and integration are becoming increasingly important in vital hospital procedures. As will be seen, Information technology is driving healthcare innovations, the benefits of which will be described in detail following the challenges associated with data analysis and integration.

Challenges and Issues

Data analysis and integration present several challenges for medical systems. First, while considering any advance in technology, one must consider the security risks it may pose to confidential information within the system.

Security

Technology has advanced to the point that many medical devices are networked and are therefore vulnerable to security risks. Pettus enforces that "any networked medical device must be reliable, scalable, and secure" (Pettus, 2017). Information security on an organization-wide scale is highly necessary, especially considering the time-sensitive and confidential information in medical systems. As Marvin correctly states, "Electronic systems across the organization must be evaluated to ensure that they are secure from unauthorized access, are properly backed up, and have appropriately tested downtime process" (Marvin, 2017). Every system inside of a medical system should be regularly evaluated and updated to ensure continuing security. For some systems, this may mean hiring a new security department alongside IT support. Implementing a new system can be daunting from a financial and administrative standpoint, however hiring cybersecurity professionals or a third party security company to monitor and enforce security could ease the process of integration and mitigate risks to vital medical systems as well as private patient information. Although this would naturally incur an expense, security is indispensable in medical systems and could save systems from being compromised.

Privacy and Confidentiality

Another challenge associated specifically with data analysis is patient concerns of privacy and confidentiality of their information. Brumen states, "Despite the regulations in place, the stories of privacy and confidentiality breaches are still frequent" (Brumen, 2013). When entering a new system, a potential or regular patient desires their information to be completely secure, however, breaches happen too much for their comfort. A patient may even be concerned that his or her data would be entering a pool of other patient data to be analyzed, and in fact, many regulations would prevent access of patient data to implement in studies or analysis without the patient's permission. Brumen tackled this challenge well by outlining, "A data analyst needs to have full access to relevant data, but full access may be denied by privacy and confidentiality of medical data legal regulations" (Brumen, 2013). Obviously, this poses a challenge, especially if the analysis and integration are conducted by a third party. One possible way to mitigate this issue is to fully automate analysis, which prevents issues with patient privacy. Another issue patients may inquire about is secure communication with their providers. When moving to a technologically savvy medical system, a patient may desire to know how they can be securely involved with their care and how they could communicate privately with their medical providers and primary care physician. Marvin provisions that "the integration of patients into the decision-making process for their care will be facilitated through EHR portals and secure messaging among care team members" (Marvin, 2017). The portal would be in the medical system's network, allowing secure, reliable access to both patients and medical providers. In this way, the patient would not only have secure access to his or her medical information, including medical history and test results, but could also participate in secure messaging with physicians. The online messaging system would be similar to email, making it easy for patients to use on a regular basis. Therefore, patient concerns for privacy and confidentiality can be resolved with the proper technological advances put in place.

Training

With new innovations in technology, a steep learning curve exists for certain users, especially older ones. If data analysis and integration are to be successfully implemented into medical systems, there must be adequate training for all new technologies. From his report, Smelcer notes, "Some clinics report that users often need between six and twelve months before they are comfortable using the new technology" (Smelcer, 2009). Especially in the ever evolving technological world, this poses a large problem, particularly if clinicians cannot keep up with new technologies being implemented into their healthcare systems. To help solve this issue, Miliard points out that "Effective and ongoing […] training of clinical personnel should be an ongoing process" (Miliard, 2015). Regular trainings would be necessary for clinicians if medical providers desire to obtain the systems necessary for data analysis and integration. In addition, some basic training or online tutorials would need to be available to patients, as well as a fully staffed IT department to assist patients regularly. Similarly to clinicians, the learning curve may take a while, especially for older patients. Therefore, effective training for both clinicians and patients would be highly necessary for migration to systems that implement data analysis and integration.

Productivity Loss

A practical challenge observed with the implementation of data analysis systems is the loss of productivity, which directly leads to making sure technology is usable from the practitioners' end. For certain doctors, technology must be utilized for their specialty, such as ophthalmologists, who have different needs than a pediatric doctor. For example, an EMR may need to look different or be zoomed in on a specific page for each doctor's perspective, such as an eye chart for the ophthalmologist since he or she has specialized tasks in relation to eyesight. To combat this issue, developers of medical technology need to create flexible technologies in order to work with multiple types of doctors. If not, it could lead to issues with productivity. Another expected complaint is that having technology lengthens the processes doctors do hourly, such as in signing into multiple computers in different exam rooms. If the system takes too long signing them in, valuable time is lost with the patient. One suggestion posed by Smelcer is to implement tablet technology into the hospital's system in order to allow clinicians to continually access data without signing in multiple times an hour (Smelcer, 2009). However, another solution may be to implement a more dynamic computer system or network to better support multiple places of work at the same time. Another practical challenge is difficulty finding pertinent information in a new system. Clinicians may have trouble learning the layout of applications, however, it is up to the developer to create multifunctioning, flexible programs for ease of use. In addition, more training would be required for practitioners and administrators, as mentioned before. As the companies and developers who create medical analysis software continue innovating and developing, these problems of usability will gradually disappear as clinicians provide feedback and the technologies improve.

Patient-Centric Practice

A concern when implementing information technologies is how a clinician provides and maintains a patient-centric practice. Sometimes in data analysis, it is difficult to retain the identity of the source of that data: patients. As with most statistical analysis, the subjects of that analysis can often be lost in the shuffle as numbers instead of people with backgrounds and future hopes. With the loss of subject, often the significance of each number decreases too. As Miliard emphasizes, "The clinical record should include the patient's story in as much detail as is required to retell their story" (Miliard, 2015). If the clinical record accurately reflects the person, statistical analysis will not lose them in the action of information examination. In addition, apprehensions have been raised over whether or not technology distracts from doctor and patient interactions, which discourages doctors from applying new technologies, such as computer-based records. Suggestions for technology to improve patient interactions could include alternative methods of input, such as passive recording technologies or speech recognition. Regardless, maintaining a human interaction while amongst technology can be difficult, hard work for clinicians. However the work pays off, as the benefits of integrated technology outweigh the challenge of preserving a patient-centric practice.

Incentives

A final challenge outlined within this chapter is associated with data containing adequate incentives for integration, analysis, and sharing among medical practitioners, especially facing the other challenges mentioned before. Soon, clinicians will have motivation to begin changing their systems in the form of the CHIP Reauthorization Act of 2018, which will be based on a Merit-based Incentive Payment System (MIPS) (Marvin, 2017). Merit-based Incentive Payment System means that this program will require measurable improvements to care quality as well as integration of health information technologies to meet its goals (Marvin, 2017). Hopefully this program will begin raising the standards for integration and sharing across medical systems as well as encourage the practitioners to continue improvements with a solidified plan. Overall, the challenges associated with data analysis and integration may seem daunting, however, "the ability to deliver the right intervention at the right time will improve as people begin to understand their own risks, monitor their health and share pertinent information with their care providers" (Berg, 2015). As the years progress, and advances in technology are improved, so should improvements in data analysis and data integration be progressed, especially in the medical profession.

Rewards and Benefits

Data analysis and integration has many rewards and benefits, regardless of the challenges they pose. The first benefit is improved diagnosis and clinical outcomes.

Improved Diagnoses and Outcomes

One of the ways that patients experience issues is due to the lack of communication between practitioners. Making use of data via technology, such as EMRs, communication is greatly benefitted. As Timm explains, "Clinicians use the shared content to make more informed medical decisions for their patients and to better coordinate care when their patients get care from multiple sources" (Timm, 2011). Information technology better enables a coordinated response to each of a patient's needs, which improves the patient's wellbeing and eases any frustration they may have over repeating themselves. This is especially important in large practices with multiple doctors interacting with one patient, and when one doctor moves from patient to patient multiple times in an hour. Through better data analysis and integration, patients will receive improved diagnoses and a coordinated treatment plan to return them to optimal health.

Preventative Diagnoses

Since data analysis involves statistics, thorough testing and observing can lead to preventative diagnoses, or being able to see data trends and pinpoint patients at risk. This type of analysis is invaluable for preventing ailments such as diabetes, heart problems, and even later stages of cancer. The goal of using predictive analysis is to improve not only an individual's health, but also improve the general population's health. For example, "With data that have already been collected, BCBSNC (Blue Cross and Shield of North Carolina) studies current healthcare needs and predicts future health issues by using predictive modeling, thereby working to prevent future health complications and improving customers' overall health" (Wills, 2014). Pinpointing at risk patients is not only beneficial to the patient, but also population health in general due to its eventual overall effect over time. People who have hereditary ailments would also be caught at earlier stages and perhaps able to mitigate their risk by actively participating in their care. In this way, analytics can help prevent medical conditions or identify them at earlier stages to begin treatment as soon as possible. In this way, data analysis and integration can improve preventative diagnoses and potentially save lives.

Clinical Documentation

Another way that data integration can benefit medical systems is in improved clinical documentation. For example, prescriptions are better when typed rather than handwritten, because clinical notes and prescriptions become easier to read and are able to be easily shared with providers and primary care physicians within the medical system, especially in a larger medical practice with multiple people interacting with one patient. This also improves the accuracy of clinical notes and documentation. Not to say that clinician notes were inaccurate before, but as Miliard states, "Where previously documented clinical information is still accurate and adds to the value of current documentation, this process [...] may improve accuracy, completeness and efficiency of documentation" (Miliard, 2015). In addition to the documentation being more accurate and efficient, the electronic records are more cohesive in retaining data from prior or current treatments, which gives clinicians a better understanding of a patient's overall health. This includes a complete list of allergies, especially to medicines, and a continuously updated list of patient prescriptions and medications. In this way, a patient is less likely to receive conflicting medications that could lead to a fatal drug interaction or overdose, or have two medications simply cancel each other out. Therefore, improved clinical documentation is imperative for improved communication, especially in large or medium sized practices, and is achieved through data integration, especially in electronic medical records.

Real-Time Applications

Data analysis and integration have endless possibilities in regards to real-time applications within the medical system. Real-time diagnoses and treatment come with the hope of preventing inpatient emergencies and saving lives. Berg points out that, "With improved data accessibility and analysis of that data, systems can deliver faster identification of high-risk members, recommend more timely interventions, and provide data-driven monitoring" (Berg, 2015). The efforts surrounding this possibility focus on the opportunity to save lives, especially for surgery inpatients and critical care inpatients. As Wills says, "Real-time analytics focuses on the recording of point readings and streaming data, but more important, it analyzes the data at the point of care to present immediate and actionable information for providers" (Wills, 2014). All being well, areas that improve on real-time data analysis can notify clinicians of immediate needs as well as continually monitor everyone and everything in the hospital's system for the quickest possible triaging, which would be especially useful in large hospitals. Consequentially, real-time analytics is a growing area for data analysis and integration, using automated systems to monitor inpatients and alert practitioners if something needs to be taken care of at the moment.

Cost Efficiency

Another benefit to data analysis and integration is the eventual cost effectiveness of it. Since transitioning into a system that effectively utilizes data costs a lot of money, a deterrent to switching is often the cost. However, in the long run, implementing a system like this saves the medical providers a huge amount of money. As Berg emphasizes, "The potential to improve outcomes and contain costs from analyzing big data in healthcare are, well, big" (Berg, 2015). Analyzing data gleaned from patients allows accurate prescriptions, consistent preemption of later stages of a disease or condition, and a better anticipation of population needs, all of which decrease the cost of operating a hospital or medical system. As mentioned before, Kaiser Permanente has saved approximately 1 billion dollars as of 2013 and have improved their disease management of cardiovascular diseases (Wills, 2014). With systems actively using preemption and management of diseases through data analysis and integration, medical practitioners can create a healthier population as well as healthy individuals.

Research

Lastly, data analytics and integration is beneficial to future research. As Wingrove pointedly states, "Data is nice but must be turned into useful information" (Wingrove, 2016). Through research, data analysis can be expanded and continue to improve, and data integration can develop further for increased usability and efficiency across healthcare platforms. To give incentives and encourage research in this area, "the

United States government has [recently] announced a Precision Medicine initiative, which includes as a part of its objectives the rapid translation of scientific knowledge generated via research programs into actionable, evidence-driven interventions aimed at improving the health of individuals and populations" (Payne, 2016). The hope of this initiative is to make use of research into data analysis and implement it in reliable, usable systems for medical professionals to use while working to heal individuals and eventually heal the population as well. Research is invaluable in any field involving technology, but even more so for the medical field due to its value in saving lives and preventing population disease. From these various instances, predominantly improved diagnosis, preventative diagnoses, accurate records of prior and current treatment, protection from drug interactions, overdoses, and allergies, real time diagnoses and treatment, a more cost effective system, and enhanced research for future improvements, data analysis and integration's benefits far outweigh the challenges to implementing them into medical systems. This makes solving those challenges even more vital for continuing improvements to data analysis and integration.

SOLUTIONS AND RECOMMENDATIONS

Proposals and Solutions

In medical systems, data analysis and integration will become increasingly important as medical data increases and information technology progresses. As technology improves, the medical system in the United States, or other countries, may rethink their stance on medical systems as individualistic in nature. If a person gets treated by a doctor in another system, the primary doctor cannot access all of the medical information gleaned from the second. For instance, if an x-ray is taken by one doctor in another system, it is likely that person will have a second x-ray taken by their own primary care physician or family doctor in order to confirm what the other doctor found, because they are in different medical systems. In another example, patients going to different doctors for a second opinion on treatment are required to go through and pay for the exact same testing process before obtaining a second verdict. One doctor's thorough testing cannot be used by another medical system, even if the same testing procedures are in place, which is likely. Considering this, the proposal by the authors is to create cooperation between medical professionals across various medical professions through predictive medical analysis and integration. This would call for "a coordinated approach: across settings and providers, all caregivers should have the same information and work toward the same goal" (Berg, 2015). In this case, medical practitioners everywhere in the medical system possess all of the information necessary for accurately treating patients, not only information from their own practice, but also from any practice the patient decides to visit. Healthcare Financial Management concludes, "We will always be limited [...] until the industry can find a way to completely integrate data across systems" (HFM, 2013). This integration would not only include medical doctors, but also other practitioners of medicine, such as dentists. In this way, the patient's profile would include all medicine practiced in order for their primary care physician could easily pinpoint areas of the patient's life that may have caused or impacted a current problem, or it could prevent a problem from happening in the first place. For instance, if a patient were to have a prescription from their dentist for after wisdom teeth surgery, the primary care physician would be aware of the surgery as well as the prescription given to the patient. Data analysis and integration on this scale would encounter various complications, even with the benefits involved, which will be highlighted.

Issues and Challenges

Fully integrating data analysis across medical systems is a daunting task which may come with hesitation and suspicion and will cause certain issues and challenges. The first to overcome is a lack of sufficient motivation, which may be the toughest obstacle to overcome. Medical systems in the United States are varied, autonomous, and individualistic, typically remaining within themselves in regards to treating patients and sharing information. Some incentives to begin a part of this process were previously stated, however those are only the beginning of possibilities for continuing progress in the areas of data analysis and integration. If a unified medical system is to exist in the future, more incentives must be given, possibly in a form similar to the initiatives before. A second complication is enforcing information and data security on a nation-wide scale while allowing information to be accessed via networks to multiple medical systems. This kind of a system would require the best security technology available as well as a new administrative department of information assurance or digital security, and it would be extremely expensive to begin initially, even if the proposal would save money as time continues. A third problem to address is patient confidentiality. If a patient's data can be accessed from multiple systems, is there truly confidentiality between the doctor and the patient? This question would have to be formally addressed and compared to the HIPPA standards for admissibility into healthcare system policies. And finally, on a practical level, a data analysis system of necessary size would be difficult to construct, update, and manage due to its complex functionality. In addition to more security professionals, healthcare systems would need to add an additional vendor or internal department specifically for the construction, regular update, and management of the data system and its components. This inclusion would also incur a rather large expense, even if the system would save time and money in the long run. In order for the healthcare system to implement an all-inclusive system across providers, there needs to be adequate incentive, security, confidentiality, and management for the purpose of maintaining the level of healthcare quality and quantity across all healthcare professions as well as maintaining patient confidentiality and assurance.

Rewards and Benefits

However, if the challenges above could be properly solved and funded, the proposal's rewards and benefits could be worth all of the trouble of integrating medical systems for several reasons. First of all, a fully integrated system has a great potential save many lives. For example, when accidents occur, patients are sent to the nearest hospital, regardless of their provider, which leads to problems for clinicians identifying injuries, allergies, medications, personal information, injury history, et cetera, so being able to quickly retrieve a patient's information could aid in identifying vital information, such as blood type for a transfusion. In addition, population health would benefit from earlier identification of at risk patients, as Berg emphasizes, "When dealing with large populations, it becomes even more important to know who can potentially benefit from intervention as a way to improve health and lower costs" (Berg, 2015). This idea directly applies to preventative diagnoses, as explained in detail before. The highest impact would likely be seen with alleviating issues regarding heart problems and diabetes, but could also lead to other trends, such as cancer prevention or mitigation of cancer at earlier stages. Another way this proposal would benefit both patients and clinicians is in comprehensive patient profiles, as previously stated in this chapter. Since some information is misplaced when moving to a different medical provider, having shared patient data completes records that might otherwise be incomplete, spanning across medical providers to reach each person in any hospital they could possibly visit in the system. This would also increase accountability with providers and enable them to view their patients' profiles comprehensibly, which would allow for better treatment and mitigation of potential disease or certain conditions. And finally, integrating shared data analysis would greatly benefit population research and disease prevention. By implementing more technology and regularly updating it, researchers can continue innovations and new cures for not only individual health, but also population health, which could decrease outbreaks or the number of people affected by the outbreak. Considering all of these benefits, implementing data analysis and integration across medical providers for a comprehensive view and access to medical information is not only beneficial to individual health, but also population health.

FUTURE RESEARCH DIRECTIONS

This chapter primarily focuses on the physical aspects of health care and medical data in terms of data analysis and integration. However, mental health is as important as physical health. In many cases, mental health issues can cause or aggravate physical illnesses. In fact, with the advance of life styles and working paces, mental issues have become more prominent and notorious in the present time. Countless studies have been conducted on the effects of stress in the workplace as well as accounting for other aspects of a modern, technologically advanced society. The authors anticipate a great deal of applied research on mental health, including data analysis and data integration. In the future, not only would data be assessed from a physical standpoint, but also from a mental health point of view in order to hone in on the causes of illnesses and diseases. Therefore, due to its necessity, electronic collection and sharing of mental health data will also be in great demand.

CONCLUSION

In conclusion, medical systems can greatly benefit from using data analysis and integration inside their daily practices. Not only will data analysis and integration aid in revolutionizing medical care but will also help future research continue developing. Benefits of data analysis and integration include: improved diagnosis, preventative diagnoses, accurate records of prior and current treatment, protection from drug interactions, overdoses, and allergies, real time diagnoses and treatment, a more cost effective system, and enhanced research for future improvements. Overcoming challenges associated with data analysis and integration is crucial to successful implementation, and is a task worthy of the effort, especially with the opportunity to save lives and create healthier populations. The challenges addressed prior include: data security, patients' privacy concerns, the learning curve for clinicians, incentives for data integration, analysis, and sharing, implementing a standard for integration and sharing, and maintaining a patient-centric practice. Clinicians would be wise to consider data analysis and integration as a requirement for modern medical systems and begin the process of upgrading their systems while initiatives are in place and before their systems with traditional relational databases is outdated. Lastly, cooperation between medical professionals across various medical professions through predictive medical analysis and integration would significantly benefit individuals as well as the general population. Striving toward this goal of technologically advanced systems that use data to analyze information and then implement it back into the medical system is a commendable aspiration for medical professionals.

REFERENCES

Berg, G. (2015, July 17). *3 ways big data is improving healthcare analytics*. Retrieved October 15, 2017, from http://www.healthcareitnews.com/blog/3-ways-big-data-improving-healthcare-analytics

Brumen, B., Heričko, M., Sevčnikar, A., Završnik, J., & Hölbl, M. (2013). Outsourcing medical data analyses: Can technology overcome legal, privacy, and confidentiality issues? *Journal of Medical Internet Research*, *15*(12), e283. doi:10.2196/jmir.2471 PMID:24342053

ECQMs. (2017). Retrieved October 23, 2017, from http://ecqi.healthit.gov/ecqms

EHR Incentives and Certification. (2015, February 6). Retrieved November 15, 2017, from http://www.healthit.gov/providers-professionals/meaningful-use-definition-objectives

Kohli, R., & Tan, S. S. (2016). Electronic Health Records: How Can Is Researchers Contribute To Transforming Healthcare? *Management Information Systems Quarterly*, *40*(3), 553–574. doi:10.25300/MISQ/2016/40.3.02

Marvin, K. C. (2017). Health Information Technology: Integration, Patient Empowerment, and Security. *American Journal of Health-System Pharmacy*, *74*(2), 36–38.

McDonald, C. (2017, September 2). *5 Big Data Trends in Healthcare for 2017*. Retrieved October 21, 2017, from http://www.7wdata.be/big-data/5-big-data-trends-in-healthcare-for-2017

Miliard, M. (2015, January 16). *12 tips for better EHR usability*. Retrieved October 21, 2017, from http://www.healthcareitnews.com/news/12-tips-better-ehr-usability

Nelson, R. (2017). Technology drives healthcare innovation. *EE: Evaluation Engineering*, *56*(3), 10–13.

Payne, P. O., Lussier, Y., Foraker, R. E., & Embi, P. J. (2016). Rethinking the role and impact of health information technology: Informatics as an interventional discipline. *BMC Medical Informatics and Decision Making*, 1640. PMID:27025583

Pettus, D. C., Vanderveen, T., Canfield, R. L., & Schad, R. (2017). Reliable and Scalable Infusion System Integration with the Electronic Medical Record. *Biomedical Instrumentation & Technology*, *51*(2), 120–129. doi:10.2345/0899-8205-51.2.120 PMID:28296444

Readying Your Data Use for Value-Based Payment. (2013). hfm. *Healthcare Financial Management*, *67*(6), 1–8.

Smelcer, J. (2009). Usability of Electronic Medical Records. *Journal of Usability Studies*, *4*(2), 70–84. doi:10.1145/ 2029976.2029989

Timm, J., Renly, S., & Farkash, A. (2011). Large scale healthcare data integration and analysis using the semantic web. *Studies in Health Technology and Informatics*, 169729–169733. PMID:21893843

Wills, M. J. (2014). Decisions through Data: Analytics in Healthcare. *Journal of Healthcare Management*, *59*(4), 254–262. doi:10.1097/00115514-201407000-00005 PMID:25154123

Wingrove, G., & McGinnis, K. (2016). Integration of Technology. *EMS World*, 14. PMID:29847040

ADDITIONAL READING

Adamson, D. (2015, April 13). Big Data in Healthcare Made Simple: Where It Stands Today and Where I... Retrieved October 13, 2017, from http://www.slideshare.net/healthcatalyst1/big-data-in-healthcare-made-simple-where-it-stands-today-and-where-its-going

Bresnick, J. (2017, August 16). How Big Data Analytics Companies Support Value-Based Healthcare. Retrieved October 10, 2017, from http://healthitanalytics.com/news/how-big-data-analytics-companies-support-value-based-healthcare

Hagland, M. (2015). Is This Population Health's Moment? Time for Data and Analytics. *Healthcare Informatics*, *32*(3), 8–15.

Kraus, J., Lausser, L., Kuhn, P., Jobst, F., Bock, M., Halanke, C., & ... Kestler, H. (2018). Big data and precision medicine: challenges and strategies with healthcare data. *International Journal of Data Science and Analytics*, (Preprints), 1 -9.

Mezghani, E., Exposito, E., Drira, K., Da Silveira, M., & Pruski, C. (2015). A Semantic Big Data Platform for Integrating Heterogeneous Wearable Data in Healthcare. *Journal of Medical Systems, 39* (12), 1 -8. doi: -015 -0344 -x doi:10.1007/ s10916

Percival, J., McGregor, C., Percival, N., & James, A. (2015). Enabling the Integration of Clinical Event and Physiological Data for Real-Time and Retrospective Analysis. *Information Systems and E-Business Management, 13* (4), 693 -711. doi: -014 -0232-9 doi:10.1007/ s10257

Vayena, E., Dzenowagis, J., Brownstein, J. S., & Sheikh, A. (2018). Policy implications of big data in the health sector. *Bulletin of the World Health Organization*, *96*(1), 66–68. doi:10.2471/BLT.17.197426 PMID:29403102

KEY TERMS AND DEFINITIONS

Big Data: Consists of large data sets that can be analyzed via computers to reveal trends, patterns, and associations, made up of five key parts: volume, variety, velocity, veracity, and value.

Biometric Wearables: Electronic devices worn/attached to a person in order to track that person's vitals.

Data Analysis: A systematic use of data to drive fact-based decision making for measurement, planning, learning, and management.

Data Integration: Implementation of data analysis into various applications.

Diagnosis: An assessment given by a medical professional of a medical condition or disease.

Electronic Medical Records (EMRs): Electronic records of data with consolidated diagnosis and treatment activities of a patient.

Information Technology: The study or use of electronic systems, specifically computers, for storing, retrieving, and sending information.

Microsensors: Small sensor technology, able to be inserted or ingested for medical use.

Personal Health Records (PHRs): A person's own medical record, primarily with only one person's medical information.

Real-Time Analytics: Analysis that takes place in the present, real time, with no need to store data before analyzing it and potentially acting on that information.

Relational Database: A collection of data organized into columns, rows, and tables, which can be connected to one another via "relations" or columns/rows that the tables have in common.

Chapter 11
Healthcare IoT Architectures, Technologies, Applications, and Issues: A Deep Insight

Karthick G. S.
Bharathiar University, India

Pankajavalli P. B.
Bharathiar University, India

ABSTRACT

The internet of things (IoT) revolution is improving the proficiency of human healthcare infrastructures, and this chapter analyzes the applications of IoT in healthcare systems with diversified aspects such as topological arrangement of medical devices, layered architecture, and platform services. This chapter focuses on advancements in IoT-based healthcare in order to identify the communication and sensing technologies enabling the smart healthcare systems. The transformation of healthcare from doctor-centric to patient-centric with the diversified applications of IoT is discussed in detail. In addition, this chapter examines the various issues to be emphasized on designing an effective IoT-based healthcare system. It also explores security in healthcare systems and the possible security threats that may be vulnerable to the security essentials. Finally, this chapter summarizes the procedure of applying machine learning techniques on healthcare streaming data which provides intelligence to the systems.

INTRODUCTION: OVERVIEW OF INTERNET OF THINGS

The idea of the IoT was originated and devised with the context of Radio Frequency Identification (RFID), which is used for tracking the objects in various domains like logistics and supply chain management. For example, Automated Teller Machines (ATMs) are interconnected to the bank network, which enables the payments with ATM cards at the point of sales depots. ATM uses the machine-to-machine (M2M) networks and these established a basement for IoT through network connected systems and data. The

DOI: 10.4018/978-1-5225-7071-4.ch011

probability of connecting the objects to the network provides tagging, tracking and reading of data from objects that goes hand in hand with greater efforts which would become a promising technology of this era called as IoT.

IoT was first coined by Kevin Ashton in 1999 and developed in analogous to Wireless Sensor Networks (WSN) (Rose et al., 2015). The term IoT refers to the physical devices that are interconnected to gather and share the data with each other via communication technology and cloud computing enables to collect, record and to analyze the data stream more accurately within short span of time. The term "Things" in IoT specifies variety of devices includes sensors, automobiles, buildings, industries, human beings, animals, plants any type of goods. WSNs are assumed to rely on wireless communication technologies whereas IoT does not assumed to rely on specific communication technology. The characteristics of wireless sensors like tiny, rugged, inexpensive and low powered renovated the IoT, facilitates the smallest objects can be integrated with different environments. IoT can be considered as an upcoming evolution of the internet which uses many existing features including machine-to-machine communication (M2M), radio frequency identification (RFID) and sensors.

IoT is defined as an ever growing technology through which computing devices, mechanical and digital machines, physical objects, animals or human beings are interconnected via communication medium provides the ability to exchange information and automate the tasks without human-interaction.

IoT is being labeled by different applications, protocols, standards and architectures. IoT is not just a technology but certainly comprising of different things like data analytics, actuators, hubs, artificial intelligence, communication, wide range of sensors, IoT nodes, gateways, networks, cloud computing, edge computing, processing, optimization, IoT platforms and so on. Connecting the physical things through networks and data stream processing increases the potentiality of IoT by adding intelligence to the systems. The common technologies driving the IoT applications are depicted in the Figure 1.

As IoT can be considered as a fully dependent on the potentials of sensors and other technologies, IoT devices must possess three basic qualities such as:

- **Sensable:** IoT devices must be able to sense and aggregate the data. For example, in healthcare field aggregating the blood glucose, pulse rate and body temperature data via sensors. The data aggregated must be self-directed.
- **Communicable:** The data aggregated must be transmitted to data centers or other devices upon specific conditions via communication medium (i.e. Wireless Technologies).
- **Actionable:** The data aggregation itself doesn't make any sense or change behavior. It must exhibit some actions. For example, if a patient's pulse rate or blood level exceeds its normal range, the IoT system must automatically send an alert message to the healthcare providers for further interventions.

INTERNET OF THINGS IN HEALTHCARE

The aim of IoT is to connect devices, information and human beings together with respect to local and global scenario. In the sky of various domain, the healthcare is the fastest domain which adopting it's infrastructure to the IoT. The application of sensory capabilities to all the medical devices, gives a pathway and transforming facilities for the whole bionetwork of doctors, patients, medical equipment's and pharmacies. The available infrastructure in hospitals for providing medical services to the patients becomes insufficient and flourishing technologies induced the medical sector to draft or reshape the way of servicing and managing medical units with the support of the IoT. The medical applications and hospitals are connected together through IoT, which allows doctors, patients and supporting staff to make use of advancements in medical sector efficiently. Mobile-based health technology use smart phone as an interface for caregivers and patients which lead to offer digitized medical care. Since this platform promptly supports digitized medical care, enables caregivers to provide better intervention and patients can have faster recovery. Digitization of the chronic disease management is highly empowered by IoT-enabled medical devices which include drug delivery systems, uninterrupted glucose monitoring system and other important physiological vital signs monitoring system.

The recent researches in IoT has opened a wide opportunities for caregivers with reduced medical expenses and also it increases the quality of service. In traditional healthcare systems, disease predictions may subject to error prone. Whereas IoT uses different sensors which highly facilitated with cross-device connectivity allows aggregating, maintaining and analyzing the real-time patient data, reduces the chance of erroneous disease prediction. IoT acquired the attention of elderly patients, individual patients suffering from chronic diseases and also the patients in need of constant medical intervention.

The uprising technologies of IoT changing the lives of humans with the advanced solutions that provides the following benefits:

- Real-time aggregating, sharing and analyzing of patients data from healthcare systems.
- The quality of medical services will increase based on the accurate data.
- Reachability of healthcare providers becomes simple and easier.
- Healthcare providers can monitor their patients regularly via remote monitoring medical systems.

Figure 1. Technologies driving IoT

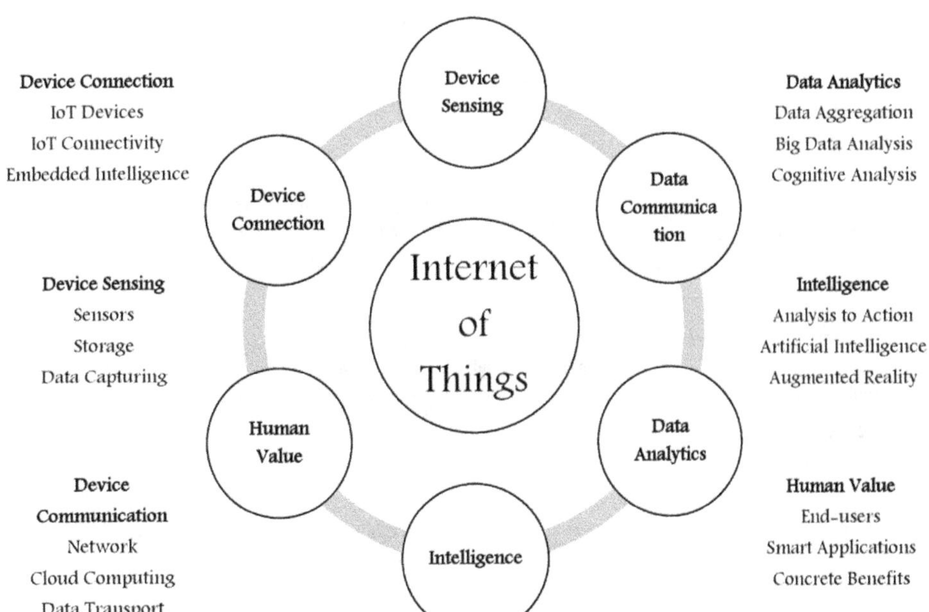

- Providing alert mechanism to send emergency messages to family members and healthcare providers on patient's emergency situations.
- Caregivers can access and analyze their patient information without any geographical restrictions.
- Providing highly-personalized and controlled data storage for individual users.

The IoT plays a major role in variety of healthcare applications ranging from monitoring chronic diseases to preventing diseases. The application of IoT in healthcare is a five step process as in Figure 2, through which the healthcare providers operates more efficiently for patient betterment.

Real-Time Monitoring

The Real-time IoT-enabled medical device collects the health data such as blood glucose, pressure, body temperature, ECG and respiratory rate. The smart medical devices make use of the communication technologies or smart phones for communicating the gathered data to cloud storage and then the authorized persons like healthcare providers, doctors or clinical assistants are allowed to access the patient's data irrespective of their place, time or device.

Figure 2. HIoT Five Step Process Model

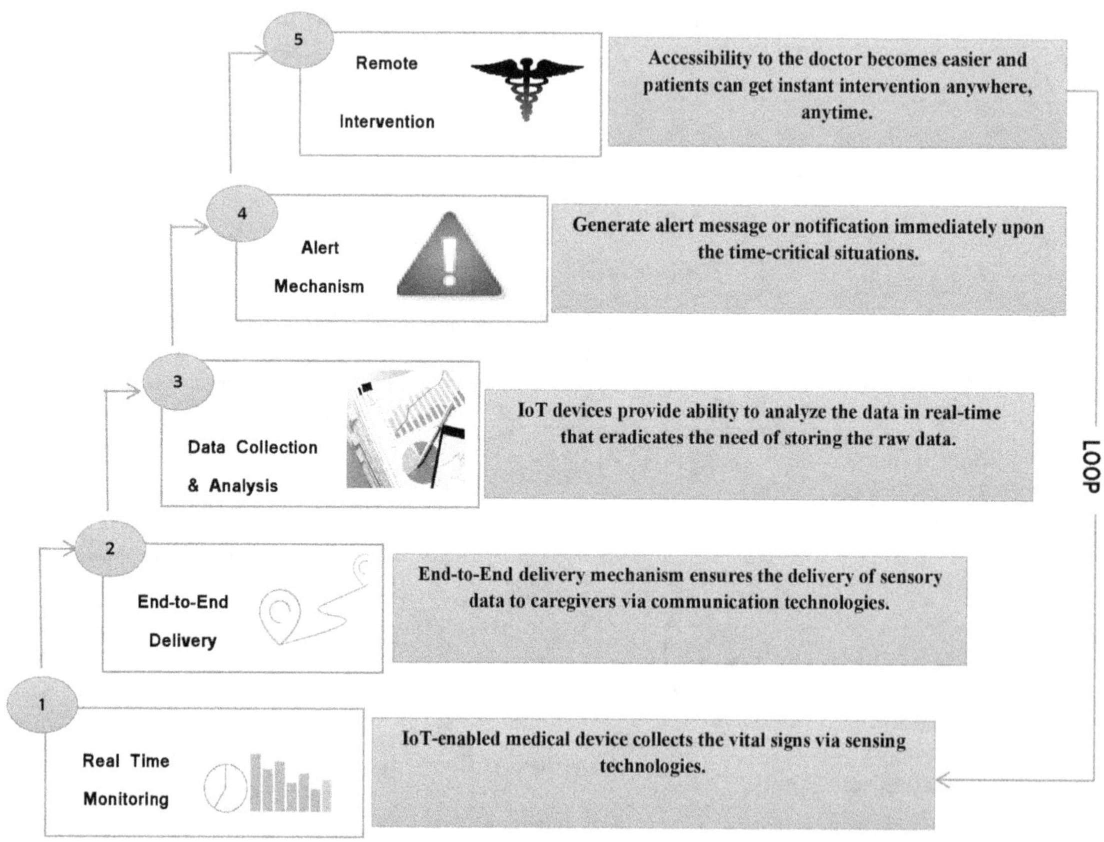

End-to-End Delivery

The effective end-to-end delivery mechanism provides high mobility solutions with respect to interoperability, device-to-device communication and data exchange. Some of the connectivity protocols like Bluetooth, Wi-Fi, ZigBee modified the way of spotting illness and health disorders. This constantly reduces the cost involved in network setup and increases the efficient use of resources.

Data Collection and Analysis

The real-time IoT-enabled medical device generates huge volume of data within a short span of time, is hard to store and maintain locally in case of cloud unavailability. It is a great challenge for healthcare providers to maintain and analyze it manually, as they receive the data generated from various devices. The IoT device with the ability of analyzing the data in real-time eradicates the need of storing the raw data. The healthcare providers are availed with accessing of analyzed reports and visual representations. Thus increases the speed of decision-making and avoid the occurrences of manual errors.

Alert Mechanism

Providing alert notification is considered as crucial event which saves the life of humans during the medical emergency situations. The real-time IoT-enabled medical device gathers the health data and transfers it to the doctors for real-time monitoring of their health status irrespective of location and time. Thus enhances the possibility of giving timely treatment and improves the accuracy of intervention made by doctors.

Remote Intervention

Accessibility to the doctor is a major issue for the patients who are in emergency condition and who needs an immediate medical assistance. IoT adds mobility to healthcare domain; physicians can check the patients and find the disorders instantaneously. It also supports automatic drug distribution based on the instant health factors through connected devices.

The drifts in healthcare domain can be divided into several categories with respect to supporting technologies like sensing, communication, analytics and intelligence. This congregates the consumer devices and healthcare devices. Recently smartphones are being designed to provide healthcare support via incorporated medical sensors and that can be called as Mobile-Health (M-Health). M-Health make use of smartphone applications and wireless communication technologies for public health monitoring and interventions. The IoT has been applied in various ways for improving the medical intelligence as showed in Table 1.

HIoT DESIGN ANATOMY

The IoT collects a huge amount of information from healthcare devices (i.e., medical equipment, sensors) which are connected to the network platform. The idea behind in connecting the clinical devices to the network platform is to give accessibility and controllability features; hence it becomes uniquely

Table 1. IoT in Human Healthcare

Nature of Applicability	Use Case
Remote Patient Monitoring	Remote Patient Monitoring enables the remote investigation of patient vital sign with the help of sensory technologies. This can be highly adoptable for chronic disease management like hypertension, diabetes, coronary heart diseases and kidney diseases.
Mobile-Health	Mobile-Health application is entirely depending upon the mobile app interface for monitoring and delivery of interventions.
Assisting-Medical devices	The devices are mainly used in tracking of patient activities, assisting surgeries and smart medical equipment's enables the doctor to give assistance.
Virtual Intervention	Virtual Intervention allows the healthcare providers to give medicine delivery, virtual therapy and consultation with the help of connected devices and multimedia solutions.
Rehabilitation System	The main aim of rehabilitation system is to provide clinical monitoring for persons who are physically challenged and independent elder patients. This system will be mostly in the form of wearable's which records the vital signs of elderly patients and give intimation or alerts to the concern healthcare providers in case of finding any abnormalities.

identifiable clinical devices. In addition, patients are exclusively monitored via smartphones and embedded devices which also uses the network as it constituents. Designing of such system is acting as a back bone for transmitting and delivering of medical data. Healthcare Internet of Things (HIoT) design has been analyzed into three different categories which includes HIoT network topology, HIoT architecture and HIoT platform as shown in Figure 3.

HIoT Network Topology

HIoT Network Topology depicts how the medical devices are organized in a network and also defines the layout for establishing communication between clinical sensors, actuators and gateways. Building the IoT-based healthcare system without network topology is merely difficult to design an efficient system. The factors to be considered on selecting the suitable network topology and protocols for IoT-enable system are power consumption, cost, reliable and communication. These factors can be carefully handled

Figure 3. HIoT Network Design Anatomy

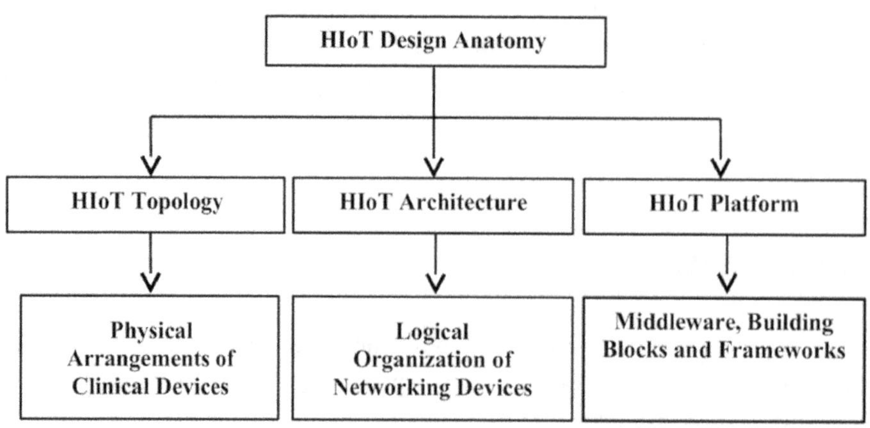

by analyzing the characteristics, abilities and performance of the network topologies include: latency, throughput, fault tolerance, scalability, range and number of hops.

The HIoT uses the network topologies based on the networking standards and this can be divided into three different topologies as shown in Figure 4.

Point-to-Point Topology

A point-to-point topology establishes a link between any two networking nodes or devices. This topology is much simpler and cost effective that exhibits the one-to-one relationship between two devices. As point-to-point topology is limited to lay a communication between two devices, it does not provide scalability and the capability of ranging is also limited to one hop. In HIoT, the sensor nodes collects real-time medical data gets directly transmitted to the network or gateway via a short range communication medium such as Bluetooth or WLAN as shown in Figure 5 (Patel et al., 2012). The point-to-point topology can able to take two forms either omnidirectional or bidirectional according to the use case. The healthcare systems which use omnidirectional form can only transfer the data to its gateway and such system cannot receive any data from other side. In bidirectional form, the data can be transmitted to the gateway and also the intervention can be delivered to the patients using the same medium i.e. via gateway to the node.

Star Topology

A star topology is composed of one central control node called hub (gateway), through which all other nodes (sensor nodes) in the network are connected. The central control node behaves like a relay for all other nodes, thus all the sensor nodes send and receive the data via central control node only. In star topology, the hub can be internal which widely uses the Wi-Fi network or external which uses public network. The start topology results in providing high throughput, consistency, reliable and low latency communication. The finding of faulty nodes will be easier, by means of isolation of distinct nodes in the network. On the other side, star topology suffers from drawbacks such as limitation in range of transmis-

Figure 4. HIoT Topologies

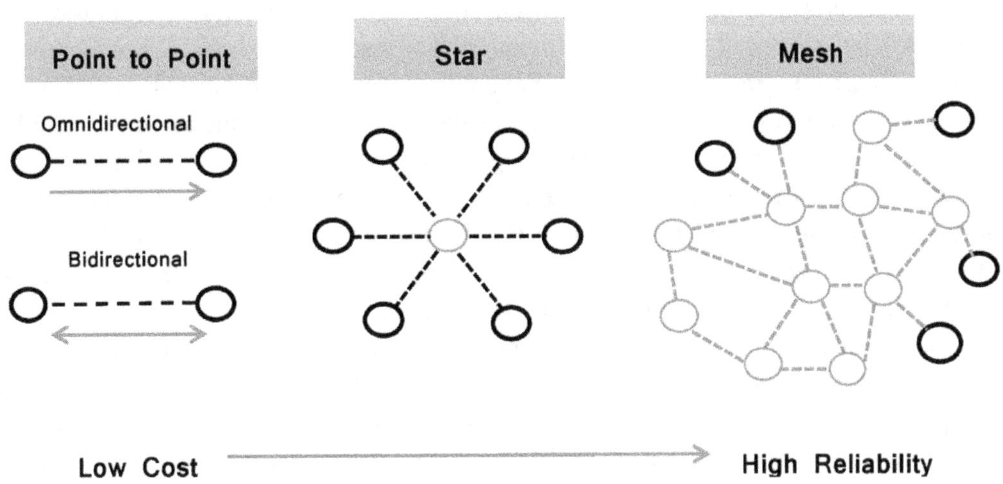

Figure 5. HIoT Point-to-Point Topology

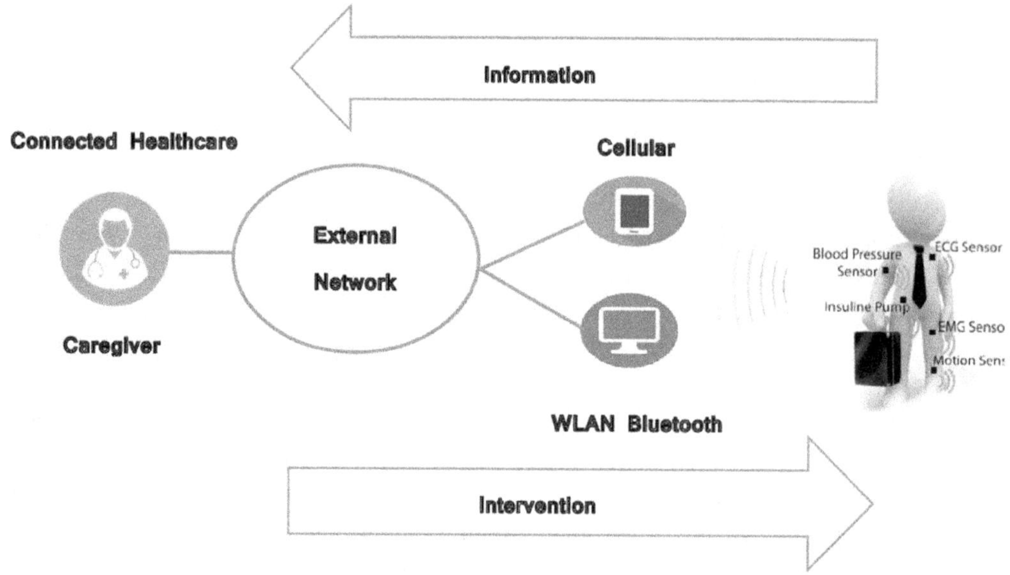

sion and in case of central control node failure, and then the entire network loses the communication with gateway.

Most of the IoT-enabled health monitoring systems is composed of medical sensor nodes, gateways, data center and healthcare providers. The vital signs of various patients made available to the doctors or caregivers for providing medical intervention from remote location any time. The star topological scenario is highly suitable for this kind of application as shown in Figure 6. The individual patient data gets transmitted to the gateway via internal network i.e. Wi-Fi. Generally gateway acts as a central control node through which various patient's medical data is being transmitted to the data center (Amir et al., 2018).

Mesh Topology

A mesh topology provides a high reliable network which composed of three different kinds of nodes: gateway node, distinct sensor nodes and router/sensor nodes. Like star topology, gateway allows the sensed data to reach the external world (i.e. data center). The distinct sensor nodes simply broadcast the data to the gateway whereas router/sensor nodes not only broadcast its own data but also it acts as a relay for other sensor nodes. In mesh network data reaches the gateway by passing through multiple router/sensor nodes. The complexity factor of mesh topology is high when compared to point-to-point and star topologies. It also suffers from high latency because it may have multiple hops to reach the gateway. This topology permits the multiple nodes to transmit the data simultaneously even under heavy traffic. Unlike star topology, in case of failure in any router/sensor node, the data transfer doesn't get affected because alternate nodes are available to carry out the task.

An IoT-enabled health monitoring system can be constructed based on mesh topology, which comprises of Body Area Network (BAN), a Wireless Personal Area Network (WPAN), a WLAN, extended gateway, application server and healthcare center as shown in Figure 7. The Body Gateway (BG) gathers the data from BAN which contains medical sensors and then forwards the data to the Base Station

Figure 6. HIoT Star Topology

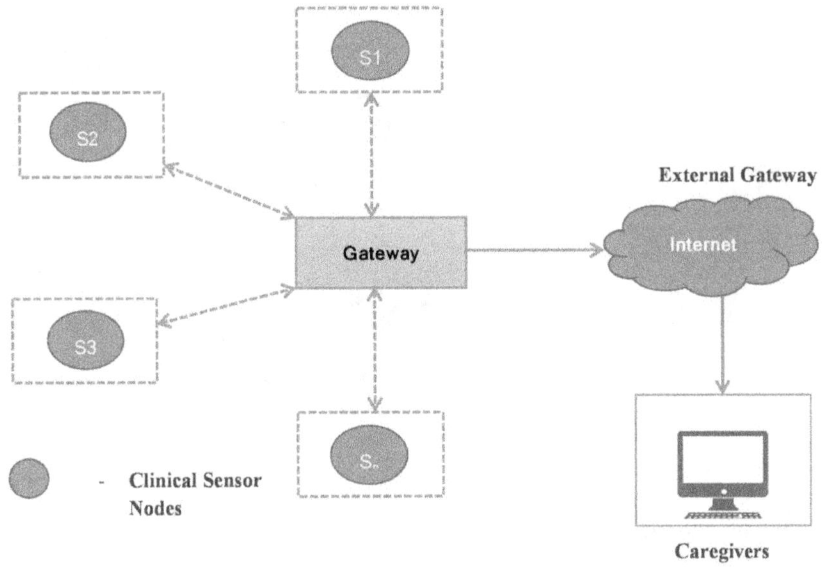

(BS) via WPAN. The BS forwards the data to the Residential Gateway (RG) through WLAN and RG is responsible for connecting BS with the public network. The healthcare providers can make use of data aggregated at health center for giving remedies to their patients (Fengou et al., 2012). There is an extended gateway that provides secured framework for accessing the patient profile database via application server.

HIoT Architecture

HIoT must concentrate on providing healthcare to the patients without any geographical limitations and also it must continuously monitor their medical data for preventing them from life time risks. This can be achieved by developing an IoT-enabled healthcare system, which incorporates five major constituents such as: sensors, network infrastructure, cloud computing, data analytics and healthcare providers. With respect to these components, HIoT architecture has been designed in Figure 8. This architecture has its own characteristic features which include:

- **Constancy:** HIoT systems are capable of providing real-time monitoring, this architecture constantly make a request to sensor nodes for trustworthy data collection. .
- **Continuity:** This provides interoperability support for communication system thus helps the network to maintain continuity in communication among end-users, nodes and links.
- **Confidentiality:** This architecture provides a scalable and secured storage in cloud which can save the real-time data and while accessing it allows the user to handle data confidentially.
- **Usability:** Data analytics is a heart of this architecture because it converts dynamic medical data into useful information which helps healthcare providers to make better decisions.

Figure 7. HIoT Mesh Topology

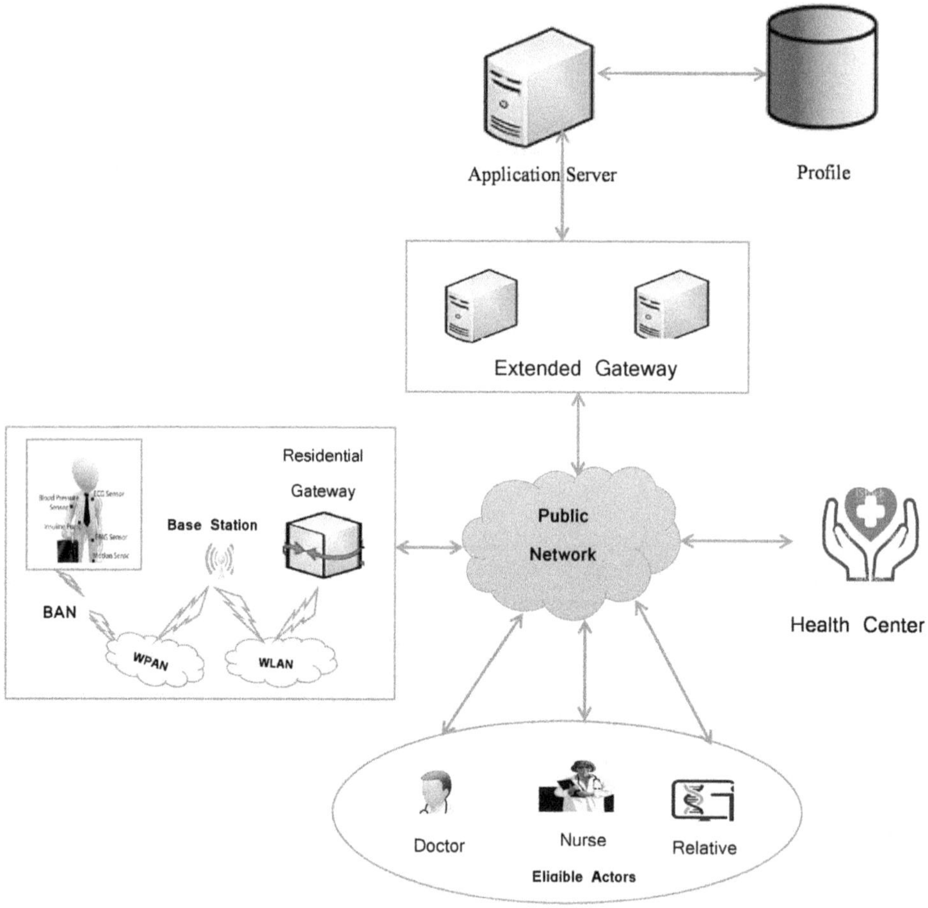

Developing HIoT systems must bind the four features together, in case of missing any one of the feature allows the system to enter into a valueless and defected system. HIoT architecture is made of four major components:

Clinical Device Layer

A device agent is incorporated into every individual medical sensor node which made them capable of processing the request. This layer registers every sensor to establish connectivity and then it can able to collect the data. Additionally, it provides various services like software up-gradation, remote accessing, troubleshooting and controlling activities. It accepts and executes the requests/commands from the middleware.

Figure 8. HIoT Architecture

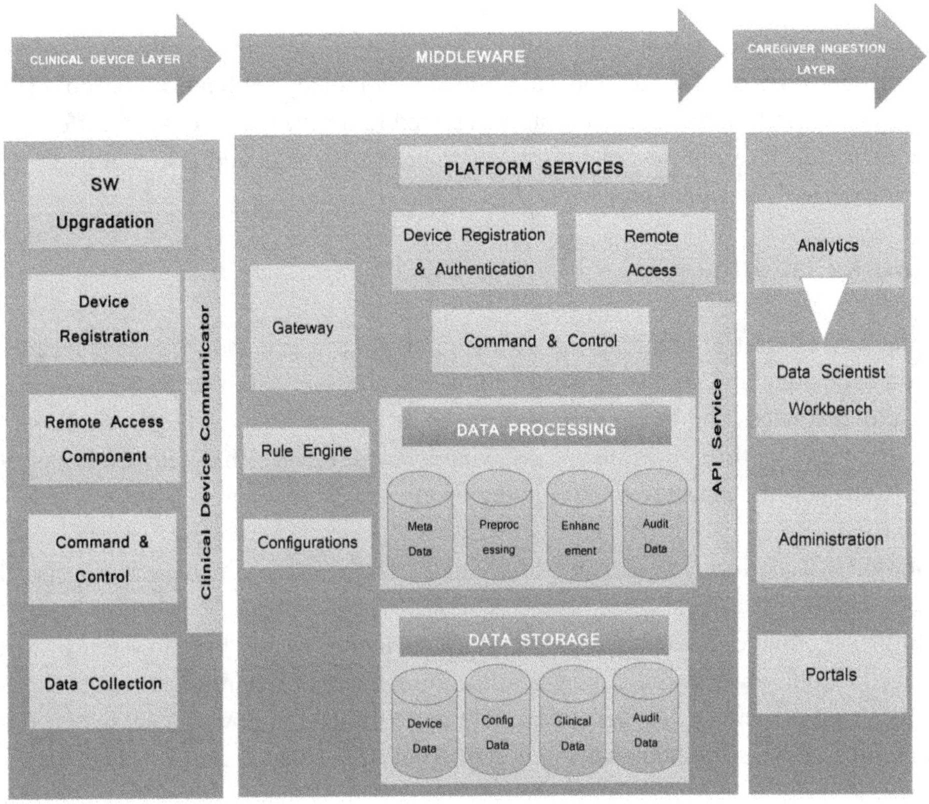

Clinical Device Communicator

A clinical device communicator also exists within every medical sensor node and tightly coupled with device agent. The responsibility of communicator is to provide connectivity between various medical devices through middleware.

Middleware

Middleware provides many services that include: gateway services, platform services, data processing services, data storage services, device configuration services and application programming interface (API) services. The gateway allows all the medical devices to communicate with each other. A platform service handles the functionalities such as device registration, authentication, remote accessing, controlling the devices on the network and requests the device agent to act according to its commands. The data processing does four jobs (i.e. metadata, preprocessing, enhancement and audit trails) in order to generate a suitable datasets for analytics. Data storage services provides four separate storage spaces for storing device data, configuration data, clinical data and audit data, in order to avoid conflicts while accessing. The API service provides a platform for end-user to access the collected data. Another important component in middleware layer is rule engine, which is a software entity that allows devices to register and configure the infrastructure.

Caregiver Ingestion Layer

The caregiver ingestion layer is where the end-users like physicians, nurses and pharmacists make use of information. This layer provides an opportunity to develop many applications based on the collected information. For example, a user interface can be created for every end-user with different access permissions and workbench can be designed for users to access the data and also facilitates the detection of diseases by means of analytical programs.

HIoT Network Platforms

The HIoT platform is a set of entities used to maintain, control and monitor the medical devices by deploying self-regulating and secure communication between devices. The platform is an application which binds cloud services and the intelligent devices. It is also called as HIoT middleware; it serves as an inter-mediator for both application layer and hardware devices. HIoT platform is entirely different from other platforms with respect to the following features:

- **Elasticity:** HIoT platforms are capable of accepting any number of end devices as per the requirements of users.
- **Flexibility:** It provides a convenient API's for developing an IoT based systems, the developers may have flexibility over coding, integration, communicating schemas and security.
- **Security:** It gives security via encryption techniques for data in flow, data at rest. It is responsible for granting access on data and ownership. It also provides isolated cloud storage for storing sensitive data.
- **Interoperability:** HIoT platform allows the integration of any hardware and software which belongs to different manufacturers significantly.

The HIoT platform ensures integration of dissimilar hardware by using communication protocols, appropriate topology and necessary software. This platform has been designed with interfaces required for feeding the medical data into storage and then used for data analytics. The HIoT platform can proficiently adopt any kind of medical devices and can be integrated with the applications. HIoT platform depicted as four-tier structure which includes: medical things, connectivity, management services, data analytics and user interface. The management services is a core tier of this platform model which securely stores the collected data via encryption techniques, manages and controls the devices, provides tools for data processing and does the adoption of communication protocols. HIoT platform model is shown in the Figure 9.

Medical Things

The medical things is the bottom most layer of HIoT platform which is analogous to the physical layer in the OSI network reference model. It consists of internet-connected physical devices like clinical sensors, medical devices, wearables and mobile applications. This can be referred as base-tier, as these medical things have ability to grasp the patient's physiological vital signs. The caregivers can monitor their patient's behavior using the data generated by these things and hence it can be otherwise called as Data Generator.

Figure 9. HIoT Platform Model

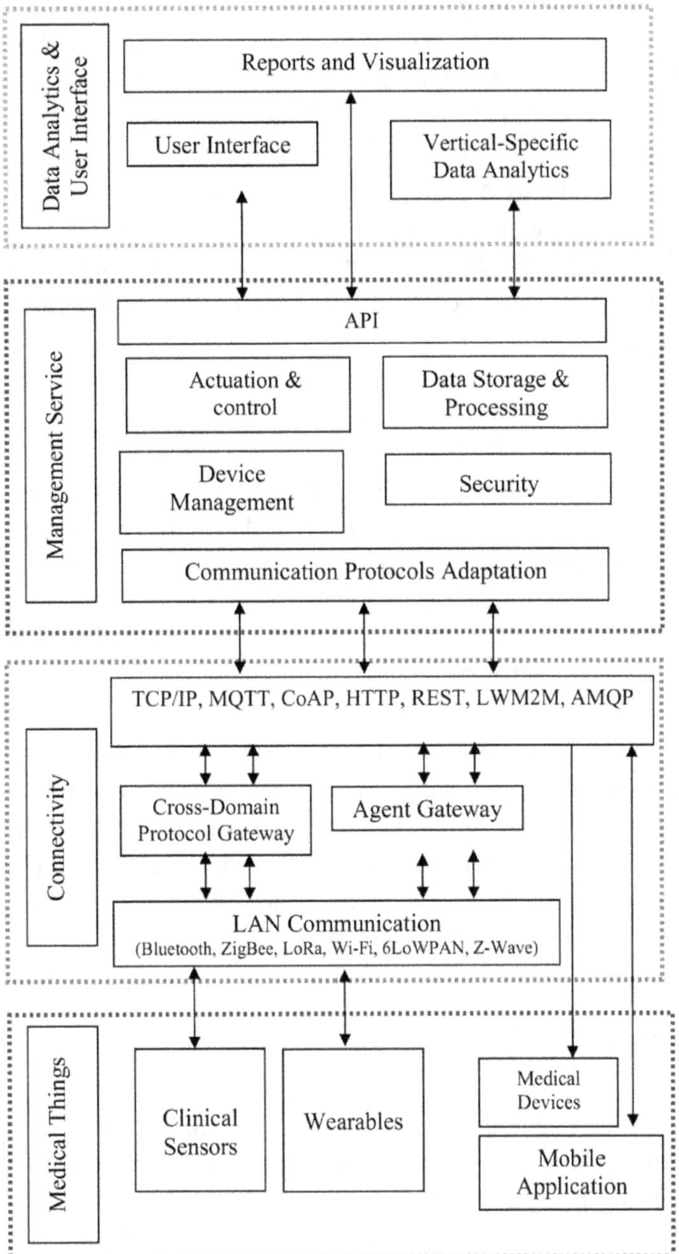

Connectivity

Connectivity is the second-tier of HIoT platform model acts as heart of IoT-enable medical devices. Like human heart maintains the body alive by circulating the blood throughout the body, this tier provides a network connection for transmitting the medical data gathered in bottom most layer to the next higher level layer. To carry out the transmission four components are involved: Local Area Network (LAN) communication, cross-domain protocol gateway, agent gateway and internet communication protocols. LAN communication is responsible for transferring the data from medical things to the gateways. Some of the commonly used communication technologies are Bluetooth, ZigBee, 6LoWPAN, Wi-Fi, Z-Wave and Low Range (LoRa) will be discussed in next section. Cross-domain protocol gateway enables the embedded systems to transfer the information between the devices which are having dissimilar security concerns. This ensures data confidentiality, data integrity and data availability without any security consequences. The agent gateway is responsible for establishing a relationship between LAN and distributed external systems. It is done by providing network policy and agent migration information. An internet communication protocol receives the medical data from gateway and forwards to the next higher layer for processing. Some of the protocols used in this case are TCP/IP, MQTT, AMQP, REST, HTTP and CoAP (*"Internet of Things Protocols and Standards"*, 2018).

Management Service

The management service is the core-tier of HIoT platform model which performs various operations such as protocol adaption, device management, security, data storage, data processing and APIs. All these functionalities have to take place at cloud infrastructure as it provides elastic resources based on usage patterns.

Data Analytics and User Interface

This is the top most tier of HIoT platform model composed of many components such as user interface, visualization, reports, vertical-specific data analytics. User interface allows the end-users (doctors or caregivers) to make use of available portals (web-based or mobile-based) to visualize the patient's medical reports. The major component is vertical-specific data analytics that offers a group of intelligence specifically designed for medical analytic applications. This enables healthcare providers to drive a better decision and conclude where to emphasis the treatment.

HIoT TECHNOLOGIES

Healthcare domain is constantly gaining the importance as much how the rate of population increases. The healthcare accessibility ratio of rural and semi-urban area is unknown. The aim of attaining the healthy population is always being a dream due to lack of technology. But now it has been made possible by improvements in sensors and communication technologies. With this great openings healthcare providers can be easily directly accessed by patients around the clock. In this section both sensor and communication technologies which improved the healthcare domain are discussed.

Communication Technologies

Communication medium is a nervous system of HIoT through which medical data transfer takes place from one end to another end. Based on the applicability of medical things and geographical constraints communication technologies has been broadly classified into two types: Short-range communications and long range communications. Most of the IoT-based health monitoring system uses the two communication technologies. The medical data transmission in HIoT systems has two relays. The first relay is for medical things to communicate with gateway requires short-range communication medium. The data collected at gateway becomes useless; until extracting high-level information for decision making. For that next relay, uses long-range communication for forwarding the data to the storage location where the caregivers can access it. Many factors has to be analyzed while selecting the short and long-range communications.

Short-range Communications

In IoT-based healthcare system, short-range communication technologies take part between medical things and internal gateways. This section discovers and compares the widely used short-range communication technologies in HIoT. In order to use short-range communications in healthcare systems it is necessary to examine the communication factors affecting human body, transmission delay, reliability. While selecting long-range communications, factors to be analyzed are reliability, error correction mechanisms, latency, delay and confidentiality. The selection of short-range communication for healthcare systems must provide strong security mechanisms for ensuring the privacy of patient's data. The communication technology with low-latency is highly preferable for health-care or time-critical IoT applications, because it may alert doctors and ambulance services during medical emergencies. If data transmission is delayed, it leads the patients to enter into the life time risks and such kind of communication technologies is not preferable. Major studies (Jara et al., 2013) (Kalsnia et al., 2012) have merited the Wi-Fi, Bluetooth, Z-Wave, ZigBee and Ultra Wide Band (UWB) as most commonly used technologies in healthcare systems. Table 2 compares the various HIoT enabling short-range communication technologies with respect to distinct parameters.

Long-Range Communications

A subset of long-range communication is low-power wide area networks (LPWAN) that are highly applicable for healthcare systems. Normally LPWAN ranges up to several kilometers which are extremely covers long distance than the coverage distance of Wi-Fi or Bluetooth. LPWAN used in healthcare devices such as remote health monitoring, rehabilitation systems operates around the clock to reduce the life time risk of patients because of interrupted connectivity. As per the study made, LPWAN is considered as a best long-range communication for transmitting data from gateway to the cloud storage for processing. Long-range communications must satisfy all the essentials as like short-range communications. In addition, high error correction mechanism is required to ensure that the data remains unaltered during transmission. Finally, availability is important feature required to transmit data at any time without any geographical restrictions. The most commonly used LPWANs are Worldwide Interoperability for Microwave Access (WiMAX), Cellular, Sigfox and LoRa. Table 3 provides the comparison of long-range communication used in HIoT with respect to their features.

Sensing Technologies

Technical improvements in sensors converted the traditional healthcare systems into modernized healthcare systems with remote monitoring capability. Sensors are identified as a key component for caregivers to monitor their patient's vital signs. Nowadays sensors are made in the form of wearables like watch,

Table 2. Short-range Communication Technologies for HIoT

Parameters	Technologies				
	Bluetooth	UWB	Wi-Fi	Z-Wave	ZigBee
Authentication	Shared Secret	CBC-MAC (CCM)	WPA2 (IEEE 802.11i)	AES-CBCMAC	CBC-MAC (Extension of CCM)
Battery Life	Days to Weeks	Hours to Days	Hours	3 Years	Months to Years
Cost	Low	Low	High	Low	Low
Data Protection	16-bit CRC	32-bit CRC	32-bit CRC	8-Bit Checksum	16-bit CRC
Data Rate	1–24 Mb/s	110 Mbits/s to 1.6 GBits/s	1 Mb/s – 6.75 Gb/s	250 kb/s	250 Kbits/s
Encryption	E0 Stream Cipher	AES Block Cipher	RC4 Stream Cipher (WEP), AES Block Cipher	AES-OFB	AES Block Cipher
Energy Consumption	Medium	Low	High	Medium	Very Low
Frequency Band	2.4 GHz	3.1 to 10.6 GHz	5-60 GHz	908.4 MHz	868/915 MHz, 2.4 GHz
Nodes	8	128	32	232+	65,000
Spreading	FHSS	DS-UWB, MB-OFDM	DSSS, CCK, OFDM	FSK	DSSS
Standard	IEEE 802.15.1	IEEE 802.15.3 (Ratified)	IEEE 802.11 a/c/b/ d/g/n	IEEE 802.11	IEEE 802.15.4
Topology	Mesh, Star, Tree	Star, P2P	Star, P2P	Mesh	P2P, Star, Tree and Mesh
Transmission Range	8m – 10m	4m – 20m	20m - 100m	100m	10m – 300m

pendant, wrist bands for the flexibility and comfort of the patient's. There are two types of sensors used widely in healthcare system: Non-invasive and Inertial sensors.

Non-Invasive Sensors

A non-invasive sensor provides a new vision to change the former techniques available for monitoring the physiological factors. It is also called as unobtrusive sensing method which enables to take physiological data without the requirement of bio fluids. Wearable based health monitoring devices popularized with the wide improvements in the field of non-invasive sensors and biosensors. These sensors can be easily fitted into the things which are used in our day to day lives. Such kind of sensors provides accurate and consistent for diagnosing the patient's disease. This section is focused on fundamental non-invasive sensors which are used for monitoring the vital signs.

Table 3. Long-range Communication Technologies for HIoT

Parameters	Technologies			
	Sigfox	LoRa	Cellular	WiMAX
Authentication	AES Encrypted / 16 bit	CCM	High Security, back by major telecoms	CBC-MAC
Battery Life	5-10 Years	Years	1 day	Months to Years
Cost	Low	High	High	High
Data Protection	128-bit CRC	128-bit CRC	---	128-bit CRC
Data Rate	100 bps	0.3–50 Kb/s	High	1 Mb/s– 1 Gb/s (Fixed)
Encryption	No Network Encryption	AES Block Cipher	CMEA	3DES, AES Block Cipher
Energy Consumption	Low	Very Low	High	Medium
Frequency Band	868/915MHz	868/900 MHz	200KHz	2-66 GHz
Nodes	50000	120	5000/Gateway	100
Spreading	UNB(Ultra Narrow Band)	Chirp Spread Spectrum (CSS)	---	OFDM
Standard	No	IEEE 802.15.4g	GSM, LTE	IEEE 802.16
Topology	Star	Star-of-Stars	Star	Radio Access Network (RAN), Mesh
Transmission Range	<9.5 Kms	< 30 Kms	<35-200Kms	< 50 Kms

Blood Pressure Sensor

Blood pressure is the rate at which blood is pumped in the arteries by the heart. This blood pressure sensor evaluates the rate of pressure into two variations – Systolic and Diastolic (pumping and relaxing). High Blood pressure (Hypertension) is considered as an important sign of heart disease and cardiovascular diseases.

Body Temperature Sensor

Body temperature is a predominant factor for diagnosing hyperthermia, stroke and fever. These sensors give accuracy results based on proximity to the human body. Hence it has been widely integrated in wearable-based health monitoring systems.

Electrocardiogram (ECG) Sensor

ECG sensor is commonly used medical test for monitoring the muscular functioning of the heart. It evaluates the abnormal cardiac rhythms and cardiac pathologies such as ischemia and palpitations. ECG sensors are capable of acquiring data even from the hand palms of the patient rather than heart.

Electroencephalogram (EEG) Sensor

EEG sensor is monitors and records the activity of the brain from the sensor electrodes placed on the scalp. It can be carried out for predicting the abnormal brain activities, tumors, seizures, dizziness and sleeping disorders by using four waves such as alpha, beta, theta and delta waves. In IoT-based healthcare systems, EEG sensors are used for capturing the driver drowsiness and stress analysis (Li.G et al., 2015) (Ha et al., 2015).

Blood Glucose Sensor

Blood glucose sensor contains electrochemical strips through which the glucose concentration in the blood can be assessed. Building a real-time blood glucose monitoring system can be highly useful for diabetes patients to manage their lift in blood glucose levels.

GSR (Galvanic Skin Response) Sensor

GSR sensor evaluates the skin conductance which acts as a symptom psychological and physiological stimulation. Hence through the evaluation of skin conductance, the emotion can be identified. GSR predicts the emotions using two electrodes that can be placed on any two fingers. GSR sensor is useful in designing a healthcare system for monitoring stress levels, as our nervous system stimulates the sweat glands to secrete more sweat on strong emotions.

Pulse Oximetry Sensors

SpO_2 sensor or pulse oximetry sensor examines the level of oxygen in the blood but it is not treated as a vital sign like blood pressure. It acts as a pointer of respiratory functions and helpful in diagnosing the hypoxia (reduced oxygen in tissues).

Pulse Sensors

Pulse sensor measure the heart beat rate and it is the most commonly monitored vital signs to predict many health disorders include cardiac arrest, vasovagal syncope and pulmonary embolisms (Zenko.J et al., 2016). This sensor is capable of reading the pulse rate at various parts of our human body such as chest, fingers and earlobes. Even though it can be read from many part of the body, accuracy of reading is more important. While analyzing the accuracy factor, it has been found that reading the pulse from earlobe and finger which attains more accurate results. Placing the pulse sensors as wearables at ears and fingers are not comfortable and it can be worthy to be in the form of wrist bands.

Respiratory Rate Sensors

Respiratory Sensor or airflow sensor calculates the inhale and exhale rates per minute and it acts as a vital sign for predicting the lung cancer, attacks, barriers in airway and tuberculosis. From the studies (Milici et al., 2017) (Varon et al., 2015), it is identified that the healthcare systems were developed for measuring respiratory rate, as it is considered to be an important factor for diagnosing many diseases.

Inertial Sensors

An inertial sensors used in healthcare systems are based on micro-electro-mechanical system (MEMS) which measures the force applied, angular rate and magnetic fields around the body. This can be achieved by integrating three different inertial sensors such as accelerometer, magnetometer and gyroscope. Many healthcare systems have been developed for regular monitoring of patients physical activities (Rand et al., 2009) (Bonnie et al., 2013). Another important inertial sensor is body position sensor, which monitors the body postures like standing, sitting and so on to predict the future health issues.

HIoT APPLICATIONS

The developing interdisciplinary applications in the field of IoT transformed the traditional way of living into smart living. Among various applications, healthcare is one of the growing technology, which provides doctors or caregivers on a pocket. It is not possible to eradicate the chronic disease in a while with the help of IoT. But the chronic diseases can be managed by doctors or caregivers with regular remote monitoring of their patients vital signs. The regular monitoring process is time consuming and costlier. IoT has changed the scenario like health check-ups from doctor-centric to patient-centric. All these have been accomplished with the applications of IoT in human healthcare domain. In this section, applications of HIoT are presented as two categories: Distributed Applications and Clustered Applications as shown in Figure 10. Distributed applications deals with the systems that focus on monitoring any single vital sign whereas clustered applications clubs two or more vital signs together.

Blood Pressure Monitoring

J.Puustjarvi et al. designed a system for monitoring and controlling the blood pressure remotely via a communication layered between patient and data center (Puustjarvi et al., 2011). A similar system has been presented in (Guan, 2013). T.J.Xin et al. developed an intelligent blood pressure monitoring along with location tracking facility (Xin et al., 2013).

Body Temperature Monitoring

Finding of common abnormalities like fever, hyperthermia and stroke is much simpler using body temperature. An IoT-enabled temperature monitoring system makes use of home-based communication to transmit collected data to remote data center is presented in (Jian et al., 2012). A TelosB mote system uses IPv6 communication between patients and caregivers for visualizing the changes in body temperature (Istepanian et al., 2011). Likewise, a system designed for recording the body temperature and uses RFID technology for sending recorded data to the storage (In Z.L, 2014).

Blood Glucose Monitoring

Diabetes is one of a metabolic disease caused due to persistent high glucose level in blood. The real-time monitoring system uses temperature sensor and non-invasive blood glucose sensor for tracking the patient's temperature and blood glucose patterns. (Z.J. Guan, 2013) presented an IoT-based utility model for sensing the blood glucose which is composed of three elements such as blood glucose collector unit, processing unit and mobile device.

ECG Monitoring

ECG is used for monitoring the activities of the heart via rhythms. (M.L.Liu et al., 2012) introduced a portable ECG monitoring system which consists of transmitter and receiver and this system identifies the cardiac problems using real-time ECG data.

GSR Monitoring

The internal and external stimuli are controlled and regulated by the sympathetic and parasympathetic nervous systems. The parasympathetic system of human body is known for preserving and restoring the energy level. The various vital signs like blood pressure, heart beat rate and sweat secretion has been driven by the sympathetic system. In many of the health monitoring system GSR is used for monitoring the stress and emotion level of humans (Critchley.H.D, 2012) (Bakker et al., 2011). A wearable-based

Figure 10. Classification of HIoT Applications

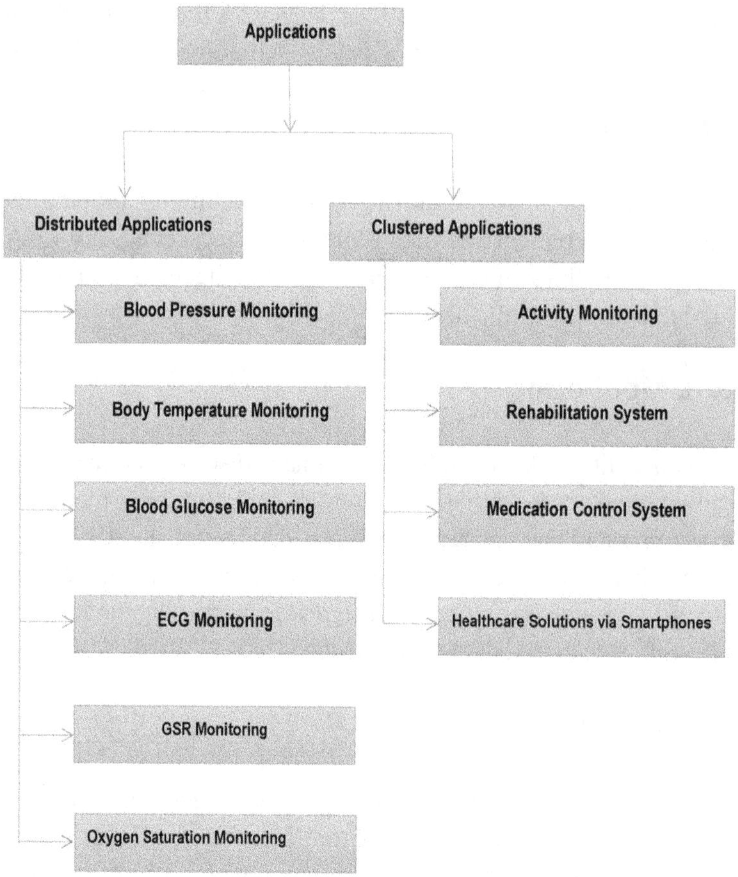

GSR monitoring device is invented and reveals the psychophysiological conditions with low power consumption (P.Bonato, 2003) (Sano et al. 2013).

Oxygen Saturation Monitoring

Oxygen Saturation Monitoring is used for evaluating the amount of oxygen present in blood. The abnormal level of oxygen in blood is a symptom for various health issues such as cardio-vascular, pulmonary diseases and anemia. A cost effective and low energy consuming pulse oximeter system is designed for monitoring the patient's oxygen level in blood (Larson et al. 2012) and also a wearable based system oxygen saturation monitoring device has been developed (Larson et al., 2011).

Activity Monitoring

The musculoskeletal diseases and fall prediction in rehabilitation system can be arrived by regular monitoring of physical movements of body parts. (S.Mulro et al., 2003) study identified that the health conditions can be revealed by the patient's walking postures and patterns. Necessity arises for a system to observe the balancing and synchronization of body parts while walking. A wearable device is developed using three inertial sensors such as an accelerometer, a magnetometer and a gyroscope for observing the limb movements of a person (Bertolotti et al., 2016). A gait-event detection device developed for measuring the angular velocity and flexion angle of legs (Bejarano et al., 2015). This device is composed of inertial and magnetic sensors along with that an adaptive algorithm has been integrated to predict the gait-event.

Rehabilitation System

The rehabilitation restores the life of differently abled persons and aged persons who all are living independently. The adoption of IoT in rehabilitation systems renovated the life of independent persons. From the studies it is identified that more number of IoT-enabled rehabilitation system has been introduced which includes rehabilitation system for prisons (Lin.D.Y, 2013), system for hemiplegic patient's (Guangnan, Z., & Penghui, L., 2012) rehabilitation system for smart city (Yue-Hong et al., 2014) and for childhood autism (Liang et al., 2011).

Medication Control System

Healthcare domain is constantly considered as a time-critical domain in which all activities have to be carried out at a right time. Likewise delaying in the medication creates a serious health issues and cause financial losses. To avoid such kind of delay in medication, an IoT-enabled medication management system is developed with intelligence (Pang et al., 2014). This gathers patient's vital signs via wearable sensors and diagnoses the disease for suggesting medicines. A similar system is also designed using an RFID tag which enables caregivers to prescribe medicines remotely (Laranjo et al., 2012).

Healthcare Solutions via Smartphones

The smartphone users are relatively high and it drives the healthcare domain to new platform where timely alerts will be possible during emergency situations. Nowadays smartphones are integrated with sensors that collect the data from smartphone users and forward it to the caregivers for real-time monitoring. Many healthcare apps are developed for diagnosing the health conditions like pulmonary disease, cough, respiratory problems, heart rate, blood pressure, oxygen saturation and diabetes.

ISSUES IN DESIGNING OF HIoT SYSTEMS

The HIoT have a significant social impact and shaping the networking strategies. Recent years many research activities are taking part towards the designing of architectures and standards but enormous amount of deployment issues to be solved globally to provide consistency and quality in treatments. The most common design issues to be considered while developing HIoT system will be discussed in this section.

Battery Life

As discussed in the section, HIoT aims to provide healthcare solutions without geographical restrictions. HIoT tends to deploy the sensors nodes at every users environment for collecting vital signs. During deployment an important issue must be carefully blended is that the battery life. The communication technologies, protocols and hardware used in the system have a direct impact on battery life. Every nodes like wearables are battery powered, which will never throw any problem in case of limited number of nodes. When it grows to millions of nodes it would increase the expenses for battery replacements. The only solution to this problem is energy harvesting which includes solar cells and piezoelectric elements.

Data Transmission Vulnerability

The regulatory bodies must ensure the security of individual's health information which is exchanged among the connected devices and stored in a centric-location. The strong access control mechanisms are not enough but every healthcare regulatory body must ensure that the patient's personal data is stored in an encrypted format. The healthcare regulatory body doesn't have any control over end-devices to ensure data security during transmission. This vulnerability increases it severity when new devices are included to the network.

Multiple Protocols and Devices Integration

When connecting the diversified devices together in a network is another barrier for implementing the IoT in healthcare. The issue arises when multiple devices are connected to share information with each other effectively is a problem. This is due to the systems connected in the network belongs to various manufacturers doesn't have any set of communication protocols and standards. The medical devices connected in IoT healthcare network suffers from lack of uniformity and thus affects the scalability.

Accuracy

The process of gathering and aggregating data via healthcare systems is useful for extracting the high level information and insights which provides better treatment to patients. The extraction of insights from large amount of healthcare data requires refined analytical programs. In particular, recognizing and categorizing valid insights becomes a critical task for caregivers when amount of data increases. This may reduce accuracy and the quality of decision made.

HIoT SECURITY AND PRIVACY ISSUES

The security in HIoT is a pain and an untidiness which annoying the journey of human between life and death. HIoT poses more risk while comparing it with other kinds of IoT smart applications. Because the connected system contains the individuals personal identical information attracts the intruders. They try to compromise the network or medical things to gain access into those medical records. In order to address the security issues, a healthcare system must comply on three crucial factors such as:

- Warranting whether the healthcare system ensures availability, accessibility and consistency (A2C),
- Adopting strong authentication and authorization mechanism, and
- Ensuring system reliability.

Figure 11 presents a Tetrahedron Security Level Model, which depicts the HIoT vulnerability with respect to users, process, things, and tools i.e. platform and applications. The medical things in HIoT are likely to suffer in the process of securing the sensors, network components, communication protocols and application platform. HIoT composed of diversified components and expandable in nature, increases the vulnerability towards human resources as represented at users node. The severity of vulnerability at process and tool nodes is relatively low when comparing it with other nodes i.e. things and users.

In this section, crucial HIoT security issues will be discussed into two factors: HIoT Security Essentials and HIoT Security Threats.

HIoT Security Essentials

The security needs for HIoT systems are analogous to the security essential standards of traditional communication circumstances. In order to attain secure HIoT systems, it becomes necessary to focus on security essentials which are specified below:

Authentication

The medical devices connected together in a network must ensure the identity of all other devices to certify the participating device is valid or not. Upon the successful verification each other's identity, both the participating devices can exchange information.

Authorization

The process of authorization allows the nodes in the network to gain access on the resources and services provided by HIoT systems. It also validates the user's access level on data while they are trying to access the medical data.

Availability

As HIoT is a time-critical application, it must allow caregivers to monitor their patient's vital signs and provide medical intervention without geographical restrictions. If availability is breached then the healthcare systems becomes useless.

Confidentiality

Confidentiality is a basic security requirement in HIoT systems, as it designed to sense and store medical information. The system must restrict the unauthorized users to access the medical data. To ensure the confidentiality data center must deploy encryption mechanisms.

Data Reliability

Every healthcare system is capable of collecting the medical data continuously and forwards it to the data center for real-time monitoring. Hence the data center content is being updated around the clock; the system must ensure that the data received at data center are very recent.

Fault Tolerance

The healthcare system must comply to work with dynamic environment for delivering the uninterrupted services even under mobility issues and component failures.

Data Integrity

The data integrity is a mechanism of ensuring that the medical information received at data center is reliable and not modified by malicious insiders during transmission. If the system is made to work on the

Figure 11. Tetrahedron Security Level Model

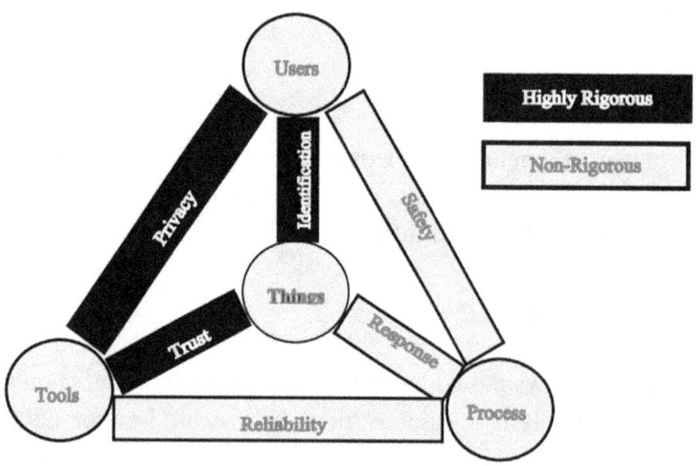

environment without encryption mechanism, then it is not sure that the medical information received is original as sent by transmitter. With the tampered information, the decision made by caregivers becomes worthless. Hence data integrity must be ensured to avoid tampering of data on transmission.

Non-Repudiation

Non-repudiation serves as an evidence of legitimacy and source of all medical information transmitted. This guarantees that the message sent or received cannot be further denied even by sender or receiver.

HIoT Security Threats

The vulnerability factors are growing parallel to increase rate of security threats with respect to HIoT devices and networks. Such threats may initiate from inside and outside of the HIoT network. When the threat originates from healthcare devices within a network, then the severity of attack is more. Figure 12 presents a HIoT Security Threat Organization Model where identified healthcare system threats are related with respect to the security essentials. The identified healthcare system threats are: Data Leakage, Denial of Service (DoS), Exploitation of Access Privilege, Repudiation, Spoofing and Tampering.

MACHINE LEARNING FOR HIoT

Machine learning is an intelligence paradigm that enables the system to build a model based on the patterns identified from the raw data and automatically uses that model to make predictions on new data as shown in Figure 13. HIoT device generate the volume of data, which grows when the number of devices increases. Intelligent analysis and processing of medical data is the key factor for developing smart medi-

Figure 12. HIoT Security Threat Organization Model

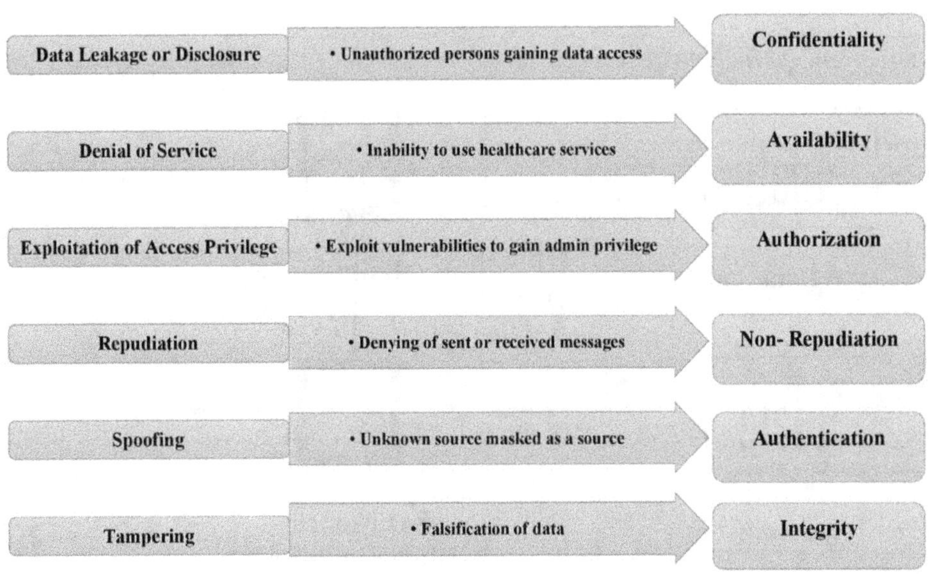

cal applications. To make the HIoT system intelligent, two important techniques must be bonded together that are: streaming data and machine learning. It is necessary to understand the needs of integrating IoT, streaming data and machine learning which brings benefits to healthcare domain. HIoT systems monitor the vital signs and when it is combined with machine learning algorithm, doctors can apply smart treatment to their patients. It improves the quality of chronic disease management at lower costs.

The process of applying streaming medical data with machine learning algorithms is presented in the Figure 14. It consists of four components that are: Health Data Source, Streaming Data Collection, Processing and Dashboard. Health Data Source is the first component which supplies a stream of data from the healthcare systems. Streaming data collection is the assembling unit where all the sensory medical data are organized. In order to make predictions on streaming health data, it is required to build an offline model. The next step is processing, which is composed of two entities: Batch Processing where an offline model is being build and Stream Processing where predictions are made based on streaming data.

In batch processing, historical medical data is used for constructing an offline-model which exhibits the normal behavior. Such model is built by applying the appropriate machine learning algorithms machine learning algorithms commonly used on streaming data are listed in Table 4). After formulation of normal behavior model, it can be validated against real-time systems to identify the variations in streaming data. Such variations are termed as anomalies.

Anomaly Detection

The anomaly detection is the basic operation which identifies the similarities in the input data. It first establishes the normal behavior pattern and then a comparison will be made with observed behavior. If there any abnormal patterns found from normal behavior, an alert will be generated. It is a part of unsupervised learning.

Healthcare systems are real-time systems, it generates the data continuously and such data will be considered as a stream which is called as window. The window comprised of last few time slot data logs. The collected data logs are analyzed to build another model for predicting the abnormality in health. This model is applied to the streaming data (online) and abnormality patterns obtained upon the observed

Figure 13. Overview of Machine Learning

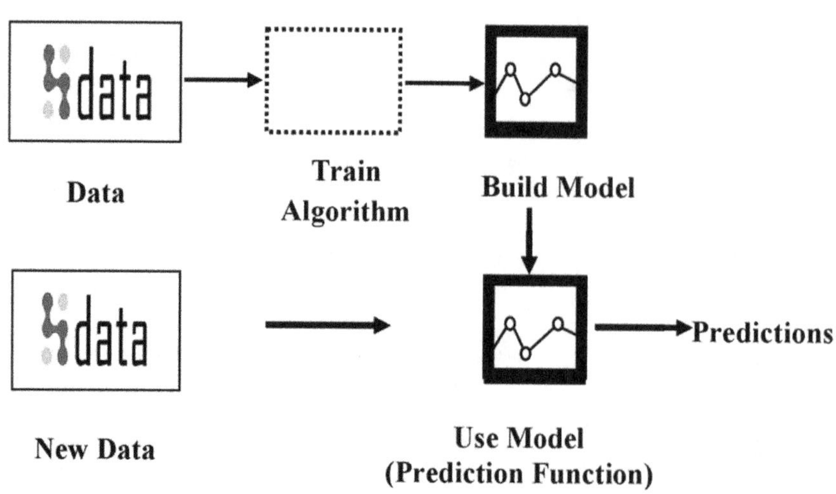

Figure 14. Application of Machine Learning Algorithm on Streaming Data

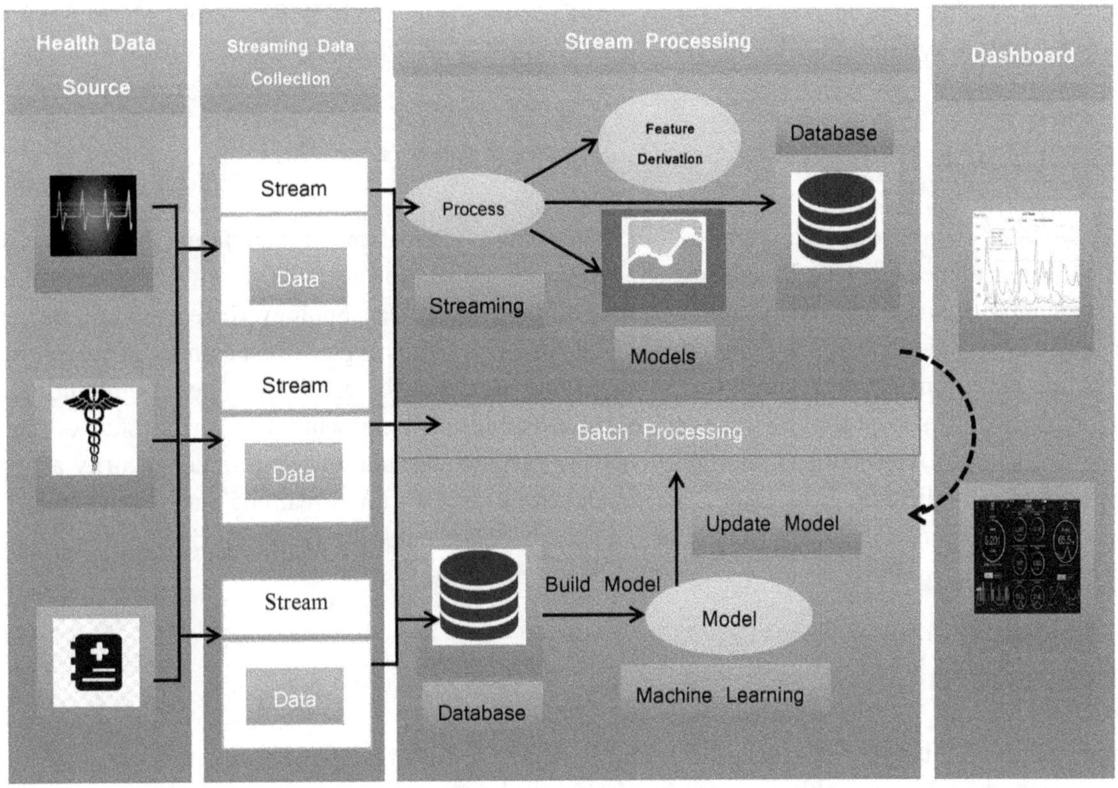

Table 4. Commonly used Machine Learning Algorithms on Streaming Data

Machine Learning Algorithm	Data Processing Tasks
K-Nearest Neighbors	Classification
Naive Bayes	Classification
Support Vector Machine	Classification
Linear Regression	Regression
Support Vector Regression	Regression
Classification and Regression Trees	Classification/Regression
Random Forests	Classification/Regression
Bagging	Classification/Regression
K-Means	Clustering
Canonical Correlation Analysis	Feature extraction
One-class Support Vector Machines	Anomaly detection

sequence. If there any abnormal patterns recognized, an alert notification is generated at dashboard region where caregivers can visualize their patient's status. Thus the machine learning algorithm made every healthcare system as intelligent system.

CONCLUSION

The HIoT design taxonomy is a primary element and acts as a backbone for facilitating the transmission and reception of medical data. The vision on wireless communication technology is available for building a healthcare system is expected to facilitate the selection of suitable technology. Recent advancements in sensing technologies and applications of IoT in healthcare systems expand the potential of IoT services for future developments. The perception on designing an effective healthcare system highlighting the major issues to be solved for providing consistent and quality in treatments. The current state of the art presented towards the security issues, discloses the various research problems under security aspects. Exploring the application of machine learning algorithm on real-time streaming data significantly improves the intelligence of healthcare systems. This chapter anticipated the major constituents of intelligent healthcare systems and promotes the universal deployment of IoT in healthcare.

REFERENCES

Amir, Rahmani, Gia, Negash, Anzanpour, Azimi, Jiang, & Liljeberg. (2018). Exploiting smart e-Health gateways at the edge of healthcare Internet-of-Things: A fog computing approach. *Future Generation Computer Systems*, *2*(78), 641–658.

Bakker, J., Pechenizkiy, M., & Sidorova, N. (2011). What's your current stress level? Detection of stress patterns from GSR sensor data. *IEEE 11th International Conference on Data Mining Workshops*, 573-580.

Bejarano, N. C., Ambrosini, E., Pedrocchi, A., Ferrigno, G., Monticone, M., & Ferrante, S. A. (2015). Novel Adaptive, Real-Time Algorithm to Detect Gait Events from Wearable Sensors. *IEEE Transactions on Neural Systems and Rehabilitation Engineering*, *23*(3), 413–422. doi:10.1109/TNSRE.2014.2337914 PMID:25069118

Bertolotti, G. M., Cristiani, A. M., Colagiorgio, P., Romano, F., Bassani, E., Caramia, N., & Ramat, S. A. (2016). Wearable and Modular Inertial Unit for Measuring Limb Movements and Balance Control Abilities. *IEEE Sensors Journal*, *16*(3), 790–797. doi:10.1109/JSEN.2015.2489381

Bonato, P. (2003). Wearable sensors/systems and their impact on biomedical engineering. *IEEE Engineering in Medicine and Biology Magazine*, *22*(3), 18–20. doi:10.1109/MEMB.2003.1213622 PMID:12845812

Bonnie, S., Basia, B., Kevin, C., Catherine, W., Jeff Coppersmith, J. H., & Rehabil Dev, J. (2013). *Bodies in motion: monitoring daily activity and exercise with motion sensors in people with chronic pulmonary diseases*. Academic Press. doi: .0045 doi:10.1682/JRRD.2003.10

Critchley, H. D. (2002). Book Review: Electro dermal Responses: What Happens in the Brain? *The Neuroscientist*, *8*(2), 132–142. doi:10.1177/107385840200800209 PMID:11954558

Fengou, Mantas, Lymberopoulos, Komnios, Fengos, Lazarou, & Nikolaos. (2012). A New Framework Architecture for Next Generation e-Health Services. *IEEE Transactions on Information Technology in Biomedicine*.

Guan, Z. J. (2013). *Internet-of-Things human body data blood pressure collecting and transmitting device*. Chinese Patent 202 821 362 U.

Guan, Z. J. (2013). *Somatic data blood glucose collection transmission device for Internet of Things*. Chinese Patent 202 838653 U.

Guangnan, Z., & Penghui, L. (2012). *IoT (Internet of Things) control system facing rehabilitation training of hemiplegic patients*. Chinese Patent 202 587045 U.

Ha. (2015). A wearable EEG-HEG-HRV multi model system with simultaneous monitoring of tES for mental health management. *IEEE Transactions on Biomedical Circuits and Systems*, *9*(6), 758–766. PMID:26742142

In, Z. L. (2014). *Patient body temperature monitoring system and device based on Internet of Things*. Chinese Patent 103 577688 A.

Internet of Things Protocols and Standards. (n.d.). Retrieved from https://www.cse.wustl.edu/~jain/cse570-15/ftp/iot_prot

Istepanian, R. S. H., Hu, S., Philip, N. Y., & Sungoor, A. (2011). The potential of Internet of m-health Things 'm-IoT' for non-invasive glucose level sensing. *Proc. IEEE Annu.*

Jara, A. J., Zamora-Izquierdo, M. A., & Skarmeta, A. F. (2013). Interconnection framework for m-Health and remote monitoring based on the Internet of Things. *IEEE Journal on Selected Areas in Communications*, *31*(9), 47–65. doi:10.1109/JSAC.2013.SUP.0513005

Jian, Z., Zhanli, W., & Zhuang, M. (2012). *Temperature measurement system and method based on home gateway*. Chinese Patent 102811 185A.

Klasnia, P., & Pratt, W. (2012). Healthcare in the pocket: Mapping the space of mobile-phone health interventions. *Journal of Biomedical Informatics*, *45*(1), 184–198. doi:10.1016/j.jbi.2011.08.017 PMID:21925288

Laranjo, Macedo, Santos, & Alexandre. (2012). Internet of Things for Medication Control: Service Implementation and Testing. *Elsevier Procedia Technology*, *5*, 777-786.

Larson, E. C., Goel, M., Boriello, G., Heltshe, S., Rosenfeld, M., & Patel, S. N. (2012). Spiro Smart: Using a microphone to measure lung function on a mobile phone. *Proc. ACM Int. Conf. Ubiquitous Comput.*, 280-289.

Larson, E. C., Lee, T., Liu, S., Rosenfeld, M., & Patel, S. N. (2011). Accurate and privacy preserving cough sensing using a low-cost microphone. *Proc. ACM Int. Conf. Ubiquitous Comput.*, 375-384.

Li, G., Lee, B. L., & Chung, W. Y. (2015). Smart watch-based wearable EEG system for driver drowsiness detection. *IEEE Sensors Journal*, *15*(12), 7169–7180. doi:10.1109/JSEN.2015.2473679

Liang, S., Zilong, Y., Hai, S., & Trinidad, M. (2011). *Childhood autism language training system and Internet-of-Things-based centralized training center.* Chinese Patent 102 184661 A.

Lin, D. Y. (2013). *Integrated Internet of Things application system for prison.* Chinese Patent 102 867236 A.

Liu, M. L., Tao, L., & Yan, Z. (2012). *Internet of Things-based electro cardio-gram monitoring system.* Chinese Patent 102 764118 A.

Milici, S., Lorenzo, J., Lazaro, A., Villarino, R., & Jirbau, D. (2017). Wireless breathing sensor based on wearable modulated frequency selective surface. *IEEE Sensors Journal, 17*(5), 1285–1292. doi:10.1109/JSEN.2016.2645766

Mulro, S., Gronley, J., & Weiss, W. (2003). Use of cluster analysis for gait pattern classification of patients in the early and late recovery phases following stroke. *Gait & Posture, 18*(1), 114–125. doi:10.1016/S0966-6362(02)00165-0 PMID:12855307

Pang, Z., Tian, J., & Chen, Q. (2014). Intelligent packaging and intelligent medicine box for medication management towards the Internet-of-Things. *16th International Conference on Advanced Communication Technology*, 352-360. 10.1109/ICACT.2014.6779193

Patel, S., Park, H., Bonato, P., Chan, L., & Rodgers, M. (2012). A Review of Wearable Sensors and Systems with Applications in Rehabilitation. *Journal of Neuro Engineering and Rehabilitation, 20*(9).

Puustjarvi, J., & Puustjarvi, L. (2011). Automating remote monitoring and information therapy: An opportunity to practice telemedicine in developing countries. *Proc. IST-Africa Conf.*, 1-9.

Rand, D., Eng, J. J., Tang, P. F., Jeng, J. S., & Hung, C. (2009). How active are people with stroke? use of accelerometers to assess physical activity. *Stroke, 40*, 163–168. doi:10.1161/STROKEAHA.108.523621

Rose, K., Eldridge, S., & Chapin, L. (2015). *The Internet of Things (IoT): An Overview –Understanding the Issues and Challenges of a More Connected World.* Internet Society.

Sano, A., Picard, & R. W. (2013). Stress Recognition Using Wearable Sensors and Mobile Phones. *Proceedings of the 2013 Humaine Association Conference on Affective Computing and Intelligent Interaction,* 671-676. 10.1109/ACII.2013.117

Varon, C., Caicedo, A., Testelmans, D., Buyse, B., & Van Huffel, S. (2015). A novel algorithm for the automatic detection of sleep apnea from single-lead ECG. *IEEE Transactions on Biomedical Engineering, 62*(9), 2269–2278. doi:10.1109/TBME.2015.2422378 PMID:25879836

Xin, T. J., Min, B., & Jie, J. (2013). *Carry-on blood pressure/pulse rate/blood oxygen monitoring location intelligent terminal based on Internet of Things.* Chinese Patent 202 875315 U.

Yue-Hong, Y., Wu, F., Jie, F. Y., Jian, L., Chao, X., & Yi, Z. (2014). *Remote medical rehabilitation system in smart city.* Chinese Patent 103488 880 A.

Zenko, J., Kos, M., & Kramberger, I. (2016). Pulse rate variability and blood oxidation content identification using miniature wearable wrist device. *Proc. Int. Conf. Syst. Signals Image Process (IWSSIP)*, 1-4.

ADDITIONAL READING

Ahmed, M. U., Begum, S., & Raad, W. (Eds.). (2017). *Internet of Things Technologies for HealthCare*. Västerås, Sweden: Springer Publisher.

Bouchard, B. (Ed.). (2017). *Smart Technologies in Healthcare*. CRC Press Publisher. doi:10.1201/9781315145686

Fengou, A., Mantas, G., Lymberopoulos, D., Komninos, N., Fengos, S., & Lazarou, N. (2013). A New Framework Architecture for Next Generation e-Health Services. *IEEE Journal of Biomedical and Health Informatics*, *1*(17), 9–18. doi:10.1109/TITB.2012.2224876 PMID:23086531

Guarda, T., Augusto, M. F., Barrionuevo, O., & Pinto, F. M. (2017). Internet of Things in Pervasive Healthcare Systems. In J. M. Machado, A. Abelha, M. F. Santos, & F. Portela (Eds.), *Next Generation Mobile and Pervasive Healthcare Solutions* (pp. 21–31). IGI Publishers.

Krohn, R., Metcalf, D., & Salber, P. (Eds.). (2017). *Connected Health: Improving Care, Safety, and Efficiency with Wearables and IoT Solution*. CRC Press Publisher.

Kvedar, J. C. (Ed.). (2015). *The Internet of Healthy Things*. Internet of Healthy Things Publisher.

Chapter 12
A Forecasting Model for Patient Arrivals of an Emergency Department in Healthcare Management Systems

Melih Yucesan
Munzur University, Turkey

Muhammet Gul
Munzur University, Turkey

Suleyman Mete
Munzur University, Turkey

Erkan Celik
Munzur University, Turkey

ABSTRACT

Emergency departments (EDs) are one of the most valuable departments of healthcare management systems. Patient arrivals at the EDs are crucial for planning of the future. Accurate forecasting of patient arrivals contributes to better organized human resources and medical devices in the EDs. Therefore, in this chapter, the authors aim to develop a hybrid model including the methods of autoregressive integrated moving average with external variables (ARIMAX) and artificial neural network (ANN) in a hospital ED. The arrival data was collected from the hospital information system of a public hospital in eastern Turkey. The model incorporates factors related to ED arrivals such as climatic and calendar variables. By the aid of the proposed model, an insight to arrangement and planning of ED resources can be provided in a better way.

DOI: 10.4018/978-1-5225-7071-4.ch012

INTRODUCTION

Forecasting can be expressed as making predictions at times when the results are not observable in the present situation. Forecasting play an important role in making short and long-term decisions (Armstrong, 2001; Qin and Shi, 2006). In all societies, the level of population access of health resources is directly related to the well-being of the community. One of the most important part of the National Health System is hospitals which has special technologies, advanced equipment and also healthcare personnel (Carvalho-Silva et al. 2017). Emergency departments (EDs) are one of the most valued parts of the healthcare management systems. It has to provide adequate, immediate and accurate healthcare management (Hoot et al. 2007). Performance determiners for service quality through EDs are related with length of stay (LOS) and waiting times, which are affected by high levels of ED arrivals (Xu et al. 2013). The number of patients who will come to the EDs and the waiting times will be one of the most important input parameters in the planning of the investments and arrangements to be made in the ED in the future (Pianykh and Rosenthal, 2015). Compared with other departments of the hospitals, the ED is clearly the more crowded than other departments (Gul et al. 2017). One of the most important factors that cannot predicted in emergency services is the time of arrival of the patients. The number of future patients which need to health care to the ED service is directly related to the various independent variables and the number of patients coming in per day in the past period (Xu et. al. 2016; Hertzum, 2017). Accurate forecasts of patient arrivals which need immediate health care contribute to better organized human resources and medical devices in EDs (Aladeemy et al. 2016).

On the other hand, time has important effects on the performance of EDs. It is measured and analyzed for suitable evaluation of ED performances. Patient arrivals are one of the important process of EDs in healthcare management systems (Gul and Guneri, 2015a). Long wait and overcrowding in ED processes is increased in recent years which directly affect the quality of ED performances. These processes have the potential to improve ED throughput and patient pleasure if these are efficiently fulfilment. Because of delay within time related processes have potential to effect overcrowding in the EDs, it gets significant must to be forecasted and known time by means of prevent from the delays. Statistical forecasting considered as an operation research technique that uses time series data and a kind of statistical formulae and data mining approaches to forecast different types of ED processes. The more researches are needed for more exact planning due to improvement of forecasting models. It helps to decrease of overcrowding linked to other hospital units and external world (Wargon et al. 2009).

In this chapter, we aim to develop a hybrid model including the methods ARIMAX and ANN for patient arrivals of a hospital ED. By the aid of the proposed model, an insight to the doctors and administrator staff for planning of ED resources will be provided in a better way. Our ultimate goal is to provide ED stakeholders with a background on the ED as healthcare management systems and a hybrid statistical forecasting method that can be practically applied to various ED processes. This chapter will contribute to the literature by the following aspects: *(i)* To the best of our knowledge, there is no studies that have used the ARIMAX-ANN hybrid model to forecast ED arrivals in Turkey, *(ii)* The model includes not only calendar factors but also climate factors and some special factors (weekend and public holidays) in forecasting ED arrivals, *(iii)* By the proposed model, it will be proved that using the ARIMAX-ANN hybridization is applicable for forecasting of ED patient arrival forecasting and helping in arrangement and planning of ED resources.

The study is structured as follows: Section 2 details related literature and background for forecasting of patient arrivals. Section 3 analyzed data source and provides detail of ARIMAX and ANN methods. In section 4, application of the hybrid approach is investigated for the case of public hospital ED arrivals in Turkey. Finally, Section 5 presents conclusion, limitations, and future remarks.

BACKGROUND

The quality of the service thanks to the EDs which is stated by waiting time and LOS, is important interest to the patient demand (Au-Yeung et al. 2009; Xu et al. 2013). When patient arrivals increase, they may lead to prolonged waits and overcrowding. A better balance among demand (patient arrivals) and ED resources (doctors, nurses, medical equipment, beds etc.) is needed to develop ED processes. If ED patient demand is accurately forecasting, it can provide managerial implication for short term and long term in order to EDs can better prepared for the coming demand variations (Xu et al. 2013). A detailed summary of papers regarding literature of ED forecasting according to data type and solution method are listed in Table1 and Table 2 respectively.

According to Table 1, five data type which are hourly, daily, weekly, monthly and yearly, were used to forecast ED patient demand in the literature. Daily data type is mostly used in the ED forecasting literature which can make more precisely forecasting.

On the other hand, literature of ED forecasting is divided according to solution method which is given in Table 2. ARIMA and SARIMA solution methods are used intensively in the literature. Details of the all papers related ED forecasting are given chronologically descending.

Rosychuk et al. (2016) forecasted monthly rates of ED presentations with chronic obstructive pulmonary disease. Xu et al. (2016) improved a hybrid ARIMA–LR approach. Butler et al. (2016) used a time-series approach to assess whether current day and previous day is correlated. Afilal et al. (2016a) estimated daily attendance at an ED using time series-based approach. Calegari et al. (2016) analyzed the performance of forecasting models in predicting the demand for medical care. Afilal et al. (2016b) studied the daily arrivals at an ED in France. Gul and Guneri (2016b) forecasted ED arrivals for short, medium

Table 1. Literature of ED patient arrival forecasting according to data type

Data Type	Studies
Daily	Xu et al. (2016); Afilal et al. (2016a); Calegari et al. (2016); Afilal et al. (2016b); Harrou et al. (2015); Zlotnik et al. (2015); Kang and Park (2015); Kadri et al. (2014); Menke et al. (2014); Xu et al. (2013); Marcilio et al. (2013); Boyle et al. (2011); Kam et al. (2010); Wargon et al. (2010); Au-Yeung et al. (2009); Sun et al. (2009); Jones et al. (2008); Jones and Joy (2002); Batal et al. (2001)
Daily, Hourly	Kim et al. (2014)
Daily, Monthly, Yearly	Gul and Guneri (2016b); Côté et al. (2013)
Hourly	Ekström et al. (2015); Chase et al. (2012); Jones et al. (2009); McCarthy et al. (2008); Morzuch and Allen (2006)
Monthly	Rosychuk et al. (2016); Rosychuk et al. (2015); Mai et al. (2015); Aboagye-Sarfo et al. (2015); Petrou (2015); Bergs et al. (2014); Rosychuk et al. (2011); Park et al. (2008); Champion et al. (2007)
Weekly	Butler et al. (2016); Aroua and Abdul-Nour (2015); Araz et al. (2014)

Table 2. Literature of ED patient arrival forecasting according to methods used

Solution Method	Studies
ANN	Gul and Guneri (2016b); Menke et al. (2014); Xu et al. (2013); Jones et al. (2008)
ARIMA	Xu et al. (2016); Afilal et al. (2016a); Mai et al. (2015); Petrou (2015); Kadri et al. (2014); Kim et al. (2014); Jones et al. (2009); Sun et al. (2009); Zibners et al. (2006); Morzuch and Allen (2006); Jones and Joy (2002)
SARIMA	Rosychuk et al. (2016); Butler et al. (2016); Calegari et al. (2016); Rosychuk et al. (2015); Aroua and Abdul-Nour (2015); Araz et al. (2014); Kim et al. (2014); Marcilio et al. (2013); Rosychuk et al. (2011); Kam et al. (2010)
Regression analysis	Gul and Guneri (2016b); Zlotnik et al. (2015); Aroua and Abdul-Nour (2015); Ekström et al. (2015); Xu et al. (2013); Côté et al. (2013); McCarthy et al. (2008); Schonwetter et al. (2008); Jones et al. (2008); Park et al. (2008); Morzuch and Allen (2006); Batal et al. (2001)
ARMA	Afilal et al. (2016b); Aboagye-Sarfo et al. (2015); Harrou et al. (2015)
Box–Jenkins	Champion et al. (2007); Zibners et al. (2006)
Exponential Smoothing	Calegari et al. (2016); Bergs et al. (2014); Jones et al. (2009); Champion et al. (2007); Morzuch and Allen (2006)

and long term considering calendar and ED specific variables. Rosychuk et al. (2015) estimated monthly patterns of asthma presentations to EDs in Alberta, Canada. Mai et al. (2015) predicted the number of ED presentations in Western Australia in the next 5 years, stratified by place of treatment, age, triage and disposition. Aboagye-Sarfo et al. (2015) developed multivariate vector-ARMA models for predicting ED demand in Western Australia (WA) and compare them to ARMA and Winters' models. Petrou (2015) proposed an ARIMA model to analyses official data from Cyprus' largest emergency room facility for three years. Harrou et al. (2015) reported the development of statistical method for enhancing detection of abnormal daily patient arrivals at the ED. Zlotnik et al. (2015) applied SVM to forecast patient visit and allocate dynamic nursing staff. Kang and Park (2015) evaluated ED patient visit variability in order to determine if the average can be used to operate EDs. Aroua and Abdul-Nour (2015) explored the capability of forecasting techniques to predict ED visits based on Major Diagnostic Categories. Ekström et al. (2015) investigated whether web site visits could be used to predict the ED attendance for the coming day. Araz et al. (2014) forecasted influenza-like–illness (ILI)-related ED visits. Kadri et al. (2014) developed models for forecasting daily attendances at a pediatrics ED. Kim et al. (2014) evaluated the predictability of patient volume in hospital medicine using a variety of known forecasting techniques. Bergs et al. (2014) evaluated an automatic forecasting algorithm to predict the number of monthly ED visits. Menke et al. (2014) designed an ANN and to test it retrospectively to determine if it may be used to predict ED volume. Xu et al. (2013) modelled ED daily patient arrivals and to quantify the relative importance of contributing variables. Marcilio et al. (2013) developed different models to forecast the daily number of ED patients according to calendar variables and ambient temperature readings. Côté et al. (2013) applied regression-based forecasting models based on data obtained from a large teaching hospital's ED. Chase et al. (2012) investigated whether ED variables could be used in mathematical models to predict a future surge in ED volume based on recent levels of use of physician capacity. Rosychuk et al. (2011) examined the monthly patterns of young children who made croup-related visits to EDs in Canada. Boyle et al. (2011) predicted and track epidemics (and, potentially, pandemics) of influenza. Kam et al. (2010) developed and evaluate time series models to predict the daily number of patients visiting the ED of a Korean hospital. Wargon et al. (2010) investigated whether mathematical models using calendar variables could identify the determinants of ED census over time in geographically close EDs. Au-Yeung et al. (2009) forecasted daily patient arrivals into an ED based on previous arrivals data. Jones et al. (2009) studied the temporal relationships between the demands for key resources in the ED and the inpatient hospital and to develop multivariate forecasting models. Sun et al. (2009) forecasted ED attendances for micro and macro level planning. McCarthy et al. (2008) developed methodology for predicting demand for ED services by characterizing ED arrivals. Schonwetter et al. (2008) devised a model to predict the probability of hospice cardiac disease patients having ED visits and/or hospitalizations after hospice admission. Jones et al. (2008) explored and evaluated the use of several statistical forecasting methods to predict daily ED patient volumes at three diverse hospital EDs. Park et al. (2008) predicted the number of patients arriving at ED and establish a forecasting model of number of ED patient arrivals Champion et al. (2007) proposed ES and Box–Jenkins methods for forecasting of ED crowding. Zibners et al. (2006) predicted the volume of patient visits to an academic pediatric ED based on short interval local weather patterns. Morzuch and Allen (2006) forecasted hourly arrivals for each day using standard Holt-Winters ES methods. Jones and Joy (2002) developed a methodology for forecasting the number of beds occupied due to emergency admissions and the number of emergency admissions. Batal et al. (2001) developed a prediction equation for the number of patients seeking urgent care.

In this chapter, we collected ED arrival data from the hospital information system of a public hospital in eastern Turkey (Trabzon province which is located in eastern black sea region). We gathered daily ED arrival data for the period of January 2015 through December 2016 (731 days) to carry out the ARIMAX-ANN hybrid model analysis. The model incorporates influencing factors related to ED arrivals, such as climate variables (e.g. maximum and minimum temperature, maximum wind speed) and calendar variables including month of the year, day of the week, public holiday and weekend.

MATERIAL AND METHODS

Data Source and Analysis

The dependent variable in this study is daily ED patient arrivals. The data between 1st January 2015 and 31th December 2016, 731 days records, was obtained from the observed ED. Patients' arrival to the ED was analyzed in terms of the month of the year, the day of the week, maximum wind speed, maximum temperature, minimum temperature, weekend and public holiday variables. The data for climatic variables is obtained from http://www.infoclimat.fr. To identify content of the data, Figure 1 shows average ED daily arrivals distribution per month (a) and per week day (b).

This figure shows that the greatest demand is in September and August (732 and 715 arrivals per day, respectively) and on Saturday and Sunday (660 and 653 arrivals per day, respectively). However, the data reflects two different years variation, we used data of the two years period. On average, there are about 604 daily arrivals to the observed hospital ED during this time period. The plot of daily arrivals (Figure 2) shows the annual seasonal fluctuations in the ED: there were more patients in January and September; there were slightly less patients in July.

Figure 1. Average number of ED arrivals per week day and per month (January 2015-December 2016)

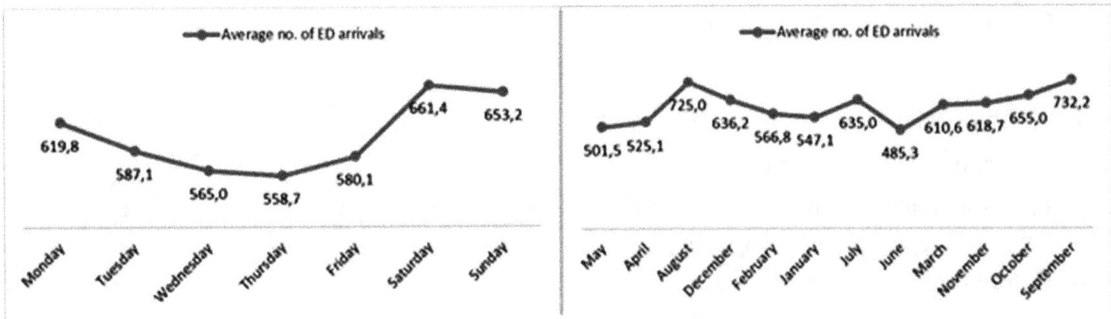

Figure 2. Daily arrivals at the observed ED through the time period

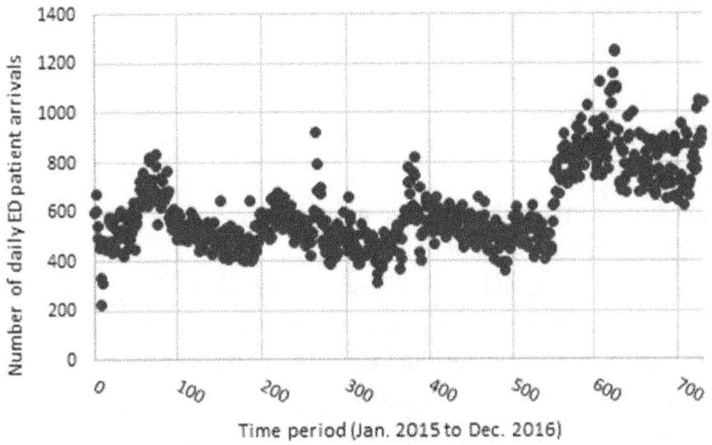

Autoregressive Integrated Moving Average With External Variables (ARIMAX)

The Box-Jenkins method is extensively used in the literature because it is simple and gives respectable results. Often this method is referred to as ARIMA method. The ARIMA method is quite diverse from the other methods because it does not enclose explanatory variables that show the tendency of the prediction series (Gahirwal, 2013). In this method, the future values of the independent variables assume that the argument will be expressed in terms of past values (Kongcharoen and Kruangpradit, 2013; Zhang, 2003).

Although ARIMA method is straightforward, it is used often because it gives respectable results. However, the ARIMA method has some drawbacks. One of them is insufficient to explain the real problems. Because only one variable is used in this method. It is possible to use explanatory variables in the ARIMAX method (Jalalkamali et al., 2015). In the ARIMAX method, instead of estimating the dependent variable Y_t with only the previous data, it is planned to estimate Y_t with both the past values and the explanatory variables X_t, thus, more accurate results are obtained compared to the ARIMA method (Cool et al., 2009; Neter et al., 1996).

Bierens (1987) has been generalized the ARIMAX method. This method was derived from the ARIMA method. ARIMAX model can be expressed as Eq 1. (Arya et al. 2015).

$$\left(1-\sum_{s}^{p}\alpha_s L_s\right)\Delta y_t = \mu + \sum_{s=1}^{q}\beta_s L^s x_t + \left(1+\sum_{s=1}^{r}\gamma_s L^s\right)e^t \tag{1}$$

where, L is the usual lag operator $\gamma_s L^s = y_{t-s}$, $\Delta y_t = y_t - y_{t-1}, \mu \in, \alpha_s \in R, \beta_s \in R^k$ and $\gamma_s \in R$ are the unknown parameters and e_t are the errors.

Lag operator creates a transformed series that consists of the differences between lagged observations in the original time series. The single lag difference operator is often denoted by the symbol first and second difference of *y* can be defined as:

$$\Delta y_t = y_t - y_{t-1}$$

$$\Delta^2 y_t = y_t - y_{t-1} - \left(y_{t-1} - y_{t-2}\right)$$

Artificial Neural Network

ANNs are algorithms which aim to solve computational processes in specific areas by using many interconnected processing elements (Gul and Guneri, 2015, 2016a, 2016b). They are mainly applied for prediction, clustering, classification, and detection of abnormal patterns (Yucesan et al. 2017; 2018). An ANN model comprises layers, presents a different number of computational elements. These computational elements are called neurons (Guneri and Gumus, 2008, 2009). Efendigil et al. (2009) depicted the model flow of an artificial neuron as consisting of input signals, weights of neurons, the linear combiner output and the threshold. Also, an activation function and an output of the neuron must be also taken into consideration. The first layer, named as ''input'' layer, is used to obtain information inside the network. The last layer, named as "output" layer, is similarly used to obtain information outside the network. The middle layers, named as "hidden" layers, are crucial for the network for conversion of certain input patterns into appropriate output patterns (Yucesan et al. 2017; 2018). Information flows through the network by linear connections and linear or nonlinear transformations. The ANN's learning can be under two different types: (1) supervised learning, (2) unsupervised learning. The error between the actual value and the predicted value is computed. A minimization procedure is then used to adjust the weights between two connection layers. There are many minimization procedures based on different algorithms, such as Quasi-Newton, Levenberg–Marquardt, gradient descent, and conjugate gradient methods. In ANN models, there is a practical problematic regarding the network architecture (the number of hidden layers and units in each layer) and network properties (the error and activation functions). The design of the hidden layer is dependent on the selected learning algorithm (Kröse et al., 1993). One of the other important aspects of an ANN model is the activation function for the hidden layer. An ANN model can include the following functions (Yucesan et al. 2017; 2018): (1) Linear function produces its input as its output; in other words, it just passes the activation level directly as the output. Its output range is [-∞,∞]. (2) Logistic function has a sigmoid curve and is calculated as follows: $F(x) = 1/(1+e^{-x})$. Its output range is [0,1]. (3) Hyperbolic tangent function also has a sigmoid curve and is calculated as follows: $F(x) = (e^x - e^{-x})/(e^x + e^{-x})$. Its output range is [-1,1].

In ANNs, two factors of learning rate and momentum are used to aid the learning of selected algorithms. They are control parameters used by several learning algorithms, which affect the weight changes. The higher learning rates cause higher weight changes during each iteration. The greater the momentum, the more the current weight change is affected by the weight change that took place during the previous iteration. To measure the performance of ANN models, network error (average train error and average test error), absolute relative error (ARE), mean square error (MSE) and mean absolute percentage error (MAPE) can be used.

The Proposed Hybrid Approach

The ARIMAX model is quite effective in clarification linear relationships. On the other hand, the ANN method gives us very acceptable results on nonlinear problems. But none of them presents good results in all cases. The number of patients coming to the ED related on many parameters. It is not possible to define precisely how these parameters affect the incoming ED. The data contains linear and non-linear parts. Therefore, hybridization of the ARIMAX and ANN methods is expected to increase the accuracy of forecasted model.

Proposed hybrid method consists of two stages. The ARIMAX model is compose in the first stage. In the second stage in addition to the explanatory variables used in the ARIMAX model and the error values obtained in the ARIMAX model are used as input variables. Necessary procedures performed in the stages are summarized below.

Step 1: The logarithm of the dependent variable or difference of dependent variable is used to decide which one should be used. First, equality (2-3) is estimated.

$$D\left(y_t^2\right) = \alpha_1 + \beta_1 y_t \tag{2}$$

$$D\log\left(y_t^2\right) = \alpha_2 + \beta_2 \log y_t \tag{3}$$

The t statistic values of β_1 and β_2 coefficients are calculated. The model with smaller t coefficient is selected. The appropriate level of difference of dependent variable is determined by the Augmented Dickey Fuller test. EViews uses model selection to determine the appropriate ARMA order. Model selection is a way of determining which type of model best fits a set of data and is often used to choose the best model from which to forecast that data. The AIC value is used for the appropriate ARMA order selection. All options are then evaluated and the model with the minimum AIC value is determined (Eviews User manual, 2017; Areekul et al. 2010).

Step 2: The factors that affect ED arrivals such as climate variables (e.g. maximum and minimum temperature, maximum wind speed) and calendar variables including month of the year, day of the week, public holiday and weekend are used as explanatory variables. In addition to these variables residuals obtained by using the ARIMAX method are also used as input variable. Mean absolute percentage error (MAPE) is used to measure the accuracy of this method. MAPE is defined as in Eq. (4)

$$MAPE = \frac{100}{n}\sum_{i=1}^{n}\left|\frac{y_i - f_i}{y_i}\right| \tag{4}$$

where f_i is as vector of n forecasting, and y_i represent of actual values.

APPLICATION OF THE APPROACH: THE CASE OF A PUBLIC HOSPITAL ED ARRIVALS

In this chapter, we develop a hybrid model to forecast daily ED patient arrivals of a public hospital ED located in Black Sea region of Turkey. In the first stage of the application of the proposed approach, an ARIMAX model is developed. We collected the daily arrival data detailed above. It includes 731 data points for the output variable corresponding to two-year data. For all of the ARIMAX modelling processes, EViews 10.0 was utilized. Specifying the ARIMAX model used for forecasting was split into three steps:

1. Transformations of the dependent variables were made, and the level of differencing was selected. Transformations of daily ED arrivals were made by differencing. The transformation of the ED arrivals was arranged based on both logarithmic and differencing manner.
2. The external independent variables such as climatic and calendar variables (as mentioned in previous sub-sections) were determined.
3. The order of the ARMA terms were selected. EViews uses model selection to determine the appropriate ARMA order. We limited the orders of AR and MA to four. Model selection is a way of determining which type of model best fits a set of data and is often used to choose the best model from which to forecast that data (EViews 10 tutorial, 2017). Akaike Information Criterion (AIC) is followed in this study. As an example, the best ARMA terms for ED patient arrivals was determined according to the AIC criteria. The results are given in Figure 3. The best ARMA term for this case is obtained as (3,4).

$$\begin{aligned}\Delta\left(ED\right) = \beta + \sum_{j=1}^{12} c_j M_{j,t} + \sum_{i=1}^{7} d_i D_{j,t} + dH_t + eT_t + fK_t + gW_t \\ + \rho_1\vartheta_{t-1} + \rho_2\vartheta_{t-2} + \rho_3\vartheta_{t-3} + \theta_1\epsilon_{t-1} + \theta_2\epsilon_{t-2} + \theta_3\epsilon_{t-3} + \theta_4\epsilon_{t-4}\end{aligned} \tag{5}$$

where ED refers to forecasted ED patient arrivals, $M_{j,t}$ month of the year, $D_{j,t}$ day of the week, H_t public holiday, T_t maximum temperature, K_t minimum temperature, and W_t maximum wind speed of the day. The remaining are the model parameters for the autoregressive and moving average terms, AR and MA variables, respectively.

Figure 3. AIC values of ARMA terms proposed for daily ED arrivals

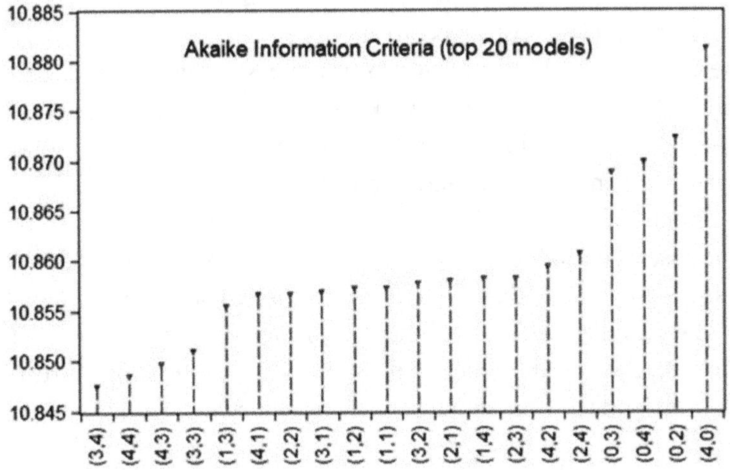

The ARIMAX-ANN hybrid model integrated the ARIMAX model with the neural network model and tested with the raw data. We built the hybrid ARIMAX-ANN model with the following input layers: (1) the dependent variables used in ARIMAX modelling, (2) the residuals of the ARIMAX model. This process is followed by data partition and normalization by [0-1] and [-1,1] normalization methods. A training and testing model based on ANN are then employed after determining the design architecture and network properties. A tangent sigmoid (tansig) transfer function and linear (purelin) transfer function are applied in hidden and output layer, respectively. Three layers which include input, hidden and output layers are constituted. The network structure for hybrid ARIMAX-ANN based daily ED patient arrival forecasting model is presented in Figure 4. While "25" in input layer represents number of inputs, "5" in hidden layer shows number of neurons with best accuracy value. "1" in output layer shows number of outputs. The accurateness of the model is directly related to the number of neurons in hidden layer. The performance indicators of R^2 and MSE are used to evaluate accurateness of the method. Finally, the best network is applied which reflects the variability better.

MATLAB is used throughout the case study. The proposed model was run under different number of hidden layer neurons. The numbers of hidden neurons are varied from 1 to 30 for evaluating the performance of the model with different neuron numbers. The performance results of the 30 experiments with different number of neurons are presented in Table 3. After the data entry to the software, it randomly selects 70:15:15 ratios for training, validation and testing. We run experiments with Bayesian

Figure 4. Network structure for the hybrid forecasting model

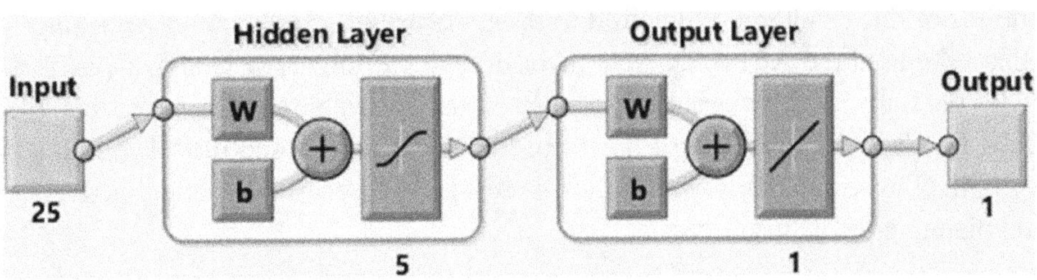

rules training. The best network and their performance measure are indicated in bold in Table 3. While R^2 value is obtained as nearly 0.87 and 0.80 for training and testing, the MSE is obtained as 0.00556295 and 0.00102972 for training and testing, respectively.

The validation performance and regression plot of the best network are presented in Figure 5. The validation performance plot demonstrates that MSE becomes minimum at epoch 138 and no significant over fitting occurs where the best validation performance has obtained. The regression plot shows network output and targets for training, testing and all are almost close because coefficient of determination is almost equal to 1 (Figure 6).

Figure 7 shows the observed and forecasted values of daily ED visits for the ARIMAX and ARIMAX-ANN hybrid models. The plots show that the lines representing each of actual and forecasted values by the hybrid model follow a similar pattern, and there is an overlapping of values in the curves compared to ARIMAX model. Also, the hybrid model could successfully forecast most turning points in patient volume. The times at which upward and downward changes in actual values were in agreement with the pattern in forecasted values.

The MAPE value of the hybrid model is calculated as 10.67% that means a reasonable result is obtained (Çelik et al., 2016). It may be noted that the MAPE of 10.67% for daily arrivals in the observed hospital ED is within the range (4.2-14.4%) reported by Wargon et al. (2009) in a review of models for forecasting the number of daily ED visits.

CONCLUSION AND FUTURE REMARKS

In this chapter, we develop a hybrid model including the methods ARIMAX and ANN for patient arrivals of a hospital ED. The model is used to forecast daily ED patient arrivals of a public hospital located in Black Sea region of Turkey. On conclusion of this model, ARIMAX-ANN hybrid model provides better results than single ARIMAX method. The MAPE value of the hybrid model is computed as 10.67% which stands in an acceptable position compared to other works in the literature.

Forecasting ED patient arrivals is important to plan the near future of hospitals. Monitoring and evaluating the ED patient arrivals enable ED stakeholders (executive, medical staff, patients etc.) to foresee future and discover the optimum method to eliminate congestion. Moreover, an accurate to recasting procedure on ED visits enables ED managers to help in rostering and planning of ED resources for a short-term period. We select the ARIMAX-ANN hybrid model suitable for the observed hospital since this method gives us effective solutions. In the proposed hybrid model, the error terms calculated with ARIMAX model and other exogenous variables create the dataset. Bayesian learning procedure was carried out in this model, and this situation boosted the learning capacity of the neural network. So, hybrid model showed a good performance in forecasting. This hybrid framework can be adapted to any other hospital ED or other departments of hospitals such as intensive care units, laboratories, outpatient clinics.

Contributions of this chapter are threefold to the literature of ED demand forecasting: (1) There is no studies that have used the ARIMAX-ANN hybrid model to forecast ED arrivals in Turkey. (2) The model includes not only calendar variables but also climatic variables and some special factors (weekend and public holidays) in forecasting ED arrivals. (3) By the proposed model, it is stated that using the ARIMAX-ANN hybridization gives applicable results to forecast ED patient arrivals and helps in rostering and planning of ED resources.

Table 3. Experiments with different number of neurons

Number of Neurons	R^2		MSE	
	Training	Testing	Training	Testing
1	0.77314	0.69676	0.00955071	0.0125557
2	0.82712	0.79466	0.00758577	0.00865238
3	0.85546	0.83533	0.00653274	0.00671282
4	0.86606	0.78672	0.00618875	0.00765746
5	**0.87208**	**0.80071**	**0.00556295**	**0.00102972**
6	0.88705	0.76757	0.00501338	0.0087996
7	0.88632	0.81431	0.00502019	0.00925002
8	0.89886	0.79342	0.0045944	0.00924863
9	0.897326	0.79125	0.00460329	0.009799994
10	0.893423	0.712149	0.00492409	0.0102792
11	0.922408	0.67288	0.00366017	0.0151907
12	0.900183	0.850982	0.00451768	0.00687299
13	0.90883	0.671497	0.00433556	0.0123047
14	0.9267901	0.627981	0.00345611	0.0159712
15	0.92159	0.627548	0.00379316	0.0148088
16	0.896273	0.792327	0.00456784	0.0140211
17	0.90257	0.90076	0.00454046	0.0123962
18	0.891392	0.744531	0.00488247	0.016547
19	0.909425	0.738509	0.00418853	0.01997
20	0.933014	0.743065	0.00308667	0.017824
21	0.915648	0.755418	0.00382864	0.0127582
22	0.898143	0.735878	0.00460142	0.019104
23	0.90717	0.741042	0.0039899	0.0150282
24	0.930847	0.71683	0.00331012	0.0134212
25	0.90514	0.664343	0.00454603	0.0105347
26	0.913575	0.7470408	0.00409671	0.00921583
27	0.91061	0.767671	0.00376246	0.0102962
28	0.89822	0.785526	0.0044415	0.0116294
29	0.9064	0.60848	0.00444791	0.016209
30	0.916263	0.706712	0.00397973	0.015644

Figure 5. The validation performance

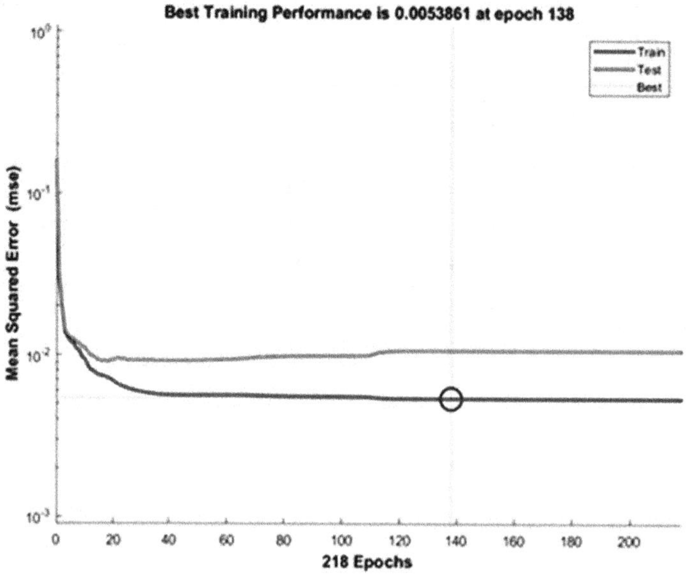

Figure 6. Regression analysis

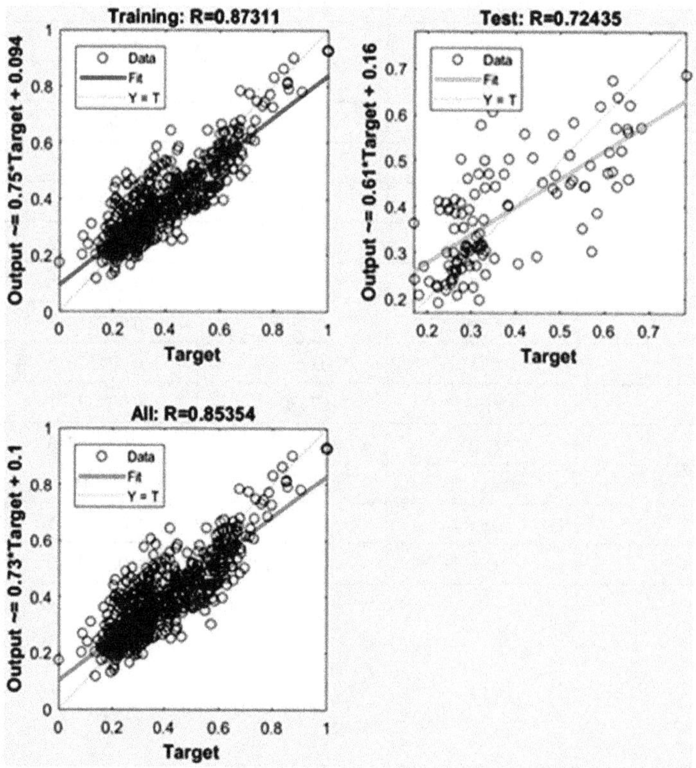

Figure 7. Actual and forecasted ED daily arrivals by ARIMAX and ARIMAX-ANN hybrid model

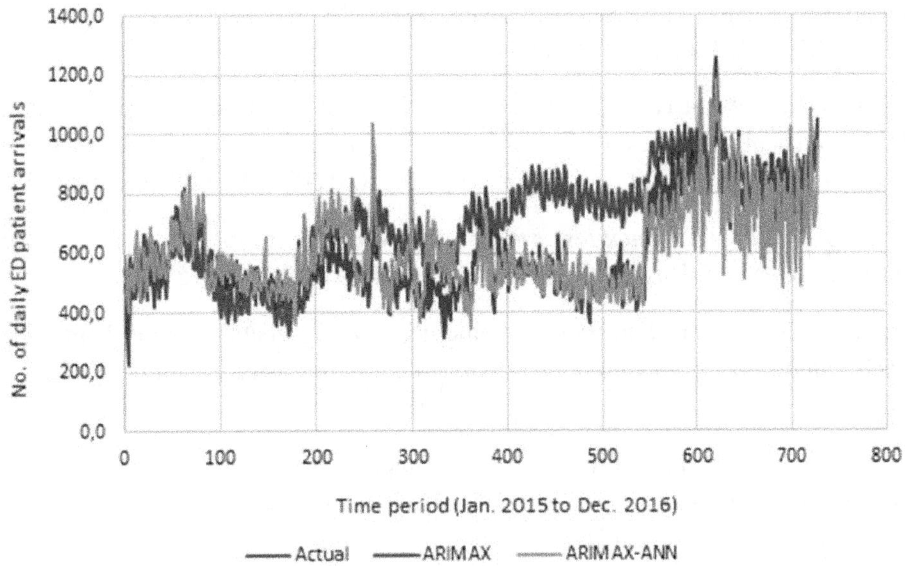

The current study has some limitations. Firstly, the application case study was implemented only for one specific ED but it can be applied to other public and private hospital EDs. Secondly, the knowledge of selecting input variables in Turkey is limited, and there are probably other important predictors we have not taken into consideration such as climatic (precip and maximum snow) and ED-specific (severity of patients) variables. In particular, other ED healthcare management and delivery processes such as patient total LOS, waiting times, boarding processes, discharge processes can be analyzed with developed hybrid model.

REFERENCES

Aboagye-Sarfo, P., Mai, Q., Sanfilippo, F. M., Preen, D. B., Stewart, L. M., & Fatovich, D. M. (2015). A comparison of multivariate and univariate time series approaches to modelling and forecasting emergency department demand in Western Australia. *Journal of Biomedical Informatics*, *57*, 62–73. doi:10.1016/j.jbi.2015.06.022 PMID:26151668

Afilal, M., Yalaoui, F., Dugardin, F., Amodeo, L., Laplanche, D., & Blua, P. (2016a). Emergency department flow: A new practical patients classification and forecasting daily attendance. *IFAC-PapersOnLine*, *49*(12), 721–726. doi:10.1016/j.ifacol.2016.07.859

Afilal, M., Yalaoui, F., Dugardin, F., Amodeo, L., Laplanche, D., & Blua, P. (2016b). Forecasting the Emergency Department Patients Flow. *Journal of Medical Systems*, *40*(7), 1–18. doi:10.100710916-016-0527-0 PMID:27272135

Aladeemy, M., Chou, C. A., Shan, X., Khasawneh, M., Srihari, K., & Poranki, S. (2016). Forecasting Daily Patient Arrivals at Emergency Department: A Comparative Study. *Proceedings of the 2016 Industrial and Systems Engineering Research Conference*.

Araz, O. M., Bentley, D., & Muelleman, R. L. (2014). Using Google Flu Trends data in forecasting influenza-like–illness related ED visits in Omaha, Nebraska. *The American Journal of Emergency Medicine*, *32*(9), 1016–1023. doi:10.1016/j.ajem.2014.05.052 PMID:25037278

Areekul, P., Senjyu, T., Toyama, H., & Yona, A. (2010). Notice of violation of IEEE publication principles a hybrid ARIMA and neural network model for short-term price forecasting in deregulated market. *IEEE Transactions on Power Systems*, *25*(1), 524–530. doi:10.1109/TPWRS.2009.2036488

Armstrong, J. S. (Ed.). (2001). *Principles of forecasting: a handbook for researchers and practitioners* (Vol. 30). Springer Science & Business Media. doi:10.1007/978-0-306-47630-3

Aroua, A., & Abdul-Nour, G. (2015). Forecast emergency room visits–a major diagnostic categories-based approach. *International Journal of Metrology and Quality Engineering*, *6*(2), 204. doi:10.1051/ijmqe/2015011

Arya, P., Paul, R. K., Kumar, A., Singh, K. N., Sivaramne, N., & Chaudhary, P. (2015). Predicting pest population using weather variables: An ARIMAX time series framework. *International Journal of Agricultural and Statistics Sciences*, *11*(2), 381–386.

Au-Yeung, S. W. M., Harder, U., McCoy, E. J., & Knottenbelt, W. J. (2009). Predicting patient arrivals to an accident and emergency department. *Emergency Medicine Journal*, *26*(4), 241–244. doi:10.1136/emj.2007.051656 PMID:19307381

Batal, H., Tench, J., McMillan, S., Adams, J., & Mehler, P. S. (2001). Predicting patient visits to an urgent care clinic using calendar variables. *Academic Emergency Medicine*, *8*(1), 48–53. doi:10.1111/j.1553-2712.2001.tb00550.x PMID:11136148

Bergs, J., Heerinckx, P., & Verelst, S. (2014). Knowing what to expect, forecasting monthly emergency department visits: A time-series analysis. *International Emergency Nursing*, *22*(2), 112–115. doi:10.1016/j.ienj.2013.08.001 PMID:24055373

Bierens, H. J. (1987). Kernel estimators of regression functions. In *Advances in econometrics: Fifth world congress* (Vol. 1, pp. 99-144). Academic Press. 10.1017/CCOL0521344301.003

Boyle, J. R., Sparks, R. S., Keijzers, G. B., Crilly, J. L., Lind, J. F., & Ryan, L. M. (2011). Prediction and surveillance of influenza epidemics. *The Medical Journal of Australia*, *194*(4), S28. PMID:21401485

Butler, M. B., Gu, H., Kenney, T., & Campbell, S. G. (2016). P017: Does a busy day predict another busy day? A time-series analysis of multi-centre emergency department volumes. *Canadian Journal of Emergency Medical Care*, *18*(S1), S83–S84. doi:10.1017/cem.2016.193

Calegari, R., Fogliatto, F. S., Lucini, F. R., Neyeloff, J., Kuchenbecker, R. S., & Schaan, B. D. (2016). Forecasting Daily Volume and Acuity of Patients in the Emergency Department. *Computational and Mathematical Methods in Medicine*. PMID:27725842

Carvalho-Silva, M., Monteiro, M. T. T., de Sá-Soares, F., & Dória-Nóbrega, S. (2017). Assessment of forecasting models for patients arrival at Emergency Department. *Operations Research for Health Care*. doi:10.1016/j.orhc.2017.05.001

Champion, R., Kinsman, L. D., Lee, G. A., Masman, K. A., May, E. A., Mills, T. M., ... Williams, R. J. (2007). Forecasting emergency department presentations. *Australian Health Review*, *31*(1), 83–90. doi:10.1071/AH070083 PMID:17266491

Chase, V. J., Cohn, A. E., Peterson, T. A., & Lavieri, M. S. (2012). Predicting emergency department volume using forecasting methods to create a "surge response" for noncrisis events. *Academic Emergency Medicine*, *19*(5), 569–576. doi:10.1111/j.1553-2712.2012.01359.x PMID:22594361

Cools, M., Moons, E., & Wets, G. (2009). Investigating the variability in daily traffic counts through use of ARIMAX and SARIMAX models: Assessing the effect of holidays on two site locations. *Transportation Research Record: Journal of the Transportation Research Board*, *2136*(1), 57–66. doi:10.3141/2136-07

Côté, M. J., Smith, M. A., Eitel, D. R., & Akçali, E. (2013). Forecasting emergency department arrivals: A tutorial for emergency department directors. *Hospital Topics*, *91*(1), 9–19. doi:10.1080/00185868.2013.757962 PMID:23428111

Efendigil, T., Önüt, S., & Kahraman, C. (2009). A decision support system for demand forecasting with artificial neural networks and neuro-fuzzy models: A comparative analysis. *Expert Systems with Applications*, *36*(3), 6697–6707. doi:10.1016/j.eswa.2008.08.058

Ekström, A., Kurland, L., Farrokhnia, N., Castrén, M., & Nordberg, M. (2015). Forecasting emergency department visits using internet data. *Annals of Emergency Medicine*, *65*(4), 436–442. doi:10.1016/j.annemergmed.2014.10.008 PMID:25487026

Gahirwal, M. (2013). *Inter Time series sales forecasting*. arXiv preprint arXiv:1303.0117

Gul, M., & Guneri, A. F. (2015a). A comprehensive review of emergency department simulation applications for normal and disaster conditions. *Computers & Industrial Engineering*, *83*, 327–344. doi:10.1016/j.cie.2015.02.018

Gul, M., & Guneri, A. F. (2015b). Forecasting patient length of stay in an emergency department by artificial neural networks. *Journal of Aeronautics and Space Technologies*, *8*(2), 43–48.

Gul, M., & Guneri, A. F. (2016a). Planning the future of emergency departments: Forecasting ED patient arrivals by using regression and neural network models, International Journal of Industrial Engineering: Theory. *Applications and Practice*, *23*(2), 137–154.

Gul, M., & Guneri, A. F. (2016b). An artificial neural network-based earthquake casualty estimation model for Istanbul city. *Natural Hazards*, *84*(3), 2163–2178. doi:10.100711069-016-2541-4

Gul, M., Yucesan, M., & Celik, E. (2017). Multi-site and multi-method forecasting modelling of hospital emergency room patient arrivals. *International Conference on Advances and Innovations in Engineering (ICAIE)*, 134-138.

Guneri, A. F., & Gumus, A. T. (2008). The usage of artificial neural networks for finite capacity planning, International Journal of Industrial Engineering: Theory. *Applications and Practice*, *15*(1), 16–25.

Guneri, A. F., & Gumus, A. T. (2009). Artificial Neural Networks for Finite Capacity Scheduling: A Comparative Study, International Journal of Industrial Engineering: Theory. *Applications and Practice*, *15*(4), 349–359.

Harrou, F., Sun, Y., Kadri, F., Chaabane, S., & Tahon, C. (2015, October). Early detection of abnormal patient arrivals at hospital emergency department. In *Industrial Engineering and Systems Management (IESM), 2015 International Conference on* (pp. 221-227). IEEE. 10.1109/IESM.2015.7380162

Hertzum, M. (2017). The Cost of Improved Overview: An Analysis of the Use of Electronic Whiteboards in Emergency Departments. In *IFIP Conference on Human-Computer Interaction* (pp. 402-410). Springer. 10.1007/978-3-319-67684-5_25

Hill, T., Marquez, L., O'Connor, M., & Remus, W. (1994). Artificial neural network models for forecasting and decision making. *International Journal of Forecasting*, *10*(1), 5–15. doi:10.1016/0169-2070(94)90045-0

Hoot, N. R., Zhou, C., Jones, I., & Aronsky, D. (2007). Measuring and forecasting emergency department crowding in real time. *Annals of Emergency Medicine*, *49*(6), 747–755. doi:10.1016/j.annemergmed.2007.01.017 PMID:17391809

Jalalkamali, A., Moradi, M., & Moradi, N. (2015). Application of several artificial intelligence models and ARIMAX model for forecasting drought using the Standardized Precipitation Index. *International Journal of Environmental Science and Technology*, *12*(4), 1201–1210. doi:10.100713762-014-0717-6

Jones, S. A., Joy, M. P., & Pearson, J. (2002). Forecasting demand of emergency care. *Health Care Management Science*, *5*(4), 297–305. doi:10.1023/A:1020390425029 PMID:12437279

Jones, S. S., Evans, R. S., Allen, T. L., Thomas, A., Haug, P. J., Welch, S. J., & Snow, G. L. (2009). A multivariate time series approach to modeling and forecasting demand in the emergency department. *Journal of Biomedical Informatics*, *42*(1), 123–139. doi:10.1016/j.jbi.2008.05.003 PMID:18571990

Jones, S. S., Thomas, A., Evans, R. S., Welch, S. J., Haug, P. J., & Snow, G. L. (2008). Forecasting daily patient volumes in the emergency department. *Academic Emergency Medicine*, *15*(2), 159–170. doi:10.1111/j.1553-2712.2007.00032.x PMID:18275446

Kadri, F., Harrou, F., Chaabane, S., & Tahon, C. (2014). Time series modelling and forecasting of emergency department overcrowding. *Journal of Medical Systems*, *38*(9), 107–127. doi:10.100710916-014-0107-0 PMID:25053208

Kam, H. J., Sung, J. O., & Park, R. W. (2010). Prediction of daily patient numbers for a regional emergency medical center using time series analysis. *Healthcare Informatics Research*, *16*(3), 158–165. doi:10.4258/hir.2010.16.3.158 PMID:21818435

Kang, S. W., & Park, H. S. (2015). Emergency department visit volume variability. *Clinical and Experimental Emergency Medicine*, *2*(3), 150–154. doi:10.15441/ceem.14.044 PMID:27752589

Kim, K., Lee, C., O'Leary, K., Rosenauer, S., & Mehrotra, S. (2014). *Predicting patient volumes in hospital medicine: A comparative study of different time series forecasting methods. Tech. rep.* Northwestern University.

Kongcharoen, C., & Kruangpradit, T. (2013). Autoregressive integrated moving average with explanatory variable (ARIMAX) model for Thailand export. *33rd International Symposium on Forecasting*, 1-8.

Kröse, B., Krose, B., van der Smagt, P., & Smagt, P. (1993). *An introduction to neural networks*. London: CRC Press.

Mai, Q., Aboagye-Sarfo, P., Sanfilippo, F. M., Preen, D. B., & Fatovich, D. M. (2015). Predicting the number of emergency department presentations in Western Australia: A population-based time series analysis. *Emergency Medicine Australasia*, *27*(1), 16–21. doi:10.1111/1742-6723.12344 PMID:25583296

Marcilio, I., Hajat, S., & Gouveia, N. (2013). Forecasting daily emergency department visits using calendar variables and ambient temperature readings. *Academic Emergency Medicine*, *20*(8), 769–777. doi:10.1111/acem.12182 PMID:24033619

McCarthy, M. L., Zeger, S. L., Ding, R., Aronsky, D., Hoot, N. R., & Kelen, G. D. (2008). The challenge of predicting demand for emergency department services. *Academic Emergency Medicine*, *15*(4), 337–346. doi:10.1111/j.1553-2712.2008.00083.x PMID:18370987

Menke, N. B., Caputo, N., Fraser, R., Haber, J., Shields, C., & Menke, M. N. (2014). A retrospective analysis of the utility of an artificial neural network to predict ED volume. *The American Journal of Emergency Medicine*, *32*(6), 614–617. doi:10.1016/j.ajem.2014.03.011 PMID:24736127

Morzuch, B. J., & Allen, P. G. (2006). *Forecasting hospital emergency department arrivals*. In *26th Annual Symposium on Forecasting*, Santander, Spain.

Neter, J., Kutner, M. H., Nachtsheim, C. J., & Wasserman, W. (1996). Applied linear statistical models, Chicago: Irwin. network modeling approach for sales forecasting. *International Journal of Production.*, *4*, 318.

Ni, Y., & Fan, F. (2011). A two-stage dynamic sales forecasting model for the fashion retail. *Expert Systems with Applications*, *38*(3), 1529–1536. doi:10.1016/j.eswa.2010.07.065

Park, J., Park, E., & Desai, Y. (2008, January). Forecasting patient load of ED at moses cone hospital. In *IIE Annual Conference. Proceedings* (p. 1). Institute of Industrial and Systems Engineers (IISE).

Petrou, P. (2015). An interrupted time-series analysis to assess impact of introduction of co-payment on emergency room visits in Cyprus. *Applied Health Economics and Health Policy*, *13*(5), 515–523. doi:10.100740258-015-0169-2 PMID:25894739

Pianykh, O. S., & Rosenthal, D. I. (2015). Can we predict patient wait time? *Journal of the American College of Radiology*, *12*(10), 1058–1066. doi:10.1016/j.jacr.2015.04.010 PMID:26435119

Qin, L. X., & Shi, Z. Z. (2006). Efficiently mining association rules from time series. *International Journal of Information Technology*, *12*(4), 30-38.

Rosychuk, R. J., Klassen, T. P., Voaklander, D. C., Senthilselvan, A., & Rowe, B. H. (2011). Seasonality patterns in croup presentations to emergency departments in Alberta, Canada: A time series analysis. *Pediatric Emergency Care*, *27*(4), 256–260. doi:10.1097/PEC.0b013e31821314b0 PMID:21490537

Rosychuk, R. J., Youngson, E., & Rowe, B. H. (2015). Presentations to Alberta emergency departments for asthma: A time series analysis. *Academic Emergency Medicine*, *22*(8), 942–949. doi:10.1111/acem.12725 PMID:26194859

Rosychuk, R. J., Youngson, E., & Rowe, B. H. (2016). Presentations to emergency departments for COPD: A time series analysis. *Canadian Respiratory Journal, 2016*, 1–9. doi:10.1155/2016/1382434 PMID:27445514

Schonwetter, R. S., Clark, L. D., Leedy, S. A., Quinn, M. J., Azer, M., & Kim, S. (2008). Predicting emergency room visits and hospitalizations among hospice patients with cardiac disease. *Journal of Palliative Medicine, 11*(8), 1142–1150. doi:10.1089/jpm.2008.0032 PMID:18980456

Sun, Y., Heng, B. H., Seow, Y. T., & Seow, E. (2009). Forecasting daily attendances at an emergency department to aid resource planning. *BMC Emergency Medicine, 9*(1), 1. doi:10.1186/1471-227X-9-1 PMID:19178716

Wargon, M., Casalino, E., & Guidet, B. (2010). From model to forecasting: A multi center study in emergency departments. *Academic Emergency Medicine, 17*(9), 970–978. doi:10.1111/j.1553-2712.2010.00847.x PMID:20836778

Wargon, M., Guidet, B., Hoang, T. D., & Hejblum, G. (2009). A systematic review of models for forecasting the number of emergency department visits. *Emergency Medicine Journal, 26*(6), 395–399. doi:10.1136/emj.2008.062380 PMID:19465606

Xu, M., Wong, T. C., & Chin, K. S. (2013). Modeling daily patient arrivals at Emergency Department and quantifying the relative importance of contributing variables using artificial neural network. *Decision Support Systems, 54*(3), 1488–1498. doi:10.1016/j.dss.2012.12.019

Xu, Q., Tsui, K. L., Jiang, W., & Guo, H. (2016). A hybrid approach for forecasting patient visits in emergency department. *Quality and Reliability Engineering International, 32*(8), 2751–2759. doi:10.1002/qre.2095

Yucesan, M., Gul, M., & Celik, E. (2017). Application of artificial neural networks using Bayesian training rule in sales forecasting for furniture industry. *Drvna industrija: Znanstveni časopis za pitanja drvne tehnologije, 68*(3), 219-228.

Yucesan, M., Gul, M., & Celik, E. (2018). Performance comparison between ARIMAX, ANN and ARIMAX-ANN hybridization in sales forecasting for furniture industry. Drvna industrija: Znanstveni časopis za pitanja drvne tehnologije. (in press)

Zhang, G. P. (2003). Time series forecasting using a hybrid ARIMA and neural network model. *Neurocomputing, 50*, 159–175. doi:10.1016/S0925-2312(01)00702-0

Zibners, L. M., Bonsu, B. K., Hayes, J. R., & Cohen, D. M. (2006). Local weather effects on emergency department visits: A time series and regression analysis. *Pediatric Emergency Care, 22*(2), 104–106. doi:10.1097/01.pec.0000199561.34475.29 PMID:16481926

Zlotnik, A., Gallardo-Antolin, A., Alfaro, M. C., Pérez, M. C. P., & Martínez, J. M. M. (2015). Emergency department visit forecasting and dynamic nursing staff allocation using machine learning techniques with readily available open-source software. *CIN: Computers, Informatics, Nursing, 33*(8), 368–377. PMID:26200901

Chapter 13
Application of Big Data in Digital Epidemiology

Sameena Naaz
Jamia Hamdard, India

Farheen Siddiqui
Jamia Hamdard, India

ABSTRACT

Epidemiology is the study of dynamics of health and disease in human population. It aims to identify the occurrence, pattern, and etiology of human diseases so that the causes of these diseases can be understood, which in turn will help in preventing their spread. In traditional epidemiology, the data is collected by various public health agencies through various means. Many times, the actual figures vary a lot from the one reported. Sometimes this difference is due to human errors, but most of the time, it is due to intentional underreporting. Big data techniques can be used to analyze this huge amount of data so as to extract useful information from it. The electronic health data is so large and complex that it cannot be processed using traditional software and hardware. It is also not possible to manage this data using traditional data management tools. This data is huge in terms of volume as well as diversity and the speed at which it is being generated. The ability to combine and analyze these different sources of data has huge impact on epidemic tracking.

INTRODCUTION

The power of technology in this era is so huge that anyone can track your whereabouts just by using your cellphone location. They can even predict where you can be at some later point of time by using various analytics. This information may be used by a security agency for nabbing the criminals. But not only this! There is a Swedish project by the name of Flowminder which tracks the movement of population during any natural disaster and can use it for the sake of relief and rescue.

This is just one of the examples of a project in the field of digital epidemiology. Epidemiology is a field which deals with the study and analysis of various patterns, their reasons and how they affect the health and disease in any geographical area or a defined population. Traditionally the data has been

DOI: 10.4018/978-1-5225-7071-4.ch013

collected from various sources by different agencies and it is analyzed using tools to get some insight into the reasons for the spread of diseases. The new field of digital epidemiology relies on collecting the data using digital techniques such as getting data from various social networking sites and then using computational methods to measure health and the spread of disease. Governments of various countries are supporting projects which use big data for digital epidemiology. Air quality data is being captured by environmental scientists from the polluted areas and then it is compared with the health status of the people living in those areas. This can give an insight into the correlation between the environmental hazards and the diseases present there. Information on sexual and social networks are gathered by Epidemiologists which helps them predict the signs of spread of diseases so that early warning signs can be issued.

Big data analytics helps in predictive modeling in healthcare sector which provide faster, better and more targeted results in digital epidemiology which helps to develop better vaccines faster. It also helps in analysis of disease patters which helps track disease outbreaks which results in faster disaster management.

The study of distribution and changes of health and disease in human population is Epidemiology. It identifies the incidence, distribution and etiology of human diseases in order to understand their causes in a better manner which in turn will help in preventing them from spreading (Green, Freedman & Gordis, 2000). Traditionally, the data was collected by various public health agencies which used to go to the hospitals, doctors and the effected people to get first-hand information. Latest work in this area is to get the data from online sources. People search for different types of information on the internet. The pattern of search in any particular area can give us some insight on their health issues. This has become possible due to increase in use of electronic devices and modern communication techniques (Eysenbach, 2009). Due to the huge size of this data various big data analytics tools are used to process it and get useful information.

The electronic health data set is so large that it cannot be managed by traditional software and hardware. The traditional data base management system also fails to manage such huge amount of data (Zenger, 2012). It is not only huge in volume but is also very diverse and extremely fast changing. These are the main reasons why we need big data techniques to handle them.

BIG DATA IN HEALTH CARE

Epidemic tracking has gone through a huge change as it can combine and analyze various sources of data. Big data initiative in the health care sector is being supported by governments of many countries. Some of the instances are: The government of Denmark is providing anonymously health as well as hospitalization data for carrying out research in the field of Big Data (Szlezak et al., 2014). They have a program which helps in better care of patients with diabetes and heart diseases by employing data analytics on the medical data available (IBM, 2013).

Swedish government is also trying to help research in Big Data analytics. Huge amount of data from lab results, healthcare centers and from ambulances carrying critically ill people or accident cases can be merged for the analytics purposes. A lot of research is going on for developing tools and techniques which can support decision making. One important area of research is the analysis of structured and unstructured data to study the effect of various drugs (Network, T.S.B.D.A., 2013).

A project on review of Big Data privacy was undertaken by the US government in January 2014. The recommendations of this work can be found in Podesta et al. (2014) and PCAST (2014). There is a World Health Organization project by the name of "Be He@lthy Be mobile" which uses the mobile devices and various wireless technologies for the study of health care. The study in the field of health care which uses mobile devices and latest communication technologies come under the domain of mHealth. A project in this domain by the name of mDiabetics is helping countries in their tryst to control, manage and prevent non-communicable diseases such as cancer, diabetes and heart disease (WHO, 2014).

The dynamics of spread of any communicable disease depends a lot on human movement. We can get the information about a person's location using mobile phone data. This data could be collected using the the mobile phone tower location used when a person makes a call. With the latest advancements in the mobile technology now all the smart phones have Global Positioning System (GPS). A person's location can be tracked using their GPS location also (Cattuto et al., 2010). All this helps in the study of mobility of human's and its influence on spread of diseases (Gonzalez, Hidalgo & Barabasi, 2008). Other wearable devices also help in tracking the social behavior (Pentland & Pentland, 2008) of a person, the work which was previously done using large-scale surveys and self reporting (Mossong et al., 2008). The self reported data and the measurements taken from social media compliment each other and helps in getting better understanding and accurate description of infectious disease dynamics. The study of disease dynamics involves collection of data from a large number of individuals, refine this data as per our requirement and then to decide upon the parameters that will be used for large scale computer simulation. In the traditional method modeling was done using population aggregates, but now with the advent of technology it is possible to use data collected from large number of individuals. This helps us in getting more variety in the data which is collected and hence better results can be achieved. Realistic models of human mobility have been developed using mobile phone (Gonzalez, Hidalgo & Barabasi, 2008). It has also been used to predict the rate at which drug resistance has increased (Lynch & Roper, 2011), to study the chances of malaria eradication (Tatem et al., 2009), and to monitor population movements in near real-time during cholera outbreak in Haiti (Bengtsson et al., 2011). Data obtained for close proximity interactions among individuals using wireless sensor network technology can be used to develop models which can help in targeted immunization strategies (Salathe et al., 2010). This method is different from the static representation of contact networks (Stehle et al., 2011) and yields better results. Worldwide spread of new emerging infectious diseases such as H1N1 can be studied using large-scale mobility (Balcam et al., 2009; Merler et al., 2011).

BioMosaic is a tool developed by Centers for Disease Control (CDC), USA and World Health Organization (WHO) to track the Ebola virus outbreak. Big Data was used to track the movement of people across US borders. BioMosaic is a tool that combined together the health data of people, population trend and movement data and used it for prediction of spread of Ebola. It has also been used for many other epidemics in the area of forecasting, targeting, testing, intervention and surveillance. CDC has also developed a new software tool, the Epi Info viral hemorrhagic fever (VHF) which helps in identifying people who are exposed to the virus faster in much lesser time as compared to the traditional reporting methods.

Researcher's and epidemiologists at Boston Children's Hospital have developed a website by the name of HealthMap which is used for disease-monitoring using big data analytics. The site collects real time data from various sources including social media, chat rooms, online news, travel sites, official records etc. and aggregates and analyses this data. The result of this analysis is used for early detection and real-time surveillance on latest health hazards.

Huge amount of data gets generated on social networking sites during outbreak of any disease. This happens as patients as well as people who are living in areas affected by these diseases share their symptoms, look for hospitals and clinics and search for various medicines on the apps. Therefore, social media plays an important role in supplying huge amount of data which can be analyzed to identify outbreaks and predict the regions where the disease can spread later on, so that preventive measures can be taken. In both the flu and Ebola epidemics data analysis was done in this manner.

Google Flu Trends is a service provided by Google which accumulates data related to influenza in 25 different countries. This web site collects data from Google search queries and aggregates it in order to predict flu activity. Google.org first launched this project in 2008 to predict outbreak of flu (Khoury & Wei, 2015). There is another project by the name of flu-prediction (Khoury & Ioannidis, 2014) launched by the institute of Cognitive Science, Osnabrück which combines social media data such as data from twitter with data from Centers for Disease Control (CDC) to develop structural models that predict the temporal and spatial spreading of the disease (Lauer, 2012)).

An ecological niche model using geographically weighted regression has been developed in Lpoeset al (2014) for prediction of H1N1 influenza in Vellore. This model based on geographically weighted regression helped in identifying high risk areas so that proper prevention steps could be implemented there. Big Data will have huge impact on the future of epidemiologic research as it collects data from a large section of population. Some of these implications have been discussed in Mooney, Westreich, and El-Sayed (2015).

National Center for Disease Control (NCDC) collects data from various Indian states through Integrated Disease Surveillance Project (IDSP). The aim of this project is to collect, compile, analyze and use data on several target diseases for surveillance so that fast response can be provided for preventing and controlling the spread these diseases in the masses. Data is collected by Syndromic Surveillance which is done by the health worker, Presumptive Surveillance which is done by the Medical Officer and Laboratory Surveillance. The health workers collect data on the water quality also. The data is collected on a weekly basis which helps to identify disease trends and seasonal outbreaks. There are Rapid Response Teams (RRT) to diagnose and control sudden outbreak of diseases. Data is collected from Major Hospitals and Infectious Disease Hospitals and is analyzed by respective State/District Surveillance Units. The status of this weekly surveillance data is further analyzed by a committee of Epidemiologists from IDSP and experts from NCDC.

There are many diseases which occur due to high level of air pollution. Some of them include Asthma and Chronic Obstructive Pulmonary Disease (COPD). In order to keep a check on these diseases air quality is being monitored by environmental scientists from the polluted areas. The data gathered from here is matched with the health care data sets to get an insight into respiratory diseases. Epidemiologists also gather information from social and sexual networks and analyze them to predict the spread of disease and create early warnings.

IMPORTANCE OF DIGITAL EPIDEMIOLOGY

The world has become a small place now. Due to easy accessibility to various places across the globe it has become very easy to travel from one corner to another. This results in ease of transmission of diseases also and so the threat of global epidemics has increased exponentially. Traditionally, data is collected manually and is analyzed to develop methods for prevention of disease outbreaks. But the response time in this manual setup is too high for a global population which keeps moving at a fast pace. Due to this the epidemics also spread from one region to another at a speed unimaginable a century ago. The viruses have also become resistant to antibiotics and this is also a major threat because traditional preventative measures are no more effective. Due to all this we need to have a new approach to disease control.

Big Data collects large sets of data from various sources such as field work, research and open web and analyzes it to develop methods to combat epidemics.

Massive data which consists of data obtained from syndromic surveillance indicators (non-medical in nature) and data from lab results and electronic health records (medical in nature) are accessed and analyzed in computational epidemiology. These two kinds of data are combined to construct flexible and dynamic system which operates in real time to provide early warnings to combat spread of diseases.

Future prediction of epidemic is difficult in India as the various factors responsible for the spread of these diseases is unmanageably scattered. Communicable as well as chronic diseases hit a large population of our country every year. The government is not able to use the available data on time due to lack of resources and such huge spread and therefore it is not possible for the Government Bodies to issue any health advisories in time. We are also not able to develop proper vaccinations and medicines to control the epidemic.

USE OF DIGITAL EPIDEMIOLOGY TO PREVENT OUTBREAK OF DENGUE IN INDIA

Dengue resurged in India at the onset of monsoon last year (2016), to put many lives at risk. Directorate of National Vector Borne Disease Control Programme (NVBDCP) is the agency which is responsible for the preventing and controlling the vector borne diseases such as Malaria, Kala azar, Dengue, Japanese Encephalitis and Chikungunya in India. According to this agency a large number of cases of Malaria, Dengue and Chikungunya occured due to heavy rainfall in many regions of the country, especially in Delhi, resulting in serious health threat.

Dengue is currently considered as the most important mosquito-borne viral disease globally (Murray, Quam & Wilder-Smith, 2013). It causes a huge amount of disease and socioeconomic burden on subtropical and tropical areas of the world (Guzman & Kouri, 2002; Gubler, 2011). Dengue is one of the major arboviral disease which has affected over 50% of the world population and approximately 50% countries in the world are dengue endemic (Gibler, 2002, 2011; WHO, 2012a, 2012b, 2013; Ferreira, 2012). There are several factors for such high rate of dengue infections and it's predicted growth. This includes evolution of news viruses, change in climatic conditions and societal factors such as population growth, rapid urbanization as well as global trade and travel (Wilder-Smith & Gubler, 2008; Astrom et al., 2012).

As no vaccine or antiviral therapy has been developed so far for dengue, so the only method to control it is through early detection and symptomatic treatment (WHO, 2009). The WHO Global Strategy for Dengue Prevention and Control, 2012–2020, talks about the necessity for better estimation of the real burden of dengue across the globe due to the current under-represented number (WHO, 2012b). Surveillance and reporting is very important for controlling dengue efficiently. Political, financial as well as research priorities will change once the impact of dengue gets quantified. This will also help in better decision making and modeling (Gubler, 2011, 2012; Shepard, Undurraga & Halasa, 2013; Bhatt et al., 2013; Beatty et al., 2010).

There has been a substantial change in the epidemiology of dengue fever in India in the past few decades. This change has occurred in terms of geographical location where it spread, severity of outbreak and the type of strain. The first reported case of dengue fever in India is from 1946 (Karamchandani, 1946). After that there were not much cases of the disease reported for the next 18 years. The first reported epidemic of dengue is from the Eastern Coast of India (Carey et al., 1966; Ramakrishnan et al., 1964; Sarkar et al., 1964; Chaudhuri, Saha & Chaudhuri, 1965; Krishnamurthy, Kasturi & Chittipantulu, 1965; Paul et al., 1965) and it occurred in the year 1963-1964. From there it spread northwards and reached Delhi in 1967 (Balaya et al., 1969)] and Kanpur in 1968 (Chaturvedi et al., 1970; Chaturvedi et al., 1970). During the same period, it also spread in the south India (Meyers et al., 1968; Ghosh, 1968) and gradually the whole country was involved. After this epidemic outbreak Dengue became endemic/ hyperendemic with all four serotypes of DV.

Good amount of work has been done on traditional epidemiology in India. Digital epidemiology has great potential to predict the future trends of spread of diseases. Methods and strategies are being developed by researchers to use digital epidemiology for monitoring and surveillance of infectious diseases. There is a need to integrate these new methods with traditional practices keeping in mind the ethical concerns about privacy.

Work on digital epidemiology for various diseases has been reported in literature, but not work has been found in the Indian sub-continent. We know that the use of social media has increased many folds in our country during the last few years. Data for research in the field of digital epidemiology can be taken from social media such as Twitter feeds (Bian et al., 2012), status updates on Facebook and other platforms, blogs (Raghupathi & Ragupathi, 2013) and web sites. Apart from these online sources of data less patient-specific data such as data available from emergency care services, data from news feeds, articles in journals of medical science etc. can all be collected in an offline mode.

APPLICATION OF BIG DATA ANALYTICS FOR DENGUE EPIDEMIOLOGY

Three main characteristics of big data that is volume, velocity and variety exist in the healthcare data (IBM, n.d.). Huge amount of health data is being generated with each passing day resulting in an tremendous volume of data. Various sources of existing healthcare data include radiology images, personal medical records, electronic submissions from Food and Drug Administration (FDA), population data, human genetics and genomic data etc. Latest technologies such as 3D imaging and genomics and biometric sensors are also generating huge volume of data.

This huge amount of data needs to be captured using some techniques for further processing in order to extract useful information. Storage of such large volume of data in another issue related to it's use in digital epidemiology. Fortunately, virtualization and cloud computing is a tool which helps us to achieve all of these (Feldman, Martin & Skotnes, 2012). The data is being created and assembled at a very fast speed in real-time and hence the velocity of the data is also quite high. There are many new challenges due to the constant flow of new data at an unprecedented rate. Tools and techniques need to be developed which can retrieve, analyze, compare and make decisions based on such fast-changing data. Analysis of such huge amount of data which has got high velocity by considering data from various sources results in the third characteristic of big data which is variety (IHTT, 2013).

With continuously changing volume, velocity and variety of health data new analytics techniques have to be developed to accommodate them. The data that was collected from electronic health records was structured in nature. But the data from digital media is unstructured in nature. Due to this variety in healthcare data: structured, unstructured and semi structured the field of digital epidemiology is both interesting and challenging.

BIG DATA ARCHITECTURAL FRAMEWORK (BDAF)

A big data analytics project in healthcare uses the same conceptual framework as any other traditional health informatics project or analytics project in any other domain. It only differs in where and how the processing is carried out. If big data is not involved, then any business intelligence tool can be used on a standalone system or a laptop for the processing of data. On the other hand, when the data is very huge it is broken down and the processing takes place simultaneously across multiple nodes. Hence, we can say that data analysis in big data uses the concept of distributed processing which has been there for decades. In the healthcare domain the available data is analyzed to gain insight which can be used for a better more informed health decision. Furthermore, we have many open source platforms such as Hadoop/MapReduce, which can be accessed over the cloud, which have been of great help for use of big data analytics in healthcare.

Although the models and algorithms used in big data analytics are similar to the one used in traditional analytics but they are not as user friendly and transparent as the later. The main reason for this is that they have evolved in an ad hoc manner mostly as an open-source development tool and platform. Although having these tools available as open source has its own advantages but it lacks support and user friendliness which a vendor provided tool possesses. The available tools are programming intensive, more complex and require a whole lot of skills.

The architectural framework of big data to be used in the healthcare domain is discussed below. The conceptual architecture of big data analytics shown in figure 1 highlights the major challenges in relation to the Big Data properties and technologies. The proposed BDAF consists of the following 4 components which together address different aspects of Big Data definition.

Data Sources

The health data that is available to us could be structured, semi-structured or unstructured. The data that can be stored and analyzed with the help of machine to extract useful information are structured data. Structured data is obtained from legacy applications, ERP and from external feeds. Semi-structured as well as unstructured data is obtained from Web Logs, Network/Application Logs, Social Media, Chat Transcripts, Emails, readings from instruments and the electronic health data. Office medical records, handwritten prescriptions, admission and discharge summary etc. also provide unstructured data.

Latest advancements in technology has resulted in many more sources of structured as well as unstructured data. These include data from fitness devices, social media records, genetics and other sources. There is a need for technological advancements which can help in capturing, storing and organizing this enormous amount of data to extract useful information.

Tools need to be developed which can combine the traditional data with new types of data both at an individual level as well as at population level. This is the strength of big data.

Apart from the medical data being generated there are other types of data which also directly or indirectly play an important role in Epidemiological study. Some of them are:

Figure 1. Conceptual architecture of big data analytics

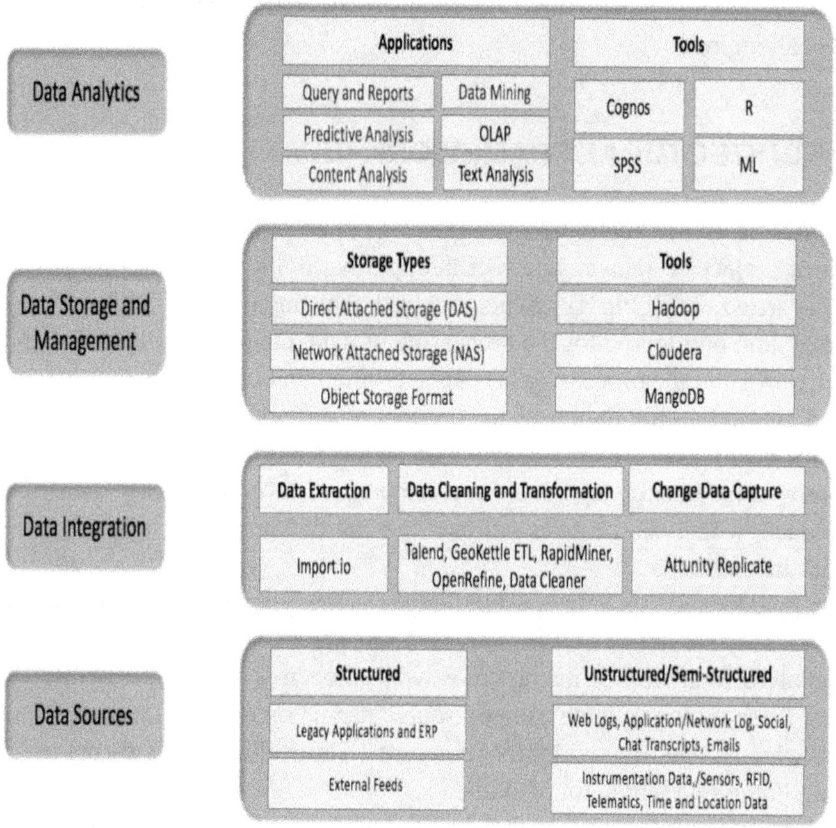

Geographic Data

Huge amount of data related physical landscapes such as roads, buildings, lakes etc. are available today from Geographic Information Systems. This information may include address of a person, work place information, routes taken by the person for commuting or may be the personal information of the person. Although people are worried about the safety of all their personal data but still they are willing to share such information. All this has resulted in new application areas and innovations both for the general public as well as for the governments.

Geostatistics is the branch of statistics which deals with the spatiotemporal and spatial datasets. In this field interpolation methods are used to build statistical models which are used for estimating and simulating spatial phenomena. The area of study could be small geographical area such as municipal level or sub-municipal level allowing studies on a fine spatial level. The geodata for Geostatistics can be collected using geographical information There are many organizations and institutions which collect these types of data for further analysis.

Real Time Media

We all know that huge amount of multimedia data is being generated in real-time which includes both recorded and live data. Users keep on sharing unlimited number of audio, pictures and video through various social networking sites such as YouTube, Flickr, Vimeo etc.

Video as well as audio conferencing is another source of generation of huge amount of data. This data could also be analyzed either in real time or by recording and analyzing it later on. Due to such huge amount of data being generated every second, it's storage and analysis requires technological advancements at a very fast pace.

Time Series

Getting the data at the right time and processing it is time is very important for real time data. Single reading of a data could be compared to an average of a sample of data or an individual data could be compared to another individual value at a different time. It is important to identify a discrete value of interest or importance from a continuous data and to analyze it properly to get the actual context and dependence on other external factors.

Network Data

Data from very large networks have connections within them and interesting information can be extracted from the structure of this connectivity. Some of the networks in this category includes biological networks (e.g. gene regulatory and metabolic nets), communication networks and social networks.

Data Integration

The data from various sources has to be pooled for the purpose of big data analytics. The data which is collected from various sources is in a 'raw' form and has to be processed or transformed. There are various methods to do this. One method is to combine service- oriented architecture with web services (middleware) (Ragupathi & Kesh, 2007). In this approach the data remains as it is in its raw form and services are used to call, extract and process the data. A different approach could be to use data warehousing in which the data from different sources is aggregated and then processed. But the drawback of this approach is that we cannot get the data in real- time. The steps of extract, transform, and load (ETL) are used here to collect data from diverse sources which is then pre-processed before being processed further. One example of a tool that can be used to extract data is Import.in. Similarly, we have various tools for data cleansing and transformation such as Talend, GeoKettle ETL, RapidMiner, OpenRefine, Data Cleaner etc.

The concept of Change Data Transfer (CDC) can be used to make the data truly "real time". This is achieved by making the data being analyzed complete and up-to-date and the analytic databases providing interactive query capabilities. The data which is being analyzed is obtained from a number of heterogeneous databases which have their set of challenges in integrating this data. The database where the data is processed is deployed on the cloud, so that also has it's own constraints.

Attunity Replicate is a tool that can be used to apply change data capture (CDC) to Big Data analytics. ETL is a batch-oriented method for data integration but CDC methods update the target analytic databases only if some change is detected in the source database.

Data Storage and Management

There are various technologies that can be used to store huge amount of data that has to be processed. Three technologies that have been discussed in this chapter are direct attached storage (DAS), network attached storage (NAS) and object storage format. In Direct Attached Storage there is direct connection between various hard disk drives (HDDs) and the servers. This approach is in accordance with the fundamental principle of Hadoop which is to move the processing to a location where the data lives, taking advantage of disk locality to optimize performance. Disk locality is the core concept used in Hadoop and virtually every description of Hadoop starts with it. But, DAS can be used only if the number of servers is limited. This type of storage is less scalable, expandable and upgradeable. Network Attached Storage (NAS) on the other hand, is a storage device that supports a network. It has a direct connection with the network, through a switch or hub via TCP/IP protocols. In NAS computation and storage takes place at different places. Here storage is shared across a number of servers by shipping data over the network in form of various files. Because NAS heavily depends on the network, so it is slower than DAS but the burden of input/output is lesser in NAS server as compared to DAS server. The third storage format is the object storage that can handle very large numbers of files. If there are very large number of files then traditional tree-like file systems become unmanageable. Object-based storage gives each file a unique identifier indexes the data with its location. Object storage systems can scale to capacity as high as billions of files, so it is the best option for companies that want to use big data to their advantage. The object storage technology is far less mature than DAS and NAS and is still evolving. Various tools are used for data management which are discussed in the next section.

Data Analytics

Some of the applications of data analytics are queries and reports, predictive analysis, content analysis, text analysis, OLAP and data mining. The main concept in all these applications is visualization. A variety of tools and techniques have been developed to analyze and visualize big data in healthcare.

TOOLS AND TECHNIQUES FOR BIG DATA ANALYSIS

Platforms

Hadoop

Hadoop (Apache platform) is an open-source platform for distributed processing of big data. It was developed in the beginning to aggregate web search indexes. It belongs to the class "NoSQL" technologies. Other tools in this class are CouchDB and MongoDB which aggregate data in unique ways. Extremely large amount of data can be processed using Hadoop. It allocates partitioned data sets to various servers (nodes), each of which solves different portions of the bigger problem and then combines them to get the final result (Borkar, Carey & Chen, 2012; Ohlhorst, 2012; Zikopoulos et al., 2013; Dean & Ghemawat, 2008). Hadoop works as a data organizer as well as an analytics tool. It has the potential harness huge amount of data which was difficult to manage and analyze till now. Hadoop can handle all the three types of data: structured, semi-structured and unstructured. But the problem with Hadoop is that although it is open source it is difficult to install, configure and administer and not many individuals with Hadoop skills are available in the market. In spite of all these associated problems companies are interested in Hadoop Distributed File System (HDFS) because it can manage and process extremes of big data for warehousing, integration and analytics at a low cost. Hadoop along with various other products layered above HDFS gives a highly scalable and high-performance platform for a wide range of applications which are data-intensive. There are many additional tools and platforms that support the Hadoop distributed platform (Zikopoulos et al., 2013; Dean & Ghemawat, 2008).

MapReduce (Singh & Reddy, 2014) is an execution engine which uses parallel processing for executing hand coded routines written in a variety of programming languages such as Java, R or Pig. MapReduce executes these routines for accessing huge file and repositories of data being managed by an HDFS cluster. By deploying MapReduce as a layer on top of HDFS we are able to obtain a high-performance analytic application which can handle huge data collections.

MapReduce breaks the entire job into two parts which are known as mappers and reducers (Lee et al., 2012). The data is read from the HDFS by the mappers, they process the data and generate some intermediate results for the reducers. Reducers use the results generated by the mappers, aggregate them and then generate the final output which finally is again written to HDFS. Several mappers and reducers run in parallel across different nodes in the cluster. A good description of MapReduce for parallel data processing is given in Deepak (2016). In 2013, Apache created YARN framework (also called MapReduce 2.0) from MapReduce. The basic MapReduce algorithm remains the same here but other processing algorithms including the ones that run interactively can be changed.

NoSQL DBMSs A NoSQL database manages data which is not relational in nature, so it need not support SQL. But the data here may be structured based on some other schema like records or value pair or may have no fixed schema. Various storage strategies may be used in NoSQL such as document stores, wide-column stores, key-value stores and graph databases (Chen & Zhang, 2014). The Hadoop family includes many other tools such as Cassandra, Hive, HBase Pig etc. some of which are discussed later on.

Spark

Spark is a paradigm developed at the University of California, Berkeley for big data processing. It overcomes the limitation of disk I/O in Hadoop (Lee et al., 2012) and hence improves the performance. The main advantage of Spark is that it can perform in-memory computations. The data can be cached in memory and in this manner, it eliminates the disk overhead problem in Hadoop for iterative tasks. Scala, Python and Java are all supported by Spark and it has been found to be 100 times faster than Hadoop MapReduce when the data can fit in the memory, and up to 10 times faster when it is on the disk. Spark can run on the YARN manager of Hadoop and can take data from HDFS

Storm

Storm (Kelly, 2013) is an open source real-time computation system which is distributed and fault-tolerant in nature. It has the power to process limitless stream of data. It differs from Hadoop as it works in real time whereas Hadoop is for batch processing. It is easy to set up Storm as compared to Hadoop and it also guarantees all the data will be processed. Some of the application areas where we can use Storm are on-line machine learning, real-time analytics, distributed RPC, ETL etc. Twitter uses Storm it to help generate its trending topics.

Drill

Apache Drill is another another platform for interactive analysis of Big Data (Malviya, Ughani & Soni, 2016). Apache Drill allows super fast ad hoc querying of giant data sets for interactive analysis and it is similar to Google's Dremel. The beauty of drill is that it can extract data from traditional databases as well as data sources such as HBase, Cassandra, MongoDB, etc. It is an excellent tool to scan petabytes of data and trillions of records in seconds and can exploit nested data. Drill is more flexible in the sense that it supports various query languages, data formats and data sources.

Statistical Languages

R

R is a freely available statistical programming language which is becoming rapidly popular as a software for data analysis, statistics and visualization. The main reasons for it's popularity are that it is cheap, powerful and works well with Hadoop. In fact, R is replacing SAS and SPSS and is preferred by the best statisticians, data scientists and analysts. Due to it's popularity we have R libraries for virtually all types of applications and this makes it even more popular as the analysts need not write new code for accessing data for their application.

Big data in cloud computing can be analyzed using R tool frame work (Mukhopadhyay et al., 2014). First thing is to identify the challenges associated with analyzing big data. Powerful business decisions are made by data scientist and business leader uses R today. The RFramework is very flexible and is available as open source. R consists of various packages that are used for analysis of data. The R Framework consists of Deploy R server, Deploy R repository and Deploy R API's. The analyst can write the scripts using R and can also upload data in files of different formats. RFramework can also be linked with other languages such as java and .NET.

Data Mining

Data mining is the term used for discovering new, interesting, and useful patterns from large data sets and applying algorithms for the extraction of hidden information. It builds an efficient predictive or descriptive model which can be used to generate new useful data (Asay, 2014). Different types of software packages can be used for data mining. Generally, Sophisticated search operations are performed in data mining which return targeted specific results. We can say that data mining is a handler that tries to dig out beneficial results from big data which is our asset.

Mahout

This Apache project is a machine learning and data mining library that is used to recognize patterns in data. It generates freely distributed machine learning algorithms which are scalable. Four data science use cases supported by Mahout are: clustering (grouping related documents together), classification (learning to match documents to categories), collaborative filtering (matching users to probable favorites) and frequent pattern matching (identifying items that typically fall into groups together).

Mahout is implemented on top of Hadoop and uses the MapReduce paradigm. It provides data science tools to find meaningful patterns from the big data sets stored on the Hadoop Distributed File System (HDFS).

Weka

Weka was developed at the University of Waikato and is a machine learning library consisting of a number of algorithms and tools for data analysis and predictive modeling. It is Java based and is capable of carrying out the various tasks of data preprocessing, clustering, classification, regression, visualization etc. which are a part of data mining.

RapidMiner

This is a stand-alone application for analysis of data. It is also used for integration with other products. RapidMiner uses Rapid-I scripting language or the R language of statistical modeling and it's learning methods are similar to that of Weka. It is written in Java and can run on multiple platform and operating system. RapidMiner can be used for machine learning, data mining, text mining and predictive analytics.

Databases / Data Warehousing

We know that we prefer NoSQL databases in big data and they are classified into the following four types each suited to different kinds of tasks:

- Document databases (or stores)
- Key-Value stores
- Wide-Column (or Distributed Column) stores
- Graph databases.

Cassandra

This is Apache's database management system which can handle huge amounts of data from various servers. It has the features of both key-value stores and distributed stores and is highly available, scalable and fault tolerant. It is also very efficient at handling bottlenecks and single points of failure. It is good for data critical applications as the data is replicated at multiple nodes using peer to peer replication.

Cassandra is being used in Facebook to power the Inbox Search feature. It is also working for eBay, Twitter, Netflix, Reddit and many more.

HBase

HBase, like Cassandra is a column-oriented key-value store (Datafloq, n.d.), built on Hadoop and is designed to support billions of messages per day. It provides a record based storage layer which helps in fast and random reads and writes to data. HBase is massively scalable, provides high throughput and low latency I/O. Because HBase is tightly integrated with the Hadoop ecosystem, so SQL queries can be used to get data for users and applications. Tools such as Apache Hive, Apache Phoenix and Cloudera Impala can be used for this purpose. It can also get data by faceted free-text search using Cloudera Search. HBase is written in Java and is modeled after Google's BigTable.

MongoDB

MongoDB is a document-oriented database which is cross-platform and is the most popular NoSQL database. The main reason for popularity of MangoDB is that it is very easy to learn (Datafloq, n.d.). It has a balanced approach that can be used for a wide variety of applications. It has the feature of horizontal scalability and can easily work with the diverse data sets due to its flexible data model. MangoDB is being used in Shutterfly's photo platform, Forbes's storage system, eBay's search suggestion and MetLife's "The Wall."

OrientDB

OrientDB is again a NoSQL DBMS which is also written in Java. It is very flexible as it is schema-less, it provides the complexity of the graph model where document records are directly related and is object oriented in nature. It can also function in schema-full and hybrid mode and is very fast.

CouchDB

CouchDB is Apache's NoSQL database which is extremely web-friendly as it uses the following components: It uses JSON for documents, JavaScript for MapReduce queries and HTTP for an API. CouchDB works well with data that does not change very frequently.

Data Aggregation

The data which is processed using big data techniques is scattered over various sources. The process of transforming this scattered data into a single source is data aggregation. The output of the aggregator is smaller than the input because the data from various sources gets combined. This makes the processing task simpler and also reduces the network traffic and increases the performance.

Sqoop

Sqoop (Spidlen et al., 2013) is an Apache product that moves bulk data between Hadoop and structured data stores. It uses MapReduce for importing and exporting data among HDFS, Hive and HBase which provides fault tolerance as well as parallel operation. Sqoop-based connector is used by Microsoft to transfer data from its SQL server databases into Hadoop.

Flume

Flume (Spidlen et al., 2013) is also an Apache product which moves data between applications and Hadoop. It can collect, aggregate and move huge amount of data log. It has a simple fault tolerant architecture based on streaming data flows which can be used for online analytic applications.

Chukwa

Chukwa (Spidlen et al., 2013) is an application built on top of MapReduce framework and Hadoop Distributed File System. It is capable of monitoring, analyzing and displaying results and is very robust and scalable.

Big Data Tools for Healthcare

Some projects specific to the use of big data in healthcare are discussed below:

GenePattern

This is a genomic analysis platform developed at the Broad Institute which has a number of free tools for gene expression analysis, SNP analysis, proteomics, RNA-sequence analysis and flow cytometry.

SpatioTemporal Epidemiological Modeler (STEM)

This is a project developed by IBM and Eclipse foundation which helps enables scientists and public health officials in creating models of emerging infectious diseases as they develop so that there spread could be controlled. IBM along with researchers from University of California, San Francisco and Johns Hopkins University developed this project to create models for spread of dengue and malaria.

This model can predict future spread pattern of the diseases by taking into account the environmental characteristics like temperature, soil conditions and precipitation. STEM helps in correlating all this data with the data of the disease and forecasts the region where the disease could spread next.

CHALLENGES ASSOCIATED WITH USE OF BIG DATA IN HEALTHCARE

There are many challenges associated with analysis of healthcare data using big data concepts. Two main challenges are the technical expertise needed and non-availability of robust and integrated security.

Expertise

Specialized skill sets are needed to process the huge amount of medical data available. But the IT experts in the hospital are only familiar with the SQL programming language and traditional data processing using RDBMS. They are not ready the learn the complexities associated with big data processing. Hence most of the work is carried out only at the research level.

Data scientists who are experts in manipulating the big data environment are employed by organizations to extract the information from it. There are very few experts available with these skill sets and are also very expensive. There is a huge demand for these data scientists specially in the banking and e-business domain.

But the situation is ought to change with the development of new tools which will help people with less-specialized skillsets to work easily with big data. Tools are being developed which can use SQL for querying. Once this happens big data can be used in a big way in the health care sector.

Polybase is a tool developed by Microsoft which uses an extended SQL syntax to query both SQL relational databases and Hadoop Distributed File System (HDFS) systems. Impala is another tool which enables the use of SQL over a Hadoop database. Use of these types of tools will help the big data analytics in healthcare in a great way.

Security

The security and privacy of patient data is of utmost importance in the healthcare sector. Health Insurance Portability and Accountability Act of 1996 (HIPAA) is an act developed in United States that provides data security and privacy provisions for safeguarding medical history of patients. HIPAA compliance is non-negotiable in healthcare. But integrated methods to manage security in big data are still not available. Till the patient information is shared only with a small group of data scientists, it is not a big issue. But once this information has to be shared by a large group of people security becomes the most important concern.

Steps have to be taken by healthcare organizations today to make the patient data secure. We know that big data runs on an open source technology with a lot of inconsistencies with regard to everything including security. The choice of big data vendors for organizations is very crucial to avoid security issues in the future.

Healthcare organizations should go for well supported, commercial software's to implement big data instead of starting with a new Apache distribution which does not consider the security aspect. Cloud-based solution like Azure HDInsight can also be used as a startup option. Cloudera is an example of a well supported secure distribution. This company has created a Hadoop environment which supports authentication, authorization, auditing and data protection. It is a Payment Card Industry (PCI) compliant environment. Other commercially available tools are also trying to ensure that they provide services which are HIPAA complaint so that they can be used in the healthcare industry.

REFERENCES

Asay, M. (2014, November 19). *MongoDB, Cassandra, and HBase -- the three NoSQL databases to watch*. Retrieved from http://www.infoworld.com

Astrom, C., Rocklov, J., Hales, S., Beguin, A., Louis, V., & Sauerborn, R. (2012). Potential distribution of dengue fever under scenarios of climate change and economic development. *EcoHealth*, *9*(4), 448–454. doi:10.100710393-012-0808-0 PMID:23408100

Balaya, S., Paul, S. D., D'Lima, L. V., & Pavri, K. M. (1969). Investigations on an outbreak of dengue in Delhi in 1967. *The Indian Journal of Medical Research*, *57*, 767–774. PMID:5805380

Balcan, D., Hu, H., Goncalves, B., Bajardi, P., Poletto, C., Ramasco, J. J., ... Vespignani, A. (2009). Seasonal transmission potential and activity peaks of the new influenza A(H1N1): A Monte Carlo likelihood analysis based on human mobility. *BMC Medicine*, *7*(1), 45. doi:10.1186/1741-7015-7-45 PMID:19744314

Beatty, M. E., Stone, A., Fitzsimons, D. W., Hanna, J. N., Lam, S. K., Vong, S., ... Margolis, H. S. (2010). Best practices in dengue surveillance: A report from the Asia-Paci c and Americas Dengue Prevention Boards. *PLoS Neglected Tropical Diseases*, *4*(11), e890. doi:10.1371/journal.pntd.0000890 PMID:21103381

Bengtsson, L., Lu, X., Thorson, A., Garfield, R., & von Schreeb, J. (2011). Improved response to disasters and outbreaks by tracking population movements with mobile phone network data: A post-earthquake geospatial study in Haiti. *PLoS Medicine*, *8*(8), e1001083. doi:10.1371/journal.pmed.1001083 PMID:21918643

Bhatt, S., Gething, P. W., Brady, O. J., Messina, J. P., Farlow, A. W., Moyes, C. L., ... Hay, S. I. (2013). The global distribution and burden of dengue. *Nature*, *496*(7446), 504–507. doi:10.1038/nature12060 PMID:23563266

Bian, J., Topaloglu, U., Yu, F., & Yu, F. (2012). *Towards Large-scale Twitter Mining for Drug-related Adverse Events*. Maui, HI: SHB. doi:10.1145/2389707.2389713

Borkar, V. R., Carey, M. J., & Chen, L. (2012). Big data platforms: What's next? *ACM Crossroads*, *19*(1), 44–49. doi:10.1145/2331042.2331057

Carey, D. E., Myers, R. M., Reuben, R., & Rodrigues, F. M. (1966). Studies on dengue in Vellore, South India. *The American Journal of Tropical Medicine and Hygiene*, *15*(4), 580–587. doi:10.4269/ajtmh.1966.15.580 PMID:5949559

Cattuto, C., Van den Broeck, W., Barrat, A., Colizza, V., Pinton, J.-F., & Vespignani, A. (2010). Dynamics of Person-to-Person Interactions from Distributed RFID Sensor Networks. *PLoS One*, *5*(7), e11596. doi:10.1371/journal.pone.0011596 PMID:20657651

Chaturvedi, U. C., Kapoor, A. K., Mathur, A., Chandra, D., Khan, A. M., & Mehrotra, R. M. L. (1970). A clinical and epidemiological study of an epidemic of febrile illness with haemorrhagic manifestations which occurred at Kanpur, India in 1968. *Bulletin of the World Health Organization*, *43*, 281–287. PMID:4249614

Chaturvedi, U. C., Mathur, A., Kapoor, A. K., Mehrotra, N. K., & Mehrotra, R. M. L. (1970). Virological study of an epidemic of febrile illness with haemorrhagic manifestations at Kanpur, India, during 1968. *Bulletin of the World Health Organization*, *43*, 289–293. PMID:5312525

Chaudhuri, R. N., Saha, T. K., & Chaudhuri, A. D. (1965). Dengue-like fever in Calcutta: Further preliminary observations. *Bulletin of the Calcutta School of Tropical Medicine*, *13*, 2–3. PMID:14281058

Datafloq. (n.d.). Retrieved from https://datafloq.com/big-data-open-source-tools/os-data-aggregation/

Dean, J., & Ghemawat, S. (2008). MapReduce: Simplified data processing on large clusters. *Communications of the ACM*, *51*(1), 107–113. doi:10.1145/1327452.1327492

Deepak. (2016). *A Critical Comparison of NOSQL Databases in the Context of Acid and Base*. Culminating Projects in Information Assurance. Paper 8.

Eysenbach, G. (2009). Infodemiology and infoveillance: Framework for an emerging set of public health informatics methods to analyze search, communication and publication behavior on the Internet. *Journal of Medical Internet Research*, *11*(1), e11. doi:10.2196/jmir.1157 PMID:19329408

Feldman, B., Martin, E. M., & Skotnes, T. (2012). *Big Data in Healthcare Hype and Hope*. Retrieved from http://www.west-info.eu/files/big-data-in- healthcare.pdf

Ferreira, G. L. (2012). Global dengue epidemiology trends. *Revista do Instituto de Medicina Tropical de São Paulo*, *54*(Suppl 18), S5–S6. doi:10.1590/S0036-46652012000700003 PMID:23011450

Ghosh, B. N. (1968). A study on the epidemic of dengue-like fever in Pondicherry (1964-65 and 1965-66). *Journal of the Indian Medical Association*, *51*, 261–264. PMID:5706900

Gonzalez, M. C., Hidalgo, C. A., & Barabasi, A.-L. (2008). Understanding individual human mobility patterns. *Nature*, *453*(7196), 779–782. doi:10.1038/nature06958 PMID:18528393

Green, M. D., Freedman, D. M., & Gordis, L. (2000). *Reference guide on epidemiology. Reference manual on scientific evidence*. Available: http://www.fjc.gov/public/pdf.nsf/lookup/sciman06.pdf/$file/sciman06.pdf

Gubler, D. J. (2002). The global emergence/resurgence of arboviral diseases as public health problems. *Archives of Medical Research*, *33*(4), 330–342. doi:10.1016/S0188-4409(02)00378-8 PMID:12234522

Gubler, D. J. (2011). Dengue, Urbanization and Globalization: The Unholy Trinity of the 21(st) Century. *Tropical Medicine and Health*, *39*(Suppl 4), 3–11. doi:10.2149/tmh.2011-S05 PMID:22500131

Gubler, D. J. (2012). The economic burden of dengue. *The American Journal of Tropical Medicine and Hygiene*, *86*(5), 743–744. doi:10.4269/ajtmh.2012.12-0157 PMID:22556068

Guzman, M. G., & Kouri, G. (2002). Dengue: An update. *The Lancet Infectious Diseases*, *2*(1), 33–42. doi:10.1016/S1473-3099(01)00171-2 PMID:11892494

IBM. (2013). *Southern Denmark Tackles Heart Disease with IBM Big Data Analytics Program*. Press Release.

IBM. (n.d.). *Big data and information management*. Retrieved from http://www-01.ibm.com/soft ware/data/bigdata/

IHTT. (2013). *Transforming Health Care through Big Data Strategies for leveraging big data in the health care industry*. Retrieved from http://ihealthtran.com/ wordpress/2013/03/iht%C2%B2-releases-big-data-research-report- download-today/

Karamchandani, P. V. (1946). Dengue group of fevers in India. *Lancet*, *1*(6386), 92–93. doi:10.1016/S0140-6736(46)91229-9 PMID:21011278

Kelly, J. (2013). *Apache drill brings sql-like, ad hoc query capabilities to big data*. Retrieved from http://wikibon.org/wiki/v/Apache-Drill-Brings-SQL-Like-Ad-Hoc-Query-Capabilities-to-Big-Data

Khoury, M. J., & Ioannidis, J. P. (2014). Big data meets public health. *Science, 3466213*(6213), 1054–1055. doi:10.1126cience.aaa2709 PMID:25430753

Khoury, M. J., & Wei, G. (2015). The future of epidemiology in the era of precision medicine: cancer, cardiovascular disease, and beyond [Web log post]. Retrieved from http://epi.grants.cancer.gov/blog/archive/2015/08-11.html

Krishnamurthy, K., Kasturi, T. E., & Chittipantulu, G. (1965). Clinical and pathological studies of an outbreak of dengue-like illness in Visakhapatnam. *The Indian Journal of Medical Research, 53*, 800–812. PMID:5830412

Lauer, M. S. (2012). Time for a creative transformation of epidemiology in the United States. *Journal of the American Medical Association, 30817*(17), 1804–1805. doi:10.1001/jama.2012.14838 PMID:23117782

Lee, K.-H., Lee, Y.-J., Choi, H., Chung, Y. D., & Moon, B. (2012). Parallel data processing with MapReduce: A survey. *SIGMOD Record, 40*(4), 11–20. doi:10.1145/2094114.2094118

Lopez, D., Gunasekaran, M., & Murugan, B. S. (2014) Spatial Big Data Analytics of Influenza Epidemic in Vellore, India. *Proceedings: IEEE International Conference on Big Data. IEEE International Conference on Big Data*, 19–24.

Lynch, C., & Roper, C. (2011). The transit phase of migration: Circulation of malaria and its multi-drug-resistant forms in Africa. *PLoS Medicine, 8*(5), e1001040. doi:10.1371/journal.pmed.1001040 PMID:21655316

Malviya, A., Udhani, A., & Soni, S. (2016). R-tool: Data analytic framework for big data. *Symposium on Colossal Data Analysis and Networking (CDAN)*. 10.1109/CDAN.2016.7570960

Merler, S., Ajelli, M., Pugliese, A., & Ferguson, N. M. (2011). Determinants of the spa- tiotemporal dynamics of the 2009 H1N1 pandemic in Europe: Implications for real- time modelling. *PLoS Computational Biology, 7*(9), e1002205. doi:10.1371/journal.pcbi.1002205 PMID:21980281

Mooney, S. J., Westreich, D. J., & El-Sayed, A. M. (2015). Epidemiology in the Era of Big Data. *Epidemiology (Cambridge, Mass.), 26*(3), 390–394. doi:10.1097/EDE.0000000000000274 PMID:25756221

Mossong, J., Hens, N., Jit, M., Beutels, P., Auranen, K., & Mikolajczak, R. (2008). Social contacts and mixing patterns relevant to the spread of infectious diseases. *PLoS Medicine, 5*(3), e74. doi:10.1371/journal.pmed.0050074 PMID:18366252

Mukhopadhyay, A., Maulik, U., Bandyopadhyay, S., & Coello, C. A. C. (2014). A survey of multiobjective evolutionary algorithms for data mining: Part I. *IEEE Transactions on Evolutionary Computation, 18*(1), 4–19. doi:10.1109/TEVC.2013.2290086

Murray, N.E.A., Quam, M.B., & Wilder-Smith, A. (2013). Epidemiology of dengue: past, present and future prospects. *Clinical Epidemiology, 5*, 299–309.

Myers, R. M., Carey, D. E., Banerjee, K., Reuben, R., & Ramamurti, D. V. (1968). Recovery of dengue type 3 virus from human serum and *Aedes aegypti* in South India. *The Indian Journal of Medical Research, 56*, 781–787. PMID:5680412

Network, T. S. B. D. A. (2013). *Big Data Analytics A Research and Innovation Agenda for Sweden*. The Swedish Big Data Analytics Network Sweden.

Ohlhorst, F. (2012). *Big Data Analytics: Turning Big Data into Big Money*. John Wiley & Sons. doi:10.1002/9781119205005

Paul, S. D., Dandawate, C. N., Banerjee, K., & Krishnamurthy, K. (1965). Virological and serological studies on an outbreak of dengue-like illness in Visakhapatnam, Andhra Pradesh. *The Indian Journal of Medical Research, 53*, 777–789. PMID:5830410

PCAST. (2014). P.s.C.o.A.o.S.a.T., Big Data and Privacy: a Technological Perspective. Washington, DC: White House.

Pentland, A., & Pentland, S. (2008). *Honest signals: how they shape our world*. Cambridge, MA: MIT Press.

Philip Chen, C. L., & Zhang, C.-Y. (2014). Data-intensive applications, challenges, techniques and technologies: A survey on Big Data. *Inform. Sci., 275*, 314–347. doi:10.1016/j.ins.2014.01.015

Podesta, J., Pritzker, P., Moniz, E. J., Holdren, J., & Zients, J. (2014). *Big data: seizing opportunities, preserving values*. Executive Office of the President. Report. Retrieved from: https://obamawhitehouse.archives.gov/sites/default/files/docs/big_data_privacy_report_may_1_2014.pdf

Raghupathi, W., & Kesh, S. (2007). Interoperable electronic health records design: towards a service-oriented architecture. *e-Service Journal, 5*, 39–57.

Raghupathi, W., & Raghupathi, V. (2013). *An Overview of Health Analytics*. Working paper.

Ramakrishanan, S. P., Gelfand, H. M., Bose, P. N., Sehgal, P. N., & Mukharjee, R. N. (1964). The epidemic of acute haemorrhagic fever, Calcutta, 163: Epidemiological inquiry. *The Indian Journal of Medical Research, 52*, 633–650. PMID:14195504

Salathe, M., Kazandjieva, M., Lee, J. W., Levis, P., Feldman, M. W., & Jones, J. H. (2010). A high- resolution human contact network for infectious disease transmission. *Proceedings of the National Academy of Sciences of the United States of America, 107*(51), 22020–22025. doi:10.1073/pnas.1009094108 PMID:21149721

Sarkar, J. K., Pavri, K. M., Chatterjee, S. N., Chakravarty, S. K., & Aanderson, C. R. (1964). Virological and serological studies of cases of haemorrhagic fever in Calcutta. *The Indian Journal of Medical Research, 52*, 684–691. PMID:14195508

Shepard, D. S., Undurraga, E. A., & Halasa, Y. A. (2013). Economic and disease burden of dengue in Southeast Asia. *PLoS Neglected Tropical Diseases, 7*(2), e2055. doi:10.1371/journal.pntd.0002055 PMID:23437406

Singh & Reddy. (2014). A survey on platforms for big data analytics. *Journal of Big Data, 1*, 8. PMID:26191487

Spidlen, Barsky, Breuer, Carr, Nazaire, Hill, … Qian. (2013). GenePattern flow cytometry suite. *Source Code for Biology and Medicine, 8*(1), 14. doi:10.1186/1751- 0473-8-14

Stehle, J., Voirin, N., Barrat, A., Cattuto, C., Colizza, V., Isella, L., ... Vanhems, P. (2011). Simulation of an SEIR infectious disease model on the dynamic contact network of conference attendees. *BMC Medicine*, *9*(1), 87. doi:10.1186/1741-7015-9-87 PMID:21771290

Szlezak, N., Evers, M., Wang, J., & Perez, L. (2014). The role of big data and advanced analytics in drug discovery, development, and commercialization. *Nature*, *95*(5), 492–495. PMID:24642713

Tatem, A. J., Qiu, Y., Smith, D. L., Sabot, O., Ali, A. S., & Moonen, B. (2009). The use of mobile phone data for the estimation of the travel patterns and imported Plasmodium falciparum rates among Zanzibar residents. *Malaria Journal*, *8*(1), 287. doi:10.1186/1475-2875-8-287 PMID:20003266

WHO. (2009). *Dengue: Guidelines for Diagnosis, Treatment, Prevention and Control.* Geneva: World Health Organization.

WHO. (2012a). *Dengue and severe dengue: Fact Sheet No 117*. Geneva: World Health Organization (WHO). Available from: http://www.who.int/mediacentre/factsheets/ fs117/en/index.html

WHO. (2012b). *Global Strategy for Dengue Prevention and Control, 2012–2020*. Geneva: WHO Press.

WHO. (2013). *TDR Global Alert and Repsonse Dengue/Dengue Haemorrhagic Fever* Geneva: World Health Organization (WHO). Available from: http://www.who. int/csr/disease/dengue/en/index.html

WHO. (2014). Mobile phones help people with diabetes to manage fasting and feasting during Ramadan. *Features 2014*.

Wilder-Smith, A., & Gubler, D. J. (2008). Geographic expansion of dengue: The impact of international travel. *The Medical Clinics of North America*, *92*(6), 1377–1390. doi:10.1016/j.mcna.2008.07.002 PMID:19061757

Zenger, B. (2012). Can Big Data Solve Healthcare's Big Problems? *HealthByte*. Retrieved from: http://www.equityhealthcare.com/docstor/EH%20Blog%20on%20Analytics.pdf

Zikopoulos, P.C., DeRoos, D., Parasuraman, K., Deutsch, T., Corrigan, D., & Giles, J. (2013). *Harness the Power of Big Data*. McGraw-Hill.

Chapter 14
Artificial Intelligence in Medical Science

Shashwati Mishra
Utkal University, India

Mrutyunjaya Panda
Utkal University, India

ABSTRACT

The use of intelligent artificial devices has solved many real-world problems and also improved the living style of human beings. The capability of providing unbiased and accurate result has also increased the demand for these devices. For getting faster and well-organized outcomes, scientists and researchers are giving more and more interest in developing such devices. Use of expert systems, concepts from nature-inspired algorithms, neural networks, genetic algorithms, fuzzy logic, internet of things are used extensively to solve various problems in science and engineering. In medical science these techniques are used for data analysis, disease diagnosis, data retrieval, object detection, pattern analysis, data management, monitoring patient health status by physicians, interactions between patients and physicians, keeping record of the medications of the patients, and so on. This chapter performs a detailed analysis on the use of intelligent devices in medical science and about the root concepts on which these devices are designed.

INTRODUCTION

Any device or machine having its own computation ability is considered as intelligent. With the advancement of technology, many intelligent devices are developed with less expense having high computational and analytical ability. These characteristics of intelligent devices have increased the demand of these devices in engineering, medical science, space research, geological survey, automobiles, traffic control and many more. The intelligent devices have the capability to learn like a human being and solve many real-world problems in an intelligent manner. In many cases, they are replacing human beings and giving more accurate and faster results than humans. Such type of systems have the ability of learning from past experience, communicating with other devices to gather and share information. The storage capacity

DOI: 10.4018/978-1-5225-7071-4.ch014

and processing speed of these devices are much higher than the human brain which has increased the popularity of these devices. These devices are used to solve many sensitive and sophisticated problems in medical field. The systems also have the capability to solve many problems using past information and data stored in the form of a knowledge base.

Intelligent systems consist of devices which are intelligent in nature and have the capability to work on software designed using the concepts from Artificial Intelligence as well as having network connectivity. Figure 1 shows the characteristics of an intelligent system.

Intelligent devices use their analytical ability on the defined set of information in the form of rules to obtain a conclusion. Humans learn from experience, machines derive new rules from existing rules using inference mechanism. Machine also have the analytical and reasoning ability like human beings. The computing capability of machine is more as compared to humans. Machine also has the ability to process different languages so that they can interact with people and can store and analyse the information stored in different languages.

Components of Artificial Intelligence

Artificial intelligence involves different sub-areas like neural network, fuzzy logic, genetic algorithm, evolutionary algorithms, natural language processing, expert systems which play a vital role in the construction of an intelligent machine. Neural networks are popularly used in object recognition, face recognition, handwritten character recognition, information retrieval, classification of information etc. Now-a-days development in neural network called deep learning techniques are used in the learning of intelligent devices. Fuzzy logic concept is used in recognizing patterns, vehicle control equipment, different electronic equipment like washing machines, air conditioners, vacuum cleaners etc. Expert systems help in medical diagnosis and monitoring, financial advice and suggestions etc. Natural Language Processing techniques are used for speech and voice recognition, analysis and interpretation. Internet of Things is a new technique which uses networking and sensor technologies to provide better healthcare facilities to the patients.

Figure 1. Characteristics of intelligent systems

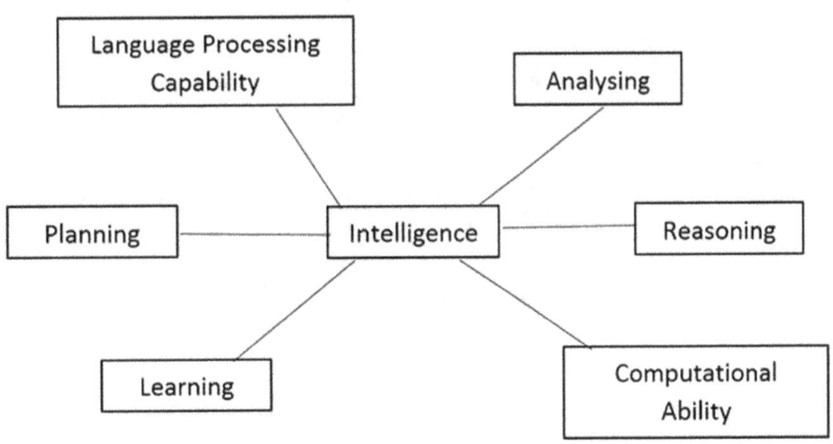

Neural Network

The concept of artificial neural network is based on the design and functioning of human brain which is the root cause of thinking, analysis, computing, reasoning power of human being. Scientists and researchers have tried to implement the same concept in the design of artificial neural network which can mimic a human brain. A typical artificial neural network consists of three layers, one input layer, one hidden layer and one output layer. Some neural networks may consist of more than one hidden layers. Each layer consists of a set of nodes and nodes in one layer are connected with the nodes in other layers through weighted links. A node in a neural network corresponds to the neurons in human brain and weighted connections are a representative of nerve synapses (Berner, E. S., 2007). A diagram of neural network having two hidden layers along with input and output layers is given in Figure 2.

Fuzzy Logic

The crisp set assumes that an object either belongs to a set or cannot be a member of the set, accordingly it assigns two possible values true (1) or false (0). The fuzzy set theory says the probability that an object is a member of a set varies between 0 and 1. Thus besides full membership value (1) and no membership value (0), it also considers partial belongingness by assigning a value between 0 and 1. Membership function also known as characteristic function is used to find the membership value of the elements in the set. The concept of membership functions is first introduced Lofti A. Zadeh in 1965. Gaussian, Triangular, Trapezoidal, Sigmoid, Generalised Bell are some examples of membership functions. Fuzzification is the process of converting a crisp set to fuzzy set and defuzzification is the process of converting a fuzzy set to crisp set.

Figure 2. Neural network

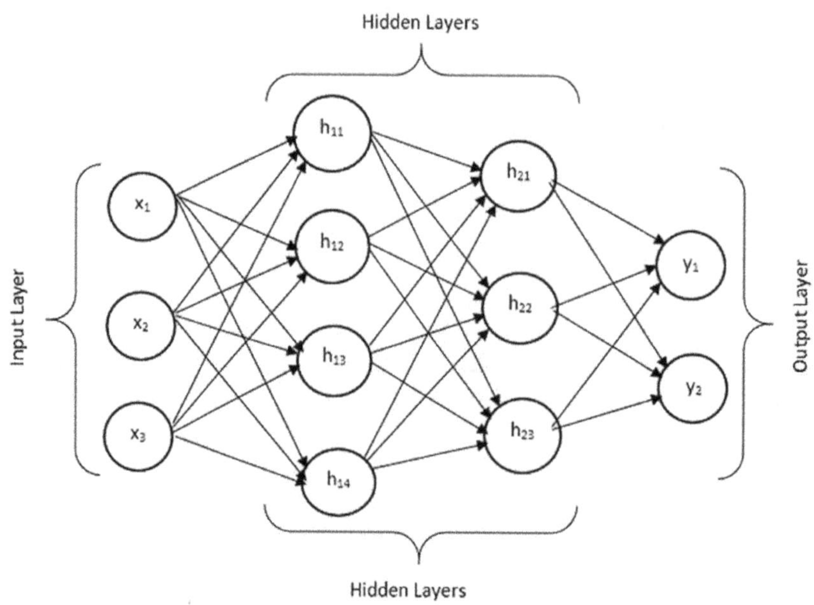

Genetic Algorithm

The concept of genetic algorithm came from the theory of evolution which is based on the concept of natural selection. Theory of evolution says during the natural selection process the fittest individual survives and participates in the natural selection process with the next generation offsprings. New generations gradually adopt to the change in environments. Like neural network it does not possess any knowledge base and tries to find out the solution from the patient data. For finding the solution of a particular problem genetic algorithm initially chooses a random set of solutions for the problem to solve. Among these solutions the best ones are selected on which crossover and mutation techniques are applied to generate next generation solutions. This process of finding solutions at different generations continues until the required solution is obtained (Berner, E. S., 2007).

Nature Inspired Algorithms

Another category of algorithms used are bio-inspired algorithms, which are inspired by biological behaviour of different species of living beings. These algorithms are basically used for solving optimization problems and use a fitness function to find the optimal value. These optimal results can be used for different types of classification and prediction problems. Some examples of bio-inspired algorithms are particle swarm optimization, ant colony optimization, cuckoo search, bat algorithm, artificial bee colony optimization, Harmony search, Firefly algorithm, Hunting search etc. (Fister Jr, I. et al., 2013).

Deep Learning

Biomedical data are heterogeneous, complex and high-dimensional in nature and comprised of different categories of data like textual data, data in the form of image and electronic format, data collected using sensors. Traditional approach use feature selection and extraction techniques to extract features from these complex set of biomedical data. Classification or clustering or prediction techniques are then applied on these set of extracted features for getting the final result. This process has now been replaced with new advanced deep learning technique. Traditional techniques generally use a linear transformation on the input data to find the relationship between the inputs for prediction and classification. To overcome the limited capability of traditional methods, machine learning techniques are used to find relationship between the input data. A learning system helps in discovering the dependency between input data. In contrast to conventional machine learning techniques, deep learning based models consist of multilayer neural network, where each layer provides a level of abstraction. As compared to a typical artificial neural network, the number of hidden layers are more in deep learning. Each layer performs some type of processing, taking input from its previous layer and giving output to the next layer. The neural network model for a given input dataset is generated through the process of learning ((Miotto, R. et al., 2017)). Deep learning techniques are used to process medical images like brain MRI scans to predict Alzheimer disease and other types of brain diseases (Liu, S. et al., 2014, April), (Brosch, T. et al., 2013, September), knee MRI to predict the probability of osteoarthritis (Prasoon, A., et al., 2013, September). Deep learning is also applied on ultrasound (Cheng, J. Z. et al., 2016) and 3D MRI (Yoo, Y. et al., 2014, September) images. Learning through deep neural network is also proved to be useful in detecting different types of skin cancer (Esteva, A., et al., 2017).

Both structured and unstructured medical records in electronic form can also be processed using deep learning techniques. Different performance measurement parameters like sensitivity, specificity, accuracy, ROC (Receiver Operating Characteristic) curve, RMSE (Root Mean Square Error) are used to evaluate the effectiveness of the model in prediction and classification. Deep learning is applied on the medical record of the patient to predict heart failure and pulmonary disease. Deep learning is also used for diagnosing a disease, predicting the disease risk, getting a suggestion regarding the required medication for a disease and predicting the future disease possibility. In mobile healthcare and genomics also deep learning is used popularly for prediction. ((Miotto, R. et al., 2017))

Though deep learning is used to develop intelligent devices to manage healthcare system, still there are a number of issues which need to be resolved. Medical data are unstructured, noisy, incomplete and heterogeneous in nature. Several factors like redundancy, data types, missing values, need to be considered for designing a deep architecture for medical data. To develop an appropriate prediction model, deep learning techniques need a huge volume of data. In healthcare system, it is very difficult to find such a huge volume of data for all types of diseases. The list of number of diseases and their variations is also large and it is very complex to understand all the disease characteristics and their variations. Generating relationships between different variants of a disease make the network complicated. Medical data is dynamic in nature; the patient disease type, disease status changes with time. Normally deep learning model considers static data as input, so handling time varying medical data is also a challenge for research community. Physicians often need to know why certain medication is predicted by deep learning technique for a disease symptom or disease as input. It is very difficult to interpret in a deep architecture because deep network does not give any information about the internal processing, why certain output is obtained from a layer, why some layer is connected with a specific layer and so on. This poor interpretability of deep learning creates a problem especially in healthcare management ((Miotto, R. et al., 2017)).

Though deep learning has so many challenges, the multilayer hierarchical learning architecture gives better prediction result integrating heterogeneous data and helps physicians in diagnosis and taking patient care ((Miotto, R. et al., 2017)).

Table 1 presents a detailed analysis on various AI techniques like neural network, fuzzy logic, genetic algorithm nature inspired computing. This proves that these approaches are used in medical science in solving different types of disease like diabetes, heart disease, eye problems, tuberculosis, cancer and many more. The techniques are applied for prediction, classification, segmentation, diagnosis etc. Neural networks basically used for prediction, classification and diagnosis. Fuzzy logic is used to generate fuzzy rules which helps in taking decision and feature selection. Genetic algorithms and nature inspired algorithms are primarily used for optimization and selection of optimal features, or optimal population to get a better result. Neuro-genetic approach gives better result in comparison to simple neural network based solution. This is possible due to the selection of optimal features or values by the use of genetic algorithm. It is also found that sometimes fuzzy-genetic approach gives better performance than neuro-genetic. The accuracy of result also depends on the type, nature and characteristics of the dataset. Advanced neural network techniques like convolutional neural network, deep neural network gave better result as compared to the traditional neural network method. Some of the characteristics of these AI components are given in table 2.

Table 1. Analysis on the use of AI techniques in medical science

Reference	Purpose	Medical Data	Method Used	Efficiency Comparison (If Any)
(Venkatesan, P., & Anitha, S., 2006)	Diagnosis	Diabetes	RBF, MLP, Classical Logistic Regression	Better performance as compared to Multilayer Perceptron and Logistic regression
(Karegowda, A. G., et al., 2011)	Diagnosis	PIMA Indian Diabetes	Genetic Algorithm and Back Propagation Network	GA optimized BPN gives better performance as compared to BPN without GA optimization
(Pappada, S. M. et al., 2008)	Glucose Concentration Prediction	Type-1 Diabetes Patients	Neural Network	-----
(Pappada, S. M. et al., 2011).	Real Time Prediction of Glucose	Insulin Dependent Patients	Feed Forward Neural Network	-----
(Jayalakshmi, T., & Santhakumaran, A., 2010)	Classification	PIMA Indian Diabetes	Artificial Neural Network	99% accuracy
(Kim, J. et al., 2018)	Genetic Prediction	Type-2 Diabetes	Deep Neural Network, Logistic Regression	DNN is a versatile tool as compared to Logistic Regression
(Ashiquzzaman, A. et al., 2018)	Prediction	PIMA Indian Diabetes	Deep Learning Neural Network	Dropout layers were used to minimize overfitting
(Ndaba, M. et al., 2018)	Type II Diabetes Classification	PIMA Indian Diabetes	Improved Generalised Regression Neural Network using enhanced k-means clustering	86% accuracy
(Ali, J. B. et al., 2018)	Blood Glucose Level Prediction (Type-1 Diabetes)	Continuous Glucose Monitoring Data	Artificial Neural Network	----------------
(Kurt, I. et al., 2008)	Coronary Artery Disease (CAD) Prediction	Dataset containing records of patients having CAD and not having CAD	Logistic Regression, Multilayer Perceptron, Classification and Regression Tree, Self-Organising Maps, Radial Basis Function	MLP gave best prediction result
(Das, R. et al., 2009)	Heart Disease Diagnosis	Cleveland heart disease database	Neural Network	89.01% accuracy
(Fidele, B. et al., 2009)	Cardiovascular Disease Prediction	Long Beach Dataset	Artificial Neural Network	---------------
(Acharya, U. R. et al., 2018)	Shockable and Non-shockable Life-threatening Ventricular Arrhythmias Identification	Electrocardiogram (ECG) Segments	Convolutional Neural Network	93.18% accuracy
(Ando, Y. et al., 2018)	Liver Transplantation Survival Prediction	United Network for Organ Sharing Database	Artificial Neural Network	-------------
(Acharya, U. R. et al., 2018)	Congestive Heart Failure Diagnosis	Electrocardiogram Signal	Deep Convolutional Neural Network	Maximum accuracy of 98.97%
(Savalia, S., et al., 2017)	Cardiovascular Disease Classification	Physiobank Database, Normal Sinus Rhythm database (NSR-DB) and MIT/BIH Arrhythmia database	Artificial Neural Network	Tachycardia, Bradycardia, first-degree Atrioventricular (AV), and second-degree Atrioventricular diseases are identified
(Zreik, M. et al., 2017).	Left Ventricle Segmentation	Cardiac CT angiography scans	Convolutional Neural Network	-------------
(Arabasadi, Z. et al., 2017)	Heart Disease Detection	Z-Alizadeh Sani dataset	Genetic Algorithm and Neural Network	93.85% accuracy
(Wachinger, C. et al., 2018).	Neuroanatomy Segmentation	T1-weighted Magnetic Resonance Images.	Deep Convolutional Neural Network	----------------
(Esteva, A. et al., 2017)	Skin Cancer Classification	Clinical images	Deep Neural Networks	---------------
(Ishioka, J. et al., 2018)	Prostate Cancer Diagnosis	Magnetic Resonance images	Convolutional Neural Network	-----------------
(Hirasawa, T. et al., 2018)	Gastric Cancer Detection	Endoscopic Images, Stomach Images	Convolutional Neural Network	---------------
(Arulmurugan, R. & Anandakumar, H., 2018)	Lung Cancer Detection	Thoracic Computed Tomography Pictures	Feed Forward Back Propagation Neural Network, Feed Forward Neural Network	Feed forward back propagation neural network gave better results (92.6% accuracy) than feed forward.

continued on following page

Table 1. Continued

Reference	Purpose	Medical Data	Method Used	Efficiency Comparison (If Any)
(Chang, K. et al., 2018)	Isocitrate dehydrogenase (IDH) Status Determination in glioma patients	MR images from Hospital of University of Pennsylvania (HUP), Brigham and Women's Hospital (BWH) and Cancer Imaging Archive (TCIA)	Residual Convolutional Neural Network	85.7% accuracy within test sets. 89.1% accuracy within test sets, considering age at diagnosis.
(Ahmed, I. O. et al., 2018)	Eye Melanoma Classification	Prediagnosed Sample Images	Artificial Neural Network	85% accuracy
(Tan, J. H. et al., 2018)	Age-related Macular Degeneration (AMD) Detection	AMD images.	Deep Convolutional Neural Network	91.17% accuracy using the blindfold and 95.45% accuracy using ten-fold cross-validation strategies.
(Sharma, M. et al., 2018)	Diabetic Retinopathy Detection	DIARETDB0 Database	Modular Feed Forward Neural Network	100% accuracy for normal retinal images and 86.67% accuracy for abnormal retinal images
(Pati, S. K. et al.,2018)	Selection of significant genes for cancer diagnosis	microarray data sets	Genetic Algorithm, Support Vector Machine Classifier	Proximity Mutation technique is used for preserving the population diversity.
(Pawar, M. M., & Talbar, S. N. 2018)	Breast Cancer Diagnosis	Mammogram image	Genetic Algorithm, Fuzzy Classifier	-------------
(Aličković, E. & Subasi, A., 2017)	Breast Cancer Diagnosis	Wisconsin Breast Cancer datasets	Genetic algorithm, Rotation forest	99.48% accuracy
(de Carvalho Filho, A. O. et al., 2017)	Lung nodules diagnosis	Image Database Consortium and Image Database Resource Initiative (LIDC-IDRI)	Genetic algorithm, SVM	92.52% accuracy
(Choubey, D. K. et al., 2017)	Classification	PIMA Indian Diabetes	Genetic algorithm, Naïve Bayes	78.6957% accuracy
(Babaoglu, İ. et al., 2010)	coronary artery disease (CAD) determination	Exercise stress testing (EST) data	Binary Particle Swarm Optimization, Genetic Algorithm, Support Vector Machine Classifier	BPSO extracts better features than GA
(Deekshatulu, B. L. & Chandra, P., 2013)	Heart Disease Classification	Weather, breast cancer, heart stalog, lymphography, hypothyroid, primary tumor from UCI repository and corporate hospitals in Andhra Pradesh	Genetic algorithm, k-nearest neighbour classifier	Accuracy varies from 75.8 to 100%
(Elveren, E. & Yumuşak, N., 2011)	Tuberculosis Disease Diagnosis	Tuberculosis dataset	Genetic algorithm, Multilayer neural network	---------------
(Sharma, P. & Saxena, K., 2017)	Heart disease risk level prediction	Cleveland dataset, UCI machine learning data	Fuzzy logic, Genetic algorithm	--------------------
(Nilashi, M. et al., 2017)	Breast Cancer Classification	Wisconsin Breast Cancer and Mammographic mass datasets	Expectation Maximization, Classification and Regression Trees, Principal Component Analysis, Fuzzy rule-based method	93.2% accuracy- WBCD 94.1% accuracy - Mammographic mass dataset
(Abood, Z. M. et al., 2017)	Red Blood Cells Classification	Collected blood samples (Baghdad city)	Fuzzy Logic	98% accuracy
(Poongothai, S. et al., 2017)	Diabetes classification	PIMA Indian diabetes	Fuzzy, Artificial Neural Network, Fuzzy Genetic, Neuro Genetic	Fuzzy Genetic hybrid approach gives the best result.
(Reddy, G. T. & Khare, N., 2017)	Heart Disease Prediction	Publicly available UCI datasets, that is, Cleveland, Hungarian and Switzerland datasets	OFBAT (Oppositional Firefly BAT algorithm, RBFL (Rule-based Fuzzy Logic)	78% accuracy
(Shrivastava, P. et al., 2017)	Parkinson's disease identification	Datasets of gait and speech of Parkinson's patients.	Particle Swarm Optimization, Genetic algorithm, Modified Cuckoo search, Binary BAT algorithm for optimal feature selection and neural network classifier	Binary BAT selects better features than others.

Table 2. Comparative study of AI techniques

Technique Used	Purpose
Neural Network	• Classification • Diagnosis • Predictions
Genetic Algorithm	• Feature Selection • Finding better population for classification and diagnosis • Optimization • Best model selection
Fuzzy Logic	• Decision making • Rule generation • Rule-based reasoning • Rule-based classification
Nature Inspired Algorithms	• Optimization • Optimal Feature Selection

Expert System

An expert system basically keeps information related to a particular area in a knowledge base and an inference engine. Such systems have the capability to take decision like an expert using the if-then rules. New rules can also be inferred from the existing system using reasoning to solve different types of problems. These systems can also be capable of giving explanation of taking a particular decision. Normally a computer program can be updated, understood by a computer professional which creates a barrier in its use by the people of other specialisations. But in an expert system the rules are written in such a way that it can be updated and understood by an expert in that field. This makes the maintenance of the system easy and flexible to use. Expert systems are widely used for planning, diagnosis, prediction, monitoring, control, design and many other purposes. Figure 3 shows the architecture of an expert system and table 3 contains information about the use of expert system in medical science.

Figure 3. Expert system architecture

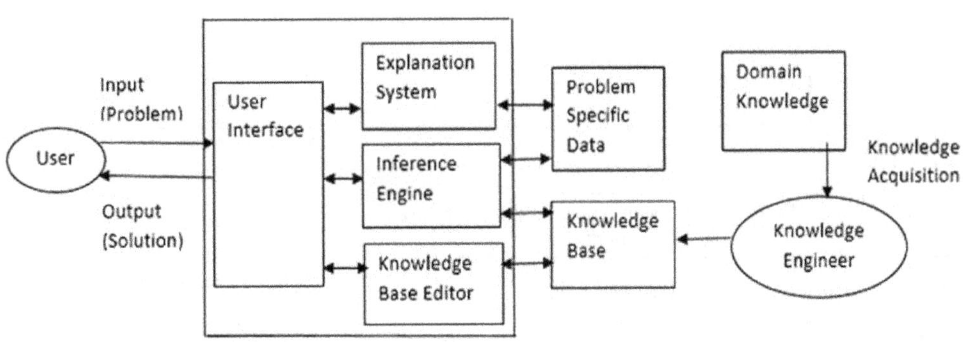

Natural Language Processing

Natural Language Processing focuses on human language data for designing an interactive system that can understand human language and can react accordingly. This requires understanding of natural language, processing of natural language data, generation of natural language symbols, speech recognition etc. Natural language processing involves steps like morphological processing, syntax analysis, semantic analysis, pragmatic analysis for the processing of natural languages (Chowdhury, G. G., 2003).

Intelligent Medical Imaging

Medical images are generated using different techniques like ultrasound, MRI, CT Scan, X-ray etc., each having different modalities. Earlier computer systems have limited storage and processing capabilities. These systems were basically concerned with storage, retrieval of medical images and called as PAC (Picture Archiving and Communication) systems which follow client-server architecture. Specialised software are developed to provide specific services to the corresponding clients. PAC systems can be used when the image is from a single department or having single modality value, but managing images having multiple modalities creates difficulty. To handle such type of images a client software is enquired which can interact and access information from each PAC server.

Like PAC systems RIS (Radiology Information) systems are also designed as a client-server system, but instead of storing image information it stores textual information. RIS systems also need a specific software for information access and it is also not possible to share information between RIS systems of different manufacturers. A PAC and RIS system cannot also exchange information between each other (Hanna, C. J., & O'connor, T. J., 2009).

Like PAC and RIS systems, some machines that are designed for specific departmental activities need specialized software for a specific application. Thus they cannot exchange and share valuable information with each other. To handle this incompatibility problem in PAC systems DICOM (Digital Imaging and Communications in Medicine) standard has been developed. This defines a set of standard datatypes and a standard set of services which use these standard datatypes. Sometimes individual variations can create problem in data interchange and interpretability. Similarly, in case of RIS systems, HL/7 standard is used for the exchange of medical data in healthcare. A PAC system also cannot exchange information with

Table 3. Expert system in medical science

Reference	Disease	Language\ Software
(Qwaider, S. R., & Abu Naser, S. S., 2017)	Ankle Fracture, Fracture of fibula, Ankle Sprain, Rheumatoid Arthritis, Rheumatic Fever, Gout, and Osteoarthritis	SL5 Expert System Language
(Abu Ghali, M. J. et al., 2017)	Teeth and gum problem	SL5 Object language for knowledge based system
(Al Rekhawi, H. A. et al., 2017)	Rickets	SL5 Object language
(Shabut, A. M. et al., 2018)	tuberculosis disease	MATLAB
(Nabahin, A. et al., 2017)	Hair loss	SL5 object
(El Agha, M. et al., 2017)	Polymyalgia Rheumatica	SL5 Object Expert System Language

a RIS system. Another important problem in medical imaging is the storage of images and information about the images is a complex process and is very expensive (Hanna, C. J., & O'connor, T. J., 2009).

Now-a-days advanced techniques are developed for providing better storage, retrieval, exchange and sharing features. Standard diagnostic tools are used in pathology, endoscopy, surgery, cardiology, ophthalmology, dentistry etc.. Due to the use of advanced image processing techniques people are getting their test reports faster as compared to earlier approaches (Hanna, C. J., & O'connor, T. J., 2009).

Internet of Things (IoT)

Internet of Things (IoT) is a new technique developed for enabling communication between physical devices and real-world objects by establishing communication network among these devices. To capture and gather the essential information sensors, cameras are used. In this busy world people neglects their health by not consulting a doctor, not taking their medication in proper time etc. Sometimes they also do not go for regular check-up. In such a scenario, IoT plays a vital role in establishing communication between the patients and the physicians. Sensors and microcontrollers are used to sense information, collect that information, then that information is sent to the cloud from where the information can be accessed by the corresponding medical professional. Patient when wants can also access own medical records from the cloud. Physicians can also monitor the health of a patient over the network with the help of portable health monitoring devices attached to the body of the patient. It also helps in providing proper medication facility to the patients in emergency condition, regular check-up of patient health condition at periodic intervals. This has also inspired the development of different apps using which healthcare facilities can be accessed through smartphones or tablets.

Sometimes patients face a lot of difficulty in getting an appointment to meet a doctor. This is because of large number of patients as compared to number of doctors. In case of emergency condition and serious health condition, many people die due to lack of proper healthcare facility. In such situations IoT based health care facility provides continuous and remote health monitoring facility, using which patients will be under the observation of physicians, physicians can monitor their patients health easily, patients can get the advice of their doctors easily, patients health check-up records can be obtained at regular intervals. (Kodali, R. K. et al., 2015, December)

In healthcare systems IoT sensor can be used for monitoring oxygen levels, heart rate (Rotariu, C., & Manta, V., 2012, September), blood sugar levels, blood pressure, body weight, cholesterol level, body temperature etc.

R. S. H. Istepanian et al. applied the Internet of Things concept for glucose level sensing and and managing diabetes (Istepanian, R. S. et al., 2011). In heart diseases many people die due to lack of proper treatment in the proper time. C. Li et al. proposed a technique to develop a pervasive monitoring system for heart disease. Their proposed system consists of data acquisition part and data transmission part and helps in sending the physical signs and environmental indicators of patients to remote centers (Li, C. et al., 2017). IoT plays a very important role in healthcare by providing real time healthcare facility and regular health updates. These huge volume of data generated by IoT devices also take the help of cloud for analysis. A cloud-centric IoT based framework for monitoring and diagnosing disease was also proposed (Verma, P. & Sood, S. K., 2018).

IoT and its applications in healthcare is represented diagrammatically in Figure 4.

Figure 4. Internet of Things and its Applications

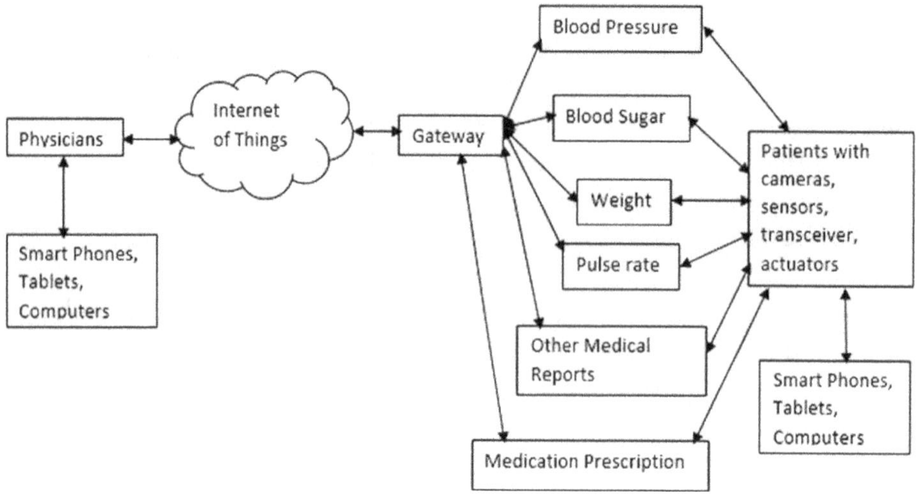

ARTIFICIAL INTELLIGENCE IN MEDICAL SCIENCE

Computer Aided Diagnosis

The 1960s was the period of automated computer diagnosis. The idea was that since computers can perform some tasks in a better way than humans, they can be used in medical field for automated diagnosis and can replace radiologists. But the approach was unsuccessful due to lack of powerful computers and advanced techniques for processing images. A new idea which came in 1980s was computer aided diagnosis which was proposed to assist radiologist to make their work simple and easy (Doi, K., 2007).

Computer aided diagnosis helps in diagnosis of abnormal body parts, detection of affected areas of body and measurement of rate of progress of a disease. Using the techniques of artificial intelligence CAD systems analyse and interpret scanned images. Interpretation results of medical images are affected by the ability and expertise of the physician. CAD systems assist physicians by providing an accurate, better and faster diagnosis. The most important components of a CAD system are the pre-processing unit, feature extraction and selection unit, region of interest extraction unit. During pre-processing step images are refined by removing noise, enhancing brightness and contrast of the image, clear diagnosis of edges of the image. This stage has great impact on the later stages of feature extraction and selection which in turn affects the final result of diagnosis (Stoitsis, J. et al, 2006). Feature extraction and selection technique uses spatial or spectral information for the extraction and selection of appropriate features. Artificial intelligence techniques like genetic algorithms, neural networks are used for feature selection and extraction. After extracting the features classification techniques like naïve Bayesian classifier, fuzzy c-means classifier, neural network based classifiers are used for classification and detection of the region of interest. Computer Aided Diagnosis systems are used for diagnosis of cancer cells (Reeves, A. P., & Kostis, W. J., 2000), tumor detection (Nattkemper, T. W. et al., 2005), (El-Dahshan, E. S. A. et al., 2014), diagnosis of brain disorders (Spetsieris, P. G. et al., 2002) and many more by using Magnetic Resonance Imaging, Computed Tomography Scan and ultrasound images.

The popularity of CAD systems is increasing day by day due to its capability of accurate and faster diagnosis which acts like a boon for radiologist. The CAD systems are developed taking concepts from machine learning and pattern recognition techniques which provides CAD systems learning, analytical, reasoning, computing capability.

In CAD results obtained using computers are used by the radiologist for comparative analysis of their results with computer outputs. A radiologist can confirm the accuracy of the results obtained by comparing with computer generated outputs. The performance of CAD is affected by the expertise, computing, analytic and decision making capability of radiologist whereas in automated computer diagnosis it totally depends on the computer. In CAD computer results can be improved by radiologist. It depends on the radiologist whether to accept or reject the results obtained using computer (Doi, K., 2007). Now-a-days CAD systems are popularly used for detection and diagnosis of diseases, cancer cells and diseased cells in different organs like brain, lungs, stomach, colon, breast, liver, chest, skin, vessels etc. (Doi, K., 2007).

Clinical Decision Support System

The aim of clinical decision support system is to provide support to physicians in making decisions. Health professionals take the help of CDSS to get a better conclusion. The patient information is given as input to the CDSS and the CDSS system uses its own knowledge base or past experience to give suggestions which can be referred by the physicians. Initially these systems were developed for diagnosis purpose, but now-a-days these systems are playing a vital role in patient care. Earlier active involvement of user was there, it was the responsibility of the user to extract important information from the information provided by the decision support system (Berner, E. S., 2007) .

A CDSS may have a knowledge-base or may not have a knowledge base. A CDSS having a knowledge base must also have an inference engine and a technique for communicating with the user. The inference engine uses inference rules for getting conclusions from the patient data using the rules and combinations present in the knowledge base. The input to the system may be given by the user directly or may be taken from the clinical patient record stored electronic format in the computer (Berner, E. S., 2007) .

Diagnostic decision support systems takes as input the disease symptoms, finds the symptoms from the knowledge base, detects the disease with the help of inference engine by using inference rules and suggest the corresponding diagnoses for the physicians. Some systems may give a single diagnosis and some may give more than one diagnosis. Medication support systems helps to provide a proper guidance for medication orders. The test reports or medication orders are given as input to the system. Knowledge base contains information regarding the way of taking medication, doses of medication. In case of any problem an alert is sent to the physicians. Some CDSS systems also control the medication orders. Current medications and newly prescribed medication is given as input to the CDSS system, the system uses the drug information present in the database and outputs the interaction of the new medicine with the old one. Accordingly it can change the order of the medicine if required. Health professionals can also provide their therapy plans as input to the CDSS system, system compares the plan with the information present in the knowledge base and informs the health professionals regarding the effectiveness of the plan. In such type of systems the knowledge base contains therapy guidelines for different types of diseases. (Berner, E. S., 2007)

Knowledge-based systems basically contain information about a specific field or problem, so they are also known as expert systems. Expert system used for patient health monitoring observes the health, pulse rate, blood pressure level, blood glucose level of a patient and informs to the physicians. It also provides reminders and warnings for the proper maintenance of regular medications of a patient. (Coiera, E., 2015)

Decision support systems can also be used for retrieving desired clinical information from a huge collection of information like web search engines. For better information retrieval decision support system must have some knowledge about the diseases, corresponding symptoms and treatments. Filtering the desired information it helps in reducing the time taken for searching the clinical information and makes the task more simple and easy. (Coiera, E., 2015)

Non-knowledge-based systems are developed using machine learning techniques which use past experience for analysis, diagnosis and pattern extraction. Genetic algorithm, artificial neural networks are some examples of non-knowledge-based systems. (Berner, E. S., 2007)

One problem with decision support systems is to keep the information in electronic format which acts as the knowledge base for the system. If sufficient information is not available, then it is difficult to design a knowledge-based decision support system. Sometimes lack of computer knowledge creates difficulty in using such type of systems. (Coiera, E., 2015)

In neural network based systems, the patient medical record is given as input in the input layer. Each node in the input layer represents a specific information of the patient. The weighted connections between nodes help in analysing the association between disease symptoms and predict the corresponding diagnosis result through output layer. Unlike knowledge based systems neural network based systems focus on a short range of symptoms which are generally associated with a single disease. Such type of systems involves two phases, one training phase and other testing phase. During training phase connection weights are decided with the help of disease symptoms as input and corresponding diagnosis as output. After designing a training model the same set of weights are used for diagnosis of the same disease taking a new set of patient symptoms as input. (Berner, E. S., 2007)

The advantages of neural network based system is that they do not need a large database or experts advice for prediction. Diagnosis process does not depend on any inference rules. But the problem with this approach is the time taken during the training phase. Interpreting the correct weights for proper diagnosis is also difficult (Berner, E. S., 2007).

Robotics

The word robot was coined from the Czech word robota, which indicates the work done by slaves forcefully. In different films, TV serials, plays and books robots are represented as mobile machines having intelligence and also having threat to humans. (Katevas, N. (Ed.), 2001)

Since 1960s the technology of using robots started in different fields like building industries, automobile technology, electronics engineering to perform difficult tasks like moving heavy loads from one place to another, assembling different parts of a device. The use of robots in medical field started in 21st century and popularly used to assist surgeons and health professionals. The advantage of using robots in healthcare is like an expert physician. These intelligent machines perform accurate and error free tasks which helps in improving the health condition of the patient. The robotics used in different fields of medical science like therapy treatments, as assistance, simulator, surgery, imaging etc.(Kim, J. et al., 2016)

Traditional robots were designed using rigid materials, so these were inflexible to external barriers and restrictions. With the increased use of robotics in medical field there is a need for robots which should have the capability to improve the environmental difficulties and should be capable of interacting with patients safely. These new generation robots are popularly known as soft robots and mainly build form non-rigid materials like gels, fluids, soft polymers and materials which can be deformed easily. Soft robots are just like living organisms and possess some characteristics to change itself for protection from obstacles just like living beings. In automobile engineering, manufacturing industry, building construction robots generally interact with hard materials. So it is better to use traditional rigid robots in such works. But in medical field a robot interacts with soft materials like sensitive organs, skin, tissues, body parts which require to be handle very carefully. So for healthcare management soft robots are better than the rigid ones.

Foot drop is an abnormal condition in which the patient cannot lift the toes or the foot from ankle. This may happen due to some disease, defect in nervous system, effect of toxic intake, abnormal anatomy etc. Patients suffering from such problem can use a soft active Ankle Foot Orthotic (AFO). In active state AFO becomes stiffen and helps the patient to raise foot. In the inactive state the AFO remains soft and helps in free movement of ankle joint. Similarly a lightweight, thin and comfortable soft hand orthotic can be used for movement of hand, wrist and fingers. Such type of devices help patients to perform their work independently without depending on a caretaker or any other person. Robots can act as assistance for taking care of elderly people and people having disability of moving from one place to another. Such robots are known as co-robots or assistive robots. (Majidi, C., 2014)

Virtual Nurses

The day service centers use robots which is capable of understanding the psychology, mental condition, emotion of patients and looks like real animals. To understand the need of patients and fulfil their requirements, such type of intelligent devices must have a processing unit, sound and vision unit, touch sensors, sensors for understanding posture, gesture and emotion. Seal robot is one such type of robots developed to help elderly persons. (Wada, K. et al., 2004) In this busy world giving time for elderly people and taking their proper care in old days (especially when they are bedridden or suffering from serious disease) is a difficult job. Working people are depending on day service centers or a servant to take care of their parents. Intelligent robots are also replacing human beings in taking care of the elderly people thereby reducing the burden of nursing people. Pets affect the emotion of its master greatly, make them happy which indirectly have a positive impact on the health of that person. A large number of study have been performed on how keeping pets affect death rate (Friedmann, E. et al., 1980), changes blood pressure level (Baun, M. M. et al., 1984), social impact of animals (Hart, L. A. et al., 1987), emotional and psychological impact of animals (Garrity, T. F. et al., 1989) etc.

In the United States Animal-Assisted Activities (AAA) and Animal-Assisted Therapy (AAT) are popularly used for in healthcare management and have a great amount of physiological, psychological and social impact. In AAA no goal is set for therapy programs, but in AAT the goal is set by nurses, doctors, physicians, health professionals, social workers with support from volunteers. Small children are more attracted towards pets like dogs and birds and are very much interested to play and interact with them. Considering these aspects therapy dogs and birds are used for small children to make them walk and speak (Kale, M., 1992), (Saldien, J. et al., 2006, September). Besides these, therapy pets are also used to reduce the stress of the people affected by AIDS (Haladay, J., 1989), because in such type of diseases stress greatly affects the immune system of the body. In some hospitals and nursing centers like in Japan do not use Animal Assisted Activities and Therapy for the treatment of patients. Though they agree that there is a positive impact of using pets, but they also assume that there is a negative impact of infection, allergy, bites etc. (Wada, K. et al., 2004)

To overcome the negative impact of using pets humans used its own creativity, scientific and technical knowledge, intelligence, thinking ability to design machines that have intelligence and that behave like pets and also looks like pets. Such pet like robots have physical bodies, have the capability to set their goals, interactive in nature, study and understand emotion of patients, give mental happiness to patients. (Wada, K. et al., 2004) Some robots used as assistants are seal robots (Wada, K. et al., 2004), Furby, AIBO (Fujita, M. and Kitano, H., 1998) etc. Various techniques used for evaluating the effect of robots on patients are study of mental state of patients through questionnaires and interactions, pathological tests, facial expressions etc.

Health Monitoring

In the telecommunication era mobile phones used widely by human beings for communication (both audio and visual), information sharing, messaging etc. The techniques of mobile computing can be combined with health care systems for communication between patients, doctors and health workers which is popularly known as mobile health monitoring system. Small, intelligent, lightweight, low-cost bio-sensor nodes are used for mobile health care which has the capability to process, communicate and sense. These nodes are designed by using advanced technologies from wireless communication, sensor networks and circuit technology. These systems are intelligent in nature and have the capability to provide feedback considering the information collected through sensors. Such type of devices are designed based on a computing mechanism considering the interaction of human and computing devices in the environment in which we work and live. This is known as pervasive computing and its application in health care is called pervasive health monitoring which enables more involvement of the human beings in maintenance of their own health perfect. Some diseases need regular check-up and routine care. But due to lack of time, unwillingness, laziness, inability to go, people neglect their regular check up and do not take the proper care of their health. A smart, intelligent, mobile system is helpful for such persons in getting information about their health status. It will also save their time and help them to maintain proper health and be fit in their busy schedule. (Shahriyar, R. et al., 2009, September)

Stress is the root cause of all type of diseases and health problems, monitoring stress levels can reduce the risk of diseases and enables a person to lead a healthy life. An intelligent sensor can be used to monitor the stress levels of a person which can be informative both for patient and health professionals. A person can get a continuous update about the change in stress levels of its own body. A physician does not need to observe the patient continuously and can get information about the stress levels of its patient when desired. E. Jovanov et al. discussed regarding monitoring stress using an intelligent wireless sensor system which is distributed in nature. Since stress level change affects heart beat rate, heart rate can be used as a quantifier to monitor stress level of an individual. This is essential for military and neuropsychological tests where heart rates are measured before and after exposure to stress. (Jovanov, E. et al., 2003)

Traditional monitors like holter monitors which are used for ECG and EEG monitoring are used for acquiring data. Advancement in communication and wireless technologies it is now possible to develop new generation intelligent monitoring systems which is capable of giving feedback, giving alert in emergency condition or contact a medical service provider. As compared to wireless local area networks, wireless wide area networks provide better mobility and better monitoring to patients. (Jovanov, E. et al., 2003)

The intelligent sensor nodes are small in size, less cost and weight and have the capability to sense, communicate and process symptoms and health factors of body. Such devices can be integrated with wireless body area networks or wireless personal area networks. A number of research is going on to maintain flexibility, security, reliability in such networks by using new developed techniques. (Milenković, A. et al., 2006)

A study says that the number of people in the age 65 years to 80 years is supposed to be more than double in 2025 than it was in 1990. In the last few years the wearable health monitoring devices are used extensively for monitoring pulse signals, activity etc. Integration of sensing technology, wireless technology and circuit technology has open the way for the use of small, integrated sensors in the human body for health monitoring, feedback and suggestions (Milenković, A. et al., 2006) .

Health monitoring systems can be divided into traditional systems and smart intelligent modern systems. These smart systems can again be grouped in three categories mobile health monitoring system, wearable health monitoring system and remote health monitoring system. A detailed study of these health monitoring systems is given by M. M. Baig and H. Gholamhosseini (Baig, M. M., & Gholamhosseini, H., 2013) .

SOME EXAMPLES OF INTELLIGENT SYSTEMS USED IN HEALTHCARE

DeepMind

DeepMind Technologies Limited is a wholly-owned subsidiary of the Google conglomerate, Alphabet Inc. which works on artificial intelligence. Royal Free London NHS (National Health Service) Foundation Trust is publicly funded British healthcare service providers (Powles, J., & Hodson, H., 2017). Google DeepMind received a proposal from Royal Free London NHS Foundation Trust to develop a software using patient record in July 2015. This was initiated by the health professionals who were part of the trust. On 18 November 2015 Royal Foundation sent millions of patient medical record to a server for processing (Powles, J., & Hodson, H., 2017).

DeepMind on 24 February 2016 declared a health project for handling acute kidney injuries with the Royal Free London NHS Foundation Trust. To handle kidney injuries which affect 40,000 people in UK in a year, DeepMind decided to develop an app called 'Streams' (Powles, J., & Hodson, H., 2017).

IBM Watson

IBM Watson is a supercomputer that has the capability to understand natural language. It takes a query in the form of natural language as input, analyses the unstructured data and gives its response. Watson is also able to learn from its success and failure, can improve its prediction process from user feedback. IBM along with some cancer care providers developed Watson to assist medical professionals in taking decisions. The clinical information is given as input to the supercomputer Watson which analyses the inputs and suggests treatment and makes prediction considering guidelines and evidence. Thus it helps in providing standardize patient care in less time which is essential both for the patients and the physicians. For providing better patient care, oncologist has to be updated with the new research findings, scientific discoveries etc. It is very difficult for oncologist to be updated with the new research findings, who handle all types of cancers (Doyle-Lindrud, S., 2015).

IBM along with Memorial Sloan Kettering Cancer Center (MSKCC) in 2012 focused on using the supercomputer in healthcare. Initially the aim was to handle breast and lung cancers by providing updated information to the computer. The health professionals of MSKCC trained the supercomputer Watson using information of 1.2 million patients collected over 20 years (Doyle-Lindrud, S., 2015). When any query is given to Watson, it first produces a number of hypotheses, analyses the data, give a rank to the answers, finds confidence levels for each possible answers and make prediction or gives suggestion. The prediction result and suggestions are also improved and updated by Watson with the change in research findings and development in medical science. Medical professionals can also ask Watson to provide information about the research findings and literature, which is used by the supercomputer for prediction and recommendation (Doyle-Lindrud, S., 2015). Though the initial attempt was for breast and lung cancer, it has been gradually improved and new programs are also added to handle other types of cancers like prostate, ovarian, bladder, colon, cervical, liver, pancreatic, kidney, uterine cancers, lymphoma, melanoma etc. (Doyle-Lindrud, S., 2015).

A pilot program was declared in October 2012 by IBM Watson at the University of Texas MD Anderson Cancer Center. Like MSKCC, Watson also takes medical data as input and gives output considering evidences and analysing the data. Watson has been designed to act as the Oncology Expert Advisor (OEA) and its accuracy is calculated by comparing the suggestions of Watson with the prediction of physicians of the university. The overall accuracy of the predictions given by the supercomputer is 82.6% (Doyle-Lindrud, S., 2015).

IBM had collaborated with WellPoint, Inc., in 2011 to develop a system called Cancer Care Quality Program for streamlining the review process of medical treatments (Doyle-Lindrud, S.,2015).

Physicians analyse the medical records, test reports of patients for diagnosing the health problems of the patient and accordingly suggest the treatment procedures. Analysing the medical records needs time and depends on the expertise of the physicians. M. Devarakonda and C.-H. Tsou proposed a technique to generate medical problem list of a patient in IBM Watson. Electronic Medical Records in the form of clinical notes or semi-structured clinical data are given as input to the system from which terms representing medical concepts are extracted (Devarakonda, M., & Tsou, C. H., 2015, January). UMLS metathesaurus, Natural Language Processing techniques, contextual and sentence structure information are used to generate Concept Unique Identifiers (CUI) for the terms. The CUIs are mapped to SNOMED CT CORE and depending on the result of mapping UMLS hierarchical movement is done. In the nest step features are generated, term frequency, confidence etc. are calculated and finally problems are grouped to generate problem list (Devarakonda, M., & Tsou, C. H., 2015, January).

Babylon Medical Consultation

Developed using the concept of Artificial Intelligence Technology, Babylon provides healthcare service on subscription. By paying a subscription fee, people can access the facilities with their mobile phones. They can monitor their health and consult medical professionals through text or video messages. Test kits for checking cholesterol, diabetes can be purchased, test reports can be sent to Babylon healthcare provider and the test results can also be accessed through mobile apps. Babylon medical consultation also provides a feature by which pre-screening the health condition of an user is possible. In 2017 a new facility was launched, which takes few seconds for appointment booking and the patient can consult through video chat within two hours of booking from any location. Through Babylon healthcare app one can see doctors, can interact with them, can make future health prediction from current health status.

AiCure App for Medication Management

AiCure company was established in 2010 with the aim to monitor patient health using new technologies, increasing life span of human beings, reducing the death rates. To develop the intelligent app advanced techniques like computer vision, predictive analysis, machine learning, deep learning are used by the company. Using intelligent techniques on smartphones it is visually confirmed that the right patient has taken the right medication on time. This interactive app can adapt to the behaviour of a patient gradually and can be customized on the basis of disease risk factors, type of disease, number of people affected by the disease etc. So, this intelligent app acts as a guide which provides visual control over the patient health by reminding patient the time of taking medicine, next clinical visit date and confirming that patient is taking the prescribed medicine .

CyberDoctor

CyberDoctor was founded in 2009 and provides doctor patient interaction through various facilities like SymptomScan, TreatmentTracker, DocLogs. SymptomScan takes patient necessary information and informs the patient about the diagnosis made by the medical professionals. TreatmentTracker informs patient about the prescribed medication, diet and lifestyle for a particular diagnosis. Through discussion physicians can improve the medication adherence of the patient. TreatmentTracker also provides facilities for clinical alerts and medication reminders. Through DocLogs doctors can share information with the patients and patients can get valuable and reliable information by just sitting at home.

Medisafe

Medisafe is also developed for solving medication non-adherence problem. It reminds the patients about their medication, educates them about their health condition and medication procedure, provides valuable tips etc. Besides this it also helps physicians in observing patient health progress.

CONCLUSION

The role of intelligent devices is a boon for society and can solve many unsolved problems effectively and efficiently. Due to this it has attracted many researchers and scientists to work on artificial intelligence and develop new techniques for solving complicated and sensitive problems. To make the use of intelligent devices successful issues like compatibility, security and privacy should be considered as very important. New advanced techniques have been developed to solve healthcare problems and to help patients in taking proper care of their health despite of their busy schedule. We hope the proposed chapter will provide detailed information about the use of artificial intelligence in medical science and their positive consequences, which will be helpful for the students and researchers of computer science and medical science. This will also attract researchers to work more on information retrieval, object detection, image and data analysis using intelligent systems which will be applicable in medical and other fields.

REFERENCES

Abood, Z. M., Karam, G. S., & Hluot, R. E. (2017, April). Classification of red blood cells disease using fuzzy logic theory. In *Current Research in Computer Science and Information Technology (ICCIT), 2017 International Conference on* (pp. 31-36). IEEE. 10.1109/CRCSIT.2017.7965558

Abu Ghali, M. J., Mukhaimer, M. N., Abu Yousef, M. K., & Abu Naser, S. S. (2017). *Expert System for Problems of Teeth and Gums. International Journal of Engineering and Information Systems.*

Acharya, U. R., Fujita, H., Oh, S. L., Hagiwara, Y., Tan, J. H., Adam, M., & Tan, R. S. (2018). Deep convolutional neural network for the automated diagnosis of congestive heart failure using ECG signals. *Applied Intelligence*, 1–12.

Acharya, U. R., Fujita, H., Oh, S. L., Raghavendra, U., Tan, J. H., Adam, M., ... Hagiwara, Y. (2018). Automated identification of shockable and non-shockable life-threatening ventricular arrhythmias using convolutional neural network. *Future Generation Computer Systems*, *79*, 952–959. doi:10.1016/j.future.2017.08.039

Ahmed, I. O., Ibraheem, B. A., & Mustafa, Z. A. (2018). Detection of Eye Melanoma Using Artificial Neural Network. *Journal of Clinical Engineering*, *43*(1), 22–28. doi:10.1097/JCE.0000000000000250

Al Rekhawi, H. A., Ayyad, A. A., & Abu Naser, S. S. (2017). *Rickets Expert System Diagnoses and Treatment. International Journal of Engineering and Information Systems.*

Ali, J. B., Hamdi, T., Fnaiech, N., Di Costanzo, V., Fnaiech, F., & Ginoux, J. M. (2018). Continuous blood glucose level prediction of Type 1 Diabetes based on Artificial Neural Network. *Biocybernetics and Biomedical Engineering.*

Aličković, E., & Subasi, A. (2017). Breast cancer diagnosis using GA feature selection and Rotation Forest. *Neural Computing & Applications*, *28*(4), 753–763. doi:10.100700521-015-2103-9

Ando, Y., Low, W. Y., & Naugler, W. (2018). Sa1512-An Artificial Neural Network Model Predicting Survival after Liver Transplantation Using the United Network for Organ Sharing Database. *Gastroenterology*, *154*(6), S-1138. doi:10.1016/S0016-5085(18)33779-X

Arabasadi, Z., Alizadehsani, R., Roshanzamir, M., Moosaei, H., & Yarifard, A. A. (2017). Computer aided decision making for heart disease detection using hybrid neural network-Genetic algorithm. *Computer Methods and Programs in Biomedicine*, *141*, 19–26. doi:10.1016/j.cmpb.2017.01.004 PMID:28241964

Arulmurugan, R., & Anandakumar, H. (2018). Early Detection of Lung Cancer Using Wavelet Feature Descriptor and Feed Forward Back Propagation Neural Networks Classifier. In *Computational Vision and Bio Inspired Computing* (pp. 103–110). Cham: Springer. doi:10.1007/978-3-319-71767-8_9

Ashiquzzaman, A., Tushar, A. K., Islam, M. R., Shon, D., Im, K., Park, J. H., ... Kim, J. (2018). Reduction of overfitting in diabetes prediction using deep learning neural network. In *IT Convergence and Security 2017* (pp. 35–43). Singapore: Springer. doi:10.1007/978-981-10-6451-7_5

Babaoglu, İ., Findik, O., & Ülker, E. (2010). A comparison of feature selection models utilizing binary particle swarm optimization and genetic algorithm in determining coronary artery disease using support vector machine. *Expert Systems with Applications*, *37*(4), 3177–3183. doi:10.1016/j.eswa.2009.09.064

Baig, M. M., & Gholamhosseini, H. (2013). Smart health monitoring systems: An overview of design and modeling. *Journal of Medical Systems*, *37*(2), 9898. doi:10.100710916-012-9898-z PMID:23321968

Baun, M. M., Bergstrom, N., Langston, N. F., & Thoma, L. (1984). Physiological effects of human/companion animal bonding. *Nursing Research*, *33*(3), 126–129. doi:10.1097/00006199-198405000-00002 PMID:6563527

Berner, E. S. (2007). Clinical decision support systems (Vol. 233). New York: Springer Science+ Business Media, LLC.

Brosch, T., & Tam, R., & Alzheimer's Disease Neuroimaging Initiative. (2013, September). Manifold learning of brain MRIs by deep learning. In *International Conference on Medical Image Computing and Computer-Assisted Intervention* (pp. 633-640). Springer. 10.1007/978-3-642-40763-5_78

Chang, K., Bai, H. X., Zhou, H., Su, C., Bi, W. L., Agbodza, E., ... Zhang, B. (2018). Residual convolutional neural network for the determination of IDH status in low-and high-grade gliomas from MR imaging. *Clinical Cancer Research*, *24*(5), 1073–1081. doi:10.1158/1078-0432.CCR-17-2236 PMID:29167275

Cheng, J. Z., Ni, D., Chou, Y. H., Qin, J., Tiu, C. M., Chang, Y. C., ... Chen, C. M. (2016). Computer-aided diagnosis with deep learning architecture: Applications to breast lesions in US images and pulmonary nodules in CT scans. *Scientific Reports*, *6*(1), 24454. doi:10.1038rep24454 PMID:27079888

Choubey, D. K., Paul, S., Kumar, S., & Kumar, S. (2017, February). Classification of Pima indian diabetes dataset using naive bayes with genetic algorithm as an attribute selection. In *Communication and Computing Systems: Proceedings of the International Conference on Communication and Computing System (ICCCS 2016)* (pp. 451-455). Academic Press.

Chowdhury, G. G. (2003). Natural language processing. *Annual Review of Information Science & Technology*, *37*(1), 51–89. doi:10.1002/aris.1440370103

Coiera, E. (2015). *Guide to health informatics*. CRC Press.

Das, R., Turkoglu, I., & Sengur, A. (2009). Effective diagnosis of heart disease through neural networks ensembles. *Expert Systems with Applications*, *36*(4), 7675–7680. doi:10.1016/j.eswa.2008.09.013

de Carvalho Filho, A. O., Silva, A. C., de Paiva, A. C., Nunes, R. A., & Gattass, M. (2017). Computer-aided diagnosis of lung nodules in computed tomography by using phylogenetic diversity, genetic algorithm, and SVM. *Journal of Digital Imaging*, *30*(6), 812–822. doi:10.100710278-017-9973-6 PMID:28526968

Deekshatulu, B. L., & Chandra, P. (2013). Classification of heart disease using k-nearest neighbor and genetic algorithm. *Procedia Technology*, *10*, 85–94. doi:10.1016/j.protcy.2013.12.340

Devarakonda, M., & Tsou, C. H. (2015, January). *Automated Problem List Generation from Electronic Medical Records in IBM Watson*. AAAI.

Doi, K. (2007). Computer-aided diagnosis in medical imaging: Historical review, current status and future potential. *Computerized Medical Imaging and Graphics*, *31*(4-5), 198–211. doi:10.1016/j.compmedimag.2007.02.002 PMID:17349778

Doyle-Lindrud, S. (2015). Watson will see you now: A supercomputer to help clinicians make informed treatment decisions. *Clinical Journal of Oncology Nursing*, *19*(1), 31–32. doi:10.1188/15.CJON.31-32 PMID:25689646

El Agha, M., Jarghon, A., & Abu Naser, S. S. (2017). *Polymyalgia Rheumatic Expert System. International Journal of Engineering and Information Systems.*

El-Dahshan, E. S. A., Mohsen, H. M., Revett, K., & Salem, A. B. M. (2014). Computer-aided diagnosis of human brain tumor through MRI: A survey and a new algorithm. *Expert Systems with Applications*, *41*(11), 5526–5545. doi:10.1016/j.eswa.2014.01.021

Elveren, E., & Yumuşak, N. (2011). Tuberculosis disease diagnosis using artificial neural network trained with genetic algorithm. *Journal of Medical Systems*, *35*(3), 329–332. doi:10.100710916-009-9369-3 PMID:20703557

Esteva, A., Kuprel, B., Novoa, R. A., Ko, J., Swetter, S. M., Blau, H. M., & Thrun, S. (2017). Dermatologist-level classification of skin cancer with deep neural networks. *Nature*, *542*(7639), 115–118. doi:10.1038/nature21056 PMID:28117445

Fidele, B., Cheeneebash, J., Gopaul, A., & Goorah, S. S. (2009). Artificial neural network as a clinical decision-supporting tool to predict cardiovascular disease. *Trends in Applied Sciences Research, 4*(1), 36-46.

Fister, I., Jr., Yang, X. S., Fister, I., Brest, J., & Fister, D. (2013). *A brief review of nature-inspired algorithms for optimization.* arXiv preprint arXiv:1307.4186

Friedmann, E., Katcher, A. H., Lynch, J. J., & Thomas, S. A. (1980). Animal companions and one-year survival of patients after discharge from a coronary care unit. *Public Health Reports*, *95*(4), 307. PMID:6999524

Fujita, M. and Kitano, H. (1998). An development of an autonomous quadruped robot for robot entertainment. Autonomous Robots, 5, 7–18.

Garrity, T. F., Stallones, L. F., Marx, M. B., & Johnson, T. P. (1989). Pet ownership and attachment as supportive factors in the health of the elderly. *Anthrozoos*, *3*(1), 35–44. doi:10.2752/089279390787057829

Haladay, J. (1989). Animal assisted therapy for PWA's – Bringing a sense of connection. *AIDS Patient Care*, 38–39.

Hanna, C. J., & O'Connor, T. J. (2009). *U.S. Patent No. 7,583,861*. Washington, DC: U.S. Patent and Trademark Office.

Hart, L. A., Hart, B. L., & Bergin, B. L. (1987). Socializing effects of service dogs for people with disabilities. *Anthrozoos*, *1*(1), 41–44. doi:10.2752/089279388787058696

Hirasawa, T., Aoyama, K., Tanimoto, T., Ishihara, S., Shichijo, S., Ozawa, T., ... Tada, T. (2018). Application of artificial intelligence using a convolutional neural network for detecting gastric cancer in endoscopic images. *Gastric Cancer, 21*(4), 653–660. doi:10.100710120-018-0793-2 PMID:29335825

Ishioka, J., Matsuoka, Y., Uehara, S., Yasuda, Y., Kijima, T., Yoshida, S., ... Kimura, T. (2018). Computer-aided diagnosis of prostate cancer on magnetic resonance imaging using a convolutional neural network algorithm. *BJU International*. doi:10.1111/bju.14397 PMID:29772101

Istepanian, R. S., Hu, S., Philip, N. Y., & Sungoor, A. (2011, August). The potential of Internet of m-health Things "m-IoT" for non-invasive glucose level sensing. In *Engineering in medicine and biology society, EMBC, 2011 annual international conference of the IEEE* (pp. 5264-5266). IEEE. 10.1109/IEMBS.2011.6091302

Jayalakshmi, T., & Santhakumaran, A. (2010). A novel classification method for diagnosis of diabetes mellitus using artificial neural networks. In *Data Storage and Data Engineering (DSDE), 2010 International Conference on* (pp. 159-163). IEEE. 10.1109/DSDE.2010.58

Jovanov, E., Lords, A. D., Raskovic, D., Cox, P. G., Adhami, R., & Andrasik, F. (2003). Stress monitoring using a distributed wireless intelligent sensor system. *IEEE Engineering in Medicine and Biology Magazine, 22*(3), 49–55. doi:10.1109/MEMB.2003.1213626 PMID:12845819

Kale, M. (1992). Kids and animals: A comforting hospital combination. *Interaction, 10*(3), 17–21.

Karegowda, A. G., Manjunath, A. S., & Jayaram, M. A. (2011). Application of genetic algorithm optimized neural network connection weights for medical diagnosis of pima Indians diabetes. *International Journal on Soft Computing, 2*(2), 15–23. doi:10.5121/ijsc.2011.2202

Katevas, N. (Ed.). (2001). *Mobile robotics in healthcare* (Vol. 7). IOS Press.

Kim, J., Gu, G. M., & Heo, P. (2016). Robotics for healthcare. In *Biomedical Engineering: Frontier Research and Converging Technologies* (pp. 489–509). Cham: Springer. doi:10.1007/978-3-319-21813-7_21

Kim, J., Kim, J., Kwak, M. J., & Bajaj, M. (2018). Genetic prediction of type 2 diabetes using deep neural network. *Clinical Genetics, 93*(4), 822–829. doi:10.1111/cge.13175 PMID:29136281

Kodali, R. K., Swamy, G., & Lakshmi, B. (2015, December). An implementation of IoT for healthcare. In Intelligent Computational Systems (RAICS), 2015 IEEE Recent Advances in (pp. 411-416). IEEE. doi:10.1109/RAICS.2015.7488451

Kurt, I., Ture, M., & Kurum, A. T. (2008). Comparing performances of logistic regression, classification and regression tree, and neural networks for predicting coronary artery disease. *Expert Systems with Applications, 34*(1), 366–374. doi:10.1016/j.eswa.2006.09.004

Li, C., Hu, X., & Zhang, L. (2017). The IoT-based heart disease monitoring system for pervasive healthcare service. *Procedia Computer Science, 112*, 2328–2334. doi:10.1016/j.procs.2017.08.265

Liu, S., Liu, S., Cai, W., Pujol, S., Kikinis, R., & Feng, D. (2014, April). Early diagnosis of Alzheimer's disease with deep learning. In *Biomedical Imaging (ISBI), 2014 IEEE 11th International Symposium on* (pp. 1015-1018). IEEE. 10.1109/ISBI.2014.6868045

Majidi, C. (2014). Soft robotics: A perspective—current trends and prospects for the future. *Soft Robotics*, *1*(1), 5–11. doi:10.1089oro.2013.0001

Milenković, A., Otto, C., & Jovanov, E. (2006). Wireless sensor networks for personal health monitoring: Issues and an implementation. *Computer Communications*, *29*(13-14), 2521–2533. doi:10.1016/j.comcom.2006.02.011

Miotto, R., Wang, F., Wang, S., Jiang, X., & Dudley, J. T. (2017). Deep learning for healthcare: Review, opportunities and challenges. *Briefings in Bioinformatics*. doi:10.1093/bib/bbx044 PMID:28481991

Nabahin, A., Abou Eloun, A., & Abu Naser, S. S. (2017). *Expert System for Hair Loss Diagnosis and Treatment. International Journal of Engineering and Information Systems.*

Nattkemper, T. W., Arnrich, B., Lichte, O., Timm, W., Degenhard, A., Pointon, L., ... Leach, M. O. (2005). Evaluation of radiological features for breast tumour classification in clinical screening with machine learning methods. *Artificial Intelligence in Medicine*, *34*(2), 129–139. doi:10.1016/j.artmed.2004.09.001 PMID:15894177

Ndaba, M., Pillay, A. W., & Ezugwu, A. E. (2018, May). An Improved Generalized Regression Neural Network for Type II Diabetes Classification. In *International Conference on Computational Science and Its Applications* (pp. 659-671). Springer, Cham. 10.1007/978-3-319-95171-3_52

Nilashi, M., Ibrahim, O., Ahmadi, H., & Shahmoradi, L. (2017). A knowledge-based system for breast cancer classification using fuzzy logic method. *Telematics and Informatics*, *34*(4), 133–144. doi:10.1016/j.tele.2017.01.007

Pappada, S. M., Cameron, B. D., & Rosman, P. M. (2008). Development of a neural network for prediction of glucose concentration in type 1 diabetes patients. *Journal of Diabetes Science and Technology*, *2*(5), 792–801. doi:10.1177/193229680800200507 PMID:19885262

Pappada, S. M., Cameron, B. D., Rosman, P. M., Bourey, R. E., Papadimos, T. J., Olorunto, W., & Borst, M. J. (2011). Neural network-based real-time prediction of glucose in patients with insulin-dependent diabetes. *Diabetes Technology & Therapeutics*, *13*(2), 135–141. doi:10.1089/dia.2010.0104 PMID:21284480

Pati, S. K., Sengupta, S., & Das, A. K. (2018). Improved Genetic Algorithm for Selecting Significant Genes in Cancer Diagnosis. In *Progress in Advanced Computing and Intelligent Engineering* (pp. 395–405). Singapore: Springer. doi:10.1007/978-981-10-6875-1_39

Pawar, M. M., & Talbar, S. N. (2018). Wavelet Statistical Feature Selection Using Genetic Algorithm with Fuzzy Classifier for Breast Cancer Diagnosis. In *Progress in Intelligent Computing Techniques: Theory, Practice, and Applications* (pp. 95–105). Singapore: Springer. doi:10.1007/978-981-10-3373-5_8

Poongothai, S., Dharuman, C., Venkatesan, P., & Campus, R. (2017). *A Comparison of Fuzzy Genetic and Neuro Genetic Hybrid Algorithm for the Classification of Diabetes Disease*. Academic Press.

Powles, J., & Hodson, H. (2017). Google DeepMind and healthcare in an age of algorithms. *Health and technology*, *7*(4), 351–367. doi:10.100712553-017-0179-1 PMID:29308344

Prasoon, A., Petersen, K., Igel, C., Lauze, F., Dam, E., & Nielsen, M. (2013, September). Deep feature learning for knee cartilage segmentation using a triplanar convolutional neural network. In *International conference on medical image computing and computer-assisted intervention* (pp. 246-253). Springer. 10.1007/978-3-642-40763-5_31

Qwaider, S. R., & Abu Naser, S. S. (2017). *Expert System for Diagnosing Ankle Diseases. International Journal of Engineering and Information Systems.*

Reddy, G. T., & Khare, N. (2017). An efficient system for heart disease prediction using hybrid OFBAT with rule-based fuzzy logic model. *Journal of Circuits, Systems, and Computers*, *26*(04), 1750061. doi:10.1142/S021812661750061X

Reeves, A. P., & Kostis, W. J. (2000). Computer-aided diagnosis for lung cancer. *Radiologia Clinica*, *38*(3), 497–509. PMID:10855257

Rotariu, C., & Manta, V. (2012, September). Wireless system for remote monitoring of oxygen saturation and heart rate. In *Computer Science and Information Systems (FedCSIS), 2012 Federated Conference on* (pp. 193-196). IEEE.

Saldien, J., Goris, K., Vanderborght, B., Verrelst, B., Van Ham, R., & Lefeber, D. (2006, September). ANTY: The development of an intelligent huggable robot for hospitalized children. *9th International Conference on Climbing and Walking Robots and the Support Technologies for Mobile Machines.*

Savalia, S., Acosta, E., & Emamian, V. (2017). Classification of Cardiovascular Disease Using Feature Extraction and Artificial Neural Networks. *The Journal of Bioscience and Medicine*, *5*(11), 64–79. doi:10.4236/jbm.2017.511008

Shabut, A. M., Tania, M. H., Lwin, K. T., Evans, B. A., Yusof, N. A., Abu-Hassan, K. J., & Hossain, M. A. (2018). An Intelligent Mobile-Enabled Expert System for Tuberculosis Disease Diagnosis in Real Time. *Expert Systems with Applications*, *114*, 65–77. doi:10.1016/j.eswa.2018.07.014

Shahriyar, R., Bari, M. F., Kundu, G., Ahamed, S. I., & Akbar, M. M. (2009, September). Intelligent mobile health monitoring system (IMHMS). In *International Conference on Electronic Healthcare* (pp. 5-12). Springer.

Sharma, M., Sharma, P., Saini, A., & Sharma, K. (2018). Modular Neural Network for Detection of Diabetic Retinopathy in Retinal Images. In *Proceedings of First International Conference on Smart System, Innovations and Computing*(pp. 363-370). Springer. 10.1007/978-981-10-5828-8_35

Sharma, P., & Saxena, K. (2017). Application of fuzzy logic and genetic algorithm in heart disease risk level prediction. *International Journal of System Assurance Engineering and Management*, *8*(2), 1109–1125. doi:10.100713198-017-0578-8

Shrivastava, P., Shukla, A., Vepakomma, P., Bhansali, N., & Verma, K. (2017). A survey of nature-inspired algorithms for feature selection to identify Parkinson's disease. *Computer Methods and Programs in Biomedicine*, *139*, 171–179. doi:10.1016/j.cmpb.2016.07.029 PMID:28187888

Spetsieris, P. G., Dhawan, V., Ma, Y., Moeller, J. R., Mentis, M. J., & Eidelberg, D. (2002). Computer aided diagnosis of functional brain disorders using PET on a PC based platform. In *Engineering in Medicine and Biology, 2002. 24th Annual Conference and the Annual Fall Meeting of the Biomedical Engineering Society EMBS/BMES Conference, 2002. Proceedings of the Second Joint* (*Vol. 2*, pp. 1107-1108). IEEE. 10.1109/IEMBS.2002.1106300

Stoitsis, J., Valavanis, I., Mougiakakou, S. G., Golemati, S., Nikita, A., & Nikita, K. S. (2006). Computer aided diagnosis based on medical image processing and artificial intelligence methods. *Nuclear Instruments & Methods in Physics Research. Section A, Accelerators, Spectrometers, Detectors and Associated Equipment*, *569*(2), 591–595. doi:10.1016/j.nima.2006.08.134

Tan, J. H., Bhandary, S. V., Sivaprasad, S., Hagiwara, Y., Bagchi, A., Raghavendra, U., ... Chua, K. C. (2018). Age-related Macular Degeneration detection using deep convolutional neural network. *Future Generation Computer Systems*, *87*, 127–135. doi:10.1016/j.future.2018.05.001

Venkatesan, P., & Anitha, S. (2006). Application of a radial basis function neural network for diagnosis of diabetes mellitus. *Current Science*, *91*(9), 1195–1199.

Verma, P., & Sood, S. K. (2018). Cloud-centric IoT based disease diagnosis healthcare framework. *Journal of Parallel and Distributed Computing*, *116*, 27–38. doi:10.1016/j.jpdc.2017.11.018

Wachinger, C., Reuter, M., & Klein, T. (2018). DeepNAT: Deep convolutional neural network for segmenting neuroanatomy. *NeuroImage*, *170*, 434–445. doi:10.1016/j.neuroimage.2017.02.035 PMID:28223187

Wada, K., Shibata, T., Saito, T., & Tanie, K. (2004). Effects of robot-assisted activity for elderly people and nurses at a day service center. *Proceedings of the IEEE*, *92*(11), 1780–1788. doi:10.1109/JPROC.2004.835378

Yoo, Y., Brosch, T., Traboulsee, A., Li, D. K., & Tam, R. (2014). Deep learning of image features from unlabeled data for multiple sclerosis lesion segmentation. In *International Workshop on Machine Learning in Medical Imaging* (pp. 117-124). Springer. 10.1007/978-3-319-10581-9_15

Zreik, M., Leiner, T., de Vos, B. D., van Hamersvelt, R. W., Viergever, M. A., & Isgum, I. (2017). *Automatic Segmentation of the Left Ventricle in Cardiac CT Angiography Using Convolutional Neural Network*. arXiv preprint arXiv:1704.05698

Compilation of References

7 . Big Data Use Cases for Healthcare. (2016, October 8). Retrieved July 24, 2017, from http://www.ingrammicroadvisor.com/data-center/7-big-data-use-cases-for-healthcare

A Cloud-based Platform: Purpose-built for Healthcare. (2018). Retrieved July 24, 2017, from http://www.usa.philips.com/healthcare/innovation/about-health-suite

Aboagye-Sarfo, P., Mai, Q., Sanfilippo, F. M., Preen, D. B., Stewart, L. M., & Fatovich, D. M. (2015). A comparison of multivariate and univariate time series approaches to modelling and forecasting emergency department demand in Western Australia. *Journal of Biomedical Informatics*, *57*, 62–73. doi:10.1016/j.jbi.2015.06.022 PMID:26151668

Abood, Z. M., Karam, G. S., & Hluot, R. E. (2017, April). Classification of red blood cells disease using fuzzy logic theory. In *Current Research in Computer Science and Information Technology (ICCIT), 2017 International Conference on* (pp. 31-36). IEEE. 10.1109/CRCSIT.2017.7965558

About HealthSuite. (2018). Retrieved April 29, 2018, from https://www.philips.co.in/healthcare/innovation/about-health-suite

Abu Ghali, M. J., Mukhaimer, M. N., Abu Yousef, M. K., & Abu Naser, S. S. (2017). *Expert System for Problems of Teeth and Gums. International Journal of Engineering and Information Systems.*

Acampora, G., Cook, D. J., Rashidi, P., & Vasilakos, V., A. (2013). A Survey on Ambient Intelligence in Health Care. *Proc IEEE Inst Electr Electron Eng.*

Accenture. (n.d.). *Pharmaceutical companies that digitize grow more*. Retrieved January 25, 2018 from https://www.accenture.com/in-en/insight-highlights-life-sciences-pharmaceutical-grow

Achanta, R., Estrada, F., Wils, P., & Süsstrunk, S. (2008, May). Salient region detection and segmentation. In *International conference on computer vision systems* (pp. 66-75). Springer. 10.1007/978-3-540-79547-6_7

Acharya, U. R., Fujita, H., Oh, S. L., Hagiwara, Y., Tan, J. H., Adam, M., & Tan, R. S. (2018). Deep convolutional neural network for the automated diagnosis of congestive heart failure using ECG signals. *Applied Intelligence*, 1–12.

Acharya, U. R., Fujita, H., Oh, S. L., Raghavendra, U., Tan, J. H., Adam, M., ... Hagiwara, Y. (2018). Automated identification of shockable and non-shockable life-threatening ventricular arrhythmias using convolutional neural network. *Future Generation Computer Systems*, *79*, 952–959. doi:10.1016/j.future.2017.08.039

Ackermann, H. (2008). Cerebellar contributions to speech production and speech perception: Psycholinguistic and neurobiological perspectives. *Trends in Neurosciences*, *31*(6), 265–272. doi:10.1016/j.tins.2008.02.011 PMID:18471906

Ackermann, H., & Riecker, A. (2010). Cerebral control of motor aspects of speech production: neurophysiological and functional imaging data. In *Speech motor control: new developments in basic and applied research* (pp. 117–134). Oxford, UK: Oxford University Press. doi:10.1093/acprof:oso/9780199235797.003.0007

Adelson, E. H., & Bergen, J. R. (1991). *The plenoptic function and the elements of early vision*. Academic Press.

Afilal, M., Yalaoui, F., Dugardin, F., Amodeo, L., Laplanche, D., & Blua, P. (2016a). Emergency department flow: A new practical patients classification and forecasting daily attendance. *IFAC-PapersOnLine*, *49*(12), 721–726. doi:10.1016/j.ifacol.2016.07.859

Afilal, M., Yalaoui, F., Dugardin, F., Amodeo, L., Laplanche, D., & Blua, P. (2016b). Forecasting the Emergency Department Patients Flow. *Journal of Medical Systems*, *40*(7), 1–18. doi:10.100710916-016-0527-0 PMID:27272135

Agostinelli, F., Anderson, M. R., & Lee, H. (2013). *Adaptive Multi-Column Deep Neural Networks with Application to Robust Image Denoising*. NIPS. Available at http://papers.nips.cc/paper/5030-adaptive-multi-column-deep-neural-networks-with-application-to-robust-image-denoising.pdf

Ahamed, N. U., Sundaraj, K., Ahmad, B., Rahman, M., Ali, A., Islam, A., & Palaniappan, R. (2013). Rehabilitation systems for physically disabled patients: A brief review of sensor-based computerised signal-monitoring systems. *Biomedical Research*, *24*(3).

Ahmed, I. O., Ibraheem, B. A., & Mustafa, Z. A. (2018). Detection of Eye Melanoma Using Artificial Neural Network. *Journal of Clinical Engineering*, *43*(1), 22–28. doi:10.1097/JCE.0000000000000250

Ai, O. C., Hariharan, M., Yaacob, S., & Chee, L. S. (2012). Classification of speech dysfluencies with MFCC and LPCC features. *Expert Systems with Applications*, *39*(2), 2157–2165. doi:10.1016/j.eswa.2011.07.065

Al Rekhawi, H. A., Ayyad, A. A., & Abu Naser, S. S. (2017). *Rickets Expert System Diagnoses and Treatment. International Journal of Engineering and Information Systems.*

Aladeemy, M., Chou, C. A., Shan, X., Khasawneh, M., Srihari, K., & Poranki, S. (2016). Forecasting Daily Patient Arrivals at Emergency Department: A Comparative Study. *Proceedings of the 2016 Industrial and Systems Engineering Research Conference*.

Ali, J. B., Hamdi, T., Fnaiech, N., Di Costanzo, V., Fnaiech, F., & Ginoux, J. M. (2018). Continuous blood glucose level prediction of Type 1 Diabetes based on Artificial Neural Network. *Biocybernetics and Biomedical Engineering*.

Aličković, E., & Subasi, A. (2017). Breast cancer diagnosis using GA feature selection and Rotation Forest. *Neural Computing & Applications*, *28*(4), 753–763. doi:10.100700521-015-2103-9

Allen-Vercoe, H. (2017). Prepare for the VR and AR healthcare revolution. *Pharmaphorum*. Retrieved February 15, 2018 from https://pharmaphorum.com/views-and-analysis/vr-ar-healthcare-pharma/

Alpaydın, E. (2012). *Introduction to machine learning*. The MIT Press.

Alsumidaie, M. (2017a). *Non-Adherence: A Direct Influence on Clinical Trial Duration and Cost*. Retrieved March 10, 2018 from http://www.appliedclinicaltrialsonline.com/non-adherence-direct-influence-clinical-trial-duration-and-cost

Alsumidaie, M. (2017b). *Technology Tips on Improving Clinical Trial Patient Adherence*. Retrieved March 10, 2018 from http://www.appliedclinicaltrialsonline.com/technology-tips-improving-clinical-trial-patient-adherence

Alwakeel, S. S., Alhalabi, B., Aggoune, H., & Alwakeel, M. (2015). A Machine Learning Based WSN System for Autism Activity Recognition. In *Machine Learning and Applications (ICMLA), 2015 IEEE 14th International Conference* (pp. 771-776). IEEE. 10.1109/ICMLA.2015.46

Alzheimer's Association. (2014). Alzheimer's Disease Facts and Figures. *Alzheimer's & Dementia*, *10*(2), 1–80. PMID:23871765

Alzubi, R., Ramzan, N., & Alzoubi, H. (n.d.). *Hybrid Feature Selection Method for Autism Spectrum Disorder SNPs.*

Amir, Rahmani, Gia, Negash, Anzanpour, Azimi, Jiang, & Liljeberg. (2018). Exploiting smart e-Health gateways at the edge of healthcare Internet-of-Things: A fog computing approach. *Future Generation Computer Systems*, *2*(78), 641–658.

Anavi, Y. (2016). *Visualizing and enhancing a deep learning framework using patients age and gender for chest x-ray image retrieval.* Available at: http://proceedings.spiedigitallibrary.org/proceeding.aspx?doi=10.1117/12.2217587

Anavi, Y. (2015). A Comparative Study for Chest Radiograph Image Retrieval Using Binary, Texture and Deep Learning Classification. *Proceedings of the 37th Annual International Conference of the IEEE Engineering in Medicine and Biology Society*, 2940–2943. 10.1109/EMBC.2015.7319008

Ando, Y., Low, W. Y., & Naugler, W. (2018). Sa1512-An Artificial Neural Network Model Predicting Survival after Liver Transplantation Using the United Network for Organ Sharing Database. *Gastroenterology*, *154*(6), S-1138. doi:10.1016/S0016-5085(18)33779-X

Ang, K. K., Chua, K. S., Phua, K. S., Wang, C., Chin, Z. Y., Kuah, C. W., ... Guan, C. (2015). A randomized controlled trial of EEG-based motor imagery brain-computer interface robotic rehabilitation for stroke. *Clinical EEG and Neuroscience*, *46*(4), 310–320. doi:10.1177/1550059414522229 PMID:24756025

Apache Avro™ 1.8.2 Documentation. (2017, August 2). Retrieved April 29, 2018, from https://avro.apache.org/docs/current/

Arabasadi, Z., Alizadehsani, R., Roshanzamir, M., Moosaei, H., & Yarifard, A. A. (2017). Computer aided decision making for heart disease detection using hybrid neural network-Genetic algorithm. *Computer Methods and Programs in Biomedicine*, *141*, 19–26. doi:10.1016/j.cmpb.2017.01.004 PMID:28241964

Araz, O. M., Bentley, D., & Muelleman, R. L. (2014). Using Google Flu Trends data in forecasting influenza-like–illness related ED visits in Omaha, Nebraska. *The American Journal of Emergency Medicine*, *32*(9), 1016–1023. doi:10.1016/j.ajem.2014.05.052 PMID:25037278

Areekul, P., Senjyu, T., Toyama, H., & Yona, A. (2010). Notice of violation of IEEE publication principles a hybrid ARIMA and neural network model for short-term price forecasting in deregulated market. *IEEE Transactions on Power Systems*, *25*(1), 524–530. doi:10.1109/TPWRS.2009.2036488

Arel, I., Rose, D. C., & Karnowski, T. P. (2010). Deep Machine Learning - A New Frontier in Artificial Intelligence Research. *IEEE Computational Intelligence Magazine*, *5*(4), 13–18. doi:10.1109/MCI.2010.938364

Armstrong, J. S. (Ed.). (2001). *Principles of forecasting: a handbook for researchers and practitioners* (Vol. 30). Springer Science & Business Media. doi:10.1007/978-0-306-47630-3

Aroua, A., & Abdul-Nour, G. (2015). Forecast emergency room visits–a major diagnostic categories-based approach. *International Journal of Metrology and Quality Engineering*, *6*(2), 204. doi:10.1051/ijmqe/2015011

Arthur.D.Little. (2016). *Impact of Digital Health on the Pharmaceutical Industry.* Retrieved March 23, 2018 from http://www.adlittle.com/sites/default/files/viewpoints/ADL_HC_2016_Digital-Health_01.pdf

Arulmurugan, R., & Anandakumar, H. (2018). Early Detection of Lung Cancer Using Wavelet Feature Descriptor and Feed Forward Back Propagation Neural Networks Classifier. In *Computational Vision and Bio Inspired Computing* (pp. 103–110). Cham: Springer. doi:10.1007/978-3-319-71767-8_9

Arya, P., Paul, R. K., Kumar, A., Singh, K. N., Sivaramne, N., & Chaudhary, P. (2015). Predicting pest population using weather variables: An ARIMAX time series framework. *International Journal of Agricultural and Statistics Sciences, 11*(2), 381–386.

Asay, M. (2014, November 19). *MongoDB, Cassandra, and HBase -- the three NoSQL databases to watch*. Retrieved from http://www.infoworld.com

Ascione, A. (n.d.). *The convergence of healthcare: when digital and medical collide*. Retrieved March 23, 2018 from http://deep-dive.pharmaphorum.com/deep-dive-future-pharma-july-2017#!/the-convergence-of-healthcare-when-digital-and-medical-collide

Ashiquzzaman, A., Tushar, A. K., Islam, M. R., Shon, D., Im, K., Park, J. H., ... Kim, J. (2018). Reduction of overfitting in diabetes prediction using deep learning neural network. In *IT Convergence and Security 2017* (pp. 35–43). Singapore: Springer. doi:10.1007/978-981-10-6451-7_5

Astrom, C., Rocklov, J., Hales, S., Beguin, A., Louis, V., & Sauerborn, R. (2012). Potential distribution of dengue fever under scenarios of climate change and economic development. *EcoHealth, 9*(4), 448–454. doi:10.100710393-012-0808-0 PMID:23408100

Atal, B., & Rabiner, L. (1976). A pattern recognition approach to voiced-unvoiced-silence classification with applications to speech recognition. *IEEE Transactions on Acoustics, Speech, and Signal Processing, 24*(3), 201–212. doi:10.1109/TASSP.1976.1162800

Atyabi, A., Li, B., Ahn, Y. A., Kim, M., Barney, E., & Shic, F. (2017). An exploratory analysis targeting diagnostic classification of AAC app usage patterns. In *Neural Networks (IJCNN), 2017 International Joint Conference* (pp. 1633-1640). IEEE. 10.1109/IJCNN.2017.7966047

Au-Yeung, S. W. M., Harder, U., McCoy, E. J., & Knottenbelt, W. J. (2009). Predicting patient arrivals to an accident and emergency department. *Emergency Medicine Journal, 26*(4), 241–244. doi:10.1136/emj.2007.051656 PMID:19307381

Auzias, G., Takerkart, S., & Deruelle, C. (2016). On the Influence of Confounding Factors in Multisite Brain Morphometry Studies of Developmental Pathologies: Application to Autism Spectrum Disorder. *IEEE Journal of Biomedical and Health Informatics, 20*(3), 810–817. doi:10.1109/JBHI.2015.2460012 PMID:26208373

Babaoglu, İ., Findik, O., & Ülker, E. (2010). A comparison of feature selection models utilizing binary particle swarm optimization and genetic algorithm in determining coronary artery disease using support vector machine. *Expert Systems with Applications, 37*(4), 3177–3183. doi:10.1016/j.eswa.2009.09.064

Bahl, L. R., Jelinek, F., & Mercer, R. L. (1990). A maximum likelihood approach to continuous speech recognition. In Readings in Speech Recognition. Elsevier.

Bahrami, K. (2016). Convolutional Neural Network for Reconstruction of 7T-like Images from 3T MRI Using Appearance and Anatomical Features. In *Deep Learning and Data Labeling for Medical Applications: First International Workshop, LABELS 2016, and Second International Workshop, DLMIA 2016, Held in Conjunction with MICCAI 2016, Athens, Greece, October 21, 2016, Proceedings*. Cham: Springer International Publishing. 10.1007/978-3-319-46976-8_5

Baig, M. M., & Gholamhosseini, H. (2013). Smart health monitoring systems: An overview of design and modeling. *Journal of Medical Systems, 37*(2), 9898. doi:10.100710916-012-9898-z PMID:23321968

Bakker, J., Pechenizkiy, M., & Sidorova, N. (2011). What's your current stress level? Detection of stress patterns from GSR sensor data. *IEEE 11th International Conference on Data Mining Workshops*, 573-580.

Balaya, S., Paul, S. D., D'Lima, L. V., & Pavri, K. M. (1969). Investigations on an outbreak of dengue in Delhi in 1967. *The Indian Journal of Medical Research*, *57*, 767–774. PMID:5805380

Balcan, D., Hu, H., Goncalves, B., Bajardi, P., Poletto, C., Ramasco, J. J., ... Vespignani, A. (2009). Seasonal transmission potential and activity peaks of the new influenza A(H1N1): A Monte Carlo likelihood analysis based on human mobility. *BMC Medicine*, *7*(1), 45. doi:10.1186/1741-7015-7-45 PMID:19744314

Bandini, L. G., Curtin, C., Phillips, S., Anderson, S. E., Maslin, M., & Must, A. (2017). Changes in food selectivity in children with autism spectrum disorder. *Journal of Autism and Developmental Disorders*, *47*(2), 439–446. doi:10.100710803-016-2963-6 PMID:27866350

Banerjee, A., Datta, S., Das, P., Konar, A., Tibarewala, & Janarthan, R. (2012). Electrooculogram based online control signal generation for wheelchair. In *Electronic System Design (ISED), 2012 International Symposium on*. IEEE.

Barchiesi, D., Giannoulis, D., Stowell, D., & Plumbley, M. D. (2015). Acoustic scene classification: Classifying environments from the sounds they produce. *IEEE Signal Processing Magazine*, *32*(3), 16–34. doi:10.1109/MSP.2014.2326181

Bar, Y. (2016). Chest pathology identification using deep feature selection with non-medical training. *Computer Methods in Biomechanics and Biomedical Engineering. Imaging & Visualization*, 1–5. Available at http://www.tandfonline.com/doi/full/10.1080/21681163.2016.1138324

Batal, H., Tench, J., McMillan, S., Adams, J., & Mehler, P. S. (2001). Predicting patient visits to an urgent care clinic using calendar variables. *Academic Emergency Medicine*, *8*(1), 48–53. doi:10.1111/j.1553-2712.2001.tb00550.x PMID:11136148

Bauer, O., Le Sourd, A. M., Nardi, G., Bourgeron, T., Olivo-Marin, J. C., Ey, E., & de Chaumont, F. (2017). Unbiased analysis of mouse social behaviour using unsupervised machine learning. In *Biomedical Imaging (ISBI 2017), 2017 IEEE 14th International Symposium* (pp. 878-881). IEEE. 10.1109/ISBI.2017.7950656

Baun, M. M., Bergstrom, N., Langston, N. F., & Thoma, L. (1984). Physiological effects of human/companion animal bonding. *Nursing Research*, *33*(3), 126–129. doi:10.1097/00006199-198405000-00002 PMID:6563527

Beatty, M. E., Stone, A., Fitzsimons, D. W., Hanna, J. N., Lam, S. K., Vong, S., ... Margolis, H. S. (2010). Best practices in dengue surveillance: A report from the Asia-Paci c and Americas Dengue Prevention Boards. *PLoS Neglected Tropical Diseases*, *4*(11), e890. doi:10.1371/journal.pntd.0000890 PMID:21103381

Bejarano, N. C., Ambrosini, E., Pedrocchi, A., Ferrigno, G., Monticone, M., & Ferrante, S. A. (2015). Novel Adaptive, Real-Time Algorithm to Detect Gait Events from Wearable Sensors. *IEEE Transactions on Neural Systems and Rehabilitation Engineering*, *23*(3), 413–422. doi:10.1109/TNSRE.2014.2337914 PMID:25069118

Bell-Berti, F., & Harris, K. S. (1981). A temporal model of speech production. *Phonetica*, *38*(1-3), 9–20. doi:10.1159/000260011 PMID:7267724

Bellifemine, F., Caire, G., & Greenwood, D. (2007). Developing Multi-Agent Systems with JADE. John Wiley & Sons Ltd.

Belongie, S., Malik, J., & Puzicha, J. (2001). Matching shapes. In *Computer Vision, 2001. ICCV 2001. Proceedings. Eighth IEEE International Conference on* (Vol. 1, pp. 454-461). IEEE. 10.1109/ICCV.2001.937552

Belongie, S., Malik, J., & Puzicha, J. (2001). Shape context: A new descriptor for shape matching and object recognition. In Advances in neural information processing systems (pp. 831-837). Academic Press.

Belongie, S., Malik, J., & Puzicha, J. (2002). Shape matching and object recognition using shape contexts. *IEEE Transactions on Pattern Analysis and Machine Intelligence*, *24*(4), 509–522. doi:10.1109/34.993558

Bengio, Y., Courville, A., & Vincent, P. (2009). *Learning Deep Architectures for AI*, Bengio, Y., Courville, A. & Vincent, P., 2012. Representation Learning: A Review and New Perspectives. *IEEE Transactions on Pattern Analysis and Machine Intelligence*, *35*(8), 1798–1828. doi:10.1109/TPAMI.2013.50 PMID:23787338

Bengtsson, L., Lu, X., Thorson, A., Garfield, R., & von Schreeb, J. (2011). Improved response to disasters and outbreaks by tracking population movements with mobile phone network data: A post-earthquake geospatial study in Haiti. *PLoS Medicine*, *8*(8), e1001083. doi:10.1371/journal.pmed.1001083 PMID:21918643

Berg, G. (2015, July 17). *3 ways big data is improving healthcare analytics*. Retrieved October 15, 2017, from http://www.healthcareitnews.com/blog/3-ways-big-data-improving-healthcare-analytics

Bergs, J., Heerinckx, P., & Verelst, S. (2014). Knowing what to expect, forecasting monthly emergency department visits: A time-series analysis. *International Emergency Nursing*, *22*(2), 112–115. doi:10.1016/j.ienj.2013.08.001 PMID:24055373

Berner, E. S. (2007). Clinical decision support systems (Vol. 233). New York: Springer Science+ Business Media, LLC.

Bertolotti, G. M., Cristiani, A. M., Colagiorgio, P., Romano, F., Bassani, E., Caramia, N., & Ramat, S. A. (2016). Wearable and Modular Inertial Unit for Measuring Limb Movements and Balance Control Abilities. *IEEE Sensors Journal*, *16*(3), 790–797. doi:10.1109/JSEN.2015.2489381

Bhatt, S., Gething, P. W., Brady, O. J., Messina, J. P., Farlow, A. W., Moyes, C. L., ... Hay, S. I. (2013). The global distribution and burden of dengue. *Nature*, *496*(7446), 504–507. doi:10.1038/nature12060 PMID:23563266

Bian, J., Topaloglu, U., Yu, F., & Yu, F. (2012). *Towards Large-scale Twitter Mining for Drug-related Adverse Events*. Maui, HI: SHB. doi:10.1145/2389707.2389713

Bierens, H. J. (1987). Kernel estimators of regression functions. In *Advances in econometrics: Fifth world congress* (Vol. 1, pp. 99-144). Academic Press. 10.1017/CCOL0521344301.003

Bogdashevsky, R., Vladimir, A., Vitaly, Y., George, B., & Harrison, S. (1999). *Speech signal processing for determining psychological or physiological characteristics using a knowledge base*. Google Patents.

Bonato, P. (2003). Wearable sensors/systems and their impact on biomedical engineering. *IEEE Engineering in Medicine and Biology Magazine*, *22*(3), 18–20. doi:10.1109/MEMB.2003.1213622 PMID:12845812

Bonnie, S., Basia, B., Kevin, C., Catherine, W., Jeff Coppersmith, J. H., & Rehabil Dev, J. (2013). *Bodies in motion: monitoring daily activity and exercise with motion sensors in people with chronic pulmonary diseases*. Academic Press. doi: .0045 doi:10.1682/JRRD.2003.10

Borkar, V. R., Carey, M. J., & Chen, L. (2012). Big data platforms: What's next? *ACM Crossroads*, *19*(1), 44–49. doi:10.1145/2331042.2331057

Boumstein, J. (2013). *The case for Outsourced Invoice Scanning and data Capture*. Academic Press.

Bourlard, H. A., & Morgan, N. (2012). *Connectionist speech recognition: a hybrid approach*. Springer Science & Business Media.

Boyle, K. C. (2016). *Occluded Edge Detection in Light Field Images for Background Removal*. Academic Press.

Boyle, J. R., Sparks, R. S., Keijzers, G. B., Crilly, J. L., Lind, J. F., & Ryan, L. M. (2011). Prediction and surveillance of influenza epidemics. *The Medical Journal of Australia*, *194*(4), S28. PMID:21401485

Brandstein, M., & Ward, D. (2013). *Microphone arrays: signal processing techniques and applications*. Springer Science & Business Media.

Bresnick, J. (2015, January 13). *How to Select a Big Data Analytics, Business Intelligence Vendor.* Retrieved July 14, 2017, from https://healthitanalytics.com/news/how-to-select-a-big-data-analytics-business-intelligence-vendor

Bresnick, J. (2015, September 18). *Healthcare Big Data Analytics Suffers from "Fragmented" Approach.* Retrieved May 26, 2017, from http://healthitanalytics.com/news/healthcare-big-data-analytics-suffers-from-fragmented-approach

Bresnick, J. (2016a). *How to Choose the Right Healthcare Big Data Analytics Tools.* Retrieved July 14, 2017, from https://healthitanalytics.com/features/how-to-choose-the-right-healthcare-big-data-analytics-tools

Bresnick, J. (2016b). *The Difference Between Big Data and Smart Data in Healthcare.* Retrieved July 14, 2017, from https://healthitanalytics.com/features/the-difference-between-big-data-and-smart-data-in-healthcare

Bresnick, J. (2016c). *The Role of Healthcare Data Governance in Big Data Analytics.* Retrieved July 14, 2017, from https://healthitanalytics.com/features/the-role-of-healthcare-data-governance-in-big-data-analytics

Bresnick, J. (2017, June 5). *Understanding the Many V's of Healthcare Big Data Analytics.* Retrieved July 20, 2018, from Health IT Analytics: https://healthitanalytics.com/news/understanding-the-many-vs-of-healthcare-big-data-analytics

Brosch, T., & Tam, R., & Alzheimer's Disease Neuroimaging Initiative. (2013, September). Manifold learning of brain MRIs by deep learning. In *International Conference on Medical Image Computing and Computer-Assisted Intervention* (pp. 633-640). Springer. 10.1007/978-3-642-40763-5_78

Brosch, T. (2016). Deep learning of brain images and its application to multiple sclerosis. In G. Wu, D. Shen, & M. R. Sabuncu (Eds.), *Machine Learning and Medical Imaging* (pp. 69–96). Elsevier. doi:10.1016/B978-0-12-804076-8.00003-7

Brown, N. (2015, September 11). *Healthcare Data Growth: An Exponential Problem.* Retrieved August 8, 2017, from http://www.nextech.com/blog/healthcare-data-growth-an-exponential-problem

Brumen, B., Heričko, M., Sevčnikar, A., Završnik, J., & Hölbl, M. (2013). Outsourcing medical data analyses: Can technology overcome legal, privacy, and confidentiality issues? *Journal of Medical Internet Research, 15*(12), e283. doi:10.2196/jmir.2471 PMID:24342053

Burkland, S. (2005). *Near Field Communication in Smartphones (Unpublished work).* Berlin Institute of Technology. Retrieved from http://citeseerx.ist.psu.edu/viewdoc/versions?doi=10.1.1.455.3514

Butler, M. B., Gu, H., Kenney, T., & Campbell, S. G. (2016). P017: Does a busy day predict another busy day? A time-series analysis of multi-centre emergency department volumes. *Canadian Journal of Emergency Medical Care, 18*(S1), S83–S84. doi:10.1017/cem.2016.193

Cabielles-Hernández, D., Pérez-Pérez, J. R., Paule-Ruiz, M., & Fernández-Fernández, S. (2017, April 1). Specialized Intervention Using Tablet Devices for Communication Deficits in Children with Autism Spectrum Disorders. *IEEE Transactions on Learning Technologies, 10*(2), 182–193. doi:10.1109/TLT.2016.2559482

Calegari, R., Fogliatto, F. S., Lucini, F. R., Neyeloff, J., Kuchenbecker, R. S., & Schaan, B. D. (2016). Forecasting Daily Volume and Acuity of Patients in the Emergency Department. *Computational and Mathematical Methods in Medicine.* PMID:27725842

Camada, M. Y., Cerqueira, J. J., & Lima, A. M. Stereotyped gesture recognition: An analysis between HMM and SVM. In *Innovations in Intelligent Systems and Applications (INISTA), 2017 IEEE International Conference* (pp. 328-333). IEEE.

Camarinha, L. M., & Vieira, W. (1999). Intelligent mobile agents in elderly care. *Robotics and Autonomous Systems, 27*(1-2), 59–75. doi:10.1016/S0921-8890(98)00083-9

Cambridge, Mass & Rochester, Minn. (2013, January 15). *Optum, Mayo Clinic Partner to Launch Optum Labs: An Open, Collaborative Research and Innovation Facility Focused on Better Care for Patients.* Retrieved April 20, 2018, from https://www.optum.com/about/news/optum-labs.html

Çamlica, Z., Tizhoosh, H. R., & Khalvati, F. (2015). Autoencoding the retrieval relevance of medical images. *5th International Conference on Image Processing, Theory, Tools and Applications 2015, IPTA 2015*, 550–555. 10.1109/IPTA.2015.7367208

Canny, J. F. (1983). *Finding edges and lines in images.* Academic Press.

Cao, Y. (2015). Medical Image Retrieval: A Multimodal Approach. *Computational Advances in Cancer Informatics, 13*(S3), 125–136. PMID:26309389

Carey, D. E., Myers, R. M., Reuben, R., & Rodrigues, F. M. (1966). Studies on dengue in Vellore, South India. *The American Journal of Tropical Medicine and Hygiene, 15*(4), 580–587. doi:10.4269/ajtmh.1966.15.580 PMID:5949559

Carneiro, G., Nascimento, J. C., & Freitas, A. (2010). *Robust left ventricle segmentation from ultrasound data using deep neu- ral networks and efficient search methods.* Isbi. Available at http://ieeexplore.ieee.org/xpls/abs_all.jsp?arnumber=5490181

Carvalho-Silva, M., Monteiro, M. T. T., de Sá-Soares, F., & Dória-Nóbrega, S. (2017). Assessment of forecasting models for patients arrival at Emergency Department. *Operations Research for Health Care.* doi:10.1016/j.orhc.2017.05.001

Castle, B. L., & Szymanski, G. (2008). Supply Chain Management on Clinical Units. In eBusiness in Healthcare (pp. 197-217). London: Springe.

Caswell, I., Shen, C., & Wang, L. (2016). *Loopy Neural Nets: Imitating Feedback Loops in the Human Brain.* Stanford.

Cattuto, C., Van den Broeck, W., Barrat, A., Colizza, V., Pinton, J.-F., & Vespignani, A. (2010). Dynamics of Person-to-Person Interactions from Distributed RFID Sensor Networks. *PLoS One, 5*(7), e11596. doi:10.1371/journal.pone.0011596 PMID:20657651

Champion, R., Kinsman, L. D., Lee, G. A., Masman, K. A., May, E. A., Mills, T. M., ... Williams, R. J. (2007). Forecasting emergency department presentations. *Australian Health Review, 31*(1), 83–90. doi:10.1071/AH070083 PMID:17266491

Chandler, D. L. (2016). Opening New Worlds for Those with Autism: Technology Is Creating Great New Possibilities for Those on Every Part of the Spectrum. *IEEE Pulse, 7*(4), 43–46. doi:10.1109/MPUL.2016.2563819 PMID:27414634

Chang, K., Bai, H. X., Zhou, H., Su, C., Bi, W. L., Agbodza, E., ... Zhang, B. (2018). Residual convolutional neural network for the determination of IDH status in low-and high-grade gliomas from MR imaging. *Clinical Cancer Research, 24*(5), 1073–1081. doi:10.1158/1078-0432.CCR-17-2236 PMID:29167275

Chase, V. J., Cohn, A. E., Peterson, T. A., & Lavieri, M. S. (2012). Predicting emergency department volume using forecasting methods to create a "surge response" for noncrisis events. *Academic Emergency Medicine, 19*(5), 569–576. doi:10.1111/j.1553-2712.2012.01359.x PMID:22594361

Chaturvedi, U. C., Kapoor, A. K., Mathur, A., Chandra, D., Khan, A. M., & Mehrotra, R. M. L. (1970). A clinical and epidemiological study of an epidemic of febrile illness with haemorrhagic manifestations which occurred at Kanpur, India in 1968. *Bulletin of the World Health Organization, 43*, 281–287. PMID:4249614

Chaturvedi, U. C., Mathur, A., Kapoor, A. K., Mehrotra, N. K., & Mehrotra, R. M. L. (1970). Virological study of an epidemic of febrile illness with haemorrhagic manifestations at Kanpur, India, during 1968. *Bulletin of the World Health Organization, 43*, 289–293. PMID:5312525

Chaudhuri, R. N., Saha, T. K., & Chaudhuri, A. D. (1965). Dengue-like fever in Calcutta: Further preliminary observations. *Bulletin of the Calcutta School of Tropical Medicine*, *13*, 2–3. PMID:14281058

Cheng, J.-Z. (2016). *Computer-Aided Diagnosis with Deep Learning Architecture: Applications to Breast Lesions in US Images and Pulmonary Nodules in CT Scans.* Nature Publishing Group. Available at: http://www.pubmedcentral.nih.gov/articlerender.fcgi?artid=4832199&tool=pmcentrez&rendertype=abstract

Cheng, J. Z., Ni, D., Chou, Y. H., Qin, J., Tiu, C. M., Chang, Y. C., ... Chen, C. M. (2016). Computer-aided diagnosis with deep learning architecture: Applications to breast lesions in US images and pulmonary nodules in CT scans. *Scientific Reports*, *6*(1), 24454. doi:10.1038rep24454 PMID:27079888

Cheung, S. C. (2015). Integrating multimedia into autism intervention. *IEEE MultiMedia*, *22*(4), 4–10. doi:10.1109/MMUL.2015.86

Choubey, D. K., Paul, S., Kumar, S., & Kumar, S. (2017, February). Classification of Pima indian diabetes dataset using naive bayes with genetic algorithm as an attribute selection. In *Communication and Computing Systems: Proceedings of the International Conference on Communication and Computing System (ICCCS 2016)* (pp. 451-455). Academic Press.

Chowdhury, G. G. (2003). Natural language processing. *Annual Review of Information Science & Technology*, *37*(1), 51–89. doi:10.1002/aris.1440370103

Ciresan, D. (2012). *Deep Neural Networks Segment Neuronal Membranes in Electron Microscopy Images*. Nips. Available at https://papers.nips.cc/paper/4741-deep-neural-networks-segment-neuronal-membranes-in-electron-microscopy-images.pdf

Cisco. (2015). *Fog Computing and the Internet of Things: Extend.* Cisco. Retrieved from https://www.cisco.com/c/dam/en_us/solutions/trends/iot/docs/computing-overview.pdf

Clinical Leader. (n.d.). *Considerations For Improving Patient Recruitment Into Clinical Trials*. Retrieved March 10, 2018 from https://www.clinicalleader.com/doc/considerations-for-improving-patient-0001

Coiera, E. (2015). *Guide to health informatics*. CRC Press.

Cools, M., Moons, E., & Wets, G. (2009). Investigating the variability in daily traffic counts through use of ARIMAX and SARIMAX models: Assessing the effect of holidays on two site locations. *Transportation Research Record: Journal of the Transportation Research Board*, *2136*(1), 57–66. doi:10.3141/2136-07

Corneli, A., Pierre, C., Hinkley, T., Lin, L., Fordyce, C. B., Hamre, G., & Roe, M. T. (2017). One and done: Reasons principal investigators conduct only one FDA-regulated drug trial. *Contemporary Clinical Trials Communications, 6*. Retrieved March 10, 2018 from https://www.sciencedirect.com/science/article/pii/S245186541630093X

Côté, M. J., Smith, M. A., Eitel, D. R., & Akçali, E. (2013). Forecasting emergency department arrivals: A tutorial for emergency department directors. *Hospital Topics*, *91*(1), 9–19. doi:10.1080/00185868.2013.757962 PMID:23428111

Crapo, J. (2017). *Big Data in Healthcare: Separating The Hype From The Reality.* Retrieved July 27, 2017, from https://www.healthcatalyst.com/healthcare-big-data-realities

Cristóbal, G., Schelkens, P., & Thienpont, H. (Eds.). (2013). *Optical and digital image processing: fundamentals and applications*. John Wiley & Sons.

Critchley, H. D. (2002). Book Review: Electro dermal Responses: What Happens in the Brain? *The Neuroscientist*, *8*(2), 132–142. doi:10.1177/107385840200800209 PMID:11954558

Crouse, M. S., Nowak, R. D., & Baraniuk, R. G. (1998). Wavelet-based statistical signal processing using hidden Markov models. *IEEE Transactions on Signal Processing*, *46*(4), 886–902. doi:10.1109/78.668544

Dansereau, D. (2016). *Lightfield toolbox v. 0.4*. Available at: http://www.mathworks.com/matlabcentral/fileexchange/49683-lightfield-toolboxv0-4

Dansereau, D. G. (2015). Light field toolbox for matlab. *Software Manual*.

Dansereau, D. G., Pizarro, O., & Williams, S. B. (2013, June). Decoding, calibration and rectification for lenselet-based plenoptic cameras. In *Computer Vision and Pattern Recognition (CVPR), 2013 IEEE Conference on* (pp. 1027-1034). IEEE. 10.1109/CVPR.2013.137

Das, R., Turkoglu, I., & Sengur, A. (2009). Effective diagnosis of heart disease through neural networks ensembles. *Expert Systems with Applications*, *36*(4), 7675–7680. doi:10.1016/j.eswa.2008.09.013

Datafloq. (n.d.). Retrieved from https://datafloq.com/big-data-open-source-tools/os-data-aggregation/

de Bruijne, M. (2016). Machine learning approaches in medical image analysis: From detection to diagnosis. *Medical Image Analysis*, *33*, 94–97. doi:10.1016/j.media.2016.06.032 PMID:27481324

de Carvalho Filho, A. O., Silva, A. C., de Paiva, A. C., Nunes, R. A., & Gattass, M. (2017). Computer-aided diagnosis of lung nodules in computed tomography by using phylogenetic diversity, genetic algorithm, and SVM. *Journal of Digital Imaging*, *30*(6), 812–822. doi:10.100710278-017-9973-6 PMID:28526968

De Meo, P., Quattrone, G., & Ursino, D. (2011). Integration of the HL7 Standard in a multiagent system to support personalized access to e-health services. *IEEE Transactions on Knowledge and Data Engineering*, *23*(8), 1244–1260. doi:10.1109/TKDE.2010.174

De Paz, J. F., Rodríguez, S., Zatoand, C., & Corchado, J. M. (2015). An Integrated System for Helping Disabled and Dependent People: AGALZ, AZTECA, and MOVI-MAS Projects. Springer International Publishing.

Dean, J., & Ghemawat, S. (2008). MapReduce: Simplified data processing on large clusters. *Communications of the ACM*, *51*(1), 107–113. doi:10.1145/1327452.1327492

Deekshatulu, B. L., & Chandra, P. (2013). Classification of heart disease using k-nearest neighbor and genetic algorithm. *Procedia Technology*, *10*, 85–94. doi:10.1016/j.protcy.2013.12.340

Deepak. (2016). *A Critical Comparison of NOSQL Databases in the Context of Acid and Base*. Culminating Projects in Information Assurance. Paper 8.

Deeplearning4j Development Team. (2016). *Deeplearning4j: Open-source distributed deep learning for the JVM*. Apache Software Foundation License 2.0. Available at: http://deeplearning4j.org

Deller, J. R. Jr, Proakis, J. G., & Hansen, J. H. (1993). *Discrete time processing of speech signals*. Prentice Hall PTR.

Devarakonda, M., & Tsou, C. H. (2015, January). *Automated Problem List Generation from Electronic Medical Records in IBM Watson*. AAAI.

Diamond, O. (2015). *Overcoming Patient Recruitment and Retention Hurdles*. Retrieved March 10, 2018 from http://medrio.com/partners/overcoming-patient-recruitment-and-retention-hurdles/

Disch, W. (2016, August 11). *How to Use Big Data to Improve Patient Engagement*. Retrieved 8 2017, from http://data-informed.com/how-to-use-big-data-to-improve-patient-engagement/

Dmitrievich, I. A. (2015). *Deep Learning in information analysis of electrocardiogram signals for disease diagnostics* (Diss.). Moscow Institute of Physics and Technology.

Doi, K. (2007). Computer-aided diagnosis in medical imaging: Historical review, current status and future potential. *Computerized Medical Imaging and Graphics, 31*(4-5), 198–211. doi:10.1016/j.compmedimag.2007.02.002 PMID:17349778

Doyle-Lindrud, S. (2015). Watson will see you now: A supercomputer to help clinicians make informed treatment decisions. *Clinical Journal of Oncology Nursing, 19*(1), 31–32. doi:10.1188/15.CJON.31-32 PMID:25689646

Dr. Shyam Kumar v Rameshbhai, Harmanbhai Kachiya, 2002 (1) CPR 320, I (2006) CPJ 16 (NC)

Eastwood, B. (2013, April 23). *6 Big Data Analytics Use Cases for Healthcare IT.* Retrieved July 24, 2017, from http://www.cio.com/article/2386531/healthcare/healthcare-6-big-data-analytics-use-cases-for-healthcare-it.html

ECMA International. (2013). *Near Field Communication-Interface and Protocol (NFCIP-1).* Retrieved from https://www.ecma-international.org/publications/files/ECMA-ST/Ecma-340.pdf

ECMA International. (2013). *Near Field Communication-Interface and Protocol (NFCIP-2).* Retrieved from https://www.ecma-international.org/publications/standards/Ecma-352.htm

ECQMs. (2017). Retrieved October 23, 2017, from http://ecqi.healthit.gov/ecqms

Efendigil, T., Önüt, S., & Kahraman, C. (2009). A decision support system for demand forecasting with artificial neural networks and neuro-fuzzy models: A comparative analysis. *Expert Systems with Applications, 36*(3), 6697–6707. doi:10.1016/j.eswa.2008.08.058

EHR Incentives and Certification. (2015, February 6). Retrieved November 15, 2017, from http://www.healthit.gov/providers-professionals/meaningful-use-definition-objectives

Ekström, A., Kurland, L., Farrokhnia, N., Castrén, M., & Nordberg, M. (2015). Forecasting emergency department visits using internet data. *Annals of Emergency Medicine, 65*(4), 436–442. doi:10.1016/j.annemergmed.2014.10.008 PMID:25487026

El Agha, M., Jarghon, A., & Abu Naser, S. S. (2017). *Polymyalgia Rheumatic Expert System. International Journal of Engineering and Information Systems.*

El-Dahshan, E. S. A., Mohsen, H. M., Revett, K., & Salem, A. B. M. (2014). Computer-aided diagnosis of human brain tumor through MRI: A survey and a new algorithm. *Expert Systems with Applications, 41*(11), 5526–5545. doi:10.1016/j.eswa.2014.01.021

Elnemr, H. A., Zayed, N. M., & Fakhreldein, M. A. (2016). Feature Extraction Techniques: Fundamental Concepts and Survey. Handbook of Research on Emerging Perspectives in Intelligent Pattern Recognition, Analysis, and Image Processing, 264–294.

Elveren, E., & Yumuşak, N. (2011). Tuberculosis disease diagnosis using artificial neural network trained with genetic algorithm. *Journal of Medical Systems, 35*(3), 329–332. doi:10.100710916-009-9369-3 PMID:20703557

Emad, O., Yassine, I. A., & Fahmy, A. S. (2015). Automatic Localization of the Left Ventricle in Cardiac MRI Images Using Deep Learning. *37th Annual International Conference of the IEEE Engineering in Medicine & Biology Society (EMBC)*, 683–686. 10.1109/EMBC.2015.7318454

Epidomiology and Genomics Research Program. (2018, April 5). Retrieved April 29, 2018, from https://epi.grants.cancer.gov/pharm/pharmacoepi_db/healthcore.html

Esteva, A., Kuprel, B., Novoa, R. A., Ko, J., Swetter, S. M., Blau, H. M., & Thrun, S. (2017). Dermatologist-level classification of skin cancer with deep neural networks. *Nature*, *542*(7639), 115–118. doi:10.1038/nature21056 PMID:28117445

EvaluatePharma. (2017, June). World Preview 2017 *Outlook to 2022*. Retrieved from http://info.evaluategroup.com/rs/607-YGS-364/images/WP17.pdf

Evolve, I. P. (2017). *Email Vulnerability in Healthcare*. Retrieved from http://www.evolveip.net/lp/email-vulnerability-healthcare

Eysenbach, G. (2009). Infodemiology and infoveillance: Framework for an emerging set of public health informatics methods to analyze search, communication and publication behavior on the Internet. *Journal of Medical Internet Research*, *11*(1), e11. doi:10.2196/jmir.1157 PMID:19329408

Farsi, A. Al, Doctor, F., Petrovic, D., Chandran, S., & Karyotis, C. (2017). *Interval Valued Data Enhanced Fuzzy Cognitive Maps: Towards an Approach for Autism Deduction in Toddlers*. doi:10.1109/FUZZ-IEEE.2017.8015702

Feldman, B., Martin, E. M., & Skotnes, T. (2012). *Big Data in Healthcare Hype and Hope*. Retrieved from http://www.west-info.eu/files/big-data-in- healthcare.pdf

Fengou, Mantas, Lymberopoulos, Komnios, Fengos, Lazarou, & Nikolaos. (2012). A New Framework Architecture for Next Generation e-Health Services. *IEEE Transactions on Information Technology in Biomedicine*.

Ferreira, G. L. (2012). Global dengue epidemiology trends. *Revista do Instituto de Medicina Tropical de São Paulo*, *54*(Suppl 18), S5–S6. doi:10.1590/S0036-46652012000700003 PMID:23011450

Fidele, B., Cheeneebash, J., Gopaul, A., & Goorah, S. S. (2009). Artificial neural network as a clinical decision-supporting tool to predict cardiovascular disease. *Trends in Applied Sciences Research*, *4*(1), 36-46.

FIPA ACL Message Structure Specification. (2013). Retrieved from http://www.fipa.org/specs/fipa00061/SC00061G.pdf

Fischer, S. (2017). Minibrain Storm: Cerebral Organoids Aren't Real Brains? But They Provide a Powerful Platform for Modeling Brain Diseases Like Zika Infection, Alzheimer's, and Even Autism. *IEEE Pulse*, *8*(3), 31–34. doi:10.1109/MPUL.2017.2680360 PMID:28534760

Fister, I., Jr., Yang, X. S., Fister, I., Brest, J., & Fister, D. (2013). *A brief review of nature-inspired algorithms for optimization*. arXiv preprint arXiv:1307.4186

Flanagan, J. L. (2013). *Speech analysis synthesis and perception*. Springer Science & Business Media.

Flatiron. (2017). *Community Oncology*. Retrieved 8 2017, from https://flatiron.com/community-oncology/

Food and Drug Administration. (2009). *Guidance for Clinical Investigators, Sponsors, and IRBs*. Retrieved March 18, 2018 from https://www.fda.gov/downloads/regulatoryinformation/guidances/ucm126572.pdf

Food and Drug Administration. (2015). *Digital Health Innovation Action Plan*. Retrieved March 7, 2018 from https://www.fda.gov/downloads/MedicalDevices/DigitalHealth/UCM568735.pdf

Food and Drug Administration. (2015). *Mobile Medical Applications: Guidance for Industry and Food and Drug Administration Staff*. Retrieved March 7, 2018 from https://www.fda.gov/downloads/MedicalDevices/.../UCM263366.pdf

Food and Drug Administration. (2016). *Use of Electronic Informed Consent*. Retrieved March 10, 2018 from https://www.fda.gov/downloads/Drugs/GuidanceComplianceRegulatoryInformation/Guidances/UCM436811.pdf

Food and Drug Administration. (n.d.). *Clinical Outcome Assessment Qualification Program.* Retrieved March 18, 2018 from https://www.fda.gov/Drugs/DevelopmentApprovalProcess/DrugDevelopmentToolsQualificationProgram/ucm284077.htm

Force v. M Ganeswara Rao. 1998 (3) CPR 251; 1998 (1) CPJ 413 (AP SCDRC).

Foundry. (n.d.). *VR? AR? MR? Sorry, I'm confused.* Retrieved February 12, 2018 from https://www.foundry.com/industries/virtual-reality/vr-mr-ar-confused

Freeman, L. M., Locke, J., Rotheram-Fuller, E., & Mandell, D. (2017). Brief Report: Examining Executive and Social Functioning in Elementary-Aged Children with Autism. *Journal of Autism and Developmental Disorders*, *47*(6), 1890–1895. doi:10.100710803-017-3079-3 PMID:28260182

Friedmann, E., Katcher, A. H., Lynch, J. J., & Thomas, S. A. (1980). Animal companions and one-year survival of patients after discharge from a coronary care unit. *Public Health Reports*, *95*(4), 307. PMID:6999524

Fujita, M. and Kitano, H. (1998). An development of an autonomous quadruped robot for robot entertainment. Autonomous Robots, 5, 7–18.

Furui, S. (1981). Cepstral analysis technique for automatic speaker verification. *IEEE Transactions on Acoustics, Speech, and Signal Processing*, *29*(2), 254–272. doi:10.1109/TASSP.1981.1163530

Gahirwal, M. (2013). *Inter Time series sales forecasting.* arXiv preprint arXiv:1303.0117

Galas, T., & Rodet, X. (1991). Generalized functional approximation for source-filter system modeling. *Second European Conference on Speech Communication and Technology.*

Gannot, S., Burshtein, D., & Weinstein, E. (2001). Signal enhancement using beamforming and nonstationarity with applications to speech. *IEEE Transactions on Signal Processing*, *49*(8), 1614–1626. doi:10.1109/78.934132

Garrity, T. F., Stallones, L. F., Marx, M. B., & Johnson, T. P. (1989). Pet ownership and attachment as supportive factors in the health of the elderly. *Anthrozoos*, *3*(1), 35–44. doi:10.2752/089279390787057829

Gartner. (n.d.). *Gartner IT Glossary: Virtual Assistant.* Retrieved March 10, 2018 from https://www.gartner.com/it-glossary/virtual-assistant-va/

Gautam, A., & Pan, X. (2016). The changing model of big pharma: Impact of key trends. *Drug Discovery Today*, *21*(3), 379–384. doi:10.1016/j.drudis.2015.10.002 PMID:26477304

Gay, S. L., & Benesty, J. (2012). *Acoustic signal processing for telecommunication.* Springer Science & Business Media.

Gershun, A. (1939). The light field. *Studies in Applied Mathematics*, *18*(1-4), 51–151.

Ghoraani, B., & Krishnan, S. (2011). Time–frequency matrix feature extraction and classification of environmental audio signals. *IEEE Transactions on Audio, Speech, and Language Processing*, *19*(7), 2197–2209. doi:10.1109/TASL.2011.2118753

Ghosh, B. N. (1968). A study on the epidemic of dengue-like fever in Pondicherry (1964-65 and 1965-66). *Journal of the Indian Medical Association*, *51*, 261–264. PMID:5706900

Gilbert, M. R., Rubinstein, L., & Lesser, G. (2016). Creating clinical trial designs that incorporate clinical outcome assessments. *Neuro-Oncology*, *18*(Suppl 2). Retrieved March 18, 2018 from https://www.ncbi.nlm.nih.gov/pmc/articles/PMC4795995/

Global Industry Analysts, Inc. (2018). *Virtual Reality (VR) in Healthcare – A Global Strategic Business Report*. Retrieved March 01, 2018 from http://www.strategyr.com/MarketResearch/Virtual_Reality_VR_In_Healthcare_Market_Trends.asp

Gondara, L. (2016). *Medical image denoising using convolutional denoising autoencoders*. Available at: http://arxiv.org/abs/1608.04667

Gonzalez, R. C., & Woods, R. E. (2002). *Digital image processing*. Academic Press.

Gonzalez, M. C., Hidalgo, C. A., & Barabasi, A.-L. (2008). Understanding individual human mobility patterns. *Nature*, *453*(7196), 779–782. doi:10.1038/nature06958 PMID:18528393

Gonzalez, R. C., Woods, R. E., & Eddins, S. L. (2009). *Digital Image Processing Using MATLAB*. Gatesmark Publishing.

Goodfellow, I., Bengio, Y., & Courville, A. (2016). *Deep Learning*. Available at: http://www.deeplearningbook.org

Gortler, S. J., Grzeszczuk, R., Szeliski, R., & Cohen, M. F. (1996, August). The lumigraph. In *Proceedings of the 23rd annual conference on Computer graphics and interactive techniques* (pp. 43-54). ACM.

Graves, A., Fernandez, S., & Schmidhuber, J. (2007). *Multi-Dimensional Recurrent Neural Networks*. Available at: http://arxiv.org/abs/0705.2011

Graves, A., Mohamed, A., & Hinton, G. (2013). Speech Recognition with Deep Recurrent Neural Networks. *IEEE International Conference on acoustics, speech and signal processing*, 3, 6645–6649. 10.1109/ICASSP.2013.6638947

Green, M. D., Freedman, D. M., & Gordis, L. (2000). *Reference guide on epidemiology. Reference manual on scientific evidence*. Available: http://www.fjc.gov/public/pdf.nsf/lookup/sciman06.pdf/$file/sciman06.pdf

Greenspan, H. (2016). *Special Section on Deep Learning in Medical Applications*. Available at: http://www.ieee-tmi.org/deep-learning-in-medical-applications.pdf

Greenspan, H., van Ginneken, B., & Summers, R. M. (2016). Guest Editorial Deep Learning in Medical Imaging : Overview and Future Promise of an Exciting New Technique. *IEEE Transactions on Medical Imaging*, *35*(5), 1153–1159. doi:10.1109/TMI.2016.2553401

Groves, P., Kayyali, B., Knott, D., & Kuiken, S. V. (2013). *The 'big data' revolution in healthcare*. McKinsey & Company.

Guan, Z. J. (2013). *Internet-of-Things human body data blood pressure collecting and transmitting device*. Chinese Patent 202 821 362 U.

Guan, Z. J. (2013). *Somatic data blood glucose collection transmission device for Internet of Things*. Chinese Patent 202 838653 U.

Guangnan, Z., & Penghui, L. (2012). *IoT (Internet of Things) control system facing rehabilitation training of hemiplegic patients*. Chinese Patent 202 587045 U.

Gubler, D. J. (2002). The global emergence/resurgence of arboviral diseases as public health problems. *Archives of Medical Research*, *33*(4), 330–342. doi:10.1016/S0188-4409(02)00378-8 PMID:12234522

Gubler, D. J. (2011). Dengue, Urbanization and Globalization: The Unholy Trinity of the 21(st) Century. *Tropical Medicine and Health*, *39*(Suppl 4), 3–11. doi:10.2149/tmh.2011-S05 PMID:22500131

Gubler, D. J. (2012). The economic burden of dengue. *The American Journal of Tropical Medicine and Hygiene*, *86*(5), 743–744. doi:10.4269/ajtmh.2012.12-0157 PMID:22556068

Guenther, C., Pierson, M., & Modi, N. (2018). In Blockchain We Trust: Transforming Life Sciences with blockchain. *Accenture Life Sciences*. Retrieved March 10, 2018 from https://www.accenture.com/t20180406T080254Z__w__/us-en/_acnmedia/PDF-71/Accenture_Blockchain_Innovations_Life_Sciences.pdf#zoom=50

Guenther, F. H. (1994). A neural network model of speech acquisition and motor equivalent speech production. *Biological Cybernetics*, *72*(1), 43–53. doi:10.1007/BF00206237 PMID:7880914

Gul, M., & Guneri, A. F. (2015a). A comprehensive review of emergency department simulation applications for normal and disaster conditions. *Computers & Industrial Engineering*, *83*, 327–344. doi:10.1016/j.cie.2015.02.018

Gul, M., & Guneri, A. F. (2015b). Forecasting patient length of stay in an emergency department by artificial neural networks. *Journal of Aeronautics and Space Technologies*, *8*(2), 43–48.

Gul, M., & Guneri, A. F. (2016a). Planning the future of emergency departments: Forecasting ED patient arrivals by using regression and neural network models, International Journal of Industrial Engineering: Theory. *Applications and Practice*, *23*(2), 137–154.

Gul, M., & Guneri, A. F. (2016b). An artificial neural network-based earthquake casualty estimation model for Istanbul city. *Natural Hazards*, *84*(3), 2163–2178. doi:10.100711069-016-2541-4

Gul, M., Yucesan, M., & Celik, E. (2017). Multi-site and multi-method forecasting modelling of hospital emergency room patient arrivals. *International Conference on Advances and Innovations in Engineering (ICAIE)*, 134-138.

Guneri, A. F., & Gumus, A. T. (2008). The usage of artificial neural networks for finite capacity planning, International Journal of Industrial Engineering: Theory. *Applications and Practice*, *15*(1), 16–25.

Guneri, A. F., & Gumus, A. T. (2009). Artificial Neural Networks for Finite Capacity Scheduling: A Comparative Study, International Journal of Industrial Engineering: Theory. *Applications and Practice*, *15*(4), 349–359.

Guo, Y. (2014). Segmenting Hippocampus from Infant Brains by Sparse Patch Matching with Deep-Learned Features. *Medical Image Computing and Computer-Assisted Intervention. MICCAI 2014: 17th International Conference, Boston, MA, USA, September 14-18, 2014, Proceedings*, 308–315. 10.1007/978-3-319-10470-6_39

Gupta, A., Ayhan, M. S., & Maida, A. S. (2013). Natural Image Bases to Represent Neuroimaging Data. *Journal of Machine Learning Research: Workshop and Conference Proceedings*, *28*(3), 977–984.

Guzman, M. G., & Kouri, G. (2002). Dengue: An update. *The Lancet Infectious Diseases*, *2*(1), 33–42. doi:10.1016/S1473-3099(01)00171-2 PMID:11892494

Ha. (2015). A wearable EEG-HEG-HRV multi model system with simultaneous monitoring of tES for mental health management. *IEEE Transactions on Biomedical Circuits and Systems*, *9*(6), 758–766. PMID:26742142

Hagoort, P., Brown, C. M., & Osterhout, L. (1999). The neurocognition of syntactic processing. In The neurocognition of language. Oxford University Press.

Haladay, J. (1989). Animal assisted therapy for PWA's – Bringing a sense of connection. *AIDS Patient Care*, 38–39.

Hanna, C. J., & O'Connor, T. J. (2009). *U.S. Patent No. 7,583,861*. Washington, DC: U.S. Patent and Trademark Office.

Hansen, M., & Holk, E. (2011). *Depth map estimation for plenoptic images*. Academic Press.

Harrington, J. (2010). *Phonetic analysis of speech corpora*. John Wiley & Sons.

Harrou, F., Sun, Y., Kadri, F., Chaabane, S., & Tahon, C. (2015, October). Early detection of abnormal patient arrivals at hospital emergency department. In *Industrial Engineering and Systems Management (IESM), 2015 International Conference on* (pp. 221-227). IEEE. 10.1109/IESM.2015.7380162

Hart, L. A., Hart, B. L., & Bergin, B. L. (1987). Socializing effects of service dogs for people with disabilities. *Anthrozoos*, *1*(1), 41–44. doi:10.2752/089279388787058696

Hasan, R., Winslett, M., & Sion, R. (2007). Requirements of Secure Storage Systems for Healthcare Records. In W. Jonker & M. Petković (Eds.), Lecture Notes in Computer Science: Vol. 4721. *Secure Data Management. SDM 2007.* Berlin: Springer. doi:10.1007/978-3-540-75248-6_12

Havaei, M., & Guizard, N. (2016). *Deep learning trends for focal brain pathology segmentation in MRI.* Available at: http://arxiv.org/abs/1607.05258

Havaei, M., Davy, A., Warde-Farley, D., Biard, A., Courville, A., Bengio, Y., ... Larochelle, H. (2016). Brain tumor segmentation with Deep Neural Networks. *Medical Image Analysis*, *35*, 18–31. doi:10.1016/j.media.2016.05.004 PMID:27310171

Hazan & Baker. (2011). Acoustic-phonetic characteristics of speech produced with communicative intent to counter adverse listening conditions. *The Journal of the Acoustical Society of America, 130*(4), 2139-2152.

Hazirbas, C., Leal-Taixé, L., & Cremers, D. (2017). *Deep Depth from Focus.* arXiv preprint arXiv:1704.01085

HealtIT.gov. (2016, November 4). *Electronic Prescribing of Controlled Substances (EPCS).* Retrieved 8 2017, from https://www.healthit.gov/opioids/epcs

Heckmann, M., Domont, X., Joublin, F., & Goerick, C. (2011). A hierarchical framework for spectro-temporal feature extraction. *Speech Communication*, *53*(5), 736–752. doi:10.1016/j.specom.2010.08.006

Heinsfeld, A. S., Franco, A. R., Craddock, R. C., Buchweitz, A., & Meneguzzi, F. (2017, August). Identification of autism spectrum disorder using deep learning and the ABIDE dataset. *NeuroImage. Clinical*, *17*, 16–23. doi:10.1016/j.nicl.2017.08.017 PMID:29034163

Hermansky, H. (1990). Perceptual linear predictive (PLP) analysis of speech. *The Journal of the Acoustical Society of America, 87*(4), 1738-1752.

Hertzum, M. (2017). The Cost of Improved Overview: An Analysis of the Use of Electronic Whiteboards in Emergency Departments. In *IFIP Conference on Human-Computer Interaction* (pp. 402-410). Springer. 10.1007/978-3-319-67684-5_25

Hill, T., Marquez, L., O'Connor, M., & Remus, W. (1994). Artificial neural network models for forecasting and decision making. *International Journal of Forecasting*, *10*(1), 5–15. doi:10.1016/0169-2070(94)90045-0

Hinton, G. (2014). Where do features come from? *Cognitive Science*, *38*(6), 1078–1101. doi:10.1111/cogs.12049 PMID:23800216

Hinton, G. E., Osindero, S., & Teh, Y.-W. W. (2006). A Fast Learning Algorithm for Deep Belief Nets. *Neural Computation*, *18*(7), 1527–1554. doi:10.1162/neco.2006.18.7.1527 PMID:16764513

Hinton, G., Bengio, Y., & Lecun, Y. (2015). *Deep Learning tutorial.* Nips.

Hirasawa, T., Aoyama, K., Tanimoto, T., Ishihara, S., Shichijo, S., Ozawa, T., ... Tada, T. (2018). Application of artificial intelligence using a convolutional neural network for detecting gastric cancer in endoscopic images. *Gastric Cancer*, *21*(4), 653–660. doi:10.100710120-018-0793-2 PMID:29335825

Hiroya, S., & Honda, M. (2004). Estimation of articulatory movements from speech acoustics using an HMM-based speech production model. *IEEE Transactions on Speech and Audio Processing*, *12*(2), 175–185. doi:10.1109/TSA.2003.822636

Honauer, K., Johannsen, O., Kondermann, D., & Goldluecke, B. (2016). A dataset and evaluation methodology for depth estimation on 4d light fields. In *Asian Conference on Computer Vision* (pp. 19-34). Springer.

Hoot, N. R., Zhou, C., Jones, I., & Aronsky, D. (2007). Measuring and forecasting emergency department crowding in real time. *Annals of Emergency Medicine*, *49*(6), 747–755. doi:10.1016/j.annemergmed.2007.01.017 PMID:17391809

Hossan, A., Memon, S., & Greggory, M. A. (2010). A novel approach for MFCC feature extraction. In *Signal Processing and Communication Systems (ICSPCS), 2010 4th International Conference on*. IEEE. 10.1109/ICSPCS.2010.5709752

Hosseini-Asl, E., Keynto, R., & El-Baz, A. (2016). *Alzheimer's Disease Diagnostics by Adaptation of 3D Convolutional Network*. Available at: http://arxiv.org/abs/1607.00455

Hristoskova, A., Sakkalis, V., & Zacharioudakis, G. (2014). *Ontology-driven monitoring of patient's vital signs enabling personalized medical detection and alert*. Personalized Medical Detection.

Hsin, C., & Danner, C. (2016). *Convolutional Neural Networks for Left Ventricle Volume Estimation*. Academic Press.

Huang, X., Acero, A., & Hon, H.W. (2001). *Spoken language processing: A guide to theory, algorithm, and system development*. Prentice Hall PTR.

Huang, X. D., Ariki, Y., & Jack, M. (1990). *Hidden Markov models for speech recognition*. New York: Columbia University Press.

Hurwitz, J., Nugent, A., Halper, F., & Kaufman, M. (2013). *Hadoop Pig and Pig Latin for Big Data*. Wiley.

Hwang, J.-N., & Hu, Y. H. (2001). *Handbook of neural network signal processing*. CRC Press.

IBM. (2013). *Southern Denmark Tackles Heart Disease with IBM Big Data Analytics Program*. Press Release.

IBM. (n.d.). *Big data and information management*. Retrieved from http://www-01.ibm.com/soft ware/data/bigdata/

Ibrahim, S., Djemal, R., & Alsuwailem, A. (2017). Electroencephalography (EEG) signal processing for epilepsy and autism spectrum disorder diagnosis. *Biocybernetics and Biomedical Engineering*, 1–11. doi:10.1016/J.BBE.2017.08.006

IDC. (2014). *The Digital Universe Driving Data Growth in Healthcare*. IDC. Retrieved August 7, 2017, from http://www.emc.com/analyst-report/digital-universe-healthcare-vertical-report-ar.pdf

IHTT. (2013). *Transforming Health Care through Big Data Strategies for leveraging big data in the health care industry*. Retrieved from http://ihealthtran.com/ wordpress/2013/03/iht%C2%B2-releases-big-data-research-report- download-today/

Implementers Forum, U. S. B. (2005). *USB 'A' Plug Form Factor (Revision 1.0)*. Retrieved from http://www.usb.org/developers/docs/devclass_docs/CCWG_A_Plug_Form_Factor_Guideline_Revision_1.0_.pdf

In, Z. L. (2014). *Patient body temperature monitoring system and device based on Internet of Things*. Chinese Patent 103 577688 A.

Intel. (n.d.). *Demystifying the Virtual Reality Landscape*. Retrieved February 12, 2018 from https://www.intel.com/content/www/us/en/tech-tips-and-tricks/virtual-reality-vs-augmented-reality.html

International Organization for Standardization. (2013). *Information Technology-Telecommunication and Information Exchange between Systems—Near Field Communication—Internface and Protocol (NFCIP-1)*. Retrieved from https://www.iso.org/standard/56692.html

International Organization for Standardization. (2016). *Identification Cards-Contactless Integrated Circuit Cards-Proximity Cards-Part 2: Radio Frequency Power and Signal Interface (ISO/IEC 14443-2:2016).* Retrieved from https://www.iso.org/standard/66288.html

Internet of Things Protocols and Standards. (n.d.). Retrieved from https://www.cse.wustl.edu/~jain/cse570-15/ftp/iot_prot

Isern, D., Sánchez, D., & Moreno, A. (2010). Agents applied in health care: A review. *International Journal of Medical Informatics*, *79*(3), 145–166. doi:10.1016/j.ijmedinf.2010.01.003 PMID:20129820

Ishioka, J., Matsuoka, Y., Uehara, S., Yasuda, Y., Kijima, T., Yoshida, S., ... Kimura, T. (2018). Computer-aided diagnosis of prostate cancer on magnetic resonance imaging using a convolutional neural network algorithm. *BJU International*. doi:10.1111/bju.14397 PMID:29772101

Isshiki, N. (1989). Physiology of speech production. In Phonosurgery. Springer.

Istepanian, R. S., Hu, S., Philip, N. Y., & Sungoor, A. (2011, August). The potential of Internet of m-health Things "m-IoT" for non-invasive glucose level sensing. In *Engineering in medicine and biology society, EMBC, 2011 annual international conference of the IEEE* (pp. 5264-5266). IEEE. 10.1109/IEMBS.2011.6091302

Istepanian, R. S. H., Hu, S., Philip, N. Y., & Sungoor, A. (2011). The potential of Internet of m-health Things 'm-IoT' for non-invasive glucose level sensing. *Proc. IEEE Annu.*

Iyer, M. (2011, April 20). Medical errors in top 10 Killers: WHO. *Times of India*.

JADE-LEAP. (n.d.). Retrieved from http://sharon.cslet.it/project/jade

Jalalkamali, A., Moradi, M., & Moradi, N. (2015). Application of several artificial intelligence models and ARIMAX model for forecasting drought using the Standardized Precipitation Index. *International Journal of Environmental Science and Technology*, *12*(4), 1201–1210. doi:10.100713762-014-0717-6

Jameson, R., Lorence, D., & Lee, J. (2012). Integrating computerized primitives and annotated video patterns: A proposed model for autism diagnosis and research. *Journal of Medical Systems*, *36*(3), 2037–2045. doi:10.100710916-011-9666-5 PMID:21537855

Jara, A. J., Zamora-Izquierdo, M. A., & Skarmeta, A. F. (2013). Interconnection framework for m-Health and remote monitoring based on the Internet of Things. *IEEE Journal on Selected Areas in Communications*, *31*(9), 47–65. doi:10.1109/JSAC.2013.SUP.0513005

Java Agent Development Framework (JADE). (n.d.). Available online: http://jade.tilab.com

Jawadekar, D. M. (2016, August 4). *Big Data and Pharmaceutical Drug Discovery*. Retrieved August 2017, from https://pharma.elsevier.com/pharma-rd/big-data-and-pharmaceutical-drug-discovery/

Jayalakshmi, T., & Santhakumaran, A. (2010). A novel classification method for diagnosis of diabetes mellitus using artificial neural networks. In *Data Storage and Data Engineering (DSDE), 2010 International Conference on* (pp. 159-163). IEEE. 10.1109/DSDE.2010.58

Jelinek, F. (1976). Continuous speech recognition by statistical methods. *Proceedings of the IEEE*, *64*(4), 532–556. doi:10.1109/PROC.1976.10159

Jian, Z., Zhanli, W., & Zhuang, M. (2012). *Temperature measurement system and method based on home gateway*. Chinese Patent 102811 185A.

Jones Day. (2018). FDA's Evolving Regulation of Artificial Intelligence in Digital Health Products. *Lexology*. Retrieved March 7, 2018 from https://www.lexology.com/library/detail.aspx?g=cf6351a3-a944-4468-9214-d141a689955e

Jones, S. A., Joy, M. P., & Pearson, J. (2002). Forecasting demand of emergency care. *Health Care Management Science, 5*(4), 297–305. doi:10.1023/A:1020390425029 PMID:12437279

Jones, S. S., Evans, R. S., Allen, T. L., Thomas, A., Haug, P. J., Welch, S. J., & Snow, G. L. (2009). A multivariate time series approach to modeling and forecasting demand in the emergency department. *Journal of Biomedical Informatics, 42*(1), 123–139. doi:10.1016/j.jbi.2008.05.003 PMID:18571990

Jones, S. S., Thomas, A., Evans, R. S., Welch, S. J., Haug, P. J., & Snow, G. L. (2008). Forecasting daily patient volumes in the emergency department. *Academic Emergency Medicine, 15*(2), 159–170. doi:10.1111/j.1553-2712.2007.00032.x PMID:18275446

Jovanov, E., Lords, A. D., Raskovic, D., Cox, P. G., Adhami, R., & Andrasik, F. (2003). Stress monitoring using a distributed wireless intelligent sensor system. *IEEE Engineering in Medicine and Biology Magazine, 22*(3), 49–55. doi:10.1109/MEMB.2003.1213626 PMID:12845819

Juang, B.-H., & Rahim, M. G. (1996). Signal bias removal by maximum likelihood estimation for robust telephone speech recognition. *IEEE Transactions on Speech and Audio Processing, 4*(1), 19. doi:10.1109/TSA.1996.481449

Junqua, J.-C. (1996). The influence of acoustics on speech production: A noise-induced stress phenomenon known as the Lombard reflex. *Speech Communication, 20*(1-2), 13–22. doi:10.1016/S0167-6393(96)00041-6

Kadri, F., Harrou, F., Chaabane, S., & Tahon, C. (2014). Time series modelling and forecasting of emergency department overcrowding. *Journal of Medical Systems, 38*(9), 107–127. doi:10.100710916-014-0107-0 PMID:25053208

Kale, M. (1992). Kids and animals: A comforting hospital combination. *Interaction, 10*(3), 17–21.

Kam, H. J., Sung, J. O., & Park, R. W. (2010). Prediction of daily patient numbers for a regional emergency medical center using time series analysis. *Healthcare Informatics Research, 16*(3), 158–165. doi:10.4258/hir.2010.16.3.158 PMID:21818435

Kanaiyalal Ramanlal Trivedi v Dr. Satyanarayan Vishwakarma 1996 (3) CPR 24 (Guj); I (1997) CPJ 332 (Guj); 1998 CCJ 690 (Guj)

Kang, S. W., & Park, H. S. (2015). Emergency department visit volume variability. *Clinical and Experimental Emergency Medicine, 2*(3), 150–154. doi:10.15441/ceem.14.044 PMID:27752589

Karamchandani, P. V. (1946). Dengue group of fevers in India. *Lancet, 1*(6386), 92–93. doi:10.1016/S0140-6736(46)91229-9 PMID:21011278

Karegowda, A. G., Manjunath, A. S., & Jayaram, M. A. (2011). Application of genetic algorithm optimized neural network connection weights for medical diagnosis of pima Indians diabetes. *International Journal on Soft Computing, 2*(2), 15–23. doi:10.5121/ijsc.2011.2202

Karl, H., & Willig, A. (2005). *Protocols and architectures for Wireless Sensor Networks*. John Wiley & Sons Ltd. doi:10.1002/0470095121

Kartakis, S. S. V. (2012). *Enhancing Health Care Delivery through Ambient Intelligence Applications*. Academic Press.

Kashanian, H., Ajami, N. B., & Deghati, M. Communication with autistic people through wearable sensors and cloud technology. In *Fuzzy and Intelligent Systems (CFIS), 2017 5th Iranian Joint Congress* (pp. 139-143). IEEE. 10.1109/CFIS.2017.8003672

Kasper, T., Carluccio, D., & Paar, C. (2007). An Embedded System for Practical Security Analysis of Contactless Smartcards. Information Security Theory and Practices. Smart Cards, Mobile and Ubiquitous Computing Systems Lecture Notes in Computer Science, 150-160. doi:10.1007/978-3-540-72354-7_13

Katevas, N. (Ed.). (2001). *Mobile robotics in healthcare* (Vol. 7). IOS Press.

Katuwal, G. J., Cahill, N. D., Baum, S. A., & Michael, A. M. (2015). The predictive power of structural MRI in Autism diagnosis. *Proceedings of the Annual International Conference of the IEEE Engineering in Medicine and Biology Society*, 4270–4273. 10.1109/EMBC.2015.7319338

Kelly, J. (2013). *Apache drill brings sql-like, ad hoc query capabilities to big data.* Retrieved from http://wikibon.org/wiki/v/Apache-Drill-Brings-SQL-Like-Ad-Hoc-Query-Capabilities-to-Big-Data

Khoury, M. J., & Wei, G. (2015). The future of epidemiology in the era of precision medicine: cancer, cardiovascular disease, and beyond [Web log post]. Retrieved from http://epi.grants.cancer.gov/blog/archive/2015/08-11.html

Khoury, M. J., & Ioannidis, J. P. (2014). Big data meets public health. *Science*, *3466213*(6213), 1054–1055. doi:10.1126cience.aaa2709 PMID:25430753

Kim, H.-K. (2013). Convergence agent model for developing u-healthcare systems. *Future Generation Computer Systems.*

Kim, J., Gu, G. M., & Heo, P. (2016). Robotics for healthcare. In *Biomedical Engineering: Frontier Research and Converging Technologies* (pp. 489–509). Cham: Springer. doi:10.1007/978-3-319-21813-7_21

Kim, J., Kim, J., Kwak, M. J., & Bajaj, M. (2018). Genetic prediction of type 2 diabetes using deep neural network. *Clinical Genetics*, *93*(4), 822–829. doi:10.1111/cge.13175 PMID:29136281

Kim, K., Lee, C., O'Leary, K., Rosenauer, S., & Mehrotra, S. (2014). *Predicting patient volumes in hospital medicine: A comparative study of different time series forecasting methods. Tech. rep.* Northwestern University.

Kim, M., Wu, G., & Shen, D. (2013). Unsupervised deep learning for hippocampus segmentation in 7.0 Tesla MR images. *Lecture Notes in Computer Science*, *8184*, 1–8.

Klasnia, P., & Pratt, W. (2012). Healthcare in the pocket: Mapping the space of mobile-phone health interventions. *Journal of Biomedical Informatics*, *45*(1), 184–198. doi:10.1016/j.jbi.2011.08.017 PMID:21925288

Kodali, R. K., Swamy, G., & Lakshmi, B. (2015, December). An implementation of IoT for healthcare. In Intelligent Computational Systems (RAICS), 2015 IEEE Recent Advances in (pp. 411-416). IEEE. doi:10.1109/RAICS.2015.7488451

Koehler, F., Winkler, S., Schieber, M., Sechtem, U., Stangl, K., Bohm, M., ... Anker, S. D. (2011). Impact of Remote Telemedical Management on Mortality and Hospitalizations in Ambulatory Patients With Chronic Heart Failure: The Telemedical Interventional Monitoring in Heart Failure Study. On behalf of the Telemedical Interventional Monitoring in Heart failure. *Circulation*, *123*(17), 1873–1880. doi:10.1161/CIRCULATIONAHA.111.018473 PMID:21444883

Kohli, R., & Tan, S. S. (2016). Electronic Health Records: How Can Is Researchers Contribute To Transforming Healthcare? *Management Information Systems Quarterly*, *40*(3), 553–574. doi:10.25300/MISQ/2016/40.3.02

Kongcharoen, C., & Kruangpradit, T. (2013). Autoregressive integrated moving average with explanatory variable (ARIMAX) model for Thailand export. *33rd International Symposium on Forecasting*, 1-8.

Kooi, T., Litjens, G., van Ginneken, B., Gubern-Mérida, A., Sánchez, C. I., Mann, R., ... Karssemeijer, N. (2017). Large scale deep learning for computer aided detection of mammographic lesions. *Medical Image Analysis*, *35*, 303–312. doi:10.1016/j.media.2016.07.007 PMID:27497072

Krishnamurthy, K., Kasturi, T. E., & Chittipantulu, G. (1965). Clinical and pathological studies of an outbreak of dengue-like illness in Visakhapatnam. *The Indian Journal of Medical Research*, *53*, 800–812. PMID:5830412

Kröse, B., Krose, B., van der Smagt, P., & Smagt, P. (1993). *An introduction to neural networks*. London: CRC Press.

Kulage, K. M., Smaldone, A. M., & Cohn, E. G. (2014). How will DSM-5 affect autism diagnosis? A systematic literature review and meta-analysis. *Journal of Autism and Developmental Disorders*, *44*(8), 1918–1932. doi:10.100710803-014-2065-2 PMID:24531932

Kuriakose, S., & Lahiri, U. (2017). Design of a Physiology-Sensitive VR-Based Social Communication Platform for Children with Autism. *IEEE Transactions on Neural Systems and Rehabilitation Engineering*, *25*(8), 1180–1191. doi:10.1109/TNSRE.2016.2613879 PMID:28114071

Kurt, I., Ture, M., & Kurum, A. T. (2008). Comparing performances of logistic regression, classification and regression tree, and neural networks for predicting coronary artery disease. *Expert Systems with Applications*, *34*(1), 366–374. doi:10.1016/j.eswa.2006.09.004

Lai, M. (2015). *Deep Learning for Medical Image Segmentation*. Available at: http://arxiv.org/abs/1505.02000

Laranjo, Macedo, Santos, & Alexandre. (2012). Internet of Things for Medication Control: Service Implementation and Testing. *Elsevier Procedia Technology*, *5*, 777-786.

Larson, E. C., Goel, M., Boriello, G., Heltshe, S., Rosenfeld, M., & Patel, S. N. (2012). Spiro Smart: Using a microphone to measure lung function on a mobile phone. *Proc. ACM Int. Conf. Ubiquitous Comput.*, 280-289.

Larson, E. C., Lee, T., Liu, S., Rosenfeld, M., & Patel, S. N. (2011). Accurate and privacy preserving cough sensing using a low-cost microphone. *Proc. ACM Int. Conf. Ubiquitous Comput.*, 375-384.

Lauer, M. S. (2012). Time for a creative transformation of epidemiology in the United States. *Journal of the American Medical Association*, *30817*(17), 1804–1805. doi:10.1001/jama.2012.14838 PMID:23117782

Lebied, M. (2017, May 24). *9 Examples of Big Data Analytics in Healthcare That Can Save People*. Retrieved July 26, 2017, from http://www.datapine.com/blog/big-data-examples-in-healthcare/

LeCun, Y., Bengio, Y., & Hinton, G. (2015). Deep learning. *Nature*, *521*(7553), 436–444. doi:10.1038/nature14539 PMID:26017442

Lee, K.-H., Lee, Y.-J., Choi, H., Chung, Y. D., & Moon, B. (2012). Parallel data processing with MapReduce: A survey. *SIGMOD Record*, *40*(4), 11–20. doi:10.1145/2094114.2094118

Le, Q. V. (2014). *A Tutorial on Deep Learning Part 1: Nonlinear Classifiers and The Backpropagation Algorithm*. Tutorial.

Leung, H., & Haykin, S. (1991). The complex backpropagation algorithm. *IEEE Transactions on Signal Processing*, *39*(9), 2101–2104. doi:10.1109/78.134446

Leventhal, R. (2014, December 4). *Report: Healthcare Data is Growing Exponentially, Needs Protection*. Retrieved August 7, 2017, from https://www.healthcare-informatics.com/news-item/report-healthcare-data-growing-exponentially-needs-protection

Leventhal, R. (2014, January 10). *Industry expert: "Big data is closer than it appears"*. Retrieved August 2017, from https://www.healthcare-informatics.com/article/how-healthcare-organizations-can-turn-big-data-smart-data

Levoy, M. (2006). Light fields and computational imaging. *Computer*, *39*(8), 46–55. doi:10.1109/MC.2006.270

Levoy, M., & Hanrahan, P. (1996, August). Light field rendering. In *Proceedings of the 23rd annual conference on Computer graphics and interactive techniques* (pp. 31-42). ACM.

Li, Q., & Huang, Y. (2010). Robust speaker identification using an auditory-based feature. In *Acoustics Speech and Signal Processing (ICASSP), 2010 IEEE International Conference on*. IEEE. 10.1109/ICASSP.2010.5495589

Liang, S., Zilong, Y., Hai, S., & Trinidad, M. (2011). *Childhood autism language training system and Internet-of-Things-based centralized training center.* Chinese Patent 102 184661 A.

Li, C., Hu, X., & Zhang, L. (2017). The IoT-based heart disease monitoring system for pervasive healthcare service. *Procedia Computer Science*, *112*, 2328–2334. doi:10.1016/j.procs.2017.08.265

Li, G., Lee, B. L., & Chung, W. Y. (2015). Smart watch-based wearable EEG system for driver drowsiness detection. *IEEE Sensors Journal*, *15*(12), 7169–7180. doi:10.1109/JSEN.2015.2473679

Lin, D. Y. (2013). *Integrated Internet of Things application system for prison*. Chinese Patent 102 867236 A.

Liu, M. L., Tao, L., & Yan, Z. (2012). *Internet of Things-based electro cardio-gram monitoring system*. Chinese Patent 102 764118 A.

Liu, S., Liu, S., Cai, W., Pujol, S., Kikinis, R., & Feng, D. (2014, April). Early diagnosis of Alzheimer's disease with deep learning. In *Biomedical Imaging (ISBI), 2014 IEEE 11th International Symposium on* (pp. 1015-1018). IEEE. 10.1109/ISBI.2014.6868045

Liu, W., Yu, X., Raj, B., Yi, L., Zou, X., & Li, M. (2015). Efficient autism spectrum disorder prediction with eye movement: A machine learning framework. In *Affective Computing and Intelligent Interaction (ACII), 2015 International Conference* (pp. 649-655). IEEE. 10.1109/ACII.2015.7344638

Liu, W., Zheng, W.-L., & Lu, B.-L. (2016). *Multimodal Emotion Recognition Using Multimodal Deep Learning*. Available at: http://arxiv.org/abs/1602.08225

Liu, Y., Zhang, P., & Hain, T. (2014). Using neural network front-ends on far field multiple microphones based speech recognition. In *Acoustics, Speech and Signal Processing (ICASSP), 2014 IEEE International Conference on*. IEEE. 10.1109/ICASSP.2014.6854663

Lo, C., Chen, C., Cheng, D., & Kung, H. (2011). Ubiquitous healthcare service system with context-awareness capability: Design and implementation. *Expert Systems with Applications*, *38*(4), 4416–4436. doi:10.1016/j.eswa.2010.09.111

Lopez, D., Gunasekaran, M., & Murugan, B. S. (2014) Spatial Big Data Analytics of Influenza Epidemic in Vellore, India. *Proceedings: IEEE International Conference on Big Data. IEEE International Conference on Big Data*, 19–24.

Louliej, A., Jabrane, Y., Said, B. A., & Ouahman, A. A. (2012). Reduction of power envelope fluctuations in ECMA-368 ultra wideband communication system. *2012 International Conference on Multimedia Computing and Systems*. 10.1109/ICMCS.2012.6320132

Lynch, C., & Roper, C. (2011). The transit phase of migration: Circulation of malaria and its multidrug-resistant forms in Africa. *PLoS Medicine*, *8*(5), e1001040. doi:10.1371/journal.pmed.1001040 PMID:21655316

Mai, Q., Aboagye-Sarfo, P., Sanfilippo, F. M., Preen, D. B., & Fatovich, D. M. (2015). Predicting the number of emergency department presentations in Western Australia: A population-based time series analysis. *Emergency Medicine Australasia*, *27*(1), 16–21. doi:10.1111/1742-6723.12344 PMID:25583296

Majidi, C. (2014). Soft robotics: A perspective—current trends and prospects for the future. *Soft Robotics*, *1*(1), 5–11. doi:10.1089oro.2013.0001

Malviya, A., Udhani, A., & Soni, S. (2016). R-tool: Data analytic framework for big data. *Symposium on Colossal Data Analysis and Networking (CDAN)*. 10.1109/CDAN.2016.7570960

Marcilio, I., Hajat, S., & Gouveia, N. (2013). Forecasting daily emergency department visits using calendar variables and ambient temperature readings. *Academic Emergency Medicine*, *20*(8), 769–777. doi:10.1111/acem.12182 PMID:24033619

marketsandmarkets.com. (2016). *Healthcare Analytics/Medical Analytics Market*. Retrieved August 7, 2017, from http://www.marketsandmarkets.com/Market-Reports/healthcare-data-analytics-market-905.html

Marr, B. (2016, February 16). *How Big Data Is Transforming Medicine*. Retrieved August 2017, from https://www.forbes.com/sites/bernardmarr/2016/02/16/how-big-data-is-transforming-medicine/#244b70277ddc

Marvin, K. C. (2017). Health Information Technology: Integration, Patient Empowerment, and Security. *American Journal of Health-System Pharmacy*, *74*(2), 36–38.

McAndrew, A. (2015). *A computational introduction to digital image processing*. Chapman and Hall/CRC.

McCarthy, J. (2015). Hospitals to triple use of cloud services. *HealthcareIT News*. Retrieved January 20,2018 from http://www.healthcareitnews.com/news/hospitals-triple-use-cloud-services

McCarthy, M. L., Zeger, S. L., Ding, R., Aronsky, D., Hoot, N. R., & Kelen, G. D. (2008). The challenge of predicting demand for emergency department services. *Academic Emergency Medicine*, *15*(4), 337–346. doi:10.1111/j.1553-2712.2008.00083.x PMID:18370987

McDonald, C. (2017, February 27). *5 Big Data Production Examples in Healthcare*. Retrieved July 24, 2017, from https://mapr.com/blog/5-big-data-production-examples-healthcare/

McDonald, C. (2017, September 2). *5 Big Data Trends in Healthcare for 2017*. Retrieved October 21, 2017, from http://www.7wdata.be/big-data/5-big-data-trends-in-healthcare-for-2017

Menke, N. B., Caputo, N., Fraser, R., Haber, J., Shields, C., & Menke, M. N. (2014). A retrospective analysis of the utility of an artificial neural network to predict ED volume. *The American Journal of Emergency Medicine*, *32*(6), 614–617. doi:10.1016/j.ajem.2014.03.011 PMID:24736127

Merler, S., Ajelli, M., Pugliese, A., & Ferguson, N. M. (2011). Determinants of the spa- tiotemporal dynamics of the 2009 H1N1 pandemic in Europe: Implications for real- time modelling. *PLoS Computational Biology*, *7*(9), e1002205. doi:10.1371/journal.pcbi.1002205 PMID:21980281

Mermelstein, P. (1973). Articulatory model for the study of speech production. *The Journal of the Acoustical Society of America, 53*(4), 1070-1082.

Mian, M., Teredesai, A., Hazel, D., Pokuri, S., & Uppala, K. (2014). In-Memory Analysis for Healthcare Big Data. *IEEE International Congress on Big Data*.

Milenković, A., Otto, C., & Jovanov, E. (2006). Wireless sensor networks for personal health monitoring: Issues and an implementation. *Computer Communications*, *29*(13-14), 2521–2533. doi:10.1016/j.comcom.2006.02.011

Miliard, M. (2015, January 16). *12 tips for better EHR usability*. Retrieved October 21, 2017, from http://www.healthcareitnews.com/news/12-tips-better-ehr-usability

Milici, S., Lorenzo, J., Lazaro, A., Villarino, R., & Jirbau, D. (2017). Wireless breathing sensor based on wearable modulated frequency selective surface. *IEEE Sensors Journal*, *17*(5), 1285–1292. doi:10.1109/JSEN.2016.2645766

Miller, A. B., & Pina, I. L. (2009). Understanding heart failure with preserved ejection fraction: Clinical importance and future outlook. *Congestive Heart Failure (Greenwich, Conn.)*, *15*(4), 186–192. doi:10.1111/j.1751-7133.2009.00063.x PMID:19627293

Miller, N. (2013). Measuring up to speech intelligibility. *International Journal of Language & Communication Disorders*, *48*(6), 601–612. doi:10.1111/1460-6984.12061 PMID:24119170

Min, S., Lee, B., & Yoon, S. (2016). Deep learning in bioinformatics. *Briefings in Bioinformatics*. doi:10.1093/bib/bbw068 PMID:27473064

Miotto, R., Wang, F., Wang, S., Jiang, X., & Dudley, J. T. (2017). Deep learning for healthcare: Review, opportunities and challenges. *Briefings in Bioinformatics*. doi:10.1093/bib/bbx044 PMID:28481991

Mnistdatasetiterator, A. (2006). *Tutorial : Deep-Belief Networks*. Academic Press.

Moeslund, T. B. (2012). *Introduction to video and image processing: Building real systems and applications*. Springer Science & Business Media. doi:10.1007/978-1-4471-2503-7

Moghimi, S., Kushki, A., Guerguerian, A. M., & Chau, T. (2013). A review of EEG-based brain-computer interfaces as access pathways for individuals with severe disabilities. *Assistive Technology*, *25*(2), 99–110. doi:10.1080/10400435.2012.723298 PMID:23923692

Mooney, S. J., Westreich, D. J., & El-Sayed, A. M. (2015). Epidemiology in the Era of Big Data. *Epidemiology (Cambridge, Mass.)*, *26*(3), 390–394. doi:10.1097/EDE.0000000000000274 PMID:25756221

Morzuch, B. J., & Allen, P. G. (2006). *Forecasting hospital emergency department arrivals*. In *26th Annual Symposium on Forecasting*, Santander, Spain.

Mossong, J., Hens, N., Jit, M., Beutels, P., Auranen, K., & Mikolajczak, R. (2008). Social contacts and mixing patterns relevant to the spread of infectious diseases. *PLoS Medicine*, *5*(3), e74. doi:10.1371/journal.pmed.0050074 PMID:18366252

Motorola. (2003). *SPI Block Guide v3.06 (S12SPIV3/D)*. Retrieved from https://opencores.org/usercontent,doc,1499360489

Mousa, D., Zayed, N., & Yassine, I. A. (2014). Automatic cardiac MRI localization method. *Proceedings of the 7th Cairo International Biomedical Engineering Conference, CIBEC 2014*, 153–157. 10.1109/CIBEC.2014.7020942

Mousa, D., Zayed, N., & Yassine, I. A. (2016). Factors Affecting the Segmentation of the Heart Ventricles in Short Axis Cardiac Perfusion MRI Images. *International Journal of Computers and Technology*, *15*(11), 7218–7226. doi:10.24297/ijct.v15i11.4376

Mukhopadhyay, A., Maulik, U., Bandyopadhyay, S., & Coello, C. A. C. (2014). A survey of multiobjective evolutionary algorithms for data mining: Part I. *IEEE Transactions on Evolutionary Computation*, *18*(1), 4–19. doi:10.1109/TEVC.2013.2290086

Mulro, S., Gronley, J., & Weiss, W. (2003). Use of cluster analysis for gait pattern classification of patients in the early and late recovery phases following stroke. *Gait & Posture*, *18*(1), 114–125. doi:10.1016/S0966-6362(02)00165-0 PMID:12855307

Murphy, K. P. (2012). *Machine Learning: A Probabilistic Perspective*. Academic Press.

Murphy, S.L. (2017). National Vital Statistics Reports - Deaths: Final Data for 2007. *National Vital Statistics Reports - Deaths: Final Data for 2015*, *66*(6).

Murray, N.E.A., Quam, M.B., & Wilder-Smith, A. (2013). Epidemiology of dengue: past, present and future prospects. *Clinical Epidemiology*, *5*, 299–309.

Murty, K. S. R., & Yegnanarayana, B. (2006). Combining evidence from residual phase and MFCC features for speaker recognition. *IEEE Signal Processing Letters*, *13*(1), 52–55. doi:10.1109/LSP.2005.860538

Myers, R. M., Carey, D. E., Banerjee, K., Reuben, R., & Ramamurti, D. V. (1968). Recovery of dengue type 3 virus from human serum and *Aedes aegypti* in South India. *The Indian Journal of Medical Research*, *56*, 781–787. PMID:5680412

Myung, I. J. (2003). Tutorial on maximum likelihood estimation. *Journal of Mathematical Psychology*, *47*(1), 90–100. doi:10.1016/S0022-2496(02)00028-7

Nabahin, A., Abou Eloun, A., & Abu Naser, S. S. (2017). *Expert System for Hair Loss Diagnosis and Treatment. International Journal of Engineering and Information Systems.*

Nair, A. P., Krishnan, S., & Saquib, Z. (2016). MFCC based noise reduction in ASR using Kalman filtering. In *Advances in Signal Processing (CASP), Conference on.* IEEE. 10.1109/CASP.2016.7746218

Nambiar, R., Sethi, A., Bhardwaj, R., & Vargheese, R. (2013). A Look at Challenges and Opportunities of Big Data Analytics in Healthcare. *IEEE International Conference on Big Data.* 10.1109/BigData.2013.6691753

Narayan, T. (2016). *Automated Left Ventricle Segmentation in Cardiac MRIs using Convolutional Neural Networks.* Deep Learning.

Nattkemper, T. W., Arnrich, B., Lichte, O., Timm, W., Degenhard, A., Pointon, L., ... Leach, M. O. (2005). Evaluation of radiological features for breast tumour classification in clinical screening with machine learning methods. *Artificial Intelligence in Medicine*, *34*(2), 129–139. doi:10.1016/j.artmed.2004.09.001 PMID:15894177

Ndaba, M., Pillay, A. W., & Ezugwu, A. E. (2018, May). An Improved Generalized Regression Neural Network for Type II Diabetes Classification. In *International Conference on Computational Science and Its Applications* (pp. 659-671). Springer, Cham. 10.1007/978-3-319-95171-3_52

Nelson, R. (2017). Technology drives healthcare innovation. *EE: Evaluation Engineering*, *56*(3), 10–13.

Neter, J., Kutner, M. H., Nachtsheim, C. J., & Wasserman, W. (1996). Applied linear statistical models, Chicago: Irwin. network modeling approach for sales forecasting. *International Journal of Production.*, *4*, 318.

Network, T. S. B. D. A. (2013). *Big Data Analytics A Research and Innovation Agenda for Sweden.* The Swedish Big Data Analytics Network Sweden.

Ng, A. (2015). *Deep Learning Tutorial.* University of Stanford. Available at: http://ufldl.stanford.edu/tutorial/supervised/ConvolutionalNeuralNetwork/

Ngo, T. A., Lu, Z., & Carneiro, G. (2016). Combining deep learning and level set for the automated segmentation of the left ventricle of the heart from cardiac cine magnetic resonance. *Medical Image Analysis*, *35*, 159–171. doi:10.1016/j.media.2016.05.009 PMID:27423113

Ng, R., Levoy, M., Brédif, M., Duval, G., Horowitz, M., & Hanrahan, P. (2005). Light field photography with a hand-held plenoptic camera. *Computer Science Technical Report CSTR*, *2*(11), 1–11.

Nie, D. (2016). Estimating CT Image from MRI Data Using 3D Fully Convolutional Networks. In *Deep Learning and Data Labeling for Medical Applications: First International Workshop, LABELS 2016, and Second International Workshop, DLMIA 2016, Held in Conjunction with MICCAI 2016, Athens, Greece, October 21, 2016, Proceedings.* Cham: Springer International Publishing. 10.1007/978-3-319-46976-8_18

Nie, D. (2016). 3D Deep Learning for Multi-modal Imaging-guided Survival Time Prediction of Brain Tumor Patients. In *Medical Image Computing and Computer-Assisted Intervention MICCAI'2016* (pp. 212–220). Springer. doi:10.1007/978-3-319-46723-8_25

Nilashi, M., Ibrahim, O., Ahmadi, H., & Shahmoradi, L. (2017). A knowledge-based system for breast cancer classification using fuzzy logic method. *Telematics and Informatics*, *34*(4), 133–144. doi:10.1016/j.tele.2017.01.007

Ni, Y., & Fan, F. (2011). A two-stage dynamic sales forecasting model for the fashion retail. *Expert Systems with Applications*, *38*(3), 1529–1536. doi:10.1016/j.eswa.2010.07.065

Ohlhorst, F. (2012). *Big Data Analytics: Turning Big Data into Big Money*. John Wiley & Sons. doi:10.1002/9781119205005

Orcutt, M. (2016, June 29). *The Rocket Fuel for Biden's "Cancer Moonshot"? Big Data.* Retrieved April 29, 2018, from https://www.technologyreview.com/s/601784/white-house-cancer-moonshot-data/

Pang, Z., Tian, J., & Chen, Q. (2014). Intelligent packaging and intelligent medicine box for medication management towards the Internet-of-Things. *16th International Conference on Advanced Communication Technology*, 352-360. 10.1109/ICACT.2014.6779193

Pappada, S. M., Cameron, B. D., & Rosman, P. M. (2008). Development of a neural network for prediction of glucose concentration in type 1 diabetes patients. *Journal of Diabetes Science and Technology*, *2*(5), 792–801. doi:10.1177/193229680800200507 PMID:19885262

Pappada, S. M., Cameron, B. D., Rosman, P. M., Bourey, R. E., Papadimos, T. J., Olorunto, W., & Borst, M. J. (2011). Neural network-based real-time prediction of glucose in patients with insulin-dependent diabetes. *Diabetes Technology & Therapeutics*, *13*(2), 135–141. doi:10.1089/dia.2010.0104 PMID:21284480

Park, J., Park, E., & Desai, Y. (2008, January). Forecasting patient load of ED at moses cone hospital. In *IIE Annual Conference. Proceedings* (p. 1). Institute of Industrial and Systems Engineers (IISE).

Patel, S., Park, H., Bonato, P., Chan, L., & Rodgers, M. (2012). A Review of Wearable Sensors and Systems with Applications in Rehabilitation. *Journal of Neuro Engineering and Rehabilitation, 20*(9).

Patil, H. K., & Seshadri, R. (2014). Big data security and privacy issues in healthcare. *IEEE International Congress on Big Data.*

Pati, S. K., Sengupta, S., & Das, A. K. (2018). Improved Genetic Algorithm for Selecting Significant Genes in Cancer Diagnosis. In *Progress in Advanced Computing and Intelligent Engineering* (pp. 395–405). Singapore: Springer. doi:10.1007/978-981-10-6875-1_39

Patnam, V. S., George, F. T., George, K., & Verma, A. Deep Learning Based Recognition of Meltdown in Autistic Kids. In *Healthcare Informatics (ICHI), 2017 IEEE International Conference* (pp. 391-396). IEEE. 10.1109/ICHI.2017.35

Paul, S. D., Dandawate, C. N., Banerjee, K., & Krishnamurthy, K. (1965). Virological and serological studies on an outbreak of dengue-like illness in Visakhapatnam, Andhra Pradesh. *The Indian Journal of Medical Research*, *53*, 777–789. PMID:5830410

Pawar, M. M., & Talbar, S. N. (2018). Wavelet Statistical Feature Selection Using Genetic Algorithm with Fuzzy Classifier for Breast Cancer Diagnosis. In *Progress in Intelligent Computing Techniques: Theory, Practice, and Applications* (pp. 95–105). Singapore: Springer. doi:10.1007/978-981-10-3373-5_8

Payan, A., & Montana, G. (2015). *Predicting Alzheimer's disease: a neuroimaging study with 3D convolutional neural networks*. Miccai.

Payne, P. O., Lussier, Y., Foraker, R. E., & Embi, P. J. (2016). Rethinking the role and impact of health information technology: Informatics as an interventional discipline. *BMC Medical Informatics and Decision Making*, 1640. PMID:27025583

PCAST. (2014). P.s.C.o.A.o.S.a.T., Big Data and Privacy: a Technological Perspective. Washington, DC: White House.

Peca, A. (2016). Robot enhanced therapy for children with autism disorders: Measuring ethical acceptability. *IEEE Technology and Society Magazine*, *35*(2), 54–66. doi:10.1109/MTS.2016.2554701

Pentland, A., & Pentland, S. (2008). *Honest signals: how they shape our world.* Cambridge, MA: MIT Press.

Petre, A. (2017). *Blockchain Use Cases in Healthcare.* Retrieved March 10, 2018 from https://www.intelligenthq.com/innovation-management/blockchain-use-cases-in-healthcare/

Petrou, P. (2015). An interrupted time-series analysis to assess impact of introduction of co-payment on emergency room visits in Cyprus. *Applied Health Economics and Health Policy*, *13*(5), 515–523. doi:10.100740258-015-0169-2 PMID:25894739

Pettus, D. C., Vanderveen, T., Canfield, R. L., & Schad, R. (2017). Reliable and Scalable Infusion System Integration with the Electronic Medical Record. *Biomedical Instrumentation & Technology*, *51*(2), 120–129. doi:10.2345/0899-8205-51.2.120 PMID:28296444

Pharmaceutical Online. (2017). *What To Expect From Artificial Intelligence In Pharma — And How To Get There.* Retrieved March,01, 2018 from https://www.pharmaceuticalonline.com/doc/what-to-expect-from-artificial-intelligence-in-pharma-and-how-to-get-there-0001

Philip Chen, C. L., & Zhang, C.-Y. (2014). Data-intensive applications, challenges, techniques and technologies: A survey on Big Data. *Inform. Sci.*, *275*, 314–347. doi:10.1016/j.ins.2014.01.015

Philips Healthcare. (2013). *Neonatal Event Review.* Retrieved from http://www.healthcare.philips.com/main/products/patient_monitoring/

Philips Healthcare. (n.d.a). *Protocol Watch Project.* Retrieved 11 05, 2013, from http://www.healthcare.philips.com/main/products/patient_monitoring/products/protocol_watch/

Philips Healthcare. (n.d.b). *Screen Trends.* Retrieved 08 10, 2015, from http://www.healthcare.philips.com/main/products/patient_monitoring/products/screentrends/index.wpd

Pianykh, O. S., & Rosenthal, D. I. (2015). Can we predict patient wait time? *Journal of the American College of Radiology*, *12*(10), 1058–1066. doi:10.1016/j.jacr.2015.04.010 PMID:26435119

Pickett, J. M. (1999). *The acoustics of speech communication: Fundamentals, speech perception theory, and technology.* Allyn & Bacon.

Plis, S.M. (2014). Deep learning for neuroimaging: A validation study. *Frontiers in Neuroscience*, *8*, 1–11.

Podder, P., Khan, T. Z., Khan, M. H., & Rahman, M. M. (2014). Comparative performance analysis of hamming, hanning and blackman window. *International Journal of Computers and Applications*, *96*(18).

Podesta, J., Pritzker, P., Moniz, E. J., Holdren, J., & Zients, J. (2014). *Big data: seizing opportunities, preserving values.* Executive Office of the President. Report. Retrieved from: https://obamawhitehouse.archives.gov/sites/default/files/docs/big_data_privacy_report_may_1_2014.pdf

Poongothai, S., Dharuman, C., Venkatesan, P., & Campus, R. (2017). *A Comparison of Fuzzy Genetic and Neuro Genetic Hybrid Algorithm for the Classification of Diabetes Disease.* Academic Press.

Povey, D., Burget, L., Agarwal, M., Akyazi, P., Feng, K., Ghoshal, A., … Thomas, S. (2010). Subspace Gaussian mixture models for speech recognition. In *Acoustics Speech and Signal Processing (ICASSP), 2010 IEEE International Conference on*. IEEE.

Powles, J., & Hodson, H. (2017). Google DeepMind and healthcare in an age of algorithms. *Health and technology, 7*(4), 351–367. doi:10.100712553-017-0179-1 PMID:29308344

Pramanik, P. K. D., & Choudhury, P. (2018). IoT Data Processing: The Different Archetypes and their Security & Privacy Assessments. In *Internet of Things (IoT) Security: Fundamentals, Techniques and Applications*. River Publishers. doi:10.4018/978-1-5225-4044-1.ch007

Pramanik, P. K. D., Upadhyay, B., Pal, S., & Pal, T. (2018). Internet of Things, Smart Sensors, and Pervasive Systems: Enabling the Connected and Pervasive Health Care. In *Healthcare Data Analytics and Management*. Elsevier.

Prasoon, A. (2014). *Deep Feature Learning and Cascaded Classifier for Large Scale Data Segmenting Cartilage in Knee MRIs*. University of Copenhagen.

Prasoon, A., Petersen, K., Igel, C., Lauze, F., Dam, E., & Nielsen, M. (2013, September). Deep feature learning for knee cartilage segmentation using a triplanar convolutional neural network. In *International conference on medical image computing and computer-assisted intervention* (pp. 246-253). Springer. 10.1007/978-3-642-40763-5_31

Pung, H., Gu, T., Xue, W., Palmes, P., Zhu, J., Ng, W., & Chung, N. (2009). *Context-aware middleware for pervasive elderly home care. IEEE J. Sel. Areas Commun.*

Puustjarvi, J., & Puustjarvi, L. (2011). Automating remote monitoring and information therapy: An opportunity to practice telemedicine in developing countries. *Proc. IST-Africa Conf.*, 1-9.

Qin, L. X., & Shi, Z. Z. (2006). Efficiently mining association rules from time series. *International Journal of Information Technology, 12*(4), 30-38.

Qinghua, Z., Guoquan, C., Zhuan, W. T., Hongyu, S., & Ningning, X., (2010). Research on home health care telemedicine service system concerned with the improvement of medical resources utilization rate and medical conditions. *The 12th International Conference on Advanced Communication Technology (ICACT), 2*, 1555-1559.

Qwaider, S. R., & Abu Naser, S. S. (2017). *Expert System for Diagnosing Ankle Diseases. International Journal of Engineering and Information Systems.*

Rabiner & Juang. (1986). An introduction to hidden Markov models. *IEEE ASSP Magazine, 3*(1), 4-16.

Rabiner, L. R., & Juang, B.-H. (1993). *Fundamentals of speech recognition*. PTR Prentice Hall.

Raghunath Raheja v The Maharashtra Medical Council and Ors AIR 1996 Bombay 198

Raghupathi, W., & Kesh, S. (2007). Interoperable electronic health records design: towards a service-oriented architecture. *e-Service Journal, 5*, 39–57.

Raghupathi, W., & Raghupathi, V. (2013). *An Overview of Health Analytics*. Working paper.

Raghupathi, W., & Raghupathi, V. (2014). Big data analytics in healthcare: promise and potential. *Health Information Science and Systems, 2*(3).

Raj, A. S., Lowney, M., & Shah, R. (2016). *Light-field database creation and depth estimation*. Dept. Computer Science, Stanford University, Technical Report.

Ramakrishanan, S. P., Gelfand, H. M., Bose, P. N., Sehgal, P. N., & Mukharjee, R. N. (1964). The epidemic of acute haemorrhagic fever, Calcutta, 163: Epidemiological inquiry. *The Indian Journal of Medical Research*, *52*, 633–650. PMID:14195504

Ramaswamy, S., & Truong, K. (2016). *Pulmonary Nodule Classification with Convolutional Neural Networks*. Academic Press.

Ramsey, L. (2015, December 23). *I tried 23andMe's new genetics test - and now I know why the company caused such a stir*. Retrieved August 2017, from http://www.businessinsider.in/I-tried-23andMes-new-genetics-test-and-now-I-know-why-the-company-caused-such-a-stir/articleshow/50302664.cms

Rand, D., Eng, J. J., Tang, P. F., Jeng, J. S., & Hung, C. (2009). How active are people with stroke? use of accelerometers to assess physical activity. *Stroke*, *40*, 163–168. doi:10.1161/STROKEAHA.108.523621

Readying Your Data Use for Value-Based Payment. (2013). hfm. *Healthcare Financial Management*, *67*(6), 1–8.

Reddy, G. T., & Khare, N. (2017). An efficient system for heart disease prediction using hybrid OFBAT with rule-based fuzzy logic model. *Journal of Circuits, Systems, and Computers*, *26*(04), 1750061. doi:10.1142/S021812661750061X

Reeves, A. P., & Kostis, W. J. (2000). Computer-aided diagnosis for lung cancer. *Radiologia Clinica*, *38*(3), 497–509. PMID:10855257

Reuters. (2014, September 25). *Your Medical Record Is worth More to Hackers than Your Credit card.* NDTV.

Revolutionizing the Healthcare Industry with Big Data, Analytics and Visualization. (2015). Retrieved August 2, 2018, from https://www.einfochips.com/whitepaper/Revolutionizing-the-Healthcare-Industry-with-Big-Data-Analytics-and-Visualization.pdf

Reynolds, D. A. (1995). Speaker identification and verification using Gaussian mixture speaker models. *Speech Communication*, *17*(1-2), 91–108. doi:10.1016/0167-6393(95)00009-D

Reynolds, D. A., Quatieri, T. F., & Dunn, R. B. (2000). Speaker verification using adapted Gaussian mixture models. *Digital Signal Processing*, *10*(1-3), 19–41. doi:10.1006/dspr.1999.0361

Rose, K., Eldridge, S., & Chapin, L. (2015). *The Internet of Things (IoT): An Overview –Understanding the Issues and Challenges of a More Connected World.* Internet Society.

Rosychuk, R. J., Klassen, T. P., Voaklander, D. C., Senthilselvan, A., & Rowe, B. H. (2011). Seasonality patterns in croup presentations to emergency departments in Alberta, Canada: A time series analysis. *Pediatric Emergency Care*, *27*(4), 256–260. doi:10.1097/PEC.0b013e31821314b0 PMID:21490537

Rosychuk, R. J., Youngson, E., & Rowe, B. H. (2015). Presentations to Alberta emergency departments for asthma: A time series analysis. *Academic Emergency Medicine*, *22*(8), 942–949. doi:10.1111/acem.12725 PMID:26194859

Rosychuk, R. J., Youngson, E., & Rowe, B. H. (2016). Presentations to emergency departments for COPD: A time series analysis. *Canadian Respiratory Journal*, *2016*, 1–9. doi:10.1155/2016/1382434 PMID:27445514

Rotariu, C., & Manta, V. (2012, September). Wireless system for remote monitoring of oxygen saturation and heart rate. In *Computer Science and Information Systems (FedCSIS), 2012 Federated Conference on* (pp. 193-196). IEEE.

Rothkoff, G., Reisman, M., Tal, N., Shani, O., Nissim-Rafinia, M., Meshorer, E., & Shifman, S. (2017). Isoform Dependent Functions of AUTS2 During Neuronal Differentiation. *European Neuropsychopharmacology*, *27*, S372–S373. doi:10.1016/j.euroneuro.2016.09.401

Rueckert, D., Glocker, B., & Kainz, B. (2016). Learning clinically useful information from images: Past, present and future. *Medical Image Analysis, 33*, 1339–1351.

Sahiner, B., Heang-Ping Chan, Petrick, N., Datong Wei, Helvie, M. A., Adler, D. D., & Goodsitt, M. M. (1996). Classification of mass and normal breast tissue: A convolution neural network classifier with spatial domain and texture images. *IEEE Transactions on Medical Imaging, 15*(5), 598–610. doi:10.1109/42.538937 PMID:18215941

Salathe, M., Kazandjieva, M., Lee, J. W., Levis, P., Feldman, M. W., & Jones, J. H. (2010). A high- resolution human contact network for infectious disease transmission. *Proceedings of the National Academy of Sciences of the United States of America, 107*(51), 22020–22025. doi:10.1073/pnas.1009094108 PMID:21149721

Saldien, J., Goris, K., Vanderborght, B., Verrelst, B., Van Ham, R., & Lefeber, D. (2006, September). ANTY: The development of an intelligent huggable robot for hospitalized children. *9th International Conference on Climbing and Walking Robots and the Support Technologies for Mobile Machines.*

Sano, A., Picard, & R. W. (2013). Stress Recognition Using Wearable Sensors and Mobile Phones. *Proceedings of the 2013 Humaine Association Conference on Affective Computing and Intelligent Interaction,* 671-676. 10.1109/ACII.2013.117

Sarkar, B. K. (2017). Big data for secure healthcare system: A conceptual design. *Complex Intelligent Systems, 3*(2), 133–151. doi:10.100740747-017-0040-1

Sarkar, J. K., Pavri, K. M., Chatterjee, S. N., Chakravarty, S. K., & Aanderson, C. R. (1964). Virological and serological studies of cases of haemorrhagic fever in Calcutta. *The Indian Journal of Medical Research, 52*, 684–691. PMID:14195508

Savalia, S., Acosta, E., & Emamian, V. (2017). Classification of Cardiovascular Disease Using Feature Extraction and Artificial Neural Networks. *The Journal of Bioscience and Medicine, 5*(11), 64–79. doi:10.4236/jbm.2017.511008

Schmidhuber, J. (2015). Deep Learning in neural networks: An overview. *Neural Networks, 61*, 85–117. doi:10.1016/j.neunet.2014.09.003 PMID:25462637

Schonwetter, R. S., Clark, L. D., Leedy, S. A., Quinn, M. J., Azer, M., & Kim, S. (2008). Predicting emergency room visits and hospitalizations among hospice patients with cardiac disease. *Journal of Palliative Medicine, 11*(8), 1142–1150. doi:10.1089/jpm.2008.0032 PMID:18980456

Schultz, T., Wand, M., Hueber, T., & Brumberg, J. S. (2017). Biosignal-based spoken communication: A survey. *IEEE/ACM Transactions on Audio, Speech, and Language Processing, 25*(12), 2257–2271.

Schwartz, R., Chow, Y., Kimball, O., & Makhoul, J. (1985). Context-dependent modeling for acoustic-phonetic recognition of continuous speech. In *Acoustics, Speech, and Signal Processing, IEEE International Conference on ICASSP'85.* IEEE. 10.1109/ICASSP.1985.1168283

Seven Big Data Examples That Have Improved Healthcare Operations. (2016, April 19). Retrieved July 24, 2017, from Ingram Micro Advisor: http://www.ingrammicroadvisor.com/data-center/seven-big-data-examples-that-have-improved-healthcare-operations

Shabut, A. M., Tania, M. H., Lwin, K. T., Evans, B. A., Yusof, N. A., Abu-Hassan, K. J., & Hossain, M. A. (2018). An Intelligent Mobile-Enabled Expert System for Tuberculosis Disease Diagnosis in Real Time. *Expert Systems with Applications, 114*, 65–77. doi:10.1016/j.eswa.2018.07.014

Shah, S. (2016, February 18). *Why patient engagement is so challenging to achieve.* Retrieved August 2, 2018, from http://www.ibmbigdatahub.com/blog/why-patient-engagement-so-challenging-achieve

Shahriyar, R., Bari, M. F., Kundu, G., Ahamed, S. I., & Akbar, M. M. (2009, September). Intelligent mobile health monitoring system (IMHMS). In *International Conference on Electronic Healthcare* (pp. 5-12). Springer.

Shaker, M. S. (2014). Cardiac MRI View Classification using Autoencoder. *7th Cairo International Biomedical Engineering Conference*, 125–128.

Sharma, M., Sharma, P., Saini, A., & Sharma, K. (2018). Modular Neural Network for Detection of Diabetic Retinopathy in Retinal Images. In *Proceedings of First International Conference on Smart System, Innovations and Computing*(pp. 363-370). Springer. 10.1007/978-981-10-5828-8_35

Sharma, P., & Saxena, K. (2017). Application of fuzzy logic and genetic algorithm in heart disease risk level prediction. *International Journal of System Assurance Engineering and Management*, *8*(2), 1109–1125. doi:10.100713198-017-0578-8

Shepard, D. S., Undurraga, E. A., & Halasa, Y. A. (2013). Economic and disease burden of dengue in Southeast Asia. *PLoS Neglected Tropical Diseases*, *7*(2), e2055. doi:10.1371/journal.pntd.0002055 PMID:23437406

Shimada, A., Nagahara, H., & Taniguchi, R. I. (2015, August). Change detection on light field for active video surveillance. In *Advanced Video and Signal Based Surveillance (AVSS), 2015 12th IEEE International Conference on* (pp. 1-6). IEEE. 10.1109/AVSS.2015.7301785

Shimada, A., Nagahara, H., & Taniguchi, R. I. (2013). Object detection based on spatiotemporal light field sensing. *Information and Media Technologies*, *8*(4), 1115–1119.

Short, E., Feil-Seifer, D., & Matarić, M. (2011). A comparison of machine learning techniques for modeling human-robot interaction with children with autism. In *Proceedings of the 6th international conference on Human-robot interaction* (pp. 251-252). ACM. 10.1145/1957656.1957756

Shrivastava, P., Shukla, A., Vepakomma, P., Bhansali, N., & Verma, K. (2017). A survey of nature-inspired algorithms for feature selection to identify Parkinson's disease. *Computer Methods and Programs in Biomedicine*, *139*, 171–179. doi:10.1016/j.cmpb.2016.07.029 PMID:28187888

Shvachko, K., Kuang, H., Radia, S., & Chansler, R. (2010). The Hadoop Distributed File System. In *IEEE 26th Symposium on Mass Storage Systems and Technologies (MSST)*. IEEE.

Singh & Reddy. (2014). A survey on platforms for big data analytics. *Journal of Big Data*, *1*, 8. PMID:26191487

Singh, A. V. (2015). *Content-Based Image Retrieval using Deep Learning*. New York: B. Thomas Golisano College of Computing and Information Sciences Rochester Institute of Technology Rochester.

Smelcer, J. (2009). Usability of Electronic Medical Records. *Journal of Usability Studies*, *4*(2), 70–84. doi:10.1145/2029976.2029989

Sohn, J. (1999). A statistical model-based voice activity detection. *IEEE Signal Processing Letters*, *6*(1), 1–3. doi:10.1109/97.736233

Soliman, S. S., & Hsue, S.-Z. (1992). Signal classification using statistical moments. *IEEE Transactions on Communications*, *40*(5), 908–916. doi:10.1109/26.141456

Spencer, L. E. (1988). Speech characteristics of male-to-female transsexuals: A perceptual and acoustic study. *Folia Phoniatrica et Logopaedica*, *40*(1), 31–42. doi:10.1159/000265881 PMID:3384379

Spetsieris, P. G., Dhawan, V., Ma, Y., Moeller, J. R., Mentis, M. J., & Eidelberg, D. (2002). Computer aided diagnosis of functional brain disorders using PET on a PC based platform. In *Engineering in Medicine and Biology, 2002. 24th Annual Conference and the Annual Fall Meeting of the Biomedical Engineering Society EMBS/BMES Conference, 2002. Proceedings of the Second Joint* (*Vol. 2*, pp. 1107-1108). IEEE. 10.1109/IEMBS.2002.1106300

Spidlen, Barsky, Breuer, Carr, Nazaire, Hill, … Qian. (2013). GenePattern flow cytometry suite. *Source Code for Biology and Medicine, 8*(1), 14. doi:10.1186/1751- 0473-8-14

Srinivasan, U., & Arunasalam, B. (2013). *Leveraging Big Data Analytics to Reduce Healthcare Costs*. IEEE Computer Society.

Stehle, J., Voirin, N., Barrat, A., Cattuto, C., Colizza, V., Isella, L., ... Vanhems, P. (2011). Simulation of an SEIR infectious disease model on the dynamic contact network of conference attendees. *BMC Medicine, 9*(1), 87. doi:10.1186/1741-7015-9-87 PMID:21771290

Stern, D. (2016). *Medical Image Computing and Computer-Assisted Intervention – MICCAI 2016*. Cham: Springer International Publishing. Available at http://link.springer.com/10.1007/978-3-319-46723-8

Stoitsis, J., Valavanis, I., Mougiakakou, S. G., Golemati, S., Nikita, A., & Nikita, K. S. (2006). Computer aided diagnosis based on medical image processing and artificial intelligence methods. *Nuclear Instruments & Methods in Physics Research. Section A, Accelerators, Spectrometers, Detectors and Associated Equipment, 569*(2), 591–595. doi:10.1016/j.nima.2006.08.134

Stowell, D., Giannoulis, D., Benetos, E., Lagrange, M., & Plumbey, M. (2015). Detection and classification of acoustic scenes and events. *IEEE Transactions on Multimedia, 17*(10), 1733–1746. doi:10.1109/TMM.2015.2428998

Su, C. J., & Chu, T. W. (2014). A Mobile Multi-Agent Information System for UbiquitousFetal Monitoring. *International Journal of Environmental Research and Public Health, 11*(1), 600–625. doi:10.3390/ijerph110100600 PMID:24452256

Su, C.-J., & Wu, C.-Y. (2011). JADE implemented mobile multi-agent based, distributed informationplatform for pervasive health care monitoring. *Applied Soft Computing, 11*(1), 315–325. doi:10.1016/j.asoc.2009.11.022

Suk, H. & Shen, D. (2015). Learning in Diagnosis of Brain Disorders. In S.-W. Lee, H. H. Bülthoff, & K.-R. Müller (Eds.), *Recent Progress in Brain and Cognitive Engineering*. Springer. Available at: http://link.springer.com/10.1007/978-94-017-7239-6

Suk, H.-I. I., Lee, S.-W., & Shen, D. (2014). Hierarchical Feature Representation and Multimodal Fusion with Deep Learning for AD/MCI Diagnosis. *NeuroImage, 101*(2), 569–582. doi:10.1016/j.neuroimage.2014.06.077 PMID:25042445

Suk, H., Lee, S.-W., & Shen, D. (2015). Latent feature representation with stacked auto-encoder for AD/MCI diagnosis. *Brain Structure & Function, 220*(2), 841–859. doi:10.100700429-013-0687-3 PMID:24363140

Sun, W., Zheng, B., & Qian, W. (2016). Computer aided lung cancer diagnosis with deep learning algorithms. In *SPIE Medical Imaging* (pp. 1–8). SPIE. Available at http://proceedings.spiedigitallibrary.org/proceeding.aspx?doi=10.1117/12.2216307

Sun, Y., Heng, B. H., Seow, Y. T., & Seow, E. (2009). Forecasting daily attendances at an emergency department to aid resource planning. *BMC Emergency Medicine, 9*(1), 1. doi:10.1186/1471-227X-9-1 PMID:19178716

Sussman, J. E., & Tjaden, K. (2012). Perceptual measures of speech from individuals with Parkinson's disease and multiple sclerosis: Intelligibility and beyond. *Journal of Speech, Language, and Hearing Research, 55*(4), 1208–1219. doi:10.1044/1092-4388(2011/11-0048) PMID:22232396

Szlezak, N., Evers, M., Wang, J., & Perez, L. (2014). The role of big data and advanced analytics in drug discovery, development, and commercialization. *Nature, 95*(5), 492–495. PMID:24642713

Tan, J. H., Bhandary, S. V., Sivaprasad, S., Hagiwara, Y., Bagchi, A., Raghavendra, U., ... Chua, K. C. (2018). Age-related Macular Degeneration detection using deep convolutional neural network. *Future Generation Computer Systems, 87*, 127–135. doi:10.1016/j.future.2018.05.001

Tapia, D. I., Abraham, A., Corchado, J. M., & Alonso, R. (2009). *Agents and ambient intelligence: case studies*. Academic Press.

Tapia, D. I., Alonso, R. S., De la Prieta, F., Zato, C., Rodríguez, S., Corchado, E., ... Corchado, J. M. (2010). SYLPH: An Ambient intelligence based platform for integrating heterogeneous wireless sensor networks. *IEEE International Conference on Fuzzy Systems (FUZZ)*, 1–8. 10.1109/FUZZY.2010.5584145

Tatem, A. J., Qiu, Y., Smith, D. L., Sabot, O., Ali, A. S., & Moonen, B. (2009). The use of mobile phone data for the estimation of the travel patterns and imported Plasmodium falciparum rates among Zanzibar residents. *Malaria Journal*, *8*(1), 287. doi:10.1186/1475-2875-8-287 PMID:20003266

TechTarget. (n.d.a). *Definition: AI (Artificial Intelligence)*. Retrieved March 01, 2018 from http://searchcio.techtarget.com/definition/AI

TechTarget. (n.d.b). *Definition: Virtual Assistant (AI assistant)*. Retrieved March 10, 2018 from http://searchcrm.techtarget.com/definition/virtual-assistant

Tekalp, A. M. (2015). *Digital video processing*. Prentice Hall Press.

Tentori, M., Escobedo, L., Hernandez, C., Matic, A., & Hayes, G. R. (2016). Pervasive Displays in Classrooms of Children with Severe Autism. *IEEE Pervasive Computing*, *15*(3), 48–57. doi:10.1109/MPRV.2016.49

TF7 Healthcare Subgroup. (2016, December 21). *Big Data Technologies in Healthcare: Needs, opportunities and challenges*. Retrieved July 24, 2017, from http://www.bdva.eu/sites/default/files/Big%20Data%20Technologies%20in%20Healthcare.pdf

Thabtah, F. (2017). *Autism Spectrum Disorder Screening : Machine Learning Adaptation and DSM-5 Fulfillment*. Academic Press.

The Data Science Bowl. (2016). *Transforming How We Diagnose Heart Disease*. Available at: https://www.kaggle.com/c/second-annual-data-science-bowl

Thomas, J. (2009). Medical records and issues in negligence. *Indian Journal of Urology*, *25*(3), 384. doi:10.4103/0970-1591.56208 PMID:19881136

Timm, J., Renly, S., & Farkash, A. (2011). Large scale healthcare data integration and analysis using the semantic web. *Studies in Health Technology and Informatics*, 169729–169733. PMID:21893843

Torii, I., Ohtani, K., & Ishii, N. (2016). Measurement of Ocular Movement Abnormality in Pursuit Eye Movement (PEM) of Autism Spectrum Children with Disability. In *Applied Computing and Information Technology/3rd Intl Conf on Computational Science/Intelligence and Applied Informatics/1st Intl Conf on Big Data, Cloud Computing, Data Science & Engineering (ACIT-CSII-BCD), 2016 4th Intl Conf* (pp. 235-240). IEEE.

Tsang, L., Kracov, D. A., Mulryne, J., Strom, L., Perkins, N., Dickinson, R., … Jones, B. (2017). The Impact of Artificial Intelligence on Medical Innovation in the European Union and United States. *Intellectual Property & Technology Law Journal*. Retrieved March 7, 2018 from https://www.arnoldporter.com/~/media/files/perspectives/publications/2017/08/the-impact-of-artificial-inteelligence-on-medical-innovation.pdf

Tumlinson, A. R., & Everett, M. J. (2015). *U.S. Patent No. 8,998,411*. Washington, DC: U.S. Patent and Trademark Office.

Turner, J. T. (2014). *Deep Belief Networks used on High Resolution Multichannel Electroencephalography Data for Seizure Detection. In AAAI Spring Symposium Series* (pp. 75–81). Bengio. Available at http://www.aaai.org/ocs/index.php/SSS/SSS14/paper/viewPDFInterstitial/7747/7787

Turola, M., & Gruppetta, S. (2013, October). 4D light field ophthalmoscope: a study of plenoptic imaging of the human retina. In *Frontiers in Optics* (pp. JW3A–36). Optical Society of America. doi:10.1364/FIO.2013.JW3A.36

Umbaugh, S. E. (2017). *Digital Image Processing and Analysis with MATLAB and CVIPtools: Applications with MATLAB® and CVIPtools*. CRC Press.

United Healthcare uses Hadoop to Detect Health Care Fraud, Waste and Abuse. (2018). Retrieved April 20, 2018, from https://mapr.com/customers/unitedhealthcare/

Uvanesh, K. (2015). *Linear and non-linear classification of EMG signals for probable applications in designing control system for assistive aids*. Academic Press.

Uvanesh, K., Nayak, S.K., Champaty, S., Thakur, G., Mohapatra, B., Tibarewala, D.N., & Pal, K. (2016). Development of a Surface EMG-Based Control System for Controlling Assistive Devices: A Study on Robotic Vehicle. *Classification and Clustering in Biomedical Signal Processing*, 335.

Uzsoy, R. (2005). *Supply-Chain Management and Health Care Delivery: Pursuing a System-Level Understanding*. Retrieved 2017, from https://www.ncbi.nlm.nih.gov/books/NBK22867/

Vaidehi, V., Vardhini, M., Yogeshwaran, H., Inbasagar, G., Bhargavi, R., & Hemalatha, C. S. (2013). Agent based health monitoring of elderly people in indoor environments using wireless sensornetworks. *Procedia Computer Science*, *19*, 64–71. doi:10.1016/j.procs.2013.06.014

Varon, C., Caicedo, A., Testelmans, D., Buyse, B., & Van Huffel, S. (2015). A novel algorithm for the automatic detection of sleep apnea from single-lead ECG. *IEEE Transactions on Biomedical Engineering*, *62*(9), 2269–2278. doi:10.1109/TBME.2015.2422378 PMID:25879836

Veaux, C., Yamagishi, J., & King, S. (2012). Using HMM-based speech synthesis to reconstruct the voice of individuals with degenerative speech disorders. *Thirteenth Annual Conference of the International Speech Communication Association.*

Venkataraman, K., Lelescu, D., Duparré, J., McMahon, A., Molina, G., Chatterjee, P., ... Nayar, S. (2013). Picam: An ultra-thin high-performance monolithic camera array. *ACM Transactions on Graphics*, *32*(6), 166. doi:10.1145/2508363.2508390

Venkatesan, P., & Anitha, S. (2006). Application of a radial basis function neural network for diagnosis of diabetes mellitus. *Current Science*, *91*(9), 1195–1199.

Venugopal, V. & Ramaswamy, S. (2016). *DeepMD: Transforming How We Diagnose Heart Disease Using Convolutional Neural Networks*. Academic Press.

Venugopal, M. (2016). Application of SMAC Technology. In P. Chakraborty & A. Nagal (Eds.), *Software Innovations in Clinical Drug Development and Safety* (pp. 90–126). Hershey, PA: IGI Global. doi:10.4018/978-1-4666-8726-4.ch006

Verma, P., & Sood, S. K. (2018). Cloud-centric IoT based disease diagnosis healthcare framework. *Journal of Parallel and Distributed Computing*, *116*, 27–38. doi:10.1016/j.jpdc.2017.11.018

Volkmar, F., Chawarska, K., & Klin, A. (2005). Autism in infancy and early childhood. *Annual Review of Psychology*, *56*(1), 315–336. doi:10.1146/annurev.psych.56.091103.070159 PMID:15709938

Wachinger, C., Reuter, M., & Klein, T. (2018). DeepNAT: Deep convolutional neural network for segmenting neuroanatomy. *NeuroImage*, *170*, 434–445. doi:10.1016/j.neuroimage.2017.02.035 PMID:28223187

Wada, K., Shibata, T., Saito, T., & Tanie, K. (2004). Effects of robot-assisted activity for elderly people and nurses at a day service center. *Proceedings of the IEEE*, *92*(11), 1780–1788. doi:10.1109/JPROC.2004.835378

Wang, K., & Kong, Y. (2016). *Diagnosis of Heart Disease via CNNs*. Available at: https://books.google.de/books?id=ms2oBgAAQBAJ

Wang, Y., Ding, N., Ahmar, N., Xiang, J., Poeppel, D., & Simon, J. Z. (2011). Sensitivity to temporal modulation rate and spectral bandwidth in the human auditory system: MEG evidence. *Journal of Neurophysiology*, *107*(8), 2033–2041. doi:10.1152/jn.00310.2011 PMID:21975451

Wanner, S., Meister, S., & Goldluecke, B. (2013, September). *Datasets and benchmarks for densely sampled 4d light fields*. VMV.

Wargon, M., Casalino, E., & Guidet, B. (2010). From model to forecasting: A multi center study in emergency departments. *Academic Emergency Medicine*, *17*(9), 970–978. doi:10.1111/j.1553-2712.2010.00847.x PMID:20836778

Wargon, M., Guidet, B., Hoang, T. D., & Hejblum, G. (2009). A systematic review of models for forecasting the number of emergency department visits. *Emergency Medicine Journal*, *26*(6), 395–399. doi:10.1136/emj.2008.062380 PMID:19465606

Wedyan, M., & Al-Jumaily, A. (2016). Upper limb motor coordination based early diagnosis in high risk subjects for Autism. In *Computational Intelligence (SSCI), 2016 IEEE Symposium Series* (pp. 1-8). IEEE. 10.1109/IRIS.2016.8066059

Weismer, G. & Kim, Y. (2010). Classification and taxonomy of motor speech disorders: What are the issues. *Speech motor control: New developments in basic and applied research*, 229-241.

WHO. (2009). *Dengue: Guidelines for Diagnosis, Treatment, Prevention and Control*. Geneva: World Health Organization.

WHO. (2012a). *Dengue and severe dengue: Fact Sheet No 117*. Geneva: World Health Organization (WHO). Available from: http://www.who.int/mediacentre/factsheets/ fs117/en/index.html

WHO. (2012b). *Global Strategy for Dengue Prevention and Control, 2012–2020*. Geneva: WHO Press.

WHO. (2013). *TDR Global Alert and Repsonse Dengue/Dengue Haemorrhagic Fever* Geneva: World Health Organization (WHO). Available from: http://www.who. int/csr/disease/dengue/en/index.html

WHO. (2014). Mobile phones help people with diabetes to manage fasting and feasting during Ramadan. *Features 2014*.

Wilder-Smith, A., & Gubler, D. J. (2008). Geographic expansion of dengue: The impact of international travel. *The Medical Clinics of North America*, *92*(6), 1377–1390. doi:10.1016/j.mcna.2008.07.002 PMID:19061757

Wills, M. J. (2014). Decisions through Data: Analytics in Healthcare. *Journal of Healthcare Management*, *59*(4), 254–262. doi:10.1097/00115514-201407000-00005 PMID:25154123

Wingrove, G., & McGinnis, K. (2016). Integration of Technology. *EMS World*, 14. PMID:29847040

Wooldridge, M. (2002). *An introduction to multi agents systems*. Sussex, UK: John Wiley & Sons Ltd.

World Health Organization. (2017). *Media centre: Facet sheets*. Retrieved 11 25, 2017, from World Health Organization (WHO): http://www.who.int/mediacentre/factsheets/en/

Wu, G., Kim, M. W., Qian, G., Yaozong, L. S., & Shen, D. (2014). *Unsupervised Deep Feature Learning for Deformable Registration of MR Brain Images*. Academic Press.

Wu, C.-S., Khoury, I., & Shah, H. (2012). Optimizing medical data quality based on multiagent web serviceframework. *IEEE Transactions on Information Technology in Biomedicine*, *16*(4), 745–757. doi:10.1109/TITB.2012.2195498 PMID:22614723

Wu, G., Kim, M., Wang, Q., Munsell, B. C., & Shen, D. (2015). Scalable High-Performance Image Registration Framework by Unsupervised Deep Feature Representations Learning. *IEEE Transactions on Biomedical Engineering*, *63*(7), 1505–1516. doi:10.1109/TBME.2015.2496253 PMID:26552069

Xin, T. J., Min, B., & Jie, J. (2013). *Carry-on blood pressure/pulse rate/blood oxygen monitoring location intelligent terminal based on Internet of Things*. Chinese Patent 202 875315 U.

Xu, M., Wong, T. C., & Chin, K. S. (2013). Modeling daily patient arrivals at Emergency Department and quantifying the relative importance of contributing variables using artificial neural network. *Decision Support Systems*, *54*(3), 1488–1498. doi:10.1016/j.dss.2012.12.019

Xu, Q., Tsui, K. L., Jiang, W., & Guo, H. (2016). A hybrid approach for forecasting patient visits in emergency department. *Quality and Reliability Engineering International*, *32*(8), 2751–2759. doi:10.1002/qre.2095

Xu, Y., & Lam, M. L. (2017). Light Field Vision for Artificial Intelligence. In *Artificial Intelligence and Computer Vision* (pp. 189–209). Cham: Springer. doi:10.1007/978-3-319-46245-5_11

Yoo, Y. (2014). *Deep Learning of Image Features from Unlabeled Data for Multiple Sclerosis Lesion Segmentation*. Mlmi. doi:10.1007/978-3-319-10581-9_15

Yücer, K., Sorkine-Hornung, A., Wang, O., & Sorkine-Hornung, O. (2016). Efficient 3D object segmentation from densely sampled light fields with applications to 3D reconstruction. *ACM Transactions on Graphics*, *35*(3), 22. doi:10.1145/2876504

Yucesan, M., Gul, M., & Celik, E. (2017). Application of artificial neural networks using Bayesian training rule in sales forecasting for furniture industry. *Drvna industrija: Znanstveni časopis za pitanja drvne tehnologije, 68*(3), 219-228.

Yucesan, M., Gul, M., & Celik, E. (2018). Performance comparison between ARIMAX, ANN and ARIMAX-ANN hybridization in sales forecasting for furniture industry. Drvna industrija: Znanstveni časopis za pitanja drvne tehnologije. (in press)

Yue-Hong, Y., Wu, F., Jie, F. Y., Jian, L., Chao, X., & Yi, Z. (2014). *Remote medical rehabilitation system in smart city*. Chinese Patent 103488 880 A.

Zenger, B. (2012). Can Big Data Solve Healthcare's Big Problems? *HealthByte*. Retrieved from: http://www.equity-healthcare.com/docstor/EH%20Blog%20on%20Analytics.pdf

Zenko, J., Kos, M., & Kramberger, I. (2016). Pulse rate variability and blood oxidation content identification using miniature wearable wrist device. *Proc. Int. Conf. Syst. Signals Image Process (IWSSIP)*, 1-4.

Zhang, G. P. (2003). Time series forecasting using a hybrid ARIMA and neural network model. *Neurocomputing*, *50*, 159–175. doi:10.1016/S0925-2312(01)00702-0

Zhang, L., Wade, J., Bian, D., Fan, J., Swanson, A., Weitlauf, A., ... Sarkar, N. (2017). Cognitive load measurement in a virtual reality-based driving system for autism intervention. *IEEE Transactions on Affective Computing.*, *8*(2), 176–189. doi:10.1109/TAFFC.2016.2582490 PMID:28966730

Zhang, S., & Metaxas, D. (2016). Large-Scale medical image analytics: Recent methodologies, applications and Future directions. *Medical Image Analysis*, *33*, 98–101. doi:10.1016/j.media.2016.06.010 PMID:27503077

Zhang, W., Li, R., Deng, H., Wang, L., Lin, W., Ji, S., & Shen, D. (2015). Deep convolutional neural networks for multi-modality isointense infant brain image segmentation. *NeuroImage*, *108*, 214–224. doi:10.1016/j.neuroimage.2014.12.061 PMID:25562829

Zhao, F., Qiao, L., Shi, F., Yap, P. T., & Shen, D. (2017). Feature fusion via hierarchical supervised local CCA for diagnosis of autism spectrum disorder. *Brain Imaging and Behavior, 11*(4), 1050–1060. doi:10.100711682-016-9587-5 PMID:27535871

Zheng, Z., Fu, Q., Zhao, H., Swanson, A. R., Weitlauf, A. S., Warren, Z. E., & Sarkar, N. (2017). Design of an Autonomous Social Orienting Training System (ASOTS) for Young Children With Autism. *IEEE Transactions on Neural Systems and Rehabilitation Engineering, 25*(6), 668–678. doi:10.1109/TNSRE.2016.2598727 PMID:28644796

Zheng, Z., Young, E. M., Swanson, A. R., Weitlauf, A. S., Warren, Z. E., & Sarkar, N. (2016). Robot-Mediated Imitation Skill Training for Children With Autism. *IEEE Transactions on Neural Systems and Rehabilitation Engineering, 24*(6), 682–691. doi:10.1109/TNSRE.2015.2475724 PMID:26353376

Zhou, X., Garcia-Romero, D., Duraiswami, R., Espy-Wilson, C., & Shamma, S. (2011). Linear versus mel frequency cepstral coefficients for speaker recognition. In *Automatic Speech Recognition and Understanding (ASRU), 2011 IEEE Workshop on.* IEEE. 10.1109/ASRU.2011.6163888

Zibners, L. M., Bonsu, B. K., Hayes, J. R., & Cohen, D. M. (2006). Local weather effects on emergency department visits: A time series and regression analysis. *Pediatric Emergency Care, 22*(2), 104–106. doi:10.1097/01.pec.0000199561.34475.29 PMID:16481926

Zikopoulos, P.C., DeRoos, D., Parasuraman, K., Deutsch, T., Corrigan, D., & Giles, J. (2013). *Harness the Power of Big Data.* McGraw-Hill.

Ziou, D., & Tabbone, S. (1998). Edge detection techniques-an overview. *Pattern Recognition and Image Analysis C/C of Raspoznavaniye Obrazov I Analiz Izobrazhenii, 8*, 537-559.

Zlotnik, A., Gallardo-Antolin, A., Alfaro, M. C., Pérez, M. C. P., & Martínez, J. M. M. (2015). Emergency department visit forecasting and dynamic nursing staff allocation using machine learning techniques with readily available open-source software. *CIN: Computers, Informatics, Nursing, 33*(8), 368–377. PMID:26200901

Zobel, M., Fritz, M., & Scholz, I. (2002, November). *Object Tracking and Pose Estimation Using Light-Field Object Models* (pp. 371–378). VMV.

Zou, J., Zhang, C., Dong, C., Fan, C., & Wen, Z. (2010). Mobile payment based on RFID-SIM Card. *2010 10th IEEE International Conference on Computer and Information Technology.*

Zreik, M., Leiner, T., de Vos, B. D., van Hamersvelt, R. W., Viergever, M. A., & Isgum, I. (2017). *Automatic Segmentation of the Left Ventricle in Cardiac CT Angiography Using Convolutional Neural Network.* arXiv preprint arXiv:1704.05698

About the Contributors

Nardjes Bouchemal is associate professor of Artificial Intelligence and Information Systems at the University of Abdelhafid Boussouf of Mila since 2010. She was born in Algeria in 1977. After a computer science graduate diploma, she completed a Master's Degree in "Artificial Intelligence and Software Engineering" (2010) and a PhD thesis in "Computer Science" at the University of Constantine2 (2015). Her research activities conducted at the "LIRE Laboratory" are focused on agents' security in ubiquitous computing, where agents are embedded in mobile restricted devices. Actually, she is motivated for using agents' and new technologies in the healthcare domain. Nardjes BOUCHEMAL is author & co-author of many publications. In 2015, she founded the IEEE NTIC Conference and was the general chair. In 2017, she was the IEEE Algerian Ambassador of IEEE Middle East Students and Young Professionals, (MESYP'17). Since 2015, she serves in the editorial board of Journal of Information Technology Research (JITR). Now, she is the editor in chief of a book project entitled: Intelligent Systems for Healthcare Management and Delivery.

* * *

Billel Boudjit received the Master degree in computer science from the University of Paris Nord -Paris 13-, Paris, France. Currently he is a software engineers in Zsoft-consulting on the new web technologies, JAVA/JEE and ANGULAR JS. His main research interests are in the areas of Complex Systems, Microservices, JAVA/JEE, ANGULAR JS, Spring, and Maven.

Imane Boussebough received the Magister and Ph.D. degrees in computer science from the University Mentouri of Constantine, Constantine, Algeria. Currently she is an assistant Professor at the University of Constantine 2. She is also a member of the software engineering and artificial intelligence research team of LIRE (Laboratoire d'Informatique REpartie) Laboratory at the University of Constantine 2 Abdelhamid Mehri. Her main research interests are in the areas of Artificial Intelligence, Complex systems, Multi-Agent systems, and Ambient Intelligence. She has written some papers on Adaptive Multi-Agent systems and her work about Adaptive Multi-Agent System: Cooperation and Structures Emergence.

Erkan Celik received BSc and MSc degree in Industrial Engineering from Selcuk University, Konya, Turkey in 2008 and 2011, respectively. He also received PhD in Industrial Engineering from Yildiz Technical University, İstanbul, Turkey in 2015. He is now Assistant Professor in Industrial Engineering from Munzur University, Tunceli, Turkey. He has published many papers in highly cited journals as Transportation Research Part E, Transportation Research Part A, Computers & Industrial Engineering,

International Journal of Production Research, European Journal of Industrial Engineering and etc. His research interests are in decision analysis, humanitarian logistic, fuzzy sets.

Issam Eddine Chaib received the Master degree in computer science from the University of Constantine 2 Abdelhamid Mehri, Constantine, Algeria. Currently, he is a computer science Ph.D. student and a member of MISC (Modélisation et Implémentation des Systèmes Complexes) Laboratory in the same university. His current research interests include Multi-Agents Systems, Wireless Sensor Networks, Adaptive Complex Systems, Context-Aware Systems, Ambient Intelligence, and Healthcare Monitoring Systems.

Pijush Kanti Dutta Pramanik has acquired a range of professional qualifications in the core and allied fields of Computer Science and Information Technology, viz. MIT, MCA, MBA (IT), MTech (CSE), and MPhil (CS). At present, he is registered as a Ph.D. candidate in the department of CSE at NIT Durgapur, India. He is actively engaged in research in the domains of the Internet of Things, Grid Computing, Fog Computing, Crowd Computing, Smartphone Computing, and Recommendation Systems. He has authored and co-authored a number of research papers and book chapters which are published by reputed publishers such as IEEE, Springer, CRC Press, Elsevier, River Publishers, InderScience Publishers, and IGI Global.

Heba A. Elnemr is an Associate Professor at Electronics Research Institute, Cairo-Egypt. She received her B. Sc. degree, M. Sc. degree and Ph.D. degree in Electronics and Communications Engineering from Faculty of Engineering, Cairo University, Egypt. She has supervised several masters and Ph. D. students in the field of Image Processing. Her research interests include pattern recognition, signal processing, biometrics, computer vision and image processing.

Karthick G.S. is a Ph.D Research Scholar in the Department of Computer Science, School of Computer Science and Engineering, Bharathiar University, Coimbatore, Tamil Nadu. He obtained Diploma in Computer Maintenance from Bharathiar University, Coimbatore, Tamil Nadu in 2014 and Bachelor of Computer Applications (B.C.A) from S.N.R Sons College (Autonomous) affiliated to Bharathiar University in 2015. He obtained Master of Science (M.Sc.) in Computer Science from Bharathiar University (UD), Coimbatore, Tamil Nadu in 2017. He has published research papers in International Journals and presented papers in International and National Conferences. His area of specializations and research interests are Wireless Sensor Networks, Internet of Things and Analysis of Algorithms.

Muhammet Gul is PhD and has been working as Assistant Professor at the Department of Industrial Engineering, Munzur University, Tunceli, Turkey. He received his MSc in Industrial Engineering from Yildiz Technical University. His research interests are in simulation modelling, healthcare system management, occupational safety and risk assessment, multi-criteria decision-making and fuzzy sets. His papers appeared in International high-cited journals such as Computers & Industrial Engineering, Knowledge-Based Systems, Applied Soft Computing, Journal of Loss Prevention in the Process Industries, Human and Ecological Risk Assessment and European Journal of Industrial Engineering.

Uvanesh Kasiviswanathan received the Diploma in Electronics and Communication Engineering (D.ECE) from Pallavan Polytechnic College, Tamil Nadu Directorate of Technical Education (TNDTE), Chennai, India, in 2010 and the B.E degree in Biomedical Engineering from Rajalakshmi Engineering College, Anna University, Chennai, India, in 2013 and the M.Tech degree in Biomedical Engineering from National Institute of Technology, Rourkela, India, in 2015. Now as a research scholar, I currently involved in "Specific Molecule/Component(s) detection System development" at Bioinstrumentation and Signal Processing Lab and also with Tissue Engineering and Biomicrofluidic Lab at School of Biomedical Engineering, Indian Institute of Technology (BHU), Varanasi, India. His research interests include Device development, Biomedical signal acquisition, processing & analysis, Bioinstrumentation, Circuit design and Biomaterials.

Abhishek Kushwaha is currently a fourth year IDD(Integrated Dual Degree) student at School of Biomedical Engineering, Indian Institute of Technology (BHU), Uttar Pradesh, India. His research interests mainly lies in Instrumentation, Circuit Design & Development, Signal Processing, Algorithmic Coding and Machine Learning. He is currently working in the field of Rehabilitative and Assistive Technology.

Ishwar Malapur is currently completing M.Tech in VLSI design and embedded system from VTU Extension Centre, UTL technologies limited, Bengaluru, Done internship in UTL technologies limited, Bengaluru. He obtained his bachelor's degree in Electronics and Communication engineering from BLDEA's Dr P G Halakatti college of Engg and Technology, Vijayapur.

Suleyman Mete, Ph.D., is an assistant professor employed at Industrial Engineering Department, Faculty of Engineering, Munzur University in Turkey. He received his Ph.D. from Gaziantep University Industrial Engineering in 2017. His research interests include optimization, assembly line balancing, disassembly line balancing, mathematical modelling, heuristics and supply chain network design.

Shashwati Mishra has completed her M.C.A from Ravenshaw University in 2009 and M. Tech from KIIT University in 2011. She has received Gold medal from Ravenshaw University and Vice Chancellor's Silver Medal from KIIT University for securing highest marks in M.C.A. and M. Tech respectively. She is presently pursuing Ph. D. in Utkal University and working as a lecturer in B.J.B. (Auto.) College, Bhubaneswar, Odisha. Her areas of interest include Data mining, Image mining, Artificial intelligence, Pattern recognition etc. She has more than 7 years of teaching experience.

Moutan Mukhopadhyay has received her B.Tech and M.Tech degrees in Computer Science and Engineering from West Bengal University of Technology, Kolkata, India. She has been working as an Assistant Professor in the department of Computer Science & Engineering at Bengal Institute of Technology. She is having more than 11 years of teaching experience in Computer Science domain. She had been involved in teaching subjects like Operating System, Object Oriented Technology, E-Commerce, Software Engineering, Data Structure etc. Her area of research interest includes Bigdata Analytic and Cloud Computing.

Sameena Naaz is working as an Assistant Professor (Senior Grade) in the Department of Computer Science and Engineering, Jamia Hamdard, New Delhi, India. She has a total experience of close to 18 years with one-year overseas experience. She received her Bachelor of Science (Computer Engg.) from Aligarh Muslim University, in 1998 and the M.Tech. Degree in Electronics with Specialization in Communication and Information Systems from Aligarh Muslim University, in 2000. She completed her Ph. D from Jamia Hamdard in the field of distributed systems in year 2014. Sameena Naaz has published several research articles in reputed International Journals and Proceedings of reputed International conferences published by IEEE and Springer. Her research interests include Distributed Systems, Big Data, Cloud Computing, Data Mining and Image Processing. She is life member of Indian Society for Technical Education (ISTE) and a member of International Association of Computer Science and Information Technology (IACSIT). She serves as reviewer of various Journals of International repute. She is also member of program committee of various reputed International conferences. She is in editorial Board of some reputed Intentional Journals in Computer Sciences.

Saurabh Pal is teaching as an Assistant Professor in the department of Computer Science & Engineering and Information Technology at Bengal Institute of Technology, Kolkata. He has more than 10 years of teaching experience in Computer Science and Engineering domain. He has received B.Sc degree from University of Calcutta, India, in 1998, M.Sc degree in IT (Information Technology) from Allahabad Agricultural Institute (Deemed University), India, in 2006, Advanced Diploma in Computer Application, Dept. of IT, Govt. of India, in 2007 and MTech. (IT) degree from Jadavpur University, India, in 2010. Presently he is pursuing Ph.D in Computer Science & Engineering from National Institute of Technology, Durgapur, India. He has published his research work in many international journals and conferences. His primary research area includes Education Technology, Mobile Computing, Context Aware Computing, Semantic Web and Natural Language Processing.

Pankajavalli Palanisamy is an Assistant Professor in the Department of Computer Science, School of Computer Science and Engineering, Bharathiar University, Coimbatore, Tamil Nadu, India. She obtained her Post Graduation MCA under Bharathiar University in 2003 and M.E., degree under Anna University in 2011and Ph.D., degree in Computer Science from Mother Teresa Women's University in the year 2013. She has published 20 papers in journals and in Conferences both at National and International level. She has received Best Teacher Award from Lions Club, Erode. Her areas of interest include Ad-hoc Networks, Wireless Sensor Networks and Internet of Things.

Mrutyunjaya Panda works as Reader in the Computer Science and Applications department of Utkal University. He has 18 years of teaching and research experience. His teaching and research domains include Data mining, Soft computing, Digital signal processing, Mobile communication, Social networking, Image processing, Wireless sensor network, Text mining etc.. He has published 70 research papers in different reputed journals and conferences. He has also written 2 text books, 3 edited books, 7 book chapters in different fields. He is a Reviewer of conferences of repute like: WICT, KES, SOCPROS, CCCS, IIMSS etc., Reviewer of Elsevier, Springer, WSEAS Transaction, Bentham Science, Wiley journals, TPC member of SOCPAR, SOCPROS, WICT series conferences, Editorial member of Inderscience Journal, Listed in Marquis Who's who in engineering in 2013, Nominated for Best Teacher award by NFED, Hyderabad.

Sasikala R. received the B.E. degree from Kongu Engineering College, Tamilnadu, India in 1994, the M.E degree from Govt. College of Technology, Coimbatore, Tamilnadu in 2003, and the Ph.D. degree from the Anna University, Chennai, Tamilnadu in 2011. She is currently an Associate Professor, Computer Networks Division in School of Computing Science and Engineering at VIT University, Vellore, Tamilnadu, India. Her research interests include Cloud Computing, Big Data, Wireless Networks, Body Sensor Networks and Optical Switching Networks.

Yessaadi Sabrina is a Ph.D. student at the University of Badji Mokhtar, in computer science department. Assistant Professor at the University Center of Mila, Algeria.

Shiru Sharma is serving as Associate professor in School of Biomedical Engineering, Indian Institute of Technology (BHU), Varanasi, India. She is associated with the school since 1997. She received B.E degree in Electrical Engineering, National Institute of Technology, Kurukshetra, India and Ph.D in Biomedical Engineering, Indian Institute of Technology (BHU), Varanasi, India. She was the topper of the batch (Gold Medallist). She is a Life member of Indian Society of Technical Education and she used to teach Network Analysis and Synthesis, Electronic Circuits, Control System, Biological Control System. Her area of research includes Biological control system, Mathematical modelling of biological system and Bio-instrumentation.

Shiru Sharma is serving as Associate professor in School of Biomedical Engineering, Indian Institute of Technology (BHU), Varanasi, India. She is associated with the school since 1997. She received B.E degree in Electrical Engineering, National Institute of Technology, Kurukshetra, India and Ph.D in Biomedical Engineering, Indian Institute of Technology (BHU), Varanasi, India. She was the topper of the batch (Gold Medallist). She is a Life member of Indian Society of Technical Education and she used to teach Network Analysis and Synthesis, Electronic Circuits, Control System, Biological Control System. Her area of research includes Biological control system, Mathematical modelling of biological system and Bio-instrumentation.

Farheen Siddiqui is an Assistant Professor at Jamia Hamdard. She has a total experience of 13 years and has done her Master of Computer Applications from Jamia Hamdard. She completed her Ph.D. in 2015 from Jamia Hamdard. Her area of interest are Web Ontology, Big Data, Data Mining and Image processing.

Manu Venugopal is a Lead Business Consultant in Life Sciences R&D at Accenture, India. With over 14 years of industry experience, his primary focus has been on driving technology solutions in the area of Pharmaceutical R&D and Medical Technology. He has worked with many of the Top 15 Life Sciences companies of the world playing the role of a functional consultant and product owner. His recent interest lies in exploring how new age technologies such as SMAC, AI, blockchain can bring about disruptive transformations in Life Sciences R&D space. He is passionate about building technology solutions and knowledge artefacts in the area of digital health.

Elizabeth Baoying Wang is a professor of Computer Science in Waynesburg University. She received her PhD degree in computer science from North Dakota State University, Master's degree from Minnesota State University of St. Cloud, and Bachelor's degree from Beijing University of Science and Technology. Her research interests include data mining, data warehouse, bioinformatics, parallel computing. As professional activities, she serves as a reviewer and/or a committee member of many international conferences and journals.

Siva Yellampalli is currently working as a Professor with VTU Extension Centre, UTL Technologies Ltd. He obtained his MS & Ph.D. from Louisiana State University. His area of research is system level design for power optimization. His area of research encompasses different research fields such as Very Large Scale Integration (VLSI), mixed signal circuits/systems development, micro-electromechanical systems (MEMS), and integrated carbon nanotube based sensors. He has published a book in the area of mixed signal design, and edited two books on carbon nanotubes. He also published multiple International Journal papers & IEEE Conference papers in these areas of research. In addition, he has delivered keynote speeches at International conferences held in Canada, Dubai & Spain. He has given many professional presentations including invited talks. He has been a consultant to a variety of industries and acts as a reviewer for technical journals and book publishers. He acted as the Student Activities Chair and Education Activities Chair, Executive Committee IEEE Bangalore Section. He is also a life member of Indian Society for Technical Education (ISTE), senior member, International Association of Computer Science and Information Technology (IACSIT), VLSI Society of India (VSI) and National Society of Collegiate Scholars (NSCS).

Melih Yucesan is PhD and has been working as Assistant Professor at the Department of Mechanical Engineering, Munzur University, Tunceli, Turkey. He received his MSc in Mechanical Engineering from Karadeniz Technical University. His research interests are in production planning, sales forecasting, multi-criteria decision-making and fuzzy sets. A recent paper was appeared in Drvna industrija: Scientific journal of wood technology about sales forecasting of furniture products by Artificial Neural Network modeling.

Nourhan Zayed was born in Giza, Egypt in 1975. She received her B.Sc. and M.Sc. degrees from the Biomedical Engineering Department at Cairo University, Egypt in 1998 and 2003 respectively. She received her Ph.D. in Electrical and Computer Engineering, University of Calgary, Calgary, Canada in 2010 where she also worked as a teaching assistant. She worked as an instructor in the Center for Adult and Continuing Education Department, American University in Cairo, Egypt in 2000- 2006. She has been with the Computer Science and Systems Department at Electronics Research Institute, Cairo, Egypt since 1999 where she is currently an Associate Professor, where she participated in many research projects and supervised a number of M.Sc and PhD students. Along her career, she received several awards and recognitions including the record for research studentship funded by the multiple sclerosis program of the Hotchkiss Brain Institute, Calgary, Alberta, Canada (2008), Scholarship for studying PhD funded by the Egyptian Government (2006-2010), The American University in Cairo selected her name to be placed in the CACE instructional affairs teaching honor roll for excellence in teaching as determined by the CACE selection criteria and students, Cairo, Egypt, (2003-2006), Scholarship in software skills development, training focus was on Oracle developer funded by Ministry of Telecommunication, Egyptian Government, Egypt (1998-1999), as well as stipends for attending and training in Montreal 2008 World Congress on treatment and research in multiple sclerosis (ACTRIMS + ECTRIMS + LACTRIMS) conference (2008) form EndMS society. She is a member of the IEEE, EMBS, ISMRM, and SPIE. Her research interests include medical imaging and in particular MRI and ultrasound, Neuroimaging, Multiple sclerosis and Optic neuritis imaging, multi-dimensional signal processing for biomedical applications, patter recognition, computer vision, and image processing.

Index

H

I

K

L

M

N

O

P

R

S

T

U

V

W

Z

www.ingramcontent.com/pod-product-compliance
Lightning Source LLC
LaVergne TN
LVHW060406300926
849162LV00006B/1362